GERONTOLOGICAL
NURSING

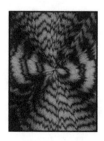

an advanced
practice approach

GERONTOLOGICAL
NURSING

an advanced
practice approach

Sheila L. Molony, MS, APRN
Geriatric Nurse Practitioner
Assistant Professor
Western Connecticut State University
Danbury, Connecticut

Christine Marek Waszynski, MS, APRN
Geriatric Nurse Practitioner and
Clinical Nurse Specialist
Founder
Advanced Practice Nursing Associates, Inc.
Rocky Hill, Connecticut

Courtney H. Lyder, ND, GNP
Associate Professor
Yale University School of Nursing
New Haven, Connecticut

Appleton & Lange
Stamford, Connecticut

Copyright © 1999 by Appleton & Lange

All rights reserved. This book, or any parts thereof, may not be used or reproduced in any manner without written permission. For information, address Appleton & Lange, Four Stamford Plaza, PO Box 120041, Stamford, Connecticut 06912-0041.

www.appletonlange.com

99 00 01 02 / 10 9 8 7 6 5 4 3 2 1

Prentice Hall International (UK) Limited, *London*
Prentice Hall of Australia Pty. Limited, *Sydney*
Prentice Hall Canada, Inc., *Toronto*
Prentice Hall Hispanoamericana, S.A., *Mexico*
Prentice Hall of India Private Limited, *New Delhi*
Prentice Hall of Japan, Inc., *Tokyo*
Simon & Schuster Asia Pte. Ltd., *Singapore*
Editora Prentice Hall do Brasil Ltda., *Rio de Janeiro*
Prentice Hall, *Upper Saddle River, New Jersey*

Library of Congress Cataloging-in-Publication Data
Gerontological nursing : an advanced practice approach / [edited by] Sheila L. Molony, Christine Marek Waszynski, Courtney H. Lyder.
    p. cm.
  Includes index.
  ISBN 0-8385-3131-8 (pbk. : alk. paper)
  1. Geriatric nursing. I. Molony, Sheila L. II.
Waszynski, Christine Marek. III. Lyder, Courtney H.
  RC954 .G4738 1999
  610.73'65—dc21
                                98-45637
                                CIP

ISBN 0-8385-3131-8

Editor-in-Chief: Sally J. Barhydt
Production Service: Rainbow Graphics, LLC
Designer: Libby Schmitz

ISBN 0-8385-3131-8

90000

9 780838 531310

PRINTED IN THE UNITED STATES OF AMERICA

CONTENTS

Preface / ix

1. WELLNESS CARE AND HEALTH MAINTENANCE / 1
   Kathleen M. Demers
   Introduction / 1
   Barriers to Preventive Care / 2
   Preventive Services Recommendations / 3

2. HEALTH PROMOTION FOR THE ELDERLY / 27
   Linda Sapio-Longo
   Introduction / 27
   Adult Learning Principles / 28
   Physical Activity / 30
   Nutrition / 33
   Smoking Cessation / 37
   Stress Management / 41
   Injury Prevention / 44
   Polypharmacy / 50

3. COGNITIVE ISSUES / 57
   Sheila L. Molony, Courtney H. Lyder, and Christine Marek Waszynski
   Introduction / 57
   Dementia / 57
   Delirium / 73
   Depression / 79
   Sleep Disorders / 79

4. TOPICS IN EYE, EAR, HEAD, AND NECK CARE / 91
   Evelyn Woodman Godwin
   Introduction / 91
   Eyes / 91
   Ears / 100
   Nose and Sinuses / 107
   Mouth / 109
   Throat and Neck / 114

5. TOPICS IN RESPIRATORY CARE / 119

Mary Frances Rooney Lewis and Margaret Campbell Haggerty

Introduction / 119
Obstructive Lung Disease / 120
Acute Diseases / 143

6. TOPICS IN CARDIOVASCULAR CARE / 161

Michele A. Marek, Janine Alfano Wilcox, and Ann E. Cocks

Introduction / 161
Coronary Heart Disease / 161
Angina / 167
Myocardial Infarction / 171
Atrial Fibrillation / 174
Hypertension / 177
Congestive Heart Failure / 183
Peripheral Vascular Disease / 188

7. TOPICS IN GASTROINTESTINAL CARE / 199

Courtney H. Lyder and Sheila L. Molony

Introduction / 199
Anorexia / 199
Gastroesophageal Reflux Disease / 202
Pepic Ulcer Disease / 204
Gastritis / 208
Gallbladder Disease / 209
Abdominal Pain / 210
Constipation / 210
Diarrhea / 216
Fecal Incontinence / 217
Diverticulitis / 218

8. NUTRITIONAL ISSUES / 221

Mary Grace Kinahan

Introduction / 221
Nutrition Management / 221
Malnutrition / 235
Eating Disorders / 244
Enteral Nutrition / 248

9. TOPICS IN GENITOURINARY CARE / 259

Catherine Canivan

Introduction / 259
Age-related Changes / 259

Pathophysiology Problems / 260
Urinary Frequency / 260
Urinary Incontinence / 261
Urinary Tract Infections / 278
Benign Prostatic Hypertrophy / 279

10. TOPICS IN MUSCULOSKELETAL CARE / 283

Geriann B. Gallagher and Ann Marie Sommer

Introduction / 283
Osteoarthritis / 283
Gout / 285
Rheumatoid Arthritis / 288
Polymyalgia Rheumatica / 293
Osteoporosis / 296
Fractures / 301

11. TOPICS IN NEUROLOGIC CARE / 311

Claudia Kling and Christine Marek Waszynski

Introduction / 311
Cerebrovascular Accident (Stroke) / 312
Parkinson's Disease / 317
Temporal Arteritis / 322
Dizziness / 322
Seizure Disorders / 333
Bell's Palsy / 339
Falls / 341

12. TOPICS IN ENDOCRINE AND HEMATOLOGIC CARE / 359

Mary Armetta and Sheila L. Molony

Introduction / 359
Diabetes / 359
Thyroid Disorders / 369
Anemias / 377

13. TOPICS IN ONCOLOGY CARE / 389

Gail A. Rogers and Joan Flaherty

Introduction / 389
Prostate Cancer / 389
Breast Cancer / 392
Lung Cancer / 395
Cervical Cancer / 396
Colorectal Cancer / 397
Skin Cancer / 400
Pain in the Elderly / 402

14. INTEGUMENTARY ISSUES / 419
Lori J. O'Connor
Introduction / 419
Integumentary Changes in Aging Skin / 419
Pruritus / 422
Dermatoses / 427
Parasitic and Fungal Conditions / 431
Stasis Dermatitis and Venous Ulceration / 437
Pressure Ulcers and Wound Management / 447
Hair / 464
Nails / 464

15. PSYCHOSOCIAL ISSUES / 473
Debbora Sutherland and Victoria L. Bourque Sklar
Introduction / 473
Grief and Loss / 474
Depression / 477
Suicide / 480
Anxiety / 485
Schizophrenia / 489
Difficult Personalities / 493
Conclusion / 495

16. SUBSTANCE ABUSE ISSUES / 505
Melissa Gorecki-Scavetta
Introduction / 505
Defining the Problem / 505
Age-related Changes / 509
Alcoholism / 510
Prescription Drug Use / 516
Nonprescription Drug Use / 523

17. NEGLECT AND ABUSE ISSUES / 529
Ann Marie DiLoreto
Introduction / 529
Age-related Changes / 530
Risk Factors / 531
Clinical Presentation of Abuse / 531
Physical Abuse/Neglect / 533
Sexual Abuse / 534
Psychologic/Emotional Abuse/Neglect / 535
Financial/Material Abuse/Neglect / 535
Clinical Management / 536

18. ETHICAL ISSUES / 545

Leslie Walker and Terrie Wetle

Introduction / 545
Core Ethical Concepts in Gerontologic Nursing / 546
Setting-specific Issues / 550
Conclusions / 555
Key Concepts / 555
Where to Go for Further Information / 555

Appendices / 559

Guided Case Studies / 583

Index / 619

CONTRIBUTORS

Mary Armetta, APRN, MSN, CDE
Adult Nurse Practitioner
Formerly of Advanced Practice Nursing
  Associates, Inc.
Rocky Hill, Connecticut

Catherine Canivan, MS, APRN, CS
Associate
Advanced Practice Nursing Associates, Inc.
Rocky Hill, Connecticut

Ann E. Cocks, RN, MSN, GNP
Associate
Advanced Practice Nursing Associates, Inc.
Rocky Hill, Connecticut

Kathleen M. Demers, MS, APRN, CS
Geriatric Nurse Practitioner
Day Kimball Hospital/Eldercare
  Program
Putnam, Connecticut

Ann Marie DiLoretto, CS, APRN
Unit Director, Psychogeriatric In-patient
  Unit
Institute of Living
Hartford, Connecticut

Joan Flaherty, RN, MSN
Staff Nurse
St. Francis Hospital and Medical Center
Hartford, Connecticut

Geriann B. Gallagher, ND, APRN
Gerontological Nurse Practitioner
Advanced Practice Nursing Associates,
  Inc.
Rocky Hill, Connecticut

Evelyn Woodman Godwin, APRN, GCNS
Associate
Advanced Practice Nursing Associates,
  Inc.
Rocky Hill, Connecticut

Melissa Gorecki-Scavetta, MSN, APRN
Nurse Therapist
Institute of Living, Hartford Hospital
Mental Health Network
Hartford, Connecticut

Margaret Campbell Haggerty, APRN
Coordinator, Pulmonary Rehabilitation
Norwalk Hospital
Norwalk, Connecticut
Assistant Clinical Professor
Yale University School of Nursing
New Haven, Connecticut

Mary Grace Kinahan, MSN, APRN, CS, CNSN
Associate
Advanced Practice Nursing Associates,
  Inc.
Rocky Hill, Connecticut

Claudia Kling, APRN
Associate
Advanced Practice Nursing Associates,
    Inc.
Rocky Hill, Connecticut

Mary Frances Rooney Lewis, APRN
Geriatric Clinical Nurse Specialist
Adult Nurse Practitioner
Advanced Practice Nursing Associates,
    Inc.
Rocky Hill, Connecticut

Michele A. Marek, APRN, MS, NP
Formerly of Advanced Practice Nursing
    Associates, Inc.
Rocky Hill, Connecticut

Lori J. O'Connor, MSN, APRN, CS
Director of Senior Wellness Services
Windham Community Memorial
    Hospital
Windham, Connecticut

Gail A. Rogers, APRN
Adult Nurse Practitioner
Oncology Clinical Nurse Specialist
Advanced Practice Nursing Associates,
    Inc.
Rocky Hill, Connecticut

Linda Sapio-Longo, RN, MSN, CS
Family Nurse Practitioner
Formerly of Advanced Practice Nursing
    Associates, Inc.
Rocky Hill, Connecticut

Victoria L. Bourque Sklar, MSN, RN
Clinical Specialist
The Center for Geriatric and Family
    Psychiatry, Inc.
Glastonbury, Connecticut

Ann Marie Sommer, RN, C, MSN, GNP
Clinical Coordinator
Metro West Medical Center Senior
    Health Center
Natick, Massachusetts

Debbora Sutherland, MS, APRN
Geriatric Nurse Practitioner
Geropsychiatric Nurse
Advanced Practice Nursing Associates, Inc.
Adult and Geriatric Nursing Services
Rocky Hill, Connecticut

Leslie Walker, MPH
Director, Braceland Center for Mental
    Health & Aging
Institute of Living, Hartford Hospital
Assistant Professor of Medicine
Assistant Professor of Community
    Medicine & Health Care
University of Connecticut
Hartford, Connecticut

Terrie Wetle, MS, PhD
Deputy Director
National Institute on Aging
National Institutes of Health
Bethesda, Maryland

Janine Alfano Wilcox, RNC, MS, APRN
Geriatric Nurse Practitioner
Formerly of Advanced Practice Nursing
    Associates, Inc.
Rocky Hill, Connecticut

PREFACE

The original idea for this book stemmed from a desire by the authors to share the lessons learned from everyday clinical practice with advanced practice nurses, health professionals, and students working with older adults. The book was intended to be a collection of case studies with "teaching points" embedded in the content. It soon became evident, however, that a substantial base of knowledge was needed to enhance the pedagogical usefulness of the teaching cases. We have tried to provide this content while leaving out core material such as pathophysiology, physical assessment, and basic pharmacology that may be found elsewhere. We have endeavored to create a clinically useful text for students and experienced practitioners seeking to extend their knowledge base in care of the geriatric client. We believe the information will be useful to nurse practitioners, clinical nurse specialists, physicians' assistants, and other clinicians who seek to expand their knowledge base in care of the older adult.

Chapters 1 and 2 present the highly valued concepts of wellness care, health promotion, and education. Older adults benefit tremendously from an approach to care that incorporates prevention into each plan of care. Chapters 3 through 14 review clinical management of commonly occurring conditions. A systems approach is used to organize the content in a manner that allows the text to be used for

quick reference, brief topical review, or in-depth study. In order to present a realistic view of the multisystem problems and influences endemic to geriatrics, we have included case studies that allow the reader to incorporate the content of each chapter into the assessment of more complex clinical scenarios. A sample case is included at the end of each chapter. Cases requiring synthesis of information are included in an appendix at the end of the book. In addition, each chapter contains information on "atypical" presentations of disease in the older adult. To assist the reader in identifying commonly occurring conditions in the integumentary system (Chapter 14), color photos are included within the chapter.

Chapters 15 through 17 follow a similar format as they review psychosocial aspects of care. The importance of considering both physiologic and psychosocial contributors to symptoms is emphasized throughout the manuscript. Clinical decision making often occurs in the context of ethical dilemmas. Chapter 18 discusses core ethical concepts in gerontologic nursing to provide a foundation for such decision making.

We use a variety of screening instruments and comprehensive assessment tools in our practice. In many cases, we have developed our own clinical guidelines and tools to facilitate diagnosis and guide our assessments. We have included these tools and tables in our text to provide the reader with readily accessible materials to aid clinical practice. In addition, clinical "pearls" and vignettes have been added to illustrate the practical application of important information.

As we edited the text, we struggled with variations in focus from medical diagnostics, procedures, and treatments to health promotion, client education, and nursing support. The role of the advanced practice nurse encompasses all these skills; therefore, we decided to allow each chapter to focus on those aspects of the role which were of greatest importance in care of the client with the presenting problem or condition. Our aim in this book as in our practices is to offer a holistic approach to care.

Our practice settings encompass acute care, long-term care, and community settings; thus, you will find the terms "client" and "patient" used interchangeably throughout the book. Whichever term is used, we regard each older adult we serve to be a partner in care and not a dependent recipient.

Our clients have been our best teachers. We hope that we can share their lessons with you.

Sheila L. Molony
Christine Marek Waszynski
Courtney H. Lyder

ACKNOWLEDGMENTS

We would like to acknowledge the following individuals who have contributed to this book through submission of clinical pearls or case studies. Others are being acknowledged for their influence, mentorship, or personal support of the authors.

Sandra Bellantonio, MD
Richard Besdire, MD
Nancy Callaghan, APRN, RN
Robert Carney
Elaine Davis, Librarian
Cristyn Franson, APRN
Laurel Halloran
Judith Hriceniak, RN, MS, PhD
Anne Kenny, MD
Linda Kowalczuk, APRN
Susan S. Krutt, MS, CCGA, FAA
Patrick Lewis
Jodi Malis, MD, MPH
Randall Molony
Doris Phillips, MD
James Walker, MD
Henry Waszynski

1

WELLNESS CARE AND HEALTH MAINTENANCE

Kathleen M. Demers

■ INTRODUCTION

In the United States, the number and percentage of older adults—persons 65 years or older—has more than tripled since 1900. Life expectancy has also increased dramatically, and people who reach the age of 65 can expect to live well into their eighties. With advancing age comes a greater risk for acute and chronic illness and related sensory, cognitive, and functional losses. Fortunately, these problems are not inevitable consequences of aging. Many can in fact be avoided, delayed, or managed better through preventive services and behaviors. The three levels of prevention and corresponding interventions are noted in Table 1–1.

The goal of preventive care in older adults is not only to decrease premature morbidity and mortality, but also to maintain function and quality of life. Measures to prevent diseases common with aging are best begun as early as possible; the older the client, the less likely that primary and secondary prevention will be effective and the greater the emphasis on tertiary prevention (Goldberg & Chavin, 1997).

In this chapter, information about routine immunizations, chemoprophylaxis, and screening strategies are presented to assist the advanced practice nurse (APN) or clinician to develop an individualized preventive care plan with each older client. Complementary health education and counseling strategies that address risk factor modification and injury prevention are discussed in Chapter 2. Other highly recommended resources related to preventive care include *The Guide to Clinical Preventive Services* (U.S. Preventive Services Task Force [USPSTF], 1996) and *Clinician's Handbook of Preventive Services* (U.S. Department of Health and Human Services [USDHHS], 1994).

TABLE 1–1.   LEVELS OF PREVENTION

Level	Purpose	Interventions
Primary prevention	To identify and reduce risk factors that predispose a person to developing a disease or disability in the future	Immunizations, chemoprophylaxis, counseling to encourage risk factor modification
Secondary prevention	Early detection of asymptomatic disease before evidence of significant organ damage or disability occurs	Screening
Tertiary prevention	When symptomatic disease is present, aims to prevent complications and further decline, as well as to maximize function	Rehabilitation, functional maintenance

■ BARRIERS TO PREVENTIVE CARE

Despite the known benefits of preventive care in the elderly, many do not receive the recommended services as often as they should. According to Kligman (1992), reasons for this include provider issues (eg, insufficient office time, lack of reimbursement, uncertainty about intervals, and disagreements with recommendations) as well as client issues (eg, fear, cost of service, belief that new symptoms are part of normal aging, and lack of a primary-care provider).

Every client contact should serve as an opportunity to deliver preventive services, especially to older persons with limited access to care (eg, homebound, rural, and low-income elderly). Fear may be reduced if the individual's concerns are explored along with the risks and benefits of the procedure. Education to dispel myths often helps the older individual realize that aging and illness are not necessarily synonymous. Identification of insurance coverage benefits and financial resources may also encourage older adults, who are often on fixed incomes, to use preventive services.

Preventive care need not be limited to office practice settings. Opportunities abound in other places such as clients' homes, workplaces, senior housing, senior centers, churches, adult day centers, hospitals, and long-term care (LTC) facilities. Preventive services can be offered wherever older people are found. Additionally, by collaborating with other community service agencies (eg, health department, visiting nurses, American Heart Association, American Cancer Society) to promote group immunization clinics, screening events, and exercise and health education programs, APNs can significantly improve access to preventive care in their community.

■ PREVENTIVE SERVICES RECOMMENDATIONS

IMMUNIZATIONS

Changes in the immune systems of older adults place them at greater risk for infectious disease. Susceptibility to infection varies directly with general health, nutritional status, and activity level. Immunizations can provide additional protection. The influenza, pneumococcal, and tetanus–diphtheria vaccines are recommended for the general older adult population. In addition to providing immunizations in the office setting, consider vaccinating elders during hospital or subacute unit stays.

Influenza

A viral respiratory illness, influenza continues to be a major cause of morbidity and mortality in the elderly. This is especially true for those in LTC facilities as well as those with chronic pulmonary and cardiovascular disorders, diabetes, renal dysfunction, hemoglobinopathies, and immunosuppression. Postinfluenza bacterial pneumonitis is a common complication of influenza infection in the elderly and has a poor prognosis (Warner, 1996).

Immunization. Vaccines against influenza are reformulated annually and are trivalent—containing inactivated viruses from three strains: two type A and one type B. Although it is only 30% to 40% effective in preventing clinical illness, the influenza vaccine usually reduces the severity of symptoms and is 80% effective in preventing death in older adults (USDHHS, 1994).

The influenza vaccine should be offered annually to all clients 65 years and older. Since it takes several weeks for antibody levels to rise after immunization, optimal administration time is between mid-October and mid-November to coincide with the start of the influenza season in December. However, the vaccine can be given as early as September and up to and even after influenza outbreaks are noted in the community.

Prior to vaccination, determine the client's allergy history and current health status. The vaccine should not be given to clients who have a history of acute allergic reactions to eggs or to those with an acute respiratory or febrile illness until after their symptoms have resolved.

The recommended dosage in adults is 0.5 mL, given intramuscularly (IM). The influenza vaccine can be administered at the same time as the pneumococcal vaccine, using a different injection site. Mild adverse reactions such as injection site soreness, fever, fatigue, and myalgia can occur but usually subside within 48 hours. Immediate allergic reactions are rare. Medicare covers the cost of vaccination.

Prophylaxis. Amantadine is 70% to 90% effective for preventing influenza type A but does not prevent influenza type B illness. It should be used during outbreaks of influenza type A for the following individuals: (1) older adults in the community who are not immunized or only recently immunized; and (2) LTC residents, regardless of immunization status, during an influenza A outbreak in the facility. The recommended dosage for adults 65 years of age or older is 100 mg daily for the duration of the influenza A activity (USDHHS, 1994). Side effects, which occur among 5% to 10% of individuals receiving amantadine, tend to decrease or resolve after 1 week of continuous use and include nervousness, anxiety, insomnia, difficulty concentrating, lightheadedness, anorexia, and nausea.

Client Education. Use every contact in the late summer and fall to encourage clients to get the influenza vaccine. Discuss possible adverse effects of the vaccine and self-care measures should they occur. Provide information regarding amantadine to clients who are unable or unwilling to receive the influenza vaccine. Frequent hand washing and crowd avoidance during the cold and influenza season offer additional protection.

Pneumonia

Pneumonia is one of the leading causes of death in the aged. Most of the community-acquired and many of the institution-acquired pneumonias are caused by *Streptococcus pneumoniae.*

Immunization. The current 23-valent pneumoccocal vaccine has a protective efficacy of approximately 60%. In some older adults, antibody levels decrease to ineffective levels 6 or more years after vaccination. Most major medical authorities agree that all persons aged 65 years and older should receive the vaccine at least once (USDHHS, 1994). Routine revaccination is not recommended but may be appropriate to consider in individuals at highest risk for morbidity and mortality from pneumococcal disease (eg, persons who are over 75 years of age, have severe chronic disease, or are immunocompromised) who were vaccinated more than 5 years earlier (USPSTF,

1996). Medicare has covered the cost of the pneumonia vaccination since 1993.

Prior to administration, determine the client's allergy history and current health status. The vaccine should not be given to clients who have allergies to any component of the vaccine (check the manufacturer's package insert for precautions). The vaccine should also not be given to clients with an acute respiratory or febrile illness until after their symptoms have resolved.

The pneumococcal vaccine can be administered at any time of the year. The recommended dosage is 0.5 mL given IM or subcutaneously (SC). Mild, local side effects such as erythema and pain at the injection site are common. Fever, myalgia, and severe local reactions are rare. Consider revaccinating older adults who received the vaccine more than 5 years earlier and who are at high risk for pneumococcal infection because of chronic illness or compromised immune systems.

Client Education. Provide instruction about pneumonia prevention including good nutrition, regular physical activity, and, as appropriate, smoking cessation. Advise older adults to receive the pneumoccocal vaccine at least once. Suggest that they discuss the need for revaccination with their health-care provider every 5 years. Prior to vaccine administration, discuss possible adverse effects and related self-care measures. Provide clients with a written record of vaccination to keep for themselves and share with other health-care providers.

Tetanus and Diphtheria

In the United States, tetanus occurs in about 60 older adults each year who are either unimmunized or incompletely immunized. The risk of mortality is greater than 30%.

Although relatively rare, diphtheria cases still occur in the United States, primarily among adults who are unimmunized or underimmunized. Up to 84% of older adults lack protective levels of antibodies against diphtheria (USDHHS, 1994).

Immunization. While conducting a health history, assess and record the client's tetanus and diphtheria immunization status, as well as any known history of serious reaction to the vaccine. A primary series of three tetanus–diphtheria (Td) vaccinations (the second 4 to 8 weeks after the first and the third 6 to 12 months after the second) should be given to adults who have never been immunized. Once the series has been received, a routine Td booster vaccine should be provided every 10 years (Advisory Committee on Immunization Practices [ACIP], 1991). The recommended adult Td dosage is 0.5 mL given IM. The Td vaccine is contraindicated in individuals who have experienced a severe reaction to previous doses. Medicare does not currently cover the cost of the vaccine for routine immunization.

Wound Management. A Td booster should be provided prophylactically if (1) the client has received fewer than three previous tetanus vaccinations; (2) vaccination status is unknown or uncertain; (3) more than 10 years have passed since the last dose for clean, minor wounds; or (4) more than 5 years have passed since the last dose for all other types of wounds (ACIP, 1991).

For contaminated or puncture wounds, avulsions, burns, or frostbite,

tetanus immune globulin (TIG) should also be given if (1) the client has received fewer than three previous tetanus vaccinations, or (2) vaccination status is unknown or uncertain. The recommended TIG dosage is 250 units given IM. Tetanus immune globulin can be given at the same time as Td, but in a different site (ACIP, 1991).

Client Education. Advise the client that mild erythema and induration at the Td and TIG injection sites are common. Other reactions such as fever and myalgias are less common; severe reactions are rare. As with other immunizations, provide clients with a written record of vaccination along with instructions regarding revaccination.

CHEMOPROPHYLAXIS

Some health problems can be prevented or delayed by chemical means. Two chemoprophylactic methods, aspirin and estrogen replacement therapy, have been noted to be beneficial in certain older adults.

Aspirin Prophylaxis

Benefits and Risks. Clinicians and researchers continue to look for ways to reduce cardiovascular disease, the leading cause of death in men and women. Studies to date have shown that although low-dose aspirin can significantly decrease the incidence of first myocardial infarction (MI) in middle-aged men and women, aspirin prophylaxis has not been shown to decrease total mortality (Manson et al., 1991; Physicians' Health Study, 1989). These same studies have shown that there may actually be an increased risk of hemorrhagic stroke and sudden death with its use. Major authorities agree that there is not enough evidence to advocate for or against routine aspirin prophylaxis for the primary prevention of MI in asymptomatic persons (USPSTF, 1996).

Prophylaxis. Those individuals most likely to obtain a preventive benefit from aspirin are clients over age 50 with risk factors for coronary artery disease. Although the optimal dosage of aspirin has not yet been determined, 325 mg taken by mouth daily or every other day is the most common regimen. Dosages above 325 mg daily offer no added protection but can increase the risk of side effects.

Aspirin is contraindicated in individuals who are allergic to aspirin, as well as those with liver, kidney, or peptic ulcer disease; a history of gastrointestinal (GI) bleeding; or a bleeding disorder. Because of the risk of hemorrhagic stroke, aspirin prophylaxis in clients whose hypertension is poorly controlled is not advised. Side effects of aspirin use are dose related and include GI upset and bleeding disorders, such as easy bruising, epistaxis, hematemesis, and melena. Although GI upset may be reduced by taking aspirin with food or by using enteric-coated aspirin, bleeding risk remains because of the systemic effects of aspirin.

Client Education. Risks and benefits of aspirin prophylaxis should always be considered and discussed with the client. Advise clients who are taking aspirin to inform their surgeon or dentist before undergoing even minor procedures, since prolonged bleeding can persist for up to 10 days after aspirin is terminated. Teach clients to identify and report any signs of bleeding or GI distress as soon as noted.

Hormone Replacement Therapy

Benefits and Risks. In their extensive review of the literature, Grady et al. (1992) concluded that numerous studies have demonstrated that hormone replacement therapy (HRT) reduces the risk of cardiovascular disease and hip fracture in postmenopausal women. Hormone replacement therapy can also provide other quality-of-life benefits after menopause by improving the common genitourinary symptoms of dryness, urgency, frequency, and incontinence. The association between HRT and Alzheimer's disease (AD) is currently being explored. At least one study (Paganini-Hill & Henderson, 1994) has suggested that HRT may reduce the risk of AD in women.

Several health risks related to HRT have been documented. The incidence of endometrial cancer increases eightfold for women with intact uteri who take unopposed estrogen for more than 8 years (Grady et al., 1992). When progestin is taken concomitantly, this risk is reduced back to a level comparable to women who are not taking estrogen.

Many women are reluctant to take estrogen because of concerns about the risk of breast cancer. Research about estrogen's effect on breast cancer incidence has been inconclusive but suggests a modest increase only among current, long-term users (> 5 years) of hormones (Colditz et al., 1995).

Estrogen and progestin can cause unpleasant side effects, including breast tenderness, endometrial bleeding, nausea, bloating, headaches, irritability, and depression. Many of these side effects abate over time or can be resolved by adjusting the dose or timing of administration (Belchetz, 1994).

Prophylaxis. At menopause and periodically afterwards, ask each woman about the presence and severity of urogenital symptoms and assess risk factors for heart disease, osteoporosis, and breast cancer. Also, determine if the client has had a hysterectomy. This information is important when considering the benefits and risks of HRT for each client.

Once a decision to provide HRT has been made, there are many options regarding types and combinations of hormones, treatment regimens, and routes of administration, which allow care to be individualized (Scharbo-DeHaan, 1996). The American College of Physicians (1992) suggest that the minimum effective dose of estrogen is 0.625 mg of conjugated estrogen or the equivalent once a day. For women who have not had a hysterectomy, adding a continuous regimen of daily progestin, such as 2.5 mg medroxyprogesterone acetate (MPA) or equivalent, or a cyclic regimen of 5 to 10 mg MPA daily for 10 to 14 days per month is recommended.

Client Education. All older women should be advised about the probable risks and benefits of HRT. Possible side effects and follow-up visits related to therapy should also be discussed. Older women should be informed about alternatives to HRT for treating perimenopausal symptoms and managing risks of osteoporosis, fractures, and heart disease.

SCREENING AND EARLY DETECTION

The use of screening tests can assist in the detection of disease and functional loss in their earliest stages. Many screening tests can be provided during the older client's periodic health visits or integrated into episodic care.

CLINICAL PEARL

Before performing or ordering screening tests, explore the client's health belief system. Some clients will decline screening because of the cost or feel strongly that they would not choose any intervention if abnormal results were found.

Blood Pressure

Although blood pressure tends to rise with age because of changes in the cardiovascular system, older adults with even mild hypertension are at elevated risk for coronary heart disease, stroke, peripheral vascular disease, renal disease, and retinopathy. Early detection and treatment is key to preventing end-organ disease.

Screening. Hypertension should never be diagnosed on the basis of a single measurement. Blood pressure is classified based on the average of two or more readings taken at different times (Table 1–2). Recommendations for follow-up, based on the initial set of blood pressure measurements, are outlined in Table 1–3.

Most authorities agree that blood pressure in adults should be measured every 1 to 2 years (American College of Physicians, 1991; National High Blood Pressure Education Program, 1990). However, because the risk of hypertension increases with age, it is prudent to

TABLE 1–2.   CLASSIFICATION OF BLOOD PRESSURE FOR ADULTS AGE 18 YEARS OR OLDER[a]

Category	Systolic (mm Hg)	Diastolic (mm Hg)
Normal[b]	< 130	< 85
High normal	130–139	85–89
Hypertension[c]		
Stage 1 (mild)	140–159	90–99
Stage 2 (moderate	160–179	100–109
Stage 3 (severe)	180–209	110–119
Stage 4 (very severe)	≥ 210	≥ 120

[a] Not taking antihypertensive drugs and not acutely ill. When systolic blood pressure (SBP) and diastolic blood pressure (DBP) fall into different categories, the higher category should be selected to classify the individual's blood pressure status. For instance, 160/92 mm Hg should be classified as stage 2, and 180/120 mm Hg should be classified as stage 4. Isolated systolic hypertension (ISH) is defined as SBP ≥ 140 mm Hg and DBP < 90 mm Hg and staged appropriately (eg, 170/85 mm Hg is defined as stage 2 ISH).

[b] Optimal blood pressure with respect to cardiovascular risk is SBP < 120 mm Hg and DBP < 80 mm Hg. However, unusually low readings should be evaluated for clinical significance.

[c] Based on the average of two or more readings taken at each of two or more visits following an initial screening.

Note: In addition to classifying stages of hypertension based on average blood pressure levels, the clinician should specify presence or absence of target-organ disease and additional risk factors. For example, a patient with diabetes and a blood pressure of 142/94 mm Hg plus left ventricular hypertrophy should be classified as "stage 1 hypertension with target-organ disease (left ventricular hypertrophy) and with another major risk factor (diabetes)." This specificity is important for risk classification and management.

Source: Joint National Committee on Detection, Evaluation, and Treatment of High Blood Pressure. (1993). The Fifth Report of the Joint National Committee on Detection, Evaluation, and Treatment of High Blood Pressure. *Arch Int Med, 153,* 154–188.

TABLE 1–3.   RECOMMENDATIONS FOR FOLLOW-UP BASED ON INITIAL SET OF BLOOD PRESSURE MEASUREMENTS FOR ADULTS AGE 18 AND OVER

Initial Screening Blood Pressure (mm Hg)[a]		Follow-up Recommended[b]
Systolic	*Diastolic*	
< 130	< 85	Recheck in 2 years
130–139	85–89	Recheck in 1 year[c]
140–159	90–99	Confirm within 2 months
160–179	100–109	Evaluate or refer to source of care within 1 month
180–209	110–119	Evaluate or refer to source of care within 1 week
≥ 210	≥ 120	Evaluate or refer to source of care immediately

[a] If the SBP and DBP categories are different, follow recommendations for the shorter time follow-up (eg, 160/85 mm Hg should be evaluated or referred to source of care within 1 month).

[b] The scheduling of follow-ups should be modified by reliable information about past blood pressure measurements, other cardiovascular risk factors, or target-organ disease.

[c] Consider providing advice about life-style modifications.

Source: Joint National Committee on Detection, Evaluation, and Treatment of High Blood Pressure. (1993). The Fifth Report of the Joint National Committee on Detection, Evaluation, and Treatment of High Blood Pressure. *Arch Int Med, 153,* 154–188.

measure blood pressure in the elderly at each visit. This is also an ideal time to assess the client for other cardiovascular risk factors (ie, family history, high cholesterol, cigarette use, diabetes mellitus, physical inactivity, and obesity).

Life-style modifications (Table 1–4) should be the treatment of choice during the first 3 to 6 months for clients with stage 1 (mild) or stage 2 (moderate) hypertension. Pharmacologic treatment may need to be added if there is inadequate response to the life-style modifications. Refer to Chapter 6 for further information on treating hypertension.

Client Education. When a high normal blood pressure or hypertension is identified, treatment is targeted at preventing morbidity and mortality by using the least intrusive means possible. Counsel all hypertensive clients to adopt appropriate life-style modifications (see Table 1–4). Although stress can raise blood pressure acutely, the literature does not currently support the use of relaxation therapies to prevent or treat hypertension, since research has not shown any significant differences in controlled studies (Joint National Committee, 1993).

CLINICAL PEARL

Clients often take a greater interest in their health status when provided with a written record of their blood pressure, pulse, and weight at each visit. A small, wallet-sized card that can be used repeatedly and shared with other providers is ideal.

Body Measurement

Many adults gain weight during midlife and often carry this extra weight into their later years. Obesity (commonly defined as 20% or more above desirable weight) puts individuals at risk for hypertension, type II diabetes mellitus, hypercholesterolemia, stroke, and heart disease, as well as some types of cancer (eg, colon, prostate, breast, ovarian, and uterine). Arthritis, back pain, gastroesophageal reflux disease (GERD), and other conditions common in older adults can also be exacerbated by excess weight.

Below-average weights are often associated with greater longevity, but in older adults low weight or loss of weight may

---

TABLE 1–4.   LIFE-STYLE MODIFICATIONS FOR HYPERTENSION CONTROL

Lose weight if overweight

Limit alcohol intake to no more than two drinks daily for men and one drink daily for women

Exercise (aerobic) regularly (three to five times a week)

Reduce sodium intake to less than 100 mmol per day (< 2.3 grams of sodium or < 6 grams of sodium chloride; 1 teaspoon of salt = 2 grams of sodium)

Maintain adequate dietary potassium, calcium, and magnesium intake

Source: Joint National Committee on Detection, Evaluation, and Treatment of High Blood Pressure. (1993). The Fifth Report of the Joint National Committee on Detection, Evaluation, and Treatment of High Blood Pressure. *Arch Int Med, 153,* 154–188.

be a sign of disease (eg, cancer or depression); loss of function (eg, inability to shop, prepare meals, or feed oneself); or loss of resources (eg, lack of income or transportation).

Screening. Height and weight should be periodically measured. Frequency is based on the clinician's judgment. When significant changes in weight are noted, a further assessment should be done to identify the cause (eg, loss of appetite, adverse medication effect, loss of finances).

Two basic methods can be used with the elderly to determine "healthy" weight. Standardized height–weight tables such as those developed by the Metropolitan Life Insurance Company (1983), based on mortality data, are commonly used but have certain limitations since body frame cannot be easily measured. In recent years, many practitioners have used calculation of body mass index (BMI) to evaluate weight since values correlate more accurately with total body fat content. The formula for calculation of BMI is:

$$\frac{\text{Weight (kilograms)}}{\text{Height}^2 \text{ (meters)}}$$

Chapter 8 presents the standard nomogram by Bray (1978) that can be used to quickly calculate BMI, along with detailed screening guidelines. The recommended cutoff points for overweight and obesity as listed on the nomogram may be more realistic for older adults since they are more liberal than those suggested by standardized weight tables. The National Academy of Sciences (1989) believes BMI age-adjusted values of 24 to 29 are acceptable for both sexes after age 65.

Client Education. Older adults who are overweight or obese should be counseled about associated health risks and encouraged to lose weight slowly through appropriate dietary changes and increased physical exercise (see later sections on nutrition and exercise for specific education strategies). Regular follow-up contact to monitor progress and reinforce counseling offers the client ongoing support, which is vital to weight loss success.

Nondieting individuals who present with a recent weight loss of 10 or more pounds in the past 6 months require a further evaluation to identify and treat causative factors. A thorough workup to rule out serious illness such as cancer, depression, and thyroid disease should be done. Referral to a dietitian for counseling to prevent further weight loss may be necessary.

Although some loss of height is normal with aging, significant and/or accelerated losses may be related to osteoporosis and vertebral fractures. This finding may offer a good opportunity to counsel the client about osteoporosis and fall prevention.

Cholesterol

Elevated serum cholesterol is a known risk factor for coronary heart disease (CHD). Lipoprotein subfractions play an important role in CHD; low-density lipoprotein (LDL) cholesterol is directly related and high-density lipoprotein (HDL) cholesterol is inversely related to CHD incidence (USDHHS, 1994).

Clinical trials performed mainly on middle-aged men have shown that lowering blood cholesterol through diet or drug therapy significantly reduces the risk of new MIs and CHD death (National Cholesterol Education Program [NCEP], 1993). However, caution must be used when applying these results to primary prevention in older men and women since the elderly and women in general have been underrepresented in cardiac research to date. Although cohort studies indicate that the risks of high cholesterol continue in both men and women up to age 75, research has not clearly demonstrated that treatment is beneficial in asymptomatic persons over age 65 (USPSTF, 1996).

Screening. For primary prevention, the NCEP (1993) advises that all adults without evidence of CHD (ie, history of MI or angina pectoris) should have a screening measurement of total cholesterol and HDL cholesterol at least once every 5 years. This can be done in a nonfasting state. Individuals with desirable total cholesterol (less than 200 mg/dL) and HDL

cholesterol levels of 35 mg/dL or greater should be given general education about CHD risk-reduction activities and advised to have a repeat screening in 5 years. Those individuals with borderline total cholesterol (200 to 239 mg/dL) along with HDL cholesterol levels of 35 mg/dL or greater and fewer than two other risk factors (Table 1–5) should be given similar education and advised to have a repeat screening in 1-2 years.

Lipoprotein analysis, which includes measurement of fasting levels of total cholesterol, total triglycerides, and HDL cholesterol, should be done in a fasting state for all individuals without CHD in any of following circumstances: (1) if the total cholesterol is 240 mg/dL or above; (2) if the total cholesterol is 200 to 239 mg/dL and the client has two or more CHD risk factors (Table 1–5); or (3) if the client has an HDL cholesterol less than 35 mg/dL (NCEP, 1993).

TABLE 1–5. CORONARY HEART DISEASE RISK FACTORS OTHER THAN LDL CHOLESTEROL

■ **POSITIVE RISK FACTORS**
Age
   Male ≥ 45 years
   Female ≥ 55 years or premature menopause without estrogen replacement therapy
Family history of premature CHD (definite myocardial infarction or sudden death in father/first-
   degree male relative < 55 years or mother/first-degree female relative < 65 years)
Current cigarette smoking
Hypertension (blood pressure ≥ 140/90 mm Hg,[a] or on antihypertensive therapy)
Low HDL cholestrol (< 35 mg/dL)
Diabetes mellitus

■ **NEGATIVE RISK FACTORS[b]**
HDL cholesterol ≥ 60 mg/dL

[a] Confirmed by measurements on several occasions.
[b] If the HDL cholesterol is ≥ 60 mg/dL, subtract one risk factor (because high HDL cholesterol levels reduce CHD risk).
Source: Adapted from National Cholesterol Education Program. (1993). Second Report of the National Cholesterol Education Program Expert Panel on Detection, Evaluation, and Treatment of High Blood Cholesterol in Adults (Adult Treatment Panel II). Bethesda, MD: National Institutes of Health, National Heart, Lung, and Blood Institute. USDHHS Pub. No. NIH 93-3095.

Interventions are then based on the LDL cholesterol level, which is calculated from the lipoprotein analysis values as follows:

$$\text{LDL cholesterol} = (\text{Total cholesterol} - \text{HDL cholesterol}) - (\text{Triglycerides}/5)$$

Individuals with desirable LDL cholesterol levels (less than 130 mg/dL) do not need further evaluation but should be counseled about general diet and exercise strategies and reevaluated at 5 years. Those with borderline high-risk LDL cholesterol (130 to 159 mg/dL) who have fewer than two other CHD risk factors should be given instruction in dietary modifications and exercise and be reevaluated in 1 year. Clients with borderline high-risk LDL cholesterol who have two or more risk factors or those with high-risk LDL cholesterol ($\geq$ 160 mg/dL) should be evaluated further clinically to determine whether a high LDL cholesterol level is secondary to another disease or drug and whether a familial lipoprotein disorder is present. Individualized Step I or Step II diet therapy and physical activity should also be prescribed for this high-risk group and continued for at least 6 months before considering drug therapy (NCEP, 1993).

Table 1–6 summarizes the classification of cholesterol levels as based on the corresponding risk for heart disease.

Because individual cholesterol levels usually plateau by age 65, continued screening may be less important for older clients without risk factors for CHD who have had desirable cholesterol levels throughout middle age. Cholesterol screening for the primary prevention of CHD is not recommended for men and women 75 years of age and older (American College of Physicians, 1996).

Client Education. Inform clients that they do not need to fast or alter their eating habits before screening for total cholesterol or HDL cholesterol. Clients undergoing lipoprotein analysis should be instructed to fast for 9 to 12 hours (NCEP, 1993).

When borderline or high-risk cholesterol is detected in clients without CHD, primary prevention is focused on education to reduce all CHD risk factors. Provide counseling to reduce dietary intake of cholesterol and saturated fat and promote weight loss in overweight individuals by eliminating excess total calories and increasing physical activity. The NCEP (1993) has developed a two-step dietary program effective for lowering

TABLE 1–6.   CLASSIFICATION OF CHOLESTEROL LEVELS BASED ON RISK OF HEART DISEASE

Risk	Total Cholesterol	LDL	HDL
High	$\geq$ 240 mg/dL	$\geq$ 160 mg/dL	< 35 mg/dL
Borderline	200–239 mg/dL	130–159 mg/dL	35–59
Desirable	< 200 mg/dL	< 130 mg/dL	$\geq$ 60 mg/dL

Source: Adapted from National Cholesterol Education Program. (1993). Second Report of the National Cholesterol Education Program Expert Panel on Detection, Evaluation, and Treatment of High Cholesterol in Adults (Adult Treatment Panel II). Bethesda, MD: National Institutes of Health, National Heart, Lung, and Blood Institute. USDHHS Pub. No. NIH 93-3095.

serum cholesterol. The involvement of a registered dietitian is often very helpful, especially when intensive dietary management is needed. The American Heart Association (1-800-AHA-USA1) is a good source for client education material.

Cancer Screening

Although the risk of cancer increases with age, many cancers can be effectively treated if detected in the early stages. Recommendations regarding the methods, frequency, and duration of cancer screening in older adults continue to evolve. The recommendations that follow are based on those suggested by the American Cancer Society (ACS) unless otherwise noted. Client education material on all types of cancer is available by contacting the ACS (1-800-ACS-2345).

Breast Cancer

Breast cancer is the most common type of cancer and the second leading cause of cancer death in women after lung cancer. Increasing age is the most influential risk factor. Over 75% of breast neoplasms occur in women older than 50 years of age (ACS, 1996).

Screening. Breast self-examination (BSE), clinical breast examination, and mammography are complementary modalities in breast cancer screening. The ACS (1997) recommends the following: (1) monthly BSE by all women; (2) annual clinical breast examination for women 40 years and older; and (3) annual mammography for women 50 years and older. Medicare will cover the cost of a screening mammogram annually.

If a suspicious mass is detected by any of these screening methods, the client should be referred to an appropriate spe-

cialist for evaluation and management. Provide ongoing emotional support through telephone or visit contact for clients experiencing anxiety about the finding.

Client Education. Instruct older women in performing BSE and encourage them to examine their breasts every month.

> ## CLINICAL PEARL
>
> Suggest to older women that they can use the day their monthly Social Security check arrives to serve as an easy reminder to do a BSE.

Many older women report that they experience breast discomfort during and several days after a mammogram that discourages them from returning for future mammograms. To reduce discomfort, advise clients to take acetaminophen or ibuprofen an hour before the mammogram and continue afterward, along with warm compresses and showers, as needed.

Cervical, Uterine, and Ovarian Cancers

Cervical cancer has a relatively slow rate of progression (8 to 9 years by some estimates) from a precancerous stage to invasive carcinoma, thereby increasing the chances that early-stage malignancies initially missed can still be detected by repeat screening (USDHHS, 1994). Risk factors for cervical cancer include early age at first intercourse, having multiple sexual partners, smoking, low socioeconomic status, and human papillomavirus infection.

The incidence of cervical cancer is low in elderly women. However, women age 65 and older present with a disproportionately high frequency of advanced-stage disease. This may be because older women are less likely to have received regular Papanicolaou (Pap) smears or pelvic examinations. According to Walsh (1992), 15% of women ages 65 to 74 and 38% of those older than age 75 have never had a Pap smear.

In older women, the risk of uterine cancer is also low but may be increased by estrogen-related exposures, including early menarche, late menopause, nulliparity, unopposed estrogen therapy, and tamoxifen use (ACS, 1997). Postmenopausal bleeding or spotting may be an early symptom of uterine cancer.

Ovarian cancer is often "silent," offering no signs, symptoms, or means of easy detection until the advanced stages. Most commonly, the woman with ovarian cancer presents with abdominal enlargement or vague digestive complaints (eg, abdominal pain, gas, distention). The risk for ovarian cancer increases with age and peaks in the eighth decade (ACS, 1997). Other risk factors include nulliparity, personal history of breast cancer, or family history of ovarian or breast cancer.

Screening. The Pap smear test affords detection of cervical cancer at its earliest stages. The ACS (1997) recommends that all women should begin having annual Pap tests at the onset of sexual activity or at 18 years of age, whichever occurs first. After a woman has had three or more consecutive, normal annual examinations, the Pap test may be performed less frequently at the discretion of the client and the clinician.

Assess an older woman's Pap smear history when deciding upon the frequency of testing. Because of cervical cancer's long preclinical interval, some authorities such as Walsh (1992) and the USPSTF (1996) suggest that Pap smears can be discontinued at age 65 if previous smears have been consistently normal. If an older woman has never received the test, Pap smears should be performed on an annual basis until three normal smears are obtained. Medicare covers the cost of the screening Pap smear once every three years.

Many clinicians also advocate ceasing Pap smears after a woman has had a hysterectomy. It is important to note that, prior to 1965, hysterectomies were commonly performed supracervically, leaving the cervix intact (Mandelblatt & Phillips, 1996). An initial speculum examination can determine whether the cervix remains.

Because the Pap test is not highly effective in detecting uterine or ovarian cancer, the ACS recommends that women age 40 and older should also have an annual pelvic exam. After menopause, the uterus and ovaries are not usually palpable; therefore, any pelvic masses detected on exam should be evaluated further.

To minimize anxiety and discomfort during the Pap test and pelvic examination, offer relaxing music and examination positions that accommodate older

CLINICAL PEARL

A small or narrow Pederson speculum is often better tolerated by older women.

clients with mobility and musculoskeletal problems. With normal aging, the vagina narrows and shortens and the mucosa becomes thinner, drier, and less elastic, making it more susceptible to trauma.

The results of the Pap smear are reported using the Bethesda System (National Cancer Institute Workshop, 1989). Although an abnormal (positive) smear in an older woman may indicate cervical dysplasia or malignancy, other conditions such as atrophic vaginitis, bacterial or monilial vaginitis, vaginal neoplasia, and, rarely, endometrial or ovarian cancer can produce abnormal smears (Mandelblatt & Phillips, 1996).

Client Education. Describe the examination steps as care is provided so that the client understands the procedure. Instruct clients to take slow, easy breaths during the Pap test and pelvic exam to promote relaxation and comfort.

Contact the client with Pap smear results and provide recommendations regarding the need for follow-up and repeat screening intervals.

Colorectal Cancer

In the United States, cancer of the colon and rectum is the fourth most common form of cancer and is the second leading cause of cancer deaths in adults (ACS, 1997). Major risk factors include a history of familial adenomatous polyposis (which is rare); familial nonpolyposis cancer syndromes; adenoma or colorectal cancer in first-degree relative(s); a personal history of adenomatous polyps, ulcerative or Crohn's colitis, colorectal cancer, or adenoma; or breast, uterine, or ovarian cancer (Cohen, 1996; USDHHS, 1994). Other risk factors include physical inactivity and a high-fat and/or low-fiber diet (ACS, 1997).

After age 50, the incidence of colorectal cancer rises significantly and peaks among individuals in their seventh decade (Cohen, 1996). Early detection of asymptomatic lesions, either benign adenomatous polyps or early-stage cancers, enables treatment that is highly curative.

Screening. In average-risk individuals, the ACS (1997) recommends annual performance of a digital rectal exam (DRE) after age 40 and a fecal occult blood (FOB) test after age 50. For the FOB test, two slide windows should be prepared by the client at home from each of three consecutive bowel movements. Slides should not be rehydrated and should be developed within 7 days of preparation (American College of Physicians, 1997). A positive result in one or more slide windows qualifies the entire test as positive and should be followed by a complete examination.

In addition to the DRE and FOB test, a flexible sigmoidoscopy examination is advised every 3 to 5 years after age 50. Individuals with a family history of colorectal cancer or other risk factors may require colonoscopy and commencement of screening at an earlier age (Cohen, 1996). Medicare will pay for one screening FOB test annually and one flexible sigmoidoscopy every 4 years for individuals over age 50.

Client Education. Testing for FOB can be facilitated by providing clients with three guaiac-impregnated cards and applicators in a self-addressed, stamped envelope (use envelopes approved by the U.S. Postal Service). Instruct the client to collect samples from three consecutive bowel movements by using a new applicator each time to obtain two samples from different sections of the stool per card. To minimize false-positive results, instruct the client to avoid red meat, raw fruits and vegetables (especially melons, radishes, turnips, and horseradish), vitamin C, aspirin, and nonsteroidal anti-inflammatory drugs (NSAIDs) for at least 48 hours prior to and during the test period. Despite earlier reports, dietary iron does not cause false-positive tests (USDHHS, 1994).

Prior to sigmoidoscopy, provide clients with information about the test to reduce anxiety. Inform clients that proper bowel preparation is essential and reinforce the scheduled regimen by assisting clients to write out the times they need to perform preparation tasks (ie, "Take first enema at 5 A.M.").

Prostate Cancer

Among American men, prostate cancer is the most common cancer (after skin cancer) and has the second highest cancer mortality rate (ACS, 1997). Yet, a significant number of men who have prostate cancer never know it.

The risk of prostate cancer increases with age, with over 80% of all prostate cancers occurring in men over age 65. Other risk factors include African-American race, family history, and, possibly, high dietary fat consumption.

The issue of whether to screen asymptomatic men remains controversial. There is no evidence to date that links early detection and treatment with reduced mortality. Although some prostate cancers grow and metastasize quickly, causing death, many others remain silently localized and are found only incidentally at autopsy. It is estimated that at least 30% of elderly men die with prostate cancer that has never become clinically evident (USDHHS, 1994). Additionally, prostate cancer treatments have not been proven to be superior to watchful waiting for localized disease and may reduce quality of life by causing impotence and incontinence.

Screening. Screening tests for prostate cancer include DRE and serum prostate-specific antigen (PSA). The value of these tests is limited since their sensitivity is variable and their specificity is low. Consequently, some men with prostate cancer will have normal tests. Others without cancer, but with prostate problems such as benign prostatic hyperplasia (BPH), will have abnormal findings and may be subjected to the expense and discomfort of transrectal ultrasound (TRUS), biopsies, or both, for no benefit.

Despite these issues, the ACS (1997) recommends that men aged 40 and over should have a DRE annually (for colorectal and prostate cancer screening). Men aged 50 and over should also have an annual PSA blood test, which may be discontinued when the client's life expectancy is less than 10 years (ACS).

Only the posterior and lateral lobes of the prostate gland are palpable during the DRE; tumors occuring in other zones may be undetectable by DRE. The prostate gland should be smooth and rubbery and have a palpable central groove. Prostate cancer typically presents as a hard, irregular nodule or asymmetry of the gland. Abnormal DRE findings warrant further testing using TRUS and/or biopsy.

The PSA is a glycoprotein that is produced by all types of prostate tissue—normal, hyperplastic, or malignant. The PSA test is falsely negative (normal) in up to

30% of men with localized prostate cancer (Small, 1993). Additionally, its low specificity limits the interpretation ability of a positive test. Most authorities and test manufacturers agree that PSA values (monoclonal tests) between 0 and 4.0 ng/mL are considered normal. Values greater than 10 ng/mL are highly indicative of prostate cancer and warrant a TRUS with biopsy. Prostate-specific antigen values between 4.1 and 10 ng/mL are difficult to interpret since the elevated level is often due to BPH rather than prostate cancer. When values fall into this "gray zone," the DRE and TRUS may help determine whether a biopsy is needed. Effective January 1, 2000, Medicare will pay for an annual prostate cancer screening test for men over age 50.

Client Education. Men 50 years of age and over should receive counseling about the known benefits, limitations, and risks associated with prostate cancer screening and treatment. The American Foundation for Urologic Disease (1-800-242-2383) has educational materials available for men on prostate disease.

Oral Cavity and Pharyngeal Cancer

The incidence of oral cavity and pharyngeal cancer increases after age 40 and is twice as likely in men as in women. Other risk factors include African-American race, use of smokeless tobacco, heavy smoking, and excessive alcohol use.

Screening. The ACS (1997) advises a yearly oral examination, which should include inspection and palpation of the lips, gingivae, buccal mucosa, palate, floor of the mouth, tongue, and pharynx. The most common location for oral malignancies is the U-shaped area under the tongue (USDHHS, 1994).

If the client is wearing dentures, offer a paper towel so these can be removed prior to the exam. Proceed systematically, from anterior to posterior, using a bright light for good visualization. Precancerous lesions tend to be flat white (leukoplakia), white–red (erythroleukoplakia), or red (erythroplakia). Any lesion, induration, ulceration, thickening, mass, or discoloration is considered abnormal and should be evaluated further.

Client Education. Instruct clients to check their oral cavity in the mirror on a regular basis and report any white or red patches, sores, or lumps that fail to resolve. Discourage the use of tobacco and alcohol.

Skin Cancer

Skin cancer is the most prevalent type of cancer in the United States, occurring most frequently in the elderly. Risk is greatest for fair-skinned individuals who have had excessive exposure to the sun, radiation, or ultraviolet light. Almost all skin cancers are curable if diagnosed and treated early.

Basal cell and squamous cell carcinomas are the most common kinds of skin cancer and occur in over 900,000 mostly white individuals per year (ACS, 1997). Both have a low risk of metastases and typically present in sun-exposed areas such as the head, neck, and arms. Characteristics of either type include an open sore that bleeds, oozes, or crusts and fails to heal within 3 weeks; an irritated, red patch that may itch or hurt; a nodule with a rolled border and central ulceration; and a pearly papule with prominent telangiectasias.

Melanoma is the most serious form of skin cancer. The ACS expects that of the 40,300 persons diagnosed with melanoma in 1997, approximately 7,300 (18%) of them will die. Risk factors for developing melanoma include having a fair complexion, excessive sun exposure, personal or family history of melanoma, presence of many pigmented nevi (moles), or any atypical nevi.

CLINICAL PEARL

To remember the signs of melanoma in a pigmented skin lesion, use the ABCD mnemonic (ACS, 1997): A—asymmetry; B—border irregularity; C—color variation; D—diameter > 0.6 cm (size of pencil eraser).

Other suspicious signs include sudden enlargement or change of a pigmented lesion; changes in surrounding skin; or development of a new pigmented lesion, especially after age 40 (USDHHS, 1994).

Screening. Early detection is important. The ACS (1997) advises that individuals aged 40 and older practice skin self-examination (SSE) monthly and have a clinical skin examination annually.

A warm environment, good lighting, and attention to respectful draping is essential during a skin examination. Thoroughly inspect all skin areas, paying particular attention to common sun-exposed areas as well as areas that clients would have difficulty examining themselves (eg, scalp, eyelids, ears, genitals, perineum, soles of feet, toe webs, and the back of the body). Any suspicious lesion should be biopsied for histologic examination.

Client Education. Skin cancer prevention should be stressed. All older clients should be advised to wear protective clothing and a sunscreen with a sun protective factor (SPF) of 15 or greater when outdoors. Compliance with using sunscreen may be increased by reminding clients that it can slow the effect of photoaging (seen as skin changes and wrinkles) and prevent drug-induced photosensitivity. Older clients should also be instructed in skin self-examination and encouraged to report any suspicious skin lesions or changes in existing moles.

Thyroid Disease

In the United States, thyroid dysfunction occurs in up to 4% of adults, with women, older adults, and individuals with a family history of thyroid disease being at greatest risk (USDHHS, 1994). In older adults, thyroid disease often manifests itself insidiously, causing atypical symptoms that are assumed to be part of normal aging. For example, hypothyroidism often presents with nonspecific symptoms such as fatigue, lethargy, memory loss, depression, and constipation. Older adults with hyperthyroidism may experience weight loss, insomnia, weakness, apathy, congestive heart failure (CHF), and atrial fibrillation.

Screening. Most authorities suggest that screening high-risk populations, such as older individuals, is prudent since early detection and treatment of subclinical disease is beneficial (USDHHS, 1994). The APN should be vigilant for subtle signs of thyroid disease during client contact. Frequency of thyroid function screening is left up to the clinician's judgment.

When screening is performed, the preferred initial test is measurement of thyroid-stimulating hormone (TSH), using a sensitive immunometric or similar assay (USPSTF, 1996). If the TSH is abnormal, the clinician should also measure free thyroxine (T_4). An elevated TSH and a depressed free T_4 suggest hypothyroidism. A suppressed TSH and elevated free T_4 are often found in hyperthyroidism. It should be noted that some medications and clinical conditions can affect the outcome of thyroid screening tests. See Chapter 12 for further information on thyroid disease evaluation.

Client Education. Inform the older client that with aging, illness often presents in vague and atypical ways. Encourage clients to report all new signs and symptoms, however insignificant, so that an appropriate evaluation can be done.

Hearing

Hearing impairment is prevalent in older adults. Over 33% of individuals aged 65 years and older have some degree of objective hearing loss (Mulrow & Lichtenstein, 1991). Although most hearing loss is related to normal aging, additional causes include exposure to regular, excessive noise; cerumen impaction; ototoxic medications; tumors; and diseases that affect sensorineural hearing.

Hearing loss can lead to miscommunication, social withdrawal, depression, and exacerbation of coexisting psychiatric illness. It may limit an aged individual's ability to perform many activities, such as driving, shopping, and using the telephone.

Because hearing impairment often progresses slowly, many older adults are not aware of the loss. Spouses and other family members may be the first to note it, but often are met with denial when they approach the hearing-affected person about the deficit. This can lead to significant stress in relationships.

Screening. Because it is quicker and less expensive than audiometry testing, the U.S. Preventive Services Task Force (1996) recommends screening older clients for hearing impairment by periodically questioning them about their hearing. Persons who perceive their hearing loss to be a problem are more likely to have further testing and accept the need for a hearing aid. Ventry and Weinstein (1983) developed a screening questionnaire (Fig. 1–1) that will facilitate this process. Audiologic referral is recommended for individuals scoring 10 or higher on this questionnaire.

If an audiometer or hand-held audioscope is used, the U.S. Department of Health and Human Services (1994) suggests presenting pure tones at 25 and 40 decibels (dB) at 1000 hertz (Hz), 2000 Hz, and 4000 Hz. Failure to respond to the 40-dB signal at any one frequency in either ear constitutes a "fail." Inability to hear any one frequency at 25 dB places an older individual at risk for hearing loss. A referral for comprehensive audiologic testing by a specialist (ie, audiologist or otolaryngologist) is indicated if the person also reports being handicapped by the hearing impairment. Annual monitoring of those persons who have failed the screening is recommended to determine whether the loss is progressive or having a further impact on their life.

	Yes (4)	Sometimes (2)	No (0)
1. Does a hearing problem cause you to feel embarrassed when meeting new people?	_____	_____	_____
2. Does a hearing problem cause you to feel frustrated when talking to members of your family?	_____	_____	_____
3. Do you have difficulty hearing when someone speaks in a whisper?	_____	_____	_____
4. Do you feel handicapped by a hearing problem?	_____	_____	_____
5. Does a hearing problem cause you difficulty when visiting friends, relatives, or neighbors?	_____	_____	_____
6. Does a hearing problem cause you to attend religious services less often than you would like?	_____	_____	_____
7. Does a hearing problem cause you to have arguments with family members?	_____	_____	_____
8. Does a hearing problem cause you difficulty when listening to TV or radio?	_____	_____	_____
9. Do you feel that any difficulty with your hearing limits your personal or social life?	_____	_____	_____
10. Does a hearing problem cause you difficulty when in a restaurant with relatives or friends?	_____	_____	_____

* Scoring: 0–8, no self-perceived handicap; 10–22, mild to moderate handicap; 24–40, significant handicap.

Figure 1–1. Hearing Handicap Inventory for the Elderly Screening Version (HHIE-S)* *(Source: Reproduced with permission from American Speech–Language–Hearing Association. From Ventry, I. M., Weinstein, B. E. [1983]. Identification of elderly people with hearing problems. Asha, 25, 37–42.)*

CLINICAL PEARL

Inspect ear canals routinely to detect cerumen impaction that may contribute to hearing loss in older adults.

Client Education. Hearing protection from regular, excessive noise (eg, in recreational and occupational settings) should be emphasized. Those with identified hearing loss should be encouraged to see a specialist rather than a hearing aid dealer to ensure comprehensive testing. Inform clients and family members about inexpensive listening aids such as amplifiers for the telephone and televi-sion that may assist hearing. The use of an inexpensive amplifier and ear phones in the clinic can facilitate communication during the visit and lead to client acceptance of such products for their own use. Refer to Chapter 4 for additional discussion on hearing loss in older adults.

Vision

The prevalence of visual impairment increases with age and poses a potentially serious problem for older people. Approximately 13% of individuals aged 65 and older and 28% of those over 85 years of age experience some degree of vision loss. Many older adults are unaware of their diminished visual acuity and up to 25% are wearing inadequate visual correction

(USDHHS, 1994). Visual disorders can pose potentially serious problems among older people, increasing the risk for falls, car accidents, and other types of injuries. Good vision is essential for functional independence in activities of daily living (eg, cooking, shopping, taking medications) and allows the older person to remain active in cherished activities such as reading, sewing, gardening, and so forth.

The most common causes of visual impairment in the elderly include presbyopia, cataract, age-related macular degeneration, and glaucoma. Early detection and treatment of these problems helps prevent further vision loss, and in most cases can lead to improved vision and quality of life.

Screening. Visual acuity can be screened using a standard Snellen wall chart at a distance of 20 feet. A passing score should be given for each line with a majority of correct responses. Each eye should be tested separately, and corrective lenses should be worn during the screening. Clients with visual acuity of 20/40 or poorer in either or both eyes should be referred to an eye-care specialist for further examination (USDHHS, 1994). Vision screening for asymptomatic older adults should be performed every 1 to 2 years. Screening for eye disease such as glaucoma using a hand-held tonometer in the primary-care setting is not recommended, since this test is relatively insensitive and nonspecific. Individuals at high risk for eye disease are best served by seeing an ophthalmologist on a regular basis for comprehensive eye examinations.

Client Education. Education emphasis includes preventing eye injury (eg, use of appropriate sunglasses to protect against damage by ultraviolet rays) and managing other disease (eg, diabetes, hypertension) that can contribute to vision loss. Any sudden changes in vision should be reported immediately. (Chapter 4 contains additional information on eye disease and vision.)

Functional Status

Perhaps the most important parameter to be screened in older adults is their functional status, since it is often the best predictor of level of independence and quality of life. Functional ability is a product of the integrated physical, cognitive, and emotional capacities of an individual. Any stress on or loss of these capacities, as occurs with illness, can lead to functional loss. For example, heart failure, depression, and dementia may interfere with an older individual's ability to bathe and dress independently. Because of the challenge of normal aging changes, sedentary lifestyles, and higher rates of acute and chronic illness, older adults are at particular risk for functional loss and decline. Functional loss is often the first sign of serious illness in the elderly.

Screening. Various tools (Katz et al., 1963; Fillenbaum, 1985) provide a formal method to screen and monitor functional ability. Most clinicians start by assessing a person's ability to meet personal care and home maintenance needs, often referred to, respectively, as the activities of daily living (ADL) and instrumental activities of daily living (IADL) as noted in Table 1–7. (See Appendix II at the back of the book for screening tools.) To screen older clients, inquire if they need any assistance in an activity or have recently experienced a change in their abilities to perform each

**TABLE 1–7.   FUNCTIONAL STATUS
SCREENING**

■ **ACTIVITIES OF DAILY LIVING (ADL)**

Eating/feeding

Bathing

Grooming

Dressing

Transferring

Ambulation

Toileting

■ **INSTRUMENTAL ACTIVITIES OF DAILY LIVING
(IADL)**

Preparing meals

Shopping

Housekeeping/yardwork

Doing laundry

Managing money and finances

Taking medications

Using the telephone

Driving/transportation

task. If possible, family members should also be interviewed, since older individuals may underreport functional problems because of embarrassment, fear, or inability to recognize deficits. In the hospital setting, physical and occupational therapists can be enlisted to screen for functional loss prior to discharge.

If a loss of function in any area is noted, further evaluation is recom-

mended to determine the possible cause. While treatment should be targeted directly at the suspected cause, support of the functional loss should be concurrently offered and in some cases may be the only intervention that can be provided. For example, the APN would treat heart failure or depression and simultaneously order home-care services for health monitoring and personal-care assistance. In the case of dementia, in which cure is not possible, efforts would focus on "prescribing" home-care resources that support function, safety, and respite.

Client Education. All older adults should be encouraged to remain physically and mentally active in order to prevent functional decline.

CLINICAL PEARL

Remind older clients "to use it or lose it."

Older clients with functional losses should be informed about resources such as adaptive equipment, clothing, home-care aides, homemakers, public transit, and home-delivered meals to help them remain independent.

 ## CASE STUDY

Mrs. Moran is a vibrant 78-year-old woman with mild arthritis who focuses on staying well so she can continue to live independently in her farm-

house with her dog and two cats. She walks two miles a day and has taken a variety of vitamin, mineral, and herb tablets daily since she read in health magazines that these supplements can improve memory, alleviate her arthritis pain, and fight off colds. She does not take any prescription medications. Past medical history includes a subtotal hysterectomy in 1959 at age 40 and a hospitalization for pneumonia 6 years ago.

Today, she presents at the office visit, reporting some recent "tiredness" when raking leaves and occasional "constipation" and "bloating." She wonders if a change in her diet would help.

On examination, Mrs. Moran's blood pressure is 160/82, weight is 120 lb, and height is 63 inches. Data from one year earlier notes blood pressure was 130/74, weight was 121 lb, and height was 64 inches. Mrs.

Moran's heart has a normal S1 and S2, with a rate of 72 beats per minute. Lungs are clear. An abdominal exam and DRE are normal. No stool is available for an FOB test. A chart review indicates that her cardiopulmonary status was the same 1 year ago during her physical examination and Pap smear. Her last mammogram was 2 years ago, and there is no record of her receiving a pneumococcal or tetanus vaccination, cholesterol test, or sigmoidoscopy in the past.

Family history reveals that her father died of an MI at age 62, and her mother had hypertension and died of a stroke at age 74. Her only brother is 72 years old and has a history of hypertension and colon cancer.

QUESTIONS

1. Considering Mrs Moran's history, presenting complaints, and exam findings, what additional screening tests and counseling should be provided?

2. What immunizations would be appropriate to provide, and when?

3. What additional prevention strategies should be considered for this client?

ANSWERS

1. Because Mrs. Moran's blood pressure elevation is a new finding today, two to three additional measures should be taken in the next month and averaged before deciding whether hypertension is present. Blood pressure counseling to reinforce her daily exercise and reduce dietary sodium use is appropriate at this time. Her weight is stable and within an acceptable range using the BMI, but she has lost one inch of height in a year, which may suggest that bone loss is taking place. She is particularly at risk for osteoporosis because of an early surgical menopause. Her daily walking should be reinforced to preserve bone mass. Counseling about the benefits and

risks of HRT, calcium requirements, and fall prevention should be offered.

Older women are at risk for thyroid disease, and Mrs. Moran's reports of fatigue and constipation may be signs of hypothyroidism. Consequently, this would be an appropriate time to order a TSH test.

Because over-the-counter (OTC) medications have potential benefits and risks, a review of Mrs. Moran's vitamin, mineral, and herb tablets should be done to identify any risks for toxicities and determine whether they may be the cause of some of her presenting complaints. She should be counseled that many of the claims made about these products have not been scientifically substantiated. Assistance to determine safe dosage levels or referral to a homeopathic healthcare provider for further consultation may be warranted.

As part of routine recommended screening, instruct Mrs. Moran to collect three stool samples at home for the annual FOB test. Provide written instructions about foods and OTC products to avoid during testing. Because of her family history of colon cancer, a colonoscopy, rather than a sigmoidoscopy, should be advised every 3 to 5 years. Both tests are timely, given her recent GI symptoms. An increase in fluids and fiber may alleviate Mrs. Moran's constipation, but she should be advised to increase fiber slowly since it can exacerbate her bloating.

A cholesterol and HDL screening should also be done now since no record of a past screening exists. Her family history of cardiovascular disease as well as her own blood pressure elevation are risk factors that should be considered when the cholesterol level is reviewed.

2. Mrs. Moran's raking activity suggests that the time of year is fall. Consequently, an influenza vaccine should be offered as long as Mrs. Moran does not have an allergy to eggs. The pneumococcal vaccine can be given at the same time, using different injection sites.

Further assessment regarding Mrs. Moran's tetanus vaccination status should be done, since the client may have received the Td vaccine in another setting (eg, emergency room or walk-in clinic). If Mrs. Moran has received the initial series, then a Td booster vaccine should be offered every 10 years. If she has never received the Td vaccine, then a primary series of three Td vaccinations should be started.

Mrs. Moran should be provided with a written record of each immunization administered during the visit. Counseling about the recommended frequency of future immunizations and additional strategies to reduce the risk of infectious illness should be provided.

3. In addition to the other prevention strategies, Mrs. Moran should be instructed in SBE and advised to get an annual clinical breast exam and mammogram. If she has not had at least three consecutive normal Pap smears

in the past, another Pap smear should be performed this year. A pelvic exam should be offered annually, even if Pap smears cease.

Because Mrs. Moran spends a significant amount of time outdoors, she is at risk for skin cancer. Instruction in skin self-examination, an annual clinical skin exam, and counseling about skin protection should be provided.

Sensory ability and functional status are vital to independent functioning and quality of life. Mrs. Moran should be advised to have a visual acuity and glaucoma test every 1 to 2 years. To identify hearing deficits, she should be questioned about her hearing ability during her annual physical exam. Functional ability should be assessed periodically by asking the client and family about her ability to perform ADL and IADL. If functional deficits are noted, counseling about community resources should be offered.

■ REFERENCES

Advisory Committee on Immunization Practices. (1991). Diphtheria, tetanus, and pertussis: Recommendations for vaccine use and other preventive measures. *MMWR, 40,* 1–28.

American Cancer Society. (1996). *Breast cancer facts and figures—1996.* Atlanta, GA: Author.

American Cancer Society. (1997). *Cancer facts & figures—1997.* Atlanta, GA: Author.

American College of Physicians. (1991). Guidelines. In Eddy, D. M. (Ed.), *Common screening tests* (pp. 396–397). Philadelphia, PA: Author.

American College of Physicians. (1992). Guidelines for counseling postmenopausal women about preventive hormone therapy. *Ann Intern Med, 117,* 1038–1041.

American College of Physicians. (1996). Clinical guideline, part 1: Guidelines for using serum cholesterol, high density lipoprotein cholesterol, and triglyceride levels as screening tests for preventing coronary heart disease in adults. *Ann Intern Med, 124,* 515–517.

American College of Physicians. (1997). Suggested technique for fecal occult blood testing and interpretation in colorectal cancer screening. *Ann Intern Med, 126,* 808–810.

Belchetz, P. E. (1994). Hormonal treatment of postmenopausal women. *N Engl J Med, 330,* 1062–1071.

Bray, G. A. (1978). Definitions, measurements and classifications of the syndromes of obesity. *Int J Obes, 2,* 99–113.

Cohen, L. (1996). Colorectal cancer: A primary case approach to screening. *Geriatrics, 51* (12), 45–50.

Colditz, G. A., Hankinson, S. E., Hunter, D. J., et al. (1995). The use of estrogens and progestins and the risk of breast cancer in postmenopausal women. *N Engl J Med, 332,* 1589–1593.

Fillenbaum, G. G. (1985). Screening the elderly: A brief instrumental activities of daily living measure. *J Am Geriatr Soc, 33,* 698–706.

Goldberg, T. H., & Chavin, S. I. (1997). Preventive medicine and screening in older adults. *J Am Geriatr Soc, 45,* 344–354.

Grady, D., Rubin, S. M., Petitti, D. B., et al. (1992). Hormone therapy to prevent disease and prolong life in postmenopausal women. *Ann Intern Med, 117,* 1016–1037.

Joint National Committee on Detection, Evaluation, and Treatment of High Blood Pressure. (1993). The Fifth Report of the Joint National Committee on Detection, Evaluation, and Treatment of High Blood Pressure. *Arch Intern Med, 153,* 154–188.

Katz, S., Ford, A. B., Moskowitz, R. W., et al. (1963). Studies of illness in the aged: The index of ADL. *JAMA, 185,* 914–919.

Kligman, E. W. (1992). Preventive geriatrics: Basic principles for primary care physicians. *Geriatrics, 47*(7), 39–50.

Mandelblatt, J., & Phillips, R. (1996). Cervical cancer: How often and why to screen older women. *Geriatrics, 51*(6), 45–48.

Manson, J. E., Stampfer, M. J., Colditz, G. A., et al. (1991). A prospective study of aspirin use and primary prevention of cardiovascular disease in women. *JAMA, 266,* 521–527.

Metropolitan Life Insurance Company. (1983). Metropolitan height and weight tables. *Statistical Bulletin Metropolitan Life Insurance Company, 64* (1), 2–9.

Mulrow, C. D., & Lichtenstein, M. J. (1991). Screening for hearing impairment in the elderly: Rationale and strategy. *J Gen Intern Med, 6,* 249–258.

National Academy of Sciences, Committee on Diet and Health, Food and Nutrition Board, Commission on Life Sciences, National Research Council. (1989). *Diet and health: Implications for reducing chronic disease risk* (pp. 564–565). Washington, DC: National Academy Press.

National Cancer Institute Workshop. (1989). The 1988 Bethesda System for reporting cervical/vaginal cytologic diagnoses. *JAMA, 262,* 931–934.

National Cholesterol Education Program. (1993). *Second report of the national cholesterol education program expert panel on detection, evaluation and treatment of high blood cholesterol in adults* (Adult treatment panel II) (USDHHS Publication No. NIH 93-3095). Bethesda, MD: National Institutes of Health; National Heart, Lung and Blood Institute.

National High Blood Pressure Education Program Working Group. (1990). Report on ambulatory blood pressure monitoring. *Arch Intern Med, 150,* 2270–2280.

Paganini-Hill, A., & Henderson, V. W. (1994). Estrogen deficiency and risk of Alzheimer's disease in women. *Am J Epidemiol, 140,* 256–261.

Physicians' Health Study Research Group, Steering Committee. (1989). Final report from the aspirin component of the ongoing physicians' health study. *N Engl J Med, 321,* 129–135.

Scharbo-DeHaan, M. (1996). Hormone replacement therapy. *Nurse Practitioner, 21* (12, Part 2 of 2), 1–28.

Small, E. J. (1993). Prostate cancer: Who to screen and what the results mean. *Geriatrics, 48*(12), 28–38.

U.S. Department of Health and Human Services. (1994). *Clinician's handbook of preventive services: Put prevention into practice.* Washington, DC: U.S. Government Printing Office.

U.S. Preventive Services Task Force. (1996). *Guide to clinical preventive services* (2nd ed.). Alexandria, VA: International Medical Publishing.

Ventry, I. M., & Weinstein, B. E. (1983). Identification of elderly people with hearing problems. *American Speech and Hearing Association, 25,* 37–42.

Walsh, J. M. (1992). Cancer screening in older adults. *West J Med, 156,* 495–500.

Warner, L. (1996). Infectious disease. In Lonergan, E. (Ed.), *Geriatrics* (pp. 123–138). Stamford, CT: Appleton & Lange.

2

HEALTH PROMOTION FOR THE ELDERLY

Linda Sapio-Longo

■ INTRODUCTION

In addition to immunizations and screening tests, assessing personal health behaviors is another component of preventive care. This factor is supported in the literature, which states that approximately one half of all deaths occurring in the United States in 1990 may be attributed to personal health behaviors such as use of tobacco, alcohol, or illicit drugs, diet and activity patterns, lack of safety belt use, and high-risk sexual behavior (McGinnis & Foege, 1993). Therefore, the associated morbidity and mortality are potentially preventable by changing personal health behavior.

The role as educator and counselor cannot be emphasized enough. It is through education and counseling that information is relayed to clients so that they have a clear understanding of the plan of care. Sadly, the role of education is often neglected because of lack of reimbursement. It has been noted that when providers expand their intervention with clients from simple warnings to brief counseling and educating sessions, they double the likelihood of changing client behavior effectively (Li et al., 1984).

The process of client education often begins when individuals have a need to know information or a skill. They may request information about promoting health or preventing disease. While it is easier to identify an opportunity for educating when the request is direct, it is much more difficult when there is no request or the client is simply not aware of the need for information.

Since learning is an active process and requires motivation, the goals of education and counseling will not be accomplished without first capturing the learner's interest. The advanced practice nurse's (APN's) intervention may vary depending on the client's presentation. Following are three examples to exemplify this. A client may present to his or her provider with no intention to change a health behavior in the near future. The APN's responsibility is to "plant the seed" by providing the client with accurate, current information on the topic at hand and to empower the client to make a choice. The client can choose to act on or disregard the information. The key is to have the client make an informed decision as to how he or she would like to proceed. The APN must support the client who has made an informed decision and follow up at appropriate intervals.

Another client may present wanting to change a behavior but be uncertain about how to begin. This client will need assistance in formulating a realistic plan of action with a measurable goal, identifying a source of social support and establishing appropriate follow-up. For example, if the client wishes to begin an exercise regime, it is not appropriate to simply encourage the client to exercise as often as possible. This would most likely result in a failed attempt because the goal is not specific, and there is no plan for support and follow-up while attempting this change. A more appropriate plan would be to begin with walking briskly with a friend at least four times a week for at least 15 minutes, with heart rate not to exceed a specified target, and return to the office in 2 weeks. At the 2-week follow-up, the APN can evaluate the client's progress and decide whether to increase the frequency, duration, and intensity of the activity.

A third client who is currently incorporating a health promotion behavior into his life style may present for a health visit. The APN's responsibility is still to assess the plan of action in relation to goal accomplishment and modify the plan as needed. Continuing support to

prevent relapse and acknowledging accomplishments is essential.

Health promotion education and counseling conducted in this way will be more effective because relevant information is presented at an appropriate point when the client may be ready to learn. Many authorities have written about adult learning principles. The APN should be knowledgeable about adult learning principles to achieve success in educating and counseling the adult client.

■ ADULT LEARNING PRINCIPLES

1. Learning is an active process, and adults prefer to participate actively (Robinson, 1979). During an education and counseling session, more of what is said will be remembered if interaction occurs versus just providing information. The APN can encourage interaction by asking about the client's concerns, offering options and asking what may be feasible in relation to time, expense, and effort.

2. Learning is promoted with progression from the known to unknown and from simple to complex (Robinson, 1979). This can be facilitated by initiating the educational session with an assessment of what the client already knows. By doing this, misconceptions can be clarified and knowledge expanded. If a complex regime must be utilized, then it is better to proceed in increments. Start with small, simple changes, and gradually adjust once

those are accomplished, until all the components of the regime are incorporated.

3. Learning is goal directed, and adults are trying to satisfy a need (Robinson, 1979). The APN's responsibility is to meet the client's need for the information he wants, as it relates to him. Although a 30-pound weight loss may be indicated to reach ideal body weight, the client wants to lose 15 pounds. The APN works with him to meet his need to lose the 15 pounds.

4. Learning that is applied immediately is retained longer (Robinson, 1979). For example, if the problem is stress management and the APN is teaching progressive relaxation techniques, provide the client with a demonstration and encourage a return demonstration. Opportunities to practice new skills will increase the rate of learning.

5. Learning must be reinforced (Robinson, 1979). Reinforcement is accomplished by repetition. The more the information is repeated, the greater the likelihood of remembering. Reinforcement can be provided via face-to-face interaction, telephone follow-up, written materials, videos, and so forth. Reinforcement increases movement toward the desired outcome. outcome.

6. Learning is facilitated when the learner is aware of his or her progress (Robinson, 1979). If clients realize that they have made progress in what they need to know or do to take care of themselves, they will experience accomplish-

ment and are often willing to then learn more (Robinson, 1979). For example, although a client desires to stop smoking and is having difficulty quitting, he has decreased the number of cigarettes smoked per day. This client may need acknowledgment of his progress and encouragement to continue to decrease the amount of cigarettes smoked per day.

7. Learning is facilitated when it relates to the individual's repertoire of experience (Robinson, 1979). This principle can be applied by asking if he knows anyone who has the same problem. Also, relating the topic to his employment experience may make it clearer to understand. For example, a plumber may understand coronary artery disease if it is related to the pipes of plumbing.

TEACHING CONSIDERATIONS FOR THE OLDER ADULT

When teaching the older adult, the adult learning principles must be kept in mind as well as some general considerations for changes that occur as part of normal aging. These changes and teaching considerations are listed in Table 2–1.

There are a number of social and behavioral theories and models that explain and predict the behavior of individuals and groups. One of the most popular and frequently cited models in preventive health behavior is the health belief model (HBM). The model addresses the relationship between a person's belief and his or her behavior.

A review of research testing the HBM suggests that the barriers and costs a

TABLE 2–1.   NORMAL AGING CHANGES AND TEACHING CONSIDERATIONS

Decrease of visual acuity	• Use contrasting print and background • Use large printed material • Utilize adequate lighting
Decrease in auditory acuity	• Decrease extraneous sounds • Speak deeper, slower, and more clearly • Assess client's understanding at intervals • Offer written materials to reinforce
Decrease in musculoskeletal agility	• Allow greater time for position changes • Assist with position changes • Allow rest periods
Decrease in reaction time	• Allow greater time for response • Do not attempt to rush client
Decrease in support system	• Offer phone call follow-up • Provide listing of support groups

client confronts are the most salient reasons for either engaging in preventive health behavior or behavior related to the illness regimen (Janz & Becker, 1984). Perceived susceptibility was a close second with perceived severity of low significance (Janz & Becker, 1984). These factors have important implications for the APN when designing health promotion programs.

CLINICAL PEARL

Overcoming perceived barriers and focusing on perceived susceptibility with minimal emphasis on the severity of the condition may lead to more successful programs.

COUNSELING FOR HEALTH PROMOTION BEHAVIORS

The following areas were chosen because they have the greatest impact on reducing morbidity and mortality in older adults. The APN must assess personal health behaviors and focus on those that need to be changed to reduce morbidity and mortality. Behavior modification is a technique that is incorporated in many of the counseling areas. Behavior modification can be used either to substitute a healthy behavior for an unhealthy one or to modify the current behavior for greater health benefit. Remember, instructions for personal health behaviors need to be as specific as other prescriptions and require follow-up for successful initiation and maintenance.

■ PHYSICAL ACTIVITY

According to the 1996 Surgeon General's report on physical activity and health, more than 60% of Americans do not exercise regularly, and, of that group, 25% do not exercise at all (U.S. Department of Health and Human Services [(USDHHS], 1996). These statistics are alarming when one considers that the importance of exercise is not a new discovery.

Why, then, is there such disparity between belief and practice? Probably because a regular physical exercise regime requires work—or does it?

Earlier guidelines recommended vigorous activity of the large muscles, such as jogging, cycling, or swimming, performed as a structured routine of at least 20 continuous minutes a day on at least three nonconsecutive days per week. The goal was to achieve a target heart rate of 60% to 90% maximum heart rate. These guidelines led many to believe that unless the intensity, duration, and frequency are achieved, there is no benefit (Blair et al., 1992).

The current physical activity recommendation is to encourage more people to be physically active to achieve health benefits. Specifically, the recommendation is that every U.S. adult should accumulate 30 minutes or more of moderate-intensity physical activity on most, preferably all, days of the week. This is the recommendation of the U.S. Surgeon General, the American College of Sports Medicine, and the Centers for Disease Control and Prevention.

This current recommendation highlights two changes from previous guidelines. The first is physical activity versus exercise. The focus on physical activity considers the fact that benefit can be gained with moderate physical activity. Physical activity may be any bodily movement of the skeletal muscles that results in energy expenditure (Casperson et al., 1985). The second major difference from previous guidelines is that the 30 minutes of moderate activity can be done either all at once or in several bouts of 8 to 10 minutes each, where the total time sums to at least 30 minutes (USDHHS, 1996; Roos, 1997).

Advanced practice nurses are in a key position to promote physical activity. The APN can motivate clients through education and role modeling, along with praise and encouragement. An important point to stress is that moderate physical activity leads to health benefits that are both physiologic and psychologic. The major benefits may include but are not limited to the following:

- Prevention of heart disease, type II diabetes, hypertension, and colon cancer
- Reduced serum triglycerides
- Increased serum high-density lipoproteins (HDLs)
- Reduced systolic and diastolic blood pressure
- Increased lean muscle mass
- Reduced body fat
- Increased bone density
- Sustained weight control or slow weight reduction
- Reduced tendency for depression and anxiety
- Increased strength and flexibility (Simon, 1995)

To determine if the client is getting adequate physical activity, the APN must review the client's daily activities and the amount of time spent each day performing these activities. Many typical daily activities produce a moderate level of energy expenditure. Examples of moderate home and leisure activities may include but are not limited to shopping with a cart, walking to mow the lawn, raking, dancing, walking 3 miles per hour, and gardening.

This assessment may reveal that the client is unknowingly meeting the current recommendation for physical activity. Others may be performing moderate-level activities but not for a sum total of 30 minutes. These individuals will need instruction to gradually increase the total time spent being active to 30 minutes a day.

Clients who are sedentary should begin first by selecting appropriate and enjoyable activities to perform. Second, they should incorporate the activity into their daily routine. The APN may be instrumental in assisting clients to identify an activity and to build this activity into their daily routine. Initially, the time spent each day should be a few minutes and, over a period of 6 weeks to 6 months (longer if necessary), gradually increase the total time to 30 minutes a day. Encourage clients to involve family and friends for support and to maintain a log to monitor progress and reward themselves. Follow-up by the provider is very important to staying on track. This can be done with regularly scheduled follow-up appointments or telephone call follow-up. Although safety is always a concern, the American College of Sports Medicine concludes that "virtually all sedentary individuals can begin a moderate exercise program safely" (Kenney et al., 1995). However, it is wise for elders with unstable conditions to be managed in conjunction with a physician.

For healthy clients desiring to begin a vigorous exercise program, the APN should refer to the guidelines for exercise testing and prescription as outlined by the American College of Sports Medicine (Kenney et al., 1995). Another resource specific to developing an exercise program for the older adult is Topp (1991). In addition, exercise physiologists, physical therapists, and physiatrists can also be invaluable resources to the APN.

Important to the successful initiation and maintenance of physical activity is a clearly defined exercise prescription that is individualized and mutually agreed upon. The following are components to be included in all exercise prescriptions:

- Mode of activity
- Duration of activity
- Frequency of activity
- Intensity of activity
- Potential symptoms to watch for and what to do

In addition, clients engaging in a sustained activity should be provided with a specific exercise routine detailing warm-up, active exercise, and cool-down period. The APN should be specific as to the duration and activity to be used for each of these, for example, 5-minute warm-up stretches, brisk walking for 10 minutes, and 10-minute cool-down stretching.

Last, if the chosen activity does not lend itself to maintaining flexibility or muscular strength, then the APN should make recommendations and provide demonstrations. A general rule to follow is strengthen what is weak and stretch what is tight. Performance of any flexibility exercise should include slow stretching of the involved muscle(s), holding a static stretch for 5 to 10 seconds (which produces a mild amount of discomfort), and repeating the procedure two to five times, at least three times per week (Topp, 1991). Jerking or bouncing movements should never be used to improve flexibility. Such movements induce muscle injury and do not contribute substantially to improved flexibility (Topp, 1991). Examples of muscular strengthening exercises are push-ups, sit-ups, arm and leg raises (with or without weights), wall pushes, and knee squats.

It is important for the APN to be innovative with the older adult who has limitations (eg, uses a walker or wheelchair). The APN can demonstrate strengthening and flexibility exercises that can be performed in a chair or in bed. Examples of these include range-of-motion exercises, lifting and lowering self using arms while sitting, and quadricep setting exercises.

Additional Resources for the Older Adult

- *Pep up Your Life: A Fitness Book for Seniors*, published by the American Association of Retired Persons, Fulfillment Services, 601 E. Street NW, Washington, DC 20049, 202-434-2277
- Richard Simmons' *Silver Foxes* (an exercise video for seniors)

■ NUTRITION

Nutrition is an important component to the maintenance of health. Nutritional status can be affected by a number of factors including inadequate nutrient intake, chronic or acute medical problems, medications, physical or cognitive impairment, low income, and social isolation. Many of these factors affect older adults, placing their nutritional health at risk. Nutritional problems of older adults can be prevented, controlled, or reversed once identified. A simple assessment tool entitled "Determine Your Nutritional Health," developed by the Nutrition Screening Initiative (NSI), can be used to identify risk factors for poor nutritional status (see Fig. 2–1).

The NSI tool is a 10-item questionnaire. This tool was designed to measure established predictors of inadequate dietary intake and nutrient deprivation rather than overconsumption of dietary lipids or other food components (Posner et al., 1993). This tool is not diagnostic, but rather provides a foundation for further nutritional problem assessment and intervention as needed.

Any education and counseling on nutrition should include the basics of food groups to choose from and recommended servings. The Food Guide Pyramid is a general guide for daily food choices. It includes the five food groups and the number of daily servings recommended from each (see Fig. 2–2). All clients should be encouraged to eat a variety of foods from each group daily for a healthful diet.

The Food Guide Pyramid is set up as a pictoral of a pyramid. The food group that needs to be consumed in the greatest quantity is at the base and graduates to the food group that needs to be consumed in the least quantity at the tip of the pyramid. The Food Guide Pyramid is easy to learn and simple to use when teaching nutrition.

The APN providing nutrition counseling needs to be aware of the amount that constitutes a serving size because the amount eaten may be more than one serving. A registered dietitian or nutrition book can be a valuable resource to this end. It is important to note that some older adults need the lowest number of servings recommended in the Food Guide Pyramid, as their caloric needs are reduced.

Also important in nutrition counseling is a review of the Dietary Guidelines for Americans. These guidelines are de-

DETERMINE YOUR NUTRITIONAL HEALTH

The Warning Signs of poor nutritional health are often overlooked. Use this checklist to find out if you or someone you know is at nutritional risk.

Read the statements below. Circle the number in the yes column for those that apply to you or someone you know. For each yes answer, score the number in the box. Total your nutritional score.

	YES
I have an illness or condition that made me change the kind and/or amount of food I eat.	2
I eat fewer than 2 meals per day.	3
I eat few fruits or vegetables, or milk products.	2
I have 3 or more drinks of beer, liquor or wine almost every day.	2
I have tooth or mouth problems that make it hard for me to eat.	2
I don't always have enough money to buy the food I need.	4
I eat alone most of the time.	1
I take 3 or more different prescribed or over-the-counter drugs a day.	1
Without wanting to, I have lost or gained 10 pounds in the last 6 months.	2
I am not always physically able to shop, cook and/or feed myself.	2
Total	

Total Your Nutritional Score. If it's —

0–2   **Good!** Recheck your nutritional score in 6 months.

3–5   **You are at moderate nutritional risk.** See what can be done to improve your eating habits and lifestyle. Your office on aging, senior nutrition program, senior citizens center or health department can help. Recheck your nutritional score in 3 months.

6 or   **You are at high nutritional risk.** Bring this checklist the next time you see your doctor, dietitian or
more   other qualified health or social service professional. Talk with them about any problems you may have. Ask for help to improve your nutritional health.

Remember that warning signs suggest risk, but do not represent diagnosis of any condition.

The Nutrition Checklist is based on the Warning Signs described below. Use the word *DETERMINE* to remind you of the Warning Signs.

Disease
Any disease, illness or chronic condition which causes you to change the way you eat or makes it hard for you to eat puts your nutritional health at risk. Four out of five adults have chronic diseases that are affected by diet. Confusion or memory loss that keeps getting worse is estimated to affect one out of five or more of older adults. This can make it hard to remember what, when or if you've eaten. Feeling sad or depressed, which happens to about one in eight older adults, can cause big changes in appetite, digestion, energy level, weight and well-being.

Eating poorly
Eating too little and eating too much both lead to poor health. Eating the same foods day after day or not eating fruit, vegetables, and milk products daily will also cause poor nutritional health. One in five adults skip meals daily. Only 13% of adults eat the minimum amount of fruit and vegetables needed. One in four older adults drink too much alcohol. Many health problems become worse if you drink more than one or two alcoholic beverages per day.

Tooth loss/mouth pain
A healthy mouth, teeth and gums are needed to eat. Missing, loose or rotten teeth or dentures which don't fit well or cause mouth sores make it hard to eat.

Economic hardship
As many as 40% of older Americans have incomes of less than $6,000 per year. Having less or choosing to spend less than $25–30 per week for food makes it very hard to get the foods you need to stay healthy.

Reduced social contact

One-third of all older people live alone. Being with people daily has a positive effect on morale, well-being and eating.

Multiple medicines

Many older Americans must take medicines for health problems. Almost half of older Americans take multiple medicines daily. Growing old may change the way we respond to drugs. The more medicines you take, the greater the chance for side effects such as increased or decreased appetite, change in taste, constipation, weakness, drowsiness, diarrhea, nausea, and others. Vitamins or minerals when taken in large doses act like drugs and can cause harm. Alert your doctor to everything you take.

Involuntary weight loss/gain

Losing or gaining a lot of weight when you are not trying to do so is an important warning sign that must not be ignored. Being overweight or underweight also increases your chance of poor health.

Needs assistance in self care

Although most older people are able to eat, one of every five have trouble walking, shopping, buying and cooking food, especially as they get older.

Elder years above age 80

Most older people lead full and productive lives. But as age increases, risk of frailty and health problems increase. Checking your nutritional health regularly makes good sense.

Figure 2–1. Determine Your Nutritional Health. *Source: Used with permission of the Nutrition Screening Initiative, Washington, DC. The Initiative is funded in part by a grant from Ross Laboratories, Columbus, OH.*

signed to decrease the incidence of hypertension, cardiovascular disease, diabetes, obesity, dental caries, and colon cancer. These guidelines, developed by the U.S. Department of Agriculture and the U.S. Department of Health and Human Services, are as follows:

1. Eat a variety of foods.
2. Maintain a healthy weight.
3. Choose a diet low in total fat (less than 30% of calories), saturated fat (less than 10% of calories), and cholesterol.
4. Choose a diet with plenty of vegetables, fruits, and grain products.
5. Use sugars only in moderation.
6. Use salt and sodium only in moderation.
7. Limit alcohol use to no more than one drink daily for women or two drinks daily for men.

Older adults may need education on how to read and use the nutrition labels, including the daily values. The APN can educate, using actual labels from products. The client's understanding can then be tested by asking him or her to perform a return demonstration of the newly learned skill.

The most common problems related to nutrition affecting the older adult are inadequate caloric intake, dehydration, constipation, osteoporosis, and anemia. Therefore, it is important to provide dietary recommendations to prevent or treat these problems.

Nutrition education and counseling for the older adult must be individualized, with careful consideration of personal factors. Some of the factors to consider are medical health, oral/dental health, level of activity, economic status, medications, living arrangements,

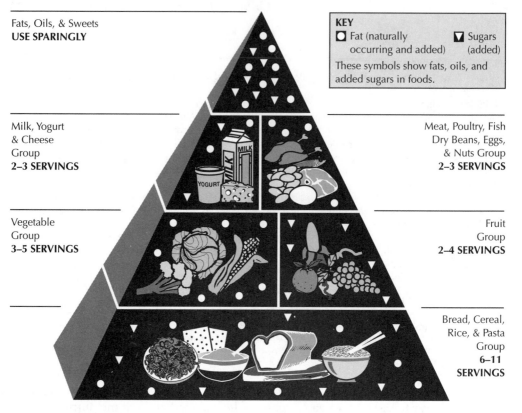

Fats, Oils, & Sweets
USE SPARINGLY

KEY
⬭ Fat (naturally occurring and added)
▼ Sugars (added)
These symbols show fats, oils, and added sugars in foods.

Milk, Yogurt & Cheese Group
2–3 SERVINGS

Meat, Poultry, Fish Dry Beans, Eggs, & Nuts Group
2–3 SERVINGS

Vegetable Group
3–5 SERVINGS

Fruit Group
2–4 SERVINGS

Bread, Cereal, Rice, & Pasta Group
6–11 SERVINGS

What Counts as a Serving?

With the Food Guide Pyramid, what counts as a "serving" may not always be a typical "helping" of what you eat. Here are some examples of servings:

Bread, Cereal, Rice & Pasta—6–11 servings recommended
Examples of one serving:
  1 slice of bread
  1 oz. of ready-to-eat cereal
  1/2 cup of cooked cereal, rice, or pasta
  3 or 4 small plain crackers

Vegetables—3–5 servings recommended
Examples of one serving:
  1 cup of raw leafy vegetables
  1/2 cup of other vegetables, cooked or chopped raw
  3/4 cup of vegetable juice

Fruits—2–4 servings recommended
Examples of one serving:
  1 medium apple, banana, or orange
  1/2 cupped of chopped, cooked, or canned fruit
  3/4 cup of fruit juice

Milk, Yogurt, and Cheese—2–3 servings recommended
Examples of one serving:
  1 cup of milk or yogurt
  1 1/2 oz. of natural cheese
  2 oz. of process cheese

Meat, Poultry, Fish, Dry Beans, Eggs, and Nuts—2–3 servings recommended
Examples of one serving:
  2–3 oz. of cooked lean meat, poultry, or fish
  1/2 cup of cooked dry beans, 1 egg, or 2 tablespoons of peanut butter = 1 oz. of lean meat

How Much Is an Ounce of Meat?

Here's a handy guide to determining how much meat, chicken, fish, or cheese weigh:
  1 ounce is the size of a match box.
  3 ounces are the size of a deck of cards.
  8 ounces are the size of a paperback book.

Figure 2–2. Food Guide Pyramid: A Guide to Daily Food Choices. *Source: U.S. Department of Agriculture/U.S. Department of Health and Human Services.*

consumption of alcohol, physical or cognitive impairment, and nutritional health.

CLINICAL PEARL

Only with a thorough assessment can appropriate, individualized education be provided and nutritional health attained.

Other Resources

- The *Nutrition Interventions Manual for Professionals Caring for Older Americans* and the "Determine Your Nutritional Health" assessment tool can be obtained from Nutritional Screening Initiative, 1010 Wisconsin Avenue NW, Suite 800, Washington, DC 20007, 202-625-1662
- American Dietetic Association, 216 West Jackson Blvd., Suite 800, Chicago, IL 60606-6995, 312-606-6995
- Consumer Nutrition Hotline of National Center for Nutrition and Dietetics, 1-800-366-1655

■ SMOKING CESSATION

Despite specific recommendations for smoking cessation, not all providers intervene with their clients who smoke. Only about one half of older smokers report that they have ever been asked by their provider about their smoking habits (USDHHS, 1990). Yet, nearly two thirds of smokers aged 50 to 74 reported in a survey that they were thinking about quitting in the next year (Rimer et al., 1990). In addition, 70% of smokers see a health-care provider at least once a year, often for a smoking-related illness (Houston, 1992). These visits could be opportunities to explore smoking habits, provide health education and materials regarding smoking cessation, assist the smoker to list reasons to quit, establish a quit date, and provide pharmacologic and behavior modification intervention.

A review of the literature does not reveal any single fail-proof method to accomplish smoking cessation. However, the main indicators of success with smoking cessation are repeated face-to-face contact with the smoker, over an extended period of time, with provider and nonprovider contacts and use of more than one modality for motivating change (Joseph & Byrd, 1989; Lennox, 1992).

Numerous studies have shown that the health-care provider can change an individual's smoking habits. This evidence makes it important that the provider at least briefly discuss smoking cessation with every smoker at every point of contact. Successful smoking cessation requires knowledge about available techniques and an appreciation of how and when to use them.

The National Cancer Institute has published four steps to smoking cessation, called the 4 A's Model (Glynn & Manley, 1990). This may serve the provider as a summary of the four key steps to smoking cessation: ask, advise, assist, and arrange follow-up. This simple mnemonic makes the steps easy to remember.

First, ask about tobacco use. Do you smoke or use smokeless tobacco? How much? For how long? Are you interested in quitting? Have you ever quit before?

For how long did you quit? What made you start again? What makes you smoke? Do you live or work with any smokers?

Second, advise all smokers to quit. Inform smokers that quitting smoking is the single most important thing they can do for their health. Emphasize the benefits of cessation. Assist clients to list at least three of the most important personal reasons they have for quitting. Instruct them to write these reasons on a card to review whenever they have an urge to smoke. Offer smoking cessation treatment at every office visit. Set a quit date with smokers and have them sign a contract with family or friends.

Third, assist smokers' quitting attempts with self-help cessation materials and, when appropriate, nicotine replacement therapy. Because smoking is a physical addiction to nicotine as well as a learned behavior, the most effective approaches must address both of these components. Pharmacologic methods are used to relieve symptoms of nicotine withdrawal, freeing the adult to focus on behavior modification (Rigotti, 1995). Pharmacologic methods available provide nicotine exposure, although at reduced and tapering doses, in a transdermal patch, a chewing gum, and a nasal spray (see Tables 2–2 through 2–4). Although there is no evidence that the nicotine replacement therapy adversely affects coronary artery or peripheral vascular disease, hypertension, or stroke, it is generally not prescribed when a history of these conditions exist (Benowitz, 1993; Hughes, 1993).

Zyban (Ibupropion) is also currently being utilized for smoking cessation as a solo therapy and also as adjunct to nicotine replacement therapy. Zyban needs to be taken daily for at least 7-12 weeks. The future success of this product is yet to be determined since studies beyond 12 weeks need to be conducted.

ANTIDEPRESSANT THERAPY

In smokers with depression or history of depression, antidepressant agents may be required. Referral for counseling and prescriptions is recommended.

TABLE 2–2.   NICOTINE REPLACEMENT THERAPY WITH NICOTINE PATCH (HABITROL, NICODERM, NICOTROL, PROSTEP)

- The nicotine patch is a transdermal system absorbed through the skin over 24 or 16 hours, depending on the brand (the 16-hour patch, Nicotrol, might be useful for clients bothered by insomnia).
- Begin patch application upon awakening on the day of quitting.
- Apply patch every morning on a dry, nonhairy area of upper arm or upper trunk.
- Rotate sites, reusing the same site no more frequently than every 7 days.
- Leave on for 24 hours (16 hours if using Nicotrol).
- Taper over 2 to 3 months (eg, 21 mg/d for 4–6 weeks, then 14 mg/d for 2–4 weeks, and finally 7 mg/d for 2–4 weeks.
- Patches are generally well tolerated; the most common side effect is local skin irritation.
- Instruct client not to smoke or use tobacco or other nicotine products while wearing the patch.
- Encourage enrollment in smoking cessation program and/or use behavior modification techniques for smoking cessation.

TABLE 2–3.   NICOTINE REPLACEMENT THERAPY WITH NICOTINE GUM (NICORETTE, OTC)

- Nicotine gum is a sugar-free chewing gum square that delivers nicotine through transbuccal absorption.
- Begin chewing gum after stopping smoking.
- After drinking any beverage or eating, wait 15 minutes before using the gum (there is decreased absorption in an acidic environment).
- Chew slowly, until there is a tingle or peppery taste, then "park" the gum against the cheek; repeat the chewing once the taste disappears.
- Each gum square lasts up to 30 minutes.
- Do not use more than 24 pieces of gum per day.
- Nicotine gum is available in 2 mg and 4 mg.
  If the client previously smoked under 25 cigarettes daily, begin with 2-mg gum.
  If the client previously smoked 25 or more cigarettes daily, begin with 4-mg gum.
- Use on a regular schedule initially (eg, one piece every 1–2 hours for 6 weeks), then begin to taper use over 2–3 months (eg, one piece every 2–4 hours for 3–4 weeks, then one piece every 4–8 hours for 3–4 weeks, then one piece every 8–12 hours for 3–4 weeks, then stop).
- Instruct client not to smoke or use tobacco or other nicotine products with nicotine gum.
- Encourage enrollment in smoking cessation program and/or use behavior modification techniques for smoking cessation.

BEHAVIOR MODIFICATION

Behavior modification strategies for smoking cessation incorporate techniques to manipulate the environmental cues that trigger or reward smoking (Rigotti, 1995). The most common behavior modification programs include self-monitoring to identify smoking cues, along with progressive restriction, aversive conditioning, positive reinforcement, deep breathing, physical exercise,

TABLE 2–4.   NICOTINE REPLACEMENT THERAPY WITH NICOTINE NASAL SPRAY (NICOTROL NS, Rx)

- This product is a nicotine aqueous nasal spray.
- Begin using after stopping smoking.
- Do not sniff, swallow, or inhale spray.
- The client should use an individualized dose based on dependence. One dose equals one spray to each nostril or two sprays total. Usually, begin with one to two doses/hr (two to four sprays/hr) to a maximum of five sprays/hr or 80 sprays/d.
- The spray may be discontinued abruptly or tapered over 3 months.
- The spray is generally well tolerated; the most common side effects are nasopharyngeal and ocular irritation.
- Instruct client not to smoke or use tobacco or other nicotine products with nicotine nasal spray.
- Encourage enrollment in smoking cessation program and/or use behavior modification techniques for smoking cessation.

and substitute activities for hands or oral stimuli.

Self-monitoring and Progressive Restriction

Individuals identify the cues that trigger smoking for them. Once these cues are identified, they are progressively avoided or modified so that they no longer trigger smoking. According to Rigotti (1995), by itself, this technique is more effective in preparing smokers to quit than in achieving long-term cessation.

Aversive Conditioning

Aversive conditioning techniques pair an unwanted act like smoking with an unpleasant stimulus to make the act less likely to occur. One example is to fill a bottle with cigarette butts and look at this bottle or smell this bottle frequently when the urge to smoke occurs. Another example is to wear a rubber band on the wrist and snap it when the urge to smoke occurs.

Positive Reinforcement

Positive reinforcement allows smokers to reward themselves when smoking is avoided. The positive reinforcement can be complemented with involvement of family or friends. Individuals may reward themselves with a treat after the initial 24 hours without smoking, then the first week, first month, and so on. They may also reward themselves with the money saved from not smoking.

Deep Breathing

The deep breathing technique is especially useful if the client smokes for relaxation and tension reduction. There are a variety of ways to utilize this technique. The first is to instruct clients when they crave a cigarette to breathe as though they are smoking (even though they are

not). Another is to instruct clients to slowly take a breath in and visualize the air entering the nasal passageway into the main bronchus, then the right and left bronchi, and finally the alveoli, enlarging the lungs. Then, exhale slowly and visualize the lungs getting smaller as the air exits the alveoli into the right and left bronchi to the main bronchi and out the mouth. This exercise should be repeated as many times as necessary to relieve the craving. Initially, instruct clients to do this at least five to ten times. Other variations incorporate deep breathing while listening to one's favorite music or imagining one is at a favorite location.

Physical Exercise

Physical exercise is especially helpful for people who smoke to reduce tension and who value the stimulating effects of nicotine. Most smokers gain some weight after stopping smoking—7 to 10 pounds is normal (Sheehan, 1995). Encourage clients to increase whatever exercise they are now doing or enjoy doing. Encourage clients to incorporate an activity like walking or stretching when a cigarette craving occurs, such as after a coffee break, lunch break, or after work. Advise clients to consult a health-care provider if they plan to embark on a new, vigorous exercise program or if they are symptomatic.

Substitute Activities for Hands or Oral Stimuli

These techniques may be important for those who smoke out of habit and those who need to have something in their hand or mouth. Assist the client in identifying items that can be substituted for a cigarette or smoking. Some examples may include toothpicks (flavored or unflavored), pens or pencils, straws or coffee stirrers, chewing gum, hard candy, or fluids like water or juices to sip throughout the day.

The last step in smoking cessation is to arrange follow-up. Follow-up is critical. Studies reveal that scheduling follow-up visits for reinforcement and encouragement increases smoking cessation rates (Kenford et al., 1994). Only after a full year of cessation can the individual be considered an ex-smoker (Rigotti, 1995). In the interim, repeat visits are essential. A suggested follow-up schedule may be once every 2 weeks for 1 month; every month for 3 months, then at 6 months, 9 months, and 1 year. Ask at every visit about the client's effort, and document cessation strategies in progress notes. Do not get discouraged if the client relapses. Praise the initial effort, explore what caused the relapse, and encourage him or her to try again.

■ STRESS MANAGEMENT

Although health risks may increase with advancing age, stress is not an inevitable consequence of older age. Stress can occur from a variety of sources, including physiologic, environmental, and situational. Stressful events can range from daily hassles and annoyances to major life changes such as death of a spouse. Furthermore, the stress response can range from restlessness or fatigue to multiple somatic complaints. It is not the amount or type of stress that is as important as the individual's perception of what is stressful and his or her ability to cope with that stressor.

The APN needs to pay attention to sources of stress, the client's reaction to stress, and his or her personal coping style. This information can be obtained at the time of the visit by asking the client about current stressors and current coping style. Additional areas to be included in the data collection are social history, including support system, psychiatric history, health habits, current medications, general appearance, and physical examination, as well as diagnostic tests to rule out underlying medical causes of the complaint.

There is no single stress management technique that works in all cases for everyone. Stress management techniques are skills that can be learned and implemented by the APN to foster health promotion.

CLINICAL PEARL

The key to successful stress management is individualizing the plan of care.

Once the source of stress is identified, the APN must assist the client to avoid, alter, or cope with the stress or stressors. Following is a listing of factors the APN needs to consider in providing stress management. Since multiple interventions may need to be implemented, the APN should always prioritize.

1. The APN should manage or refer for any medication or disease etiologies.
2. If acute situational anxiety is present, it may be necessary to implement pharmacotherapeutics or to refer to a specialist.

3. If the client has a negative coping technique, the APN must assist the client to identify and use a positive coping technique that is realistic for him or her.

4. If the client has poor health habits, the APN must assist the client to modify health habits to:
   - Achieve a healthful diet
   - Limit alcohol use

Practice is to be done while sitting in a chair with your back straight, head on a line with your back, both feet on the floor and hands resting on your lap. Each muscle is to be tightened, held in tightened position for 15–20 seconds, and then slowly let go while studying the difference between tension and relaxation.

Forehead. Wrinkle up your forehead by arching your eyebrows and creasing your forehead, hold the tension, and then slowly let go of the tension.

Eyes. Squeeze your eyes together tightly, hold the tension, and then slowly let go of the tension.

Nose. Wrinkle up your nose and spread your nostrils, hold the tension, and then slowly let go of the tension.

Face. Put a forced smile on your face and spread your face, hold the tension, and then slowly let go of the tension.

Tongue. Push your tongue hard against the roof of your mouth, hold the tension, and then slowly let go of the tension.

Jaws. Clench your jaws together tightly, hold the tension, and then slowly let go of the tension.

Lips. Pucker up your lips and spread them, hold the tension, and then slowly let go of the tension.

Neck. Tighten the muscles of your neck by pulling your chin in and shrugging up your shoulders, hold the tension, and then slowly let go of the tension.

Right Arm. Tense your right arm and hand by stretching it out in front of you and clenching your fist tightly, hold the tension, and then slowly let go of the tension.

Left Arm. Tense your left arm and hand by stretching it out in front of you, and then slowly let go of the tension.

Right Leg. Extend your right leg in front of you (at the height of the chair seat), tense your thigh and leg by pointing your toes inward toward your face, hold the tension, and then slowly let go of the tension.

Left Leg. Extend your left leg in front of you, tense your thigh and leg by pointing your toes inward toward your face, hold the tension, and then slowly let go of the tension.

Upper Back. Tense your back muscles by sitting slightly forward in the chair, bending your elbows and trying to get them to touch each other behind your back, hold the tension, and then slowly let go of the tension.

Chest. Tense your chest muscles by pulling your stomach in and thrusting your chest upward and outward, hold the tension, and then slowly let go of the tension.

Stomach. Tense your stomach muscles making them hard by pushing your stomach out, hold the tension, and then slowly let go of the tension.

Buttocks and Thighs. Tense your buttocks and thighs by placing your feet squarely on the floor, pointing your toes into the floor and forcing your heels to remain on the floor while pushing forward, hold the tension, and then slowly let go of the tension.

Practice should be engaged in twice daily for a period of 12–15 minutes. Mastery of the technique is after 2–4 weeks of twice daily practice.

Figure 2–3. Progressive Deep Muscle Relaxation. *Source: Reprinted with permission from Goroll, A. H., May, L. A., & Mulley, A. (1995). Primary care medicine: Office evaluation and management of the adult patient (p. 1031): Philadelphia: J. B. Lippincott.*

Practice is to be done while sitting in a soft, comfortable chair with your eyes closed. As attention is called to specific groups of muscles, try to *visualize* and *feel* the relaxation of those muscles. Try to let *happen* what is being suggested. Repeat each formula 2–3 times.

My forehead and scalp feel heavy, limp, loose, and relaxed.

My eyes and nose feel heavy, limp, loose, and relaxed.

My face and jaws feel heavy, limp, loose, and relaxed.

My neck, shoulders, and back feel heavy, limp, loose, and relaxed.

My arms and hands feel heavy, limp, loose, and relaxed.

My chest, solar plexus, and the central part of my body feel quiet, calm, comfortable, and relaxed.

My stomach feels heavy, limp, loose, and relaxed.

My buttocks, thighs, calves, ankles, and toes feel quiet, heavy, limp, loose, and relaxed.

My whole body feels quiet, heavy, limp, and relaxed.

Practice should be engaged in twice daily for a period of 6–8 minutes. Mastery of the technique is after 1–3 weeks of twice daily practice.

Figure 2–4. Autogenic Training. *Source: Reprinted with permission from Goroll, A. H., May, L. A., & Mulley, A. (1995). Primary care medicine: Office evaluation and management of the adult patient (p. 1032). Philadelphia: J. B. Lippincott.*

- Obtain regular physical activity
- Quit smoking
- Obtain adequate sleep and rest

5. If the stress is related to a lack of support system, the APN can assist the client to identify sources of suport among family and friends or refer to an appropriate support group.

6. If the stress is related to time management, the APN can assist the client to identify daily activities that are essential versus those that are an overextension of self or nonproductive time. In addition, the client can be encouraged to attend time management courses at a community college or adult education program. Self-help books on time management are also available (Lakein, 1974).

7. If the stress is related to a lack of assertiveness, the APN can provide counseling for assertiveness or encourage the client to attend assertiveness courses at community colleges. Self-help books on assertiveness are also available (Jakobowski and Lange, 1978).

8. If the stressor causes muscular tension, the APN can teach appropriate stretching exercises or refer the client for massage therapy or physical therapy.

9. If the stressor cannot be avoided or altered, relaxation techniques can be used. There are a variety of relaxation techniques, including biofeedback, meditation, yoga, massage therapy, progressive deep muscle relaxation, autogenic training, and diaphragmatic breathing. The latter three are easy to learn and can be used immediately by the client without incurring a cost or requiring equipment.

For progressive deep muscle relaxation, see Fig. 2–3; for autogenic training, see

While sitting or lying down with a pillow at the small of your back
1. Breathe in slowly and deeply by pushing your stomach out.
2. Say the word "relax" silently to yourself prior to exhaling.
3. Exhale slowly, letting your stomach come in.
4. Repeat entire procedure 10 times consecutively, with emphasis on slow, deep breaths.

Practice should take place 5 times per day, 10 consecutive diaphragmatic breaths each sitting. Time for mastery is after 1–2 weeks of daily practice.

Figure 2–5. Diaphragmatic Breathing. *Source: Reprinted with permission from Goroll, A. H., May, L. A., & Mulley, A. (1995).* Primary care medicine: Office evaluation and management of the adult patient *(p. 1032): Philadelphia: J. B. Lippincott.*

Fig. 2–4; for diaphagmatic breathing, see Fig. 2–5.

Successful stress management is a process that takes place over a period of time. It is not unusual for clients to have multiple stressors and need to utilize several stress management techniques. The APN can be most helpful by encouraging one change at a time and follow-up to monitor progress.

▪ INJURY PREVENTION

The most common unintentional injuries resulting in morbidity and mortality in the older adult involve motor vehicle accidents (MVAs), falls, and home-related accidents and polypharmacy. The APN is in an excellent position to screen and counsel the older adult to prevent these problems and thus reduce the associated morbidity and mortality. Older adults are at risk for all of these unintentional injuries, considering some of the normal changes that occur in aging. These changes include decrease in peripheral vision and visual acuity, slowed neurologic response, decrease in musculoskeletal agility, and decrease in renal function and hepatic metabolism. In the older adult, there is also an increased incidence of physical and cognitive impairment and chronic illness requiring multiple medications, which can cause further impairment. All of these factors place the older adult at increased risk for unintentional injuries.

In addition, the older adult may not be aware of these deficits so concerns may not be raised by the client. If the family is available, it is best for the APN to ask the family for their insight. Nonetheless, routine visits or health screenings are excellent times for the APN to assess the older adult for any physical or cognitive changes and review medications to thus provide appropriate counseling.

MOTOR VEHICLE ACCIDENTS

Motor vehicle accidents are the leading cause of death from unintentional injury for those aged 65 to 74 and second for those 75 and older (falls are first) (Mayhew, 1991). Another factor to consider is that adults older than 55 years account for more than 20% of the driving population in the United States today, and their numbers are projected to increase to 39% by 2050 (Waller, 1992). Considering the increase in numbers of older adults, the morbidity and mortality associated with MVAs will increase if older adults at risk are not identified and interventions implemented.

It is important to note that many times the older adult may not recognize or recall any deficits, and therefore the APN should involve family in the assessment whenever possible. A review of some basic considerations to prevent injuries related to MVAs should be provided to all older adults. First, older adults should be asked if they always wear a seatbelt properly in the car. If not, advise them to always wear a seatbelt, and provide a review of proper application. Second, older drivers should be asked if they perform routine vehicle maintenance. If not, the APN can stress the importance of routine maintenance in the prevention of injury. Third, older adults should be asked if they have received any traffic violations; been involved in recent accidents or near misses; experienced any difficulty driving, especially at night; or gotten lost. If so, the frequency and severity of those events should be evaluated and may be a clue to identifying unsafe drivers. Finally, the older driver should be asked about alcohol use as well as current medication usage. The APN should evaluate the potential of any of the medications to affect driving. Advice should be provided to refrain from driving after drinking alcohol or while taking medications that may affect the older driver.

Obviously, age alone should not be the only consideration as to whether an individual is safe to drive, because many older adults are experienced, safe drivers. However, some may have a deterioration in perception, cognition, or coordination—the skills that are necessary for safe driving (Carr, 1993). Therefore, it is important to assess older adults relative to these three skills to decide

whether they are safe to drive. An additional resource is the American Medical Association's guidelines for medical clearance of the older driver (Doeg & Engelberg, 1986).

Assessing perception involves an evaluation of vision, hearing, sensation, and range of motion. Visual acuity should be measured for both near and far vision as well as peripheral vision. Carr (1993) reports that the older adult with visual acuity less than 20/40 with correction or poor peripheral vision should be referred to an ophthalmologist for evaluation and treatment. If the visual impairment cannot be corrected, the ophthalmologist will often suggest driving restriction. It is important to note that most states require vision testing at the time of license renewal.

Hearing acuity should also be evaluated. However, since hearing impairment has not been shown to increase MVAs, older drivers should not be restricted based on isolated hearing impairment (Booker, 1978).

Sensory neuropathy could impair use of foot controls. Therefore, it should be tested by applying a light touch or pinprick to lower extremities (Carr, 1993). An impairment of range of motion, especially in cervical mobility, should also be assessed. When possible, attempt to correct any problems identified or at least prevent further decline.

A cognitive assessment should include testing attention span, concentration, intelligence, judgment, learning ability, memory, orientation, problem solving, psychomotor ability, and social intactness (McDougall, 1990). The Mini-Mental State Exam is a reliable and valid screening tool that can be used to assess some parameters of cognition.

CLINICAL PEARL

The APN might also use questions about hypothetical driving situations to further assess problem solving (eg, what would you do at a blinking yellow light?; if you got lost?).

An assessment of coordination is important to ascertain ability to maneuver the automobile. This assessment should include an evaluation of muscle strength, joint mobility of extremities, and cerebellar intactness. The APN can demonstrate appropriate exercises to improve mobility and function or may refer the client to a specialist.

After a thorough assessment, the APN can decide whether the older adult is able to drive safely, whether modifications need to be considered, or whether he or she should stop driving. Some modifications may include shorter trips, fewer trips, non–rush-hour driving, daytime driving only, and slower roadways (Carr, 1993). The APN must individualize these decisions. If the APN feels uncomfortable in making a determination, the following sources identified by Carr (1993) may help:

- An occupational therapist may evaluate perception and provide cognitive and road testing.
- A neurologist or neuropsychologist can often help clients with neurologic disorders.
- Private driving schools can monitor and test basic road skills.
- State departments of motor vehicles can retest older drivers and may have a driving improvement office

that makes special recommendations to drivers with medical impairments.

In addition, the American Association of Retired Persons (AARP) offers a driver education program, 55 Alive/Mature Driving, that meets the needs of drivers over the age of 50 (AARP, 1992).

If the older driver must stop driving, the APN must assist the client to identify alternate modes of transportation. If the older adult disagrees with the recommendation to stop driving, the APN should recruit the support of family members and document his or her recommendation and interventions. In addition, the APN may contact the state department of motor vehicles (DMV) with concerns. The DMV may contact the individual and suspend his or her license until retested.

The importance of assessing driving risks cannot be emphasized enough. Drivers at risk not only endanger themselves but also any passengers, as well as other drivers and pedestrians. The APN should assess, advise, and support older adults to make necessary adjustments to reduce the risk of injury for all.

HOUSEHOLD INJURIES

Falls are the leading cause of unintentional injury in the older adult. About 30% of persons aged 65 and older who are living at home will fall each year; this rate rises to 50% in those over age 80 (Tinetti, 1990). In addition, significant morbidity and mortality are associated with falls. Approximately 15% of falls result in physical injury serious enough to warrant medical attention, such as muscle sprain, soft-tissue injury, and fractures (Tinetti & Speechley, 1989). Falls represent the leading cause of accidental deaths among adults older than 65 years (Baker & Harvey, 1985). In addition, falls often lead to a fear of falling, which can decrease mobility and independence.

The causes of falls in older adults are usually multifactorial. There may be both intrinsic and extrinsic factors. The intrinsic factors associated with falls include physical or cognitive impairment, poor vision, and postural instability. The extrinsic factors include environmental factors (eg, poor lighting, wet or slippery floors, cluttered pathways, unstable furniture, low beds or toilets, inappropriate shoe wear or assistive devices) and medications. The use of four or more drugs or the use of psychoactive and antihypertensive drugs is associated with an increased risk of falling (Tibbitts, 1996; Svensson et al., 1991). These are all factors that can be avoided or closely monitored to prevent falls.

In providing education and counseling to prevent falls, the APN should assess older adults for these factors and identify those at risk for falling. Tideiksaar (1996) presents seven basic steps for mobility screening, which can be used with older adults. Additionally, the APN's interventions to prevent falls in the older adult may include the following:

1. Identify and treat disorders that may affect the client's balance, including diabetes or conditions of the heart, nervous system, musculoskeletal system, and thyroid.
2. Evaluate for visual, hearing, or other sensory deficits.
3. Evaluate the use of calcium supplementation and hormone replacement therapy (HRT) for women, because osteoporosis is a risk factor for fractures associated with falls.
4. Provide behavioral instruction and training (eg, avoid sudden changes in position, instruct how to fall safely).
5. Evaluate medications including their side effects, interactions, and how they may affect coordination and balance.
6. Educate the client on strengthening and flexibility exercises.
7. Limit alcohol intake. Even a little alcohol can further disturb already impaired balance and reflexes.
8. Assess nighttime temperature in the home, making sure it is not lower than 65°F. Prolonged exposure to cold may cause body temperature to drop, leading to dizziness and falling.
9. Assess the adequacy of footwear and assistive devices. Instruct the client to avoid wearing only socks or smooth-soled shoes or slippers that may lead to slipping and falling.
10. Evaluate the home environment.

CLINICAL PEARL

Tai Chi, a Chinese martial art that focuses on slow and graceful movements, can reduce the risk of falling and maintain strength in older persons.

The National Safety Council (1982) developed a Home Safety Checklist for Older Adults (see Fig. 2–6). This check-

Place a check mark next to each question if the answer is yes. Use this checklist to correct all hazards in the home.

Housekeeping

_____ Do you clean up spills as soon as they occur?

_____ Do you keep floors and stairways clean and free of clutter?

_____ Do you put away books, magazines, sewing supplies, and other objects as soon as you are through with them and never leave them on floors or stairways?

_____ Do you store frequently used items on shelves that are within easy reach?

Floors

_____ Do you keep everyone from walking on freshly washed floors before they are dry?

_____ If you wax floors, do you apply 2 thin coats and buff each thoroughly or use self-polishing wax?

_____ Do all area rugs have nonslip backings?

_____ Have you eliminated small rugs at the tops and bottoms of stairways?

_____ Are all carpet edges tacked down?

_____ Are rugs and carpets free of curled edges, worn spots, and rips?

_____ Have you chosen rugs and carpets with short, dense pile?

_____ Are rugs and carpets installed over good-quality, medium-thick pads?

Lighting

_____ Do you have light switches near every doorway?

_____ Do you have enough good lighting to eliminate shadowy areas?

_____ Do you have a lamp or light switch within easy reach of every bed?

_____ Do you have night lights in your bathrooms and in hallways leading from bedrooms to bathrooms?

_____ Are all stairways well lit with light switches at both top and bottom?

Bathrooms

_____ Do you use a rubber mat or nonslip decals in tubs and showers?

_____ Do you have a grab bar securely anchored over each tub and shower?

_____ Do you have a nonslip rug on all bathroom floors?

_____ Do you keep soap in easy-to-reach receptacles?

Traffic Lanes

_____ Can you walk across every room in your home, and from one room to another, without detouring around furniture?

_____ Is the traffic lane from your bedroom to the bathroom free of obstacles?

_____ Are telephone and appliance cords kept away from areas where people walk?

Stairways

_____ Do securely fastened handrails extend the full length of the stairs on each side of the stairways?

_____ Do the handrails stand out from the walls so you can get a good grip?

_____ Are handrails distinctly shaped so you are alerted when you reach the end of a stairway?

_____ Are all stairways in good condition, with no broken, sagging, or sloping steps?

_____ Are all stairway carpeting and metal edges securely fastened and in good condition?

_____ Have you replaced any single-level steps with gradually rising ramps or made sure such steps are well lighted?

Ladders and Step Stools

_____ Do you always use a step stool or ladder that is tall enough for the job?

_____ Do you always set up your ladder or step stool on a firm, level base that is free of clutter?

_____ Before you climb a ladder or step stool, do you always make sure it is fully open and that the stepladder spreaders are locked?

_____ When you use a ladder or step stool, do you face the steps and keep your body between the side rails?

_____ Do you avoid standing on the top step of a step stool or climbing beyond the second step from the top on a stepladder?

Place a check mark next to each question if the answer is yes. Use this checklist to correct all hazards in the home.

Outdoor Areas

_____ Are walks and driveways in your yard and other areas free of breaks?
_____ Are lawns and gardens free of holes?
_____ Do you put away garden tools and hoses when they are not in use?
_____ Are outdoor areas kept free of rocks, loose boards, and other tripping hazards?
_____ Do you keep outdoor walkways, steps, and porches free of wet leaves and snow?
_____ Do you sprinkle icy outdoor areas with deicers as soon as possible after a snowfall or freeze?
_____ Do you have mats at doorways for people to wipe their feet on?
_____ Do you know the safest way of walking when you can't avoid walking on a slippery surface?

Footwear

_____ Do your shoes have soles and heels that provide good traction?
_____ Do you avoid walking in stocking feet and wear house slippers that fit well and don't fall off?
_____ Do you wear low-heeled oxfords, loafers, or good-quality sneakers when you work in your house or yard?
_____ Do you replace boots or galoshes when their soles or heels are worn too smooth to keep you from slipping on wet or icy surfaces?

Personal Precautions

_____ Are you always alert for unexpected hazards, such as out-of-place furniture?
_____ If young children visit or live in your home, are you alert for children playing on the floor and toys left in your path?
_____ If you have pets, are you alert for sudden movements across your path and pets getting underfoot?
_____ When you carry packages, do you divide them into smaller loads and make sure they do not obstruct your vision?
_____ When you reach or bend, do you hold onto a firm support and avoid throwing your head back or turning it too far?
_____ Do you always move deliberately and avoid rushing to answer phone or doorbell?
_____ Do you take time to get your balance when you change position from lying down to sitting and from sitting to standing?
_____ Do you keep yourself in good condition with moderate exercise, good diet, adequate rest, and regular medical checkups?
_____ If you wear glasses, is your prescription up to date?
_____ Do you know how to reduce injury in a fall?
_____ If you live alone, do you have daily contact with a friend or neighbor?

Figure 2–6. Home Safety Checklist for Older Adults. *Source: Reprinted with permission of National Safety Council, Itasca, IL © 1982.*

list can be used to identify risk factors in the home. Once risk factors are identified, the APN can individualize the environmental improvements that should be made to prevent falls. The APN may need to identify community resources to provide financial and technical assistance to make safety repairs.

Other leading causes of unintentional injury and death in persons over 65 include asphyxiation by choking as well as injury from fires and burns. The APN can prevent injury and death from these factors as well. By identifying those at risk, the APN can provide preventive education as well as appropriate interventions.

Those at risk for choking include older adults with poor dentition, use of sedative drugs, dementia, and reduced motor coordination. Interventions the APN may implement include referring those with poor dentition for correct denture fit, evaluating medications and adjusting accordingly, and evaluating the consistency of foods eaten and adjusting as needed. In addition, the APN can train or refer those caring for the older adult in the use of the Heimlich maneuver and cardiopulmonary resuscitation (CPR).

Regarding injury and death associated with fires and burns, the APN must also identify risk factors and provide appropriate preventive education. This education may include but is not limited to the following:

- Install and maintain smoke detectors in the home.
- Test smoke detectors monthly and change batteries at least twice a year, in spring and autumn.
- Safely store matches and lighters.
- Avoid smoking near bedding or upholstery.
- Wear nonflammable sleepwear.
- Set hot water temperatures to no greater than 120°F to 130°F.

Preventing injuries through education and counseling is certainly within the APN's scope of practice. Considering the associated morbidity and mortality associated with the unintentional injuries described above, the APN should make injury prevention education and counseling an essential component of care for the individual, family and community. This is a tremendous challenge but the rewards are promising for the APN as well as the older adult.

■ POLYPHARMACY

Polypharmacy is the use of multiple medications to relieve symptoms of health deviation or symptoms resulting from drug therapy. Because older adults tend to have more illnesses, they also tend to consume more medications, leading to problems of polypharmacy. In addition, adverse drug reactions increase with age since renal and hepatic function decrease with age.

Adults aged 65 years and older consume 30% of all prescription medication. Nonprescription medication use among this age group is seven times that of the general population (USDHHS, 1994). For these reasons, the APN should assess the use of prescription and nonprescription medication by older adults regularly. In addition, the APN should evaluate for unnecessary or inappropriate medication use by the older adult.

To assist with tracking the older client's medication usage, flow sheets should be used to document prescription and nonprescription medications, including dosage, frequency, purpose, and duration of use. Clients also should be asked about vitamin products, nutritional supplements, and homeopathic or alternative medicines. These products are not considered over-the-counter (OTC) medications by the Food and Drug Administration (FDA) or the nonprescription drug industry and therefore have not met the same safety and efficacy requirements as OTC medications. Alcohol use and recreational substance use should be assessed as well.

The APN should advise clients to keep an up-to-date list of medications with dosage and frequency in their wallet so it is available for review at office visits or hospital admissions. When conducting a medication review, the APN should consider the following:

- Review whether the client is taking medication appropriately.
- Review the side effects and adverse effects of each medication, as well as symptoms of toxicity.
- Review drug–disease interaction and drug–drug interaction, as well as drug–food considerations.
- Avoid combinations of medications that augment side effects.
- Avoid medications that duplicate therapy.
- Use monotherapy to manage multiple diseases or illnesses when possible.
- Avoid drugs that can exacerbate the client's other medical conditions.
- Keep the dosage schedule simple and the number of pills as low as possible.
- Consider nonpharmacologic methods when possible (eg, increase fiber and water intake and delete laxative or stool softener).
- When a new medication is needed, consideration should be given to starting with as little as half the usual adult dosage unless an initial high plasma concentration is needed, as with antibiotics and certain cardiac medications.
- Obtain serum drug levels regularly to monitor therapeutic levels when applicable.
- Avoid medications that are metabolized in the liver or kidney in clients with impaired liver or kidney function.
- Use caution in prescribing medications with central nervous system effects, anticholinergic side effects, or long half-lives.

- When a client develops a new problem after starting a new medication, always consider the possibility that the problem could be related to the medication (Colley & Lucas, 1993; Resnick, 1996; USDHHS, 1994).

Many drugs that are commonly prescribed for young to middle-aged adult clients are inappropriate for use with older adults. Lee (1996) has listed some of the drugs to avoid and the problems associated with their use in older adults (see Table 2–5).

In addition, thorough client education cannot be overemphasized. The following are some points for the APN to consider in client education:

- The brand and generic names of the medication
- Purpose of the medication
- Dosage, frequency, and duration of the medication
- Side effects of the medication and whether these should subside with use
- Symptoms of adverse effects or toxicity to watch for and what to do
- Whether to take medication with food or on an empty stomach
- Whether to avoid alcoholic beverages or any foods
- To consult a pharmacist or healthcare provider before taking any OTC medication

By conducting regular medication reviews and providing thorough client education, many of the problems of polypharmacy can be avoided. Taking the time initially for careful consideration of a medication choice can avoid potential danger to older clients. A geriatric specialist or pharmacist can be a valuable resource to the APN in this regard.

TABLE 2–5.   UNDESIRABLE DRUGS FOR OLDER PATIENTS

Drug	Problem
■ **LONG-ACTING BENZODIAZEPINES**	
Diazepam (Valium), chlordiazepoxide (Librium), flurazepam (Dalmane)	Produce daytime hangover-like effect due to prolonged duration of action; shorter-acting benzodiazepines are considered safer
Mebrobamate (Equanil, Miltown)	Accumulates with repeated dosing; shorter-acting benzodiazepines are considered safer
Pentobarbital (Nembutal), secobarbital (Seconal)	Accumulate with repeated dosing; shorter-acting benzodiazepines are considered safer
Amitriptyline (Elavil)	Has potent anticholinergic side effects
Indomethacin (Indocin)	Headaches are more common than with other nonsteroidal anti-inflammatory agents; may also worsen depression
Chlorpropamide (Diabinese)	Causes prolonged hypoglycemia
Propoxyphene (Darvon)	Metabolite, norpropoxyphene, can cause arrhythmias, particularly in patients with impaired renal function
Pentazocine (Talwin)	Can cause seizures, hallucinations, or arrhythmias when taken in large doses
Cyclandelate (Cyclospasmol)	Ineffective as dementia treatment
Isoxsuprine (Vasodilan)	Ineffective as dementia treatment
■ **MUSCLE RELAXANTS**	
Cyclobenzaprine (Flexeril), orphenadrine (Norflex), methocarbamol (Robaxin), carisoprodol (Soma)	Potential for central nervous system toxicity is greater than potential benefit
Trimethobenzamide (Tigan)	Less effective than alternative agents; may cause drowsiness and other adverse effects
Dipyridamole (Persantine)	Efficacy unproven

Source: Lee, M (1996). Drugs and the elderly: Do you know the risk? (1996). *AJN, 96*(7), 30. Used with permission of Lippincott-Raven Publishers.

CASE STUDY

Mr. Thomas is a 65-year-old retired factory worker who is currently hospitalized with pneumonia and has not seen a health provider for over 10 years. He presented with complaints of chest pain, cough, and shortness of breath (SOB) of 3 days' duration prior to admission. He smokes two packs of cigarettes a day, drinks four beers a day, gets very little exercise, and is at least 25 pounds overweight. His father died of a myocardial infarc-

tion (MI) at age 63, and his mother, still living at age 86, has diabetes. During the discharge exam, decreased breath sounds are noted. His blood pressure (BP) is 150/94, and he experiences SOB with moderate exertion. He complains that he wants a cigarette since he has not had one for 3 days, and he is in denial regarding the seriousness of cardiovascular risk factors.

QUESTIONS

1. What are the cardiovascular risk factors for this client?
2. What approach might the APN use to counsel Mr. Thomas regarding cardiovascular risk factor reduction?
3. What might be some other interventions the APN can consider?

ANSWERS

1. Mr. Thomas' cardiovascular risk factors include male sex, increasing age, overweight, sedentary life style, history of smoking, mild hypertension, and family history of MI and diabetes.
2. The APN may begin by "planting the seed." This can be accomplished by stating the cardiovascular risk factors affecting Mr. Thomas and describing which factors can be reduced or elimi-

nated with life-style changes and behavior modification (ie, decrease weight, increase physical activity, limit salt, decrease cholesterol and fat intake, and stop smoking). The APN should remember that according to the HBM, overcoming barriers and costs are the most important factors for clients followed by perceived susceptibility. Therefore, the APN can stress that no equipment or added costs are required to make the changes listed above, with the exception of pharmacologic treatment for smoking cessation. The APN can explore community resources for the client. In addition, the APN can stress that the client is susceptible to cardiovascular disease because of the multiple risk factors identified above.

3. Other interventions the APN can consider are as follows:

- Provide Pneumovax (pneumococeal vaccine) before discharge, considering the client's age.
- Initiate aspirin prophalaxis 325 mg PO qd.
- Assess client's tetanus and diphtheria (Td) immunization status and provide initial vaccination of Td booster if needed.
- Schedule a wellness follow-up office visit to monitor progress and check BP, reevaluate respiratory assessment, check cholesterol profile, check prostate, check stool for occult blood, check oral cavity since alcohol and smoking are risk factors, assess smoking history and assist with smoking cessation, assess weight and prescribe exercise, and assess stress management techniques.
- Suggest outpatient dietary counseling for weight loss and hypertension.

■ REFERENCES

American Association of Retired Persons. (1992). *55 alive/mature driving.* Washington, DC: Author.

Baker, S. P., & Harvey, A. H. (1985). Fall injuries in the elderly. *Clin Geriatr Med, 1,* 501–508.

Benowitz, N. L. (1993). Nicotine replacement therapy: What has been accomplished—Can we do better? *Drugs, 2,* 157–170.

Blair, S. N., Kohl, H. W., Gordon, N. F., & Paffenbarger, R. S. (1992). How much physical activity is good for health? *Annual Review of Public Health, 13,* 99–126.

Booker, H. R. (1978). Effects of visual and auditory impairment in driving performance. *Hum Factors, 20,* 307–320.

Carr, D. B. (1993). Assessing older drivers for physical and cognitive impairment. *Geriatrics, 48*(5), 46–48, 51.

Casperson, C. J., Powell, K. E., & Christenson, G. M. (1985). Physical activity, exercise and physical fitness: Definitions and distinctions for health related research. *Public Health Rep, 100,* 126–131.

Colley, C. A., & Lucas, L. M. (1993). Polypharmacy: The cure becomes the disease. *J Gen Intern Med, 8,* 278–283.

Doeg, T. C., & Engelberg, A. L. (Eds.). (1986). *Medical conditions affecting drivers.* Chicago: American Medical Association.

Glynn, T. J., & Manley, M. (1990). *How to help your patients stop smoking: A National Cancer Institute manual for physicians* (NIH Publication No. 90-3064). Bethesda, MD: U.S. Department of Health and Human Services, Public Health Service, National Institutes of Health, National Cancer Institute.

Houston, T. P. (1992). Smoking cessation in office practice. *Primary Care, 19,* 493–507.

Hughes, J. R. (1993). Risk/benefit assessment of nicotine preparations on smoking cessation. *Drug Saf, 8,* 49–56.

Jakobowski, P., & Lange, A. T. (1978). *The assertive opinion: Your rights and responsibilities.* Champaign, IL: Research Press.

Janz, N. K., & Becker, M. H. (1984). The health belief model: A decade later. *Health Educ Q, 11*(1), 1–47.

Joseph, A. M., & Byrd, J. C. (1989). Smoking cessation in practice. *Primary Care, 16,* 83–98.

Kenford, L., Fiore, M. C., Jorenby, D. E., et al. (1994). Predicting smoking cessation: Who will quit with and without the nicotine patch. *JAMA, 271,* 589–594.

Kenney, W. L., Humphrey, R. H., & Bryant, C. X. (Eds.). (1995). *American college of sports medicine guidelines for exercise testing and prescription* (5th ed.). Baltimore: Williams & Wilkins.

Lakein, A. (1974). *How to get control of your time and life.* New York: Signet.

Lee, M. (1996). Drugs and the elderly: Do you know the risks? *Am J Nurs, 96,* 25–31.

Lennox, A. S. (1992). Determinants of outcome in smoking cessation. *Br J Gen Pract, 42*, 247–252.

Li, V. C., Kim, Y. J., Ewart, C. K., et al. (1984). Effects of physician counseling on the smoking behavior of asbestos-exposed workers. *Prev Med, 13*, 462–476.

Mayhew, M. S. (1991). Strategies for promoting safety and preventing injury. *Nurs Clin North Am, 26*, 885–893.

McDougall, G. (1990). A review of screening instruments for assessing cognition and mental status in older adults. *Nurse Pract, 15*(11), 18–28.

McGinnis, J. M., & Foege, W. H. (1993). Actual causes of death in the United States. *JAMA, 270*, 2207–2212.

National Safety Council. (1982). *Home safety checklist for older adults.* Itasca, IL: Author.

Posner, B. M., Jette, A. M., Smith, K. W., & Miller, D. R. (1993). Nutrition and health risks in the elderly: The nutrition screening initiative. *Am J Public Health, 83*, 972–977.

Resnick, N. M. (1996). Geriatric medicine. In Tierney, L. M., McPhee, S. J., & Papadakis, M. A. (Eds.), *Current medical diagnosis and treatment* (pp. 52–53). Stamford, CT: Appleton & Lange.

Rigotti, N. (1995). Smoking cessation. In Goroll, A. H., May, L. A., & Mulley, A. G. Jr. (Eds.), *Primary care medicine: Office evaluation and management of the adult patient* (pp. 300–308). Philadelphia: J. B. Lippincott.

Rimer, B. K., Orleans, C. T., Keintz, M. K., et al. (1990). The older smoker: Status, challenges and opportunities for intervention. *Chest, 97*, 547–553.

Robinson, R. D. (1979). *An introduction to helping adults learn and change.* Milwaukee: Omnibook Co.

Roos, R. J. (1997). The surgeon general's report: A prime resource for exercise advocated. *Physician Sports Med, 25*, 127–131.

Sheehan, K. (1995). Smoking cessation. In Star, W., Lommel, L., & Shannon, M. (Eds.), *Women's primary health care: Protocols for practice* (pp. 14:55–14:60). Washington, DC: American Nurses Publishing.

Simon, H. B. (1995). Exercise and prevention of cardiovascular disease. In Gorroll, A. H., May, L. A., & Mulley, A. G. Jr. (Eds.), *Primary care medicine: Office evaluation and management of the adult patient* (pp. 81–88). Philadelphia: J. B. Lippincott.

Svensson, M. L., Rundgren, A., Larsson, M., & Landahl, S. (1991). Accidents in the institutionalized elderly: A risk analysis. *Aging, 3*, 181–192.

Tibbitts, G. M. (1996). Patients who fall: How to predict and prevent injuries. *Geriatrics, 51*(9), 24–31.

Tideiksaar, R. (1996). Preventing falls: How to identify risk factors, reduce complications. *Geriatrics, 51*(2), 43–46, 49.

Tinetti, M. E. (1990). Falls. In Cassel, C. K., Riesenberg, D. E., Sorenson, L. B., & Walsh, J. R. (Eds.), *Geriatric medicine,* (2nd ed) (pp. 528–534). New York: Springer-Verlag.

Tinetti, M. E., & Speechley, M. (1989). Prevention of falls among the elderly. *N Engl J Med, 320*, 1055–1059.

Topp, R. (1991). Development of an exercise program for older adults: Pre-exercise testing, exercise prescription and program maintenance. *Nurse Pract, 16*(10), 16–27.

U.S. Department of Agriculture & U.S. Department of Health and Human Services. (1990). *Dietary guidelines for Americans* (Bulletin No. 232). Washington, DC: Authors.

U.S. Department of Health and Human Services. (1990). *Smoking and health: A national status report* (DHHS Publication No. [CDC] 87-8396). Bethesda, MD: Public Health Service, Centers for Disease Control and Center for Health Promotion and Education.

U.S. Department of Health and Human Services. (1994). *Clinician's handbook of preventive services: Put prevention into practice.* Washington, DC: U.S. Government Printing Office.

U.S. Department of Health and Human Services. (1996). *Physical activity and health: A report of the surgeon general.* Atlanta: DHHS; Centers for Disease Control and Prevention; National Center for Chronic Disease Prevention and Health Promotion.

Waller, P. F. (1992). The older driver. *Hum Factors, 33,* 499–505.

3

COGNITIVE ISSUES

Sheila L. Molony • Courtney H. Lyder • Christine Marek Waszynski

■ INTRODUCTION

Confusion is a common clinical entity in the older adult and was recognized as a valid focus of nursing concern in Mary Opal Wolanin and Theresa Phillip's text, *Confusion: Prevention and Care* (1981). More recently, nursing researchers have attempted to define and refine nursing's understanding of this clinical entitiy (Neelon et al., 1987; Foreman, 1989; 1994; Vermeersch 1990). This chapter focuses on disorders of cognitive function and sleep disturbances, each of which may impair intellectual functioning severely enough to affect activities of daily living, work, and social and personal relationships. The advanced practice nurse's skill in the assessment of these conditions will not only benefit the older adult in terms of appropriate diagnosis, but will inform the plan of care in a way that allows caregivers to optimize the client's strengths, provide support for known deficits, and improve function.

■ DEMENTIA

Dementia is the most prevalent neurologic disorder in older adults. It is estimated that dementia affects approximately 10% to 20% of older adults 65 years of age and older (Cohen & Eisdorfer, 1986). The prevalence of dementia increases exponentially with age (approximately doubling every 5 years). Dementia affects only 1% of 65-year-olds; however, it affects 30% to 40% of 85-year-olds (Katzman & Kawas, 1994; Jorm et al., 1987).

Dementia is defined as a permanent progressive decline in cognitive function. Although Alzheimer-type dementia is the most commonly diagnosed dementia, there are other types of dementias (see Table 3–1). There is no definitive test for dementia; therefore, a thorough assessment is critical when evaluating older adults with cognitive impairment.

TABLE 3–1.   DIFFERENTIAL DIAGNOSIS OF VARIOUS TYPES OF DEMENTIA

■ **FACTORS**

Usual age of onset
: **Depressive disorders:** Any age
: **Vascular dementia:** 55–70 years; average, 65 years
: **Alzheimer's disease, senile onset:** 70+ years; average, 75 years
: **Alzheimer's disease, presenile onset:** 50–60 years; average, 56 years
: **Pick's disease:** 50–60 years; average, 50 years

Sex distribution
: **Depressive disorders:** Early life: more women
:   Late life: more men
: **Vascular dementia:** Men:women = 3:1
: **Alzheimer's disease, senile onset:** Men:women = 2:3
: **Alzheimer's disease, presenile onset:** Men:women = 2:3
: **Pick's disease:** Men:women = 2:3

Duration
: **Depressive disorders:** Varies from weeks to years
: **Vascular dementia:** Varies from days to many years; average, 4 years
: **Alzheimer's disease, senile onset:** Varies from months to years; average, 5 years
: **Alzheimer's disease, presenile onset:** Average, 4 years
: **Pick's disease:** Average, 4 years

Mode of onset
: **Depressive disorders:** Gradual or sudden; precipitating stress often apparent
: **Vascular dementia:** Gradual or acute
: **Alzheimer's disease, senile onset:** Insidious
: **Alzheimer's disease, presenile onset:** More sudden, less gradual
: **Pick's disease:** Slow and insidious

Course
: **Depressive disorders:** Self-limited, but tendency to recur
: **Vascular dementia:** Intermittent, fluctuating
: **Alzheimer's disease, senile onset:** Slowly or rapidly progressive
: **Alzheimer's disease, presenile onset:** Rapidly progressive
: **Pick's disease:** Progressive and fatal

Prognosis
: **Depressive disorders:** Responsive to drugs or electroconvulsive therapy
: **Vascular dementia:** Varies depending on multiple factors
: **Alzheimer's disease, senile onset:** Poor (in moderate or severe cases)
: **Alzheimer's disease, presenile onset:** Very poor
: **Pick's disease:** Very poor

Outcome
: **Depressive disorders:** Usually recovery; sometimes suicide or regression to paranoid level
: **Vascular dementia:** Death from cardiovascular accident, heart disease, or infection
: **Alzheimer's disease (both senile and presenile onset) and Pick's disease:** Death from general organ failure; infection

Hereditary and precipitating factors
: **Depressive disorders:** Involution; previous history of depression
: **Vascular dementia:** Some familial tendency
: **Alzheimer's disease, senile onset:** Multiple genetically determined factors
: **Alzheimer's disease, presenile onset:** Multifactorial inheritance, genetic factors causing premature aging
: **Pick's disease:** Degenerative process

TABLE 3–1.   DIFFERENTIAL DIAGNOSIS OF VARIOUS TYPES OF DEMENTIA (CONT.)

■ **FACTORS (CONT.)**

Signs of brain damage

Depressive disorders: None
Vascular dementia: Diffuse or focal
Alzheimer's disease, senile onset: Diffuse, generalized
Alzheimer's disease, presenile onset: Diffuse, generalized, more severe than in senile onset
Pick's disease: Circumscribed atrophy; frontal, temporal, or parietal lobes

Impairment of higher cortical functions

Depressive disorders: No structural impairment
Vascular dementia: Some isolated impairments (eg, aphasia, apraxia, agnosia)
Alzheimer's disease, senile onset: Progressive dementia
Alzheimer's disease, presenile onset: Involvement of cerebral associative areas; transcortical aphasia, apraxia, agnosia, etc.
Pick's disease: Focal cortical impairments (eg, motor or sensory aphasia)

Neuromuscular

Depressive disorders: Psychomotor retardation or agitation
Vascular dementia: Paralyses, minor extrapyramidal signs
Alzheimer's disease, senile onset: Tremors, uncertain gait, variable muscular rigidity, incontinence
Alzheimer's disease, presenile onset: Transient or progressive paresis, unsteady gait, increased muscle tone, occasional tremors, incontinence
Pick's disease: Primitive reflexes, extrapyramidal signs, attacks of muscular hypotonia, incontinence

Seizures

Depressive disorders: None
Vascular dementia: Epileptiform attacks
Alzheimer's disease, senile onset: Rare
Alzheimer's disease, presenile onset: Occasional
Pick's disease: Rare

Medical

Depressive disorders: Physiologic concomitants of depression (sleep, appetite, weight, energy)
Vascular dementia: Common history of cardiovascular accident; headaches, dizziness, and syncope (in 50%); transient ischemic attacks; arteriosclerosis in heart, kidney, legs, etc.
Alzheimer's disease (both senile and presenile onset) and Pick's disease: Infections, contractures, fractures, decubitus ulcers

■ **NEUROPATHOLOGY**

Macroscopic

Depressive disorders: None characteristic
Vascular dementia: Large or small areas of softening and hemorrhage
Alzheimer's disease, senile onset: Diffused generalized shrinkage of brain, especially gray matter; dilated ventricles; internal hydrocephalus
Alzheimer's disease, presenile onset: General cerebral atrophy, dilated ventricles, internal hydrocephalus
Pick's disease: Circumscribed lobar atrophy, mostly orbitofrontal or temporal

(Continues)

TABLE 3–1.   DIFFERENTIAL DIAGNOSIS OF VARIOUS TYPES OF DEMENTIA (CONT.)

■ **NEUROPATHOLOGY (CONT.)**

Microscopic   **Depressive disorders:** None characteristic

Vascular dementia: Granular atrophy of cortex diffusely with hypertensive cardiovascular disease; destruction of neurons, nerve fibers, and glia; focal neuronal and selective cortical degeneration. Secondary gliosis; senile plaques, not typical

Alzheimer's disease, senile onset: Neuronal degeneration and shrinking; most damage in upper layers of cortex; deposition of lipofuscin and intracellular fibrils. Moderate gliosis, especially in outer layer of cortex. Senile plaques

Alzheimer's disease, presenile onset: Diffuse loss of neurons, especially in cortex layers 3 and 5; disturbed cortical layers. Neuron degeneration: pyknosis; granulovascular bodies; Alzheimer's neurofibrillary change. Gliosis more severe than in senile onset. Senile plaques throughout cortex

Pick's disease: Progressive atrophy of neurons; no predilection for cortical layers; neuron degeneration; increased pigment pyknosis; swollen cells; argyrophilic cytoplasmic inclusions. Gliosis prominent. Senile plaques rare

Vascular   **Depressive disorders:** None

Vascular dementia: Large arteries: atherosclerosis
Small vessels: endothelial proliferation, medical hypertrophy, and intima hyalinization

Alzheimer's disease, senile onset: Endothelial degeneration; medial fibrosis; adventitial proliferation; vascular loops

Alzheimer's disease, presenile onset: Degenerative changes of endothelial and adventitial cells

Pick's disease: Endothelial proliferation; hyaline degeneration

■ **PSYCHIATRIC SYMPTOMOLOGY**

Orientation   **Depressive disorders:** Intact, except in depressive stupor

Vascular dementia: Episodes of acute confusion; lucid intervals

Alzheimer's disease (both senile and presenile onset) and Pick's disease: Progressive disorientation in all spheres; loss of time perspective

Perception   **Depressive disorders:** Occasional auditory hallucinations

Vascular dementia: Auditory and visual during acute exacerbations

Alzheimer's disease, senile onset: Various types of hallucinations in advanced stages

Alzheimer's disease, presenile onset: Occasional hallucinations

Pick's disease: Occasional hallucinations

Intellect and thought   **Depressive disorders:** No mental impairment; delusions consistent with affect; insight varies

Vascular dementia: Lacunar types of intellectual deficit; delusions: rare; insight present in early stages

TABLE 3–1.   DIFFERENTIAL DIAGNOSIS OF VARIOUS TYPES OF DEMENTIA (CONT.)

■ **PSYCHIATRIC SYMPTOMOLOGY (CONT.)**

Alzheimer's disease, senile onset: Progressive, generalized dementia; delusions depend on degree of regression and premorbid personality; no insight

Alzheimer's disease, presenile onset: Progressive dementia and loss of abstraction; aphasia, alexia, agnosia, asymbolia, agraphia, apraxia; no insight

Pick's disease: Frontal lobe syndrome: progressive loss of abstraction; Aphasic syndrome: aphasia, alexia, etc. Alogic syndrome: agnosia, apraxia, etc.; no insight

Memory

Depressive disorders: Transient memory problems due to central nervous system slowing

Vascular dementia: Varying deficits of recent and remote memory, of retention and recall; confabulations: rare

Alzheimer's disease, senile onset: Progressive impairments of all memory functions; confabulations of presbyophrenic type

Alzheimer's disease, presenile onset: Progressive impairment of all memory functions; confabulations: rare

Pick's disease: Progressive impairment of all memory functions; confabulations: common

Affect

Depressive disorders: Depression, guilt, low self-esteem

Vascular dementia: Emotional lability, anxiety and depression, later blunting of affect

Alzheimer's disease, senile onset: Depends on subtype: simple: apathy; depressed: agitated; delirious: anxious; paranoid: hostile; presbyophrenic: shallow euphoria

Alzheimer's disease, presenile onset: Variable at first, later apathy

Pick's disease: Apathy and indifference

Psychomotor

Depressive disorders: Retardation, sometimes agitation

Vascular dementia and Alzheimer's disease, senile onset: Hypoactive or hyperactive or restless agitation

Alzheimer's disease, presenile onset: Hyperactive, repetitive, primitive motor behavior, extrapyramidal signs

Pick's disease: Hypo- or hyperkinetic, primitive reflexes, stereotyped activity, preservation, echolalia, logoclony

Personality changes

Depressive disorders: Transient regressive changes

Vascular dementia: Regressive changes are intermittent or slowly progressive

Alzheimer's disease (both senile and presenile onset) and Pick's disease: Progressive deterioration of social behavior and personal habits

Source: Adapted from Verwoerdt, A. *Clinical geropsychiatry* (2nd ed.) (pp. 72–76). Baltimore: Williams & Wilkins, 1981; with permission.

AGE-RELATED CHANGES

The brain is probably the least understood organ of the body. Nonetheless, there are some structural changes that occur with the aging process. There is a decline in neurons in both the brain and spinal cord. These neuronal losses appear in the amygdala, hippocampus, neocortex, anterior thalamus, basal forebrain cholinergic system, and monoaminergic brain stem systems (ie, locus ceruleus) (Kattman, & Kawas, 1994). It is important to note that neuronal losses may not affect brain function. However, loss of neurons coupled with decreases in nerve conduction and peripheral nerve function does affect the autonomic nervous system (Matteson et al., 1997).

CLINICAL PRESENTATION

The presentation of dementia can be determined based on clinical symptomatology. There are several scales that identify stages of dementia. The Global Deterioration Scale, which classifies symptoms into seven levels of cognitive functioning, is one of the most comprehensive scales (Table 3–2).

The *Diagnostic and Statistical Manual IV* (DSM-IV) is used by both the psychiatric and psychologic communities to diagnose dementia (American Psychiatric Association, 1994). According to the DSM-IV, the older adult must exhibit impaired memory in addition to abnormalities in either language, praxis, perceptual recognition, or executive function in order to meet the criteria for dementia. These changes must represent a decrease in previous functioning and be severe enough to cause either occupational or social disability. Moreover, dementia can-

not be diagnosed if the changes are present exclusively during delirium (see Table 3–3). The reader is referred to the DSM-IV for a complete description of the dementia diagnosis.

.... *vignette* ....

Mrs. Gerard, an 86-year-old woman, had become increasingly forgetful in the past year. She lived with her husband of 50 years in the same two-story house. She had much difficulty when her husband would ask her multiple questions or request complex tasks. Mrs. Gerard loved to cook for her husband, children, and grandchildren. In the past year, Mrs. Gerard began to forget how to prepare recipes she had memorized 60 years ago. She also started to forget the names of her grandchildren and needed frequent prompting by her husband. Mrs. Gerard became paranoid as she began to misplace her personal belongings. As her paranoia increased, her sleep patterns began to fluctuate. She started to sleep for 2- to 3-hour periods. Unable to sleep, she would wander around her house most of the night looking for objects that she had misplaced. In the past month, she left the stove unattended and forgot it was on.

ASSESSMENT

History

A complete history is critical in attempting to determine whether the dementia is potentially reversible. The interview should be obtained from both the older adult and primary caregivers. History taking should focus on the presence and progression of any suspicious symptoms, such as those outlined in the Global De-

TABLE 3–2. GLOBAL DETERIORATION SCALE*

Level	Cognitive Functioning
1 No cognitive decline	No subjective complaints of memory deficit. No memory deficit evident on clinical interview.
2 Very mild cognitive decline	Subjective complaints of memory deficit, most frequently in following areas: (a) forgetting location of objects; (b) forgetting familiar names. No objective evidence of memory deficit on clinical interview or in employment or social situations. Appropriate concern with respect to symptomatology.
3 Mild cognitive decline	Earliest clear-cut deficits. Manifestations in more than one of the following areas: (a) patient may have gotten lost when traveling to an unfamiliar loction; (b) co-workers become aware of patient's relatively poor performance; (c) work- and name-finding deficit becomes evident to intimates; (d) patient may read a passage or a book and retain relatively little material; (e) patient may demonstrate decreased facility in remembering names upon introduction to new people; (f) patient may have lost or misplaced an object of value; (g) concentration deficit may be evident in clinical testing.
4 Moderate cognitive decline	Clear-cut deficit on careful clinical interview. Deficit manifest in the following areas: (a) decreased knowledge of current and recent events; (b) may exhibit some deficit in memory of personal history; (c) concentration deficit elicited on serial subtractions; (d) decreased ability to travel, handle finances, etc. Frequently no deficit in following areas: (a) orientation to time and person; (b) recognition of familir persons and faces; (c) ability to travel to familiar locations. Inability to perform complex tasks. Denial is dominant defense mechanism. Flattening of affect and withdrawal from challenging situations occur.
5 Moderately severe cognitive decline	Patient can no longer survive without some assistance. Patient is unable during interview to recall a major relevant aspect of his or her current life (eg, an address or telephone number of many years, the names of close family members such as grandchildren, the name of the high school or college from which he or she graduated). Frequently some disorientation to time (date, day of week, season, etc.) or to place. An educated person may have difficulty counting back from 40 by 4s or from 20 by 2s.

(*Continues*)

TABLE 3–2.   GLOBAL DETERIORATION SCALE* (CONT.)

Level	Cognitive Functioning
5 Moderately severe cognitive decline (cont.)	Persons at this stage retain knowledge of many major facts regarding themselves and others. They invariably know their own names and generally know their spouse's and children's names. They require no assistance with toileting and eating but may have some difficulty choosing the proper clothing to wear and may occasionally clothe themselves improperly (eg, put shoes on the wrong feet).
6 Severe cognitive decline	May occasionally forget the name of a spouse upon whom they are entirely dependent for survival. Will be largely unaware of all recent events and experiences in their lives. Retain some knowledge of their past lives but this is very sketchy. Generally unaware of their surroundings, the year, the season, etc. May have difficulty counting from 10, both backward and, sometimes, forward. Will require some assistance with activities of daily living (eg, may become incontinent), will require travel assistance but occasionally will display ability to familiar locations. Diurnal rhythm frequently disturbed. Almost always recall their own name. Frequently continue to be able to distinguish from unfamiliar persons in their environment.
	Personality and emotional changes occur. These are quite variable and include: (a) delusional behavior (eg, patients may accuse spouse of being an impostor; may talk to imaginary figures in the environment, or to their own reflection in the mirror); (b) obsessive symptoms (eg, person may continually repeat simple cleaning activities); (c) anxiety symptoms, agitation, and even previously nonexistent violent behavior may occur; (d) cognitive abulia (ie, loss of willpower because an individual cannot carry a thought long enough to determine a purposeful course of action).
7 Very severe cognitive decline	All verbal abilities are lost. Frequently, there is no speech at all—only grunting. Incontinent of urine; requires assistance toileting and feeding. Loose basic psychomotor skills (eg, ability to walk). The brain appears to no longer be able to tell the body what to do.
	Generalized and cortical neurological signs and symptoms are frequently present.

* Compared with a normal individual of the same age and sex, rate the subject's level of cognitive functioning.
Source: Adapted from Reisberg, B., Ferris, S. H., de Leon M. J., & Crook, T. (1982). The global deterioration scale for assessment of primary degenerative dementia. *Am J Psych, 139*(9), 1136–1139; with permission.

TABLE 3–3.   DSM-IV DIAGNOSIS OF DEMENTIA OF THE ALZHEIMER'S TYPE

A. The development of multiple cognitive deficits manifested by both
  1. Memory impairment (impaired ability to learn new information or to recall previously learned information)
  2. One (or more) of the following cognitive disturbances:
    a. Aphasia (language disturbance)
    b. Apraxia (impaired ability to carry out motor activities despite intact motor function)
    c. Agnosia (failure to recognize or identify objects despite intact sensory function)
    d. Disturbance in executive function (ie, planning, organizing, sequencing, abstracting)

B. The cognitive deficits in criteria A1 and A2 each cause significant impairment in social or occupational functioning and represent a significant decline from a previous level of functioning.

C. The course is characterized by gradual onset and continuing cognitive decline.

D. The cognitive deficits in criteria A1 and A2 are not due to any of the following:
  1. Other central nervous system conditions that cause progressive deficits in memory and cognition (eg, cerebrovascular disease, Parkinson's disease, Huntington's disease, subdural hematoma, normal-pressure hydrocephalus, brain tumor)
  2. Systemic conditions that are known to cause dementia (eg, hypothyroidism, hypercalcemia, neurosyphilis, human immunodeficiency virus [HIV] infection)
  3. Substance-induced conditions

E. The deficits do not occur exclusively during the course of a delirium.

F. The disturbance is not better accounted for by another axis I disorder (eg, major depressive disorder, schizophrenia).

Source: Adapted from American Psychiatric Association. (1994). *Diagnostic and statistical manual of mental disorders* (4th ed.) (pp. 142–143). Washington, DC: Author; with permission.

terioration Scale (Table 3–2) or those listed in Table 3–3, that may indicate dementia. The interview may also reveal a history of giving up challenging activities related to work, recreation, and social and community involvement. The clinician should explore the circumstances surrounding this narrowing of involvement. Difficulties with medication taking and evidence of poor judgment should also be assessed. It is often helpful to "map" the progression of symptoms to document the chronology, acuity of onset, progression, duration, and sequencing of symptoms (Fig. 3–1).

History taking should also identify symptoms consistent with delirium or depression. While delirium and depression represent reversible causes of cognitive impairment, it is important to follow the older adult over time after these conditions resolve since as many as 50% may eventually demonstrate signs of dementia which was presumably present in a subclinical stage at the earlier presentation (Small et al., 1997). Table 3–4 identifies other common reversible etiologies that may contribute to cognitive impairment.

Physical Examination

The physical examination should include a comprehensive physical and neurologic examination. A mental status examination should also be completed. The Folstein Mini-Mental State Exam (MMSE) (see Ap-

TABLE 3–4. COMMON ETIOLOGIES OF DEMENTIA

Degenerative disorders
  Alzheimer's disease
  Frontotemporal dementias
  Lewy body dementia
  Parkinson's disease
  Huntington's disease
  Other movement disorder with dementia
Vascular dementia
  Atherosclerosis
  Arteriosclerosis
  Vasculitis
  Embolic disorders
  Mixed vascular degenerative dementia
Myelin disorders
  Multiple sclerosis
Toxic encephalopathies
  Medication induced
  Substance-abuse related, including alcohol
  Occupational exposure
  Environmental exposure
  Radiation therapy
Metabolic encephalopathies
  Thyroid disease
  Vitamin B_{12} deficiency
  Systemic illness with central nervous system
    effects
  Hereditary errors of metabolism
Traumatic disorders
  Traumatic encephalopathy
  Dementia pugilistica (boxer's dementia)
  Subdural hematomas
Infectious and transmissible conditions
  HIV encephalopathy
  Creutzfeldt–Jakob disease
  Meningitis (chronic)
  Encephalitis (chronic)
  Postencephalitic dementia
  Progressive multifocal leukoencephalopathy
Neoplastic and paraneoplastic disorders
  Brain tumors, primary
  Brain tumors, metastatic
  Paraneoplastic encephalopathy
Hydrocephalic
  Obstructive, communicating (including nor-
    mal pressure hydrocephalus)
  Obstructive, noncommunicating
  Depression related

■ COMMONLY USED MEDICATIONS THAT MAY CAUSE COGNITIVE OR AFFECTIVE CHANGE IN THE ELDERLY
Alcohol
Beta blockers, especially propranolol (Inderal)
Antihypertensive agents
  Beta blockers (see above)
  Methyldopa
  Reserpine
  Clonidine
  Diuretics
Neuroleptics
  Haloperidol (Haldol)
  Chlorpromazine (Thorazine)
  Thioridazine (Mellaril)
  Fluphenazine (Prolixin)
  Perphenazine (Trilafon)
  Loxapine (Loxitane)
  Molindone (Moban)
  Thiothixene (Navene)
  Trifluoperazine (Stelazine)
Benzodiazepines
  Diazepam (Valium)
  Flurazepam (Dalmane)
  Clorazepate (Tranxene)
  Chlordiazepoxide (Librium)
  Prazepam (Centrax)
  Alprazolam (Xanax)
  Halazepam (Paxipam)
  Triazolam (Halcion)
  Temazepam (Restoril)
  Oxazepam (Serax)
  Lorazepam (Ativan)
Antiseizure medications
  Barbiturates
  Carbamazepine (Tegretol)
  Phenytoin (Dilantin)
  Phenobarbital
Antihistamines
Cimetidine
Steroids
Procainamide
Disopyramide
Quinidine
Atropine and other anticholinergic agents (eg, benztropine, trihexyphenidyl, diphenhy-dramine, etc.)

Source: Adapted with permission from Jenike MA. (1988). Depression and other psychiatric disorders. In Albert, M. S., & Moss, M. (Eds.). *Geriatric neuropsychology* (pp. 115–144). New York, Guilford Press.

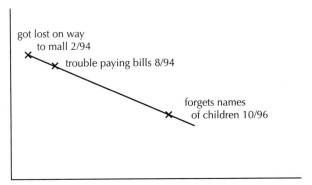

A. Progression: Slow, Gradual Decline Consistent With Dementia

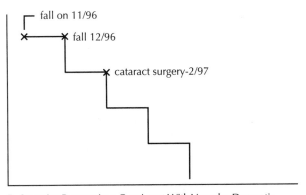

B. Stepwise Progression: Consistent With Vascular Dementia

Figure 3–1. "Map" of the Presence and Progression of Symptoms of Dementia

pendix A) is probably the most widely used tool to determine cognitive impairment (Folstein et al., 1975) Mangino & Middlemiss (1997) have modified the MMSE. Care should be exercised in interpreting the MMSE as it is affected by educational level. Use of age and education-specific cutoff scores may improve the sensitivity of the tool (Tangalos et al., 1996; Crum et al, 1993). Screening tools are best used to provide a baseline for monitoring the course of the impairment over time and to plan individualized interventions based on known deficits and abilities (Agostinelli et al., 1994). A functional assessment tool such as the Instrumental Activities of Daily Living Scale (Lawton & Brody, 1969), or the Functional Activities Questionnaire (Pfeiffer et al., 1982; Costa, P. et al., 1996) will elucidate the impact of cognitive impairments on daily function and assist in the identification of early impairments (Appendix B).

Diagnostic Studies

Laboratory tests such as complete blood count (CBC), urinalysis (UA), serum electrolytes, and blood urea nitrogen

(BUN)/creatinine should be obtained to rule out underlying infections. Stool samples for occult blood, vitamin B_{12}, and folate levels; thyroid-stimulating hormone (TSH) and free thyroid index; rapid plasma reagin (RPR) for syphilis; and human immunodeficiency virus (HIV) and liver function tests may also be obtained. Additional diagnostics studies (if indicated after initial lab results) include electroencephalography (EEG), positron emission tomography (PET), computerized tomography (CT), or magnetic resonance imaging (MRI).

CLINICAL MANAGEMENT

Pharmacologic Measures

There is no cure for dementia. Management of dementia should consist of both pharmacologic and nonpharmacologic interventions. A new classification of drugs known as memory-enhancement drugs have been developed with mixed reviews. They purport to slow the decline of intellectual function and, in some cases, raise the individual's level of cognitive ability upon initiation of the drug. The two drugs that have been approved for use with dementia patients are tacrine (Cognex) and donepezil (Aricept) (U.S. Department of Veterans Affairs and University Healthsystem Consortium, 1997). Tacrine is usually initiated at 30 mg/d and then titrated up to 160 mg/d. It is usually titrated 40 mg/d every 6 weeks as tolerated. The best results of this medication are noted at the higher doses of 120 mg/d to 160 mg/d. Tacrine is metabolized in the liver and can affect its function; thus, the advanced practice nurse should obtain a liver function test every week for the first 4 months. Many older adults are unable to tolerate this medication due to gastrointestinal side effects and liver toxicity.

Donepezil is usually initiated at 5 mg for several weeks and then titrated up to 10 mg/d. The best results of this medication are also noted at the higher doses of 10 mg/d. The benefits of donepezil are that it can be administered in a single dose, it does not appear to have adverse effects on the liver, and it appears to be tolerated well by most older adults. There have been case reports of syncopal episodes and nightmares in some individuals.

The primary focus of managing the demented older adult is the management of underlying health or behavioral problems. Quite often, dementia-related behavioral problems occur due to underlying health problems. Medications may also be used to manage behavioral problems. Table 3–5 identifies some of the most common behavioral problems and possible medicatons that may be used to minimize these behavioral problems.

Nonpharmacologic Measures

The treatment of dementia should focus on anticipatory guidance and support, community referral, frequent health assessment, and educating caregivers about behavior management. Advance directives, conservatorship, and long-term care planning should be discussed early in the illness trajectory. Figure 3–2 presents a therapeutic approach to behavior management. Treatment focuses on supporting physiologic, social, and emotional functioning while reducing environmental stressors. Strategies include developing an environment that provides visual and tactile clues to the demented older adult. The advanced practice nurse should be cognizant of

TABLE 3–5.   DRUGS COMMONLY USED TO TREAT BEHAVIORAL SYMPTOMS IN DEMENTIA PATIENTS

Behavior	Agent*	Initial Dose	Daily Dosage Range
Agitation	Haloperidol	0.5 mg	0.5–3 mg
	Trazodone	50 mg	50–300 mg
	Carbamazepine	200 mg	200–800 mg
Psychosis	Haloperidol	0.5 mg	0.5–3 mg
	Risperidone	0.5 mg	0.5–6 mg
Depression	Sertraline	50 mg	50–200 mg
	Nortriptyline	25 mg	25–150 mg
Anxiety	Lorazepam	0.5 mg	0.5–6 mg
	Buspirone	15 mg	15–60 mg
Insomnia	Trazodone	25 mg	25–300 mg
	Temazepam	15 mg	15–30 mg

* The agents listed in this chart are widely used. In many cases, other agents in the same class of drugs may have equal efficacy.

Source: Reprinted with permission from the University Health System Consortium, *Dementia identification and assessment: Guidelines for primary care practitioners,* March 1997.

correcting all sensory deficits that may impact confusional states. The use of signs visualizing the bathroom (commode) and bedroom (bed) and providing familiar objects to older adults may also be very helpful in orienting them to their environment. The advanced practice nurse should also encourage caregivers to follow a routine schedule to decrease anxiety and confusion. Caregivers should be encouraged to provide "meaningful" activities that the demented older adult may be able to engage in (eg, a retired housekeeper may be given an assignment to sweep; a retired graphic artist may be given an assignment to design a greeting card). Caregivers should be encouraged to contact the American Alzheimer's Association (1-800-272-3900) for information on the disease and to identify support groups within their respective communities.

Management of Behaviors Associated with Dementia

1. Consider all possible causes for the behavior. Rule out medical or psychiatric illness. Consider the possible role of environmental stressors. Use a behavior log to help identify causes/precipitants/patterns.
2. Identify the human needs the person is trying to meet or the human needs that must be considered in any intervention. Consider needs for food, water, elimination, sleep, oxygen, sex, relaxation, stimulation, privacy, activity, safety, security, belongingness, affection, prestige, sense of value, and sense of meaning.
3. Plan approaches that address the causes and needs listed above. Use the following guiding principles:
   - *Communication*—Use   therapeutic

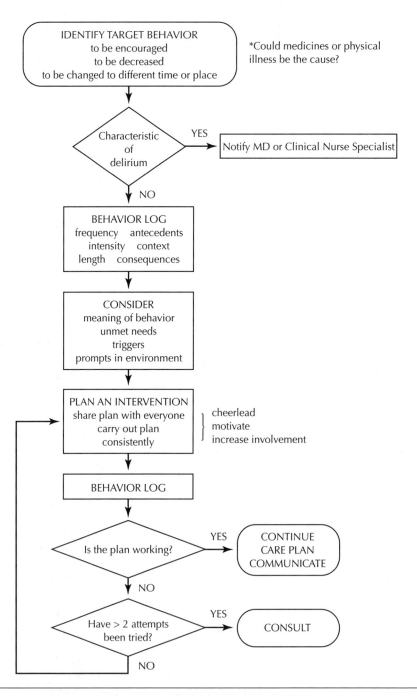

Figure 3–2. Management of Behaviors Associated With Dementia

communication techniques; give limited choices, one-step commands; use a gentle, warm, and reassuring voice; validate feelings; use distraction and redirection, praise and reward, eye contact, supportive touch; listen; avoid rushing; keep sense of humor and fun; use client's preferred name.

- *Environment*—Eliminate environmental stressors; promote structure, routine, predictability, sense of familiarity; use furniture, paths, door alarms, textures, sounds; play music to promote warmth, safety, and appropriate stimulation and activity; provide orienting cues and prompts to desired behavior.
- *Continuity*—Find out as much as possible about client's premorbid personality, life, and routine, and continue these aspects (bath and meal routines, schedules, occupational routines and props, important roles, etc.).
- *Expectations*—Accept all behavior that is not dangerous; lower expectations; plan for known behaviors/events/exacerbations(eg, frequent nighttime awakening); increase failure-free activities.
- *Individual needs*—Meet with all caregivers and share unique aspects of this individual's wants and needs (eg, likes dancing, gets upset with messy activities, eats well when sitting at small table with two friends, soothed by certain foods); use behavior log to identify unique needs; use results of MMSE to plan individualized interventions (Agostinelli et al., 1994).
- *Eliminate barriers to function*—Screen

for depression, medical illness, sensory impairment, unmet physiologic needs, discomfort; reduce physical or chemical restraints; scrutinize medicines; avoid overfatigue and stressors; maximize vision and hearing.

- *Use brainstorming and creativity*—Meet with group of involved caregivers and brainstorm several ideas to promote improved function; use creativity and imagination (eg, no-rinse shampoo, towel bath, duplicates of favorite outfits, audiotape of loved one reassuring or videotape of favorite TV show or sporting event).
- *Consult and collaborate*—Consult with colleagues and peers for ideas on behavior management; consult with clinical experts in dementia care; refer to geriatrician, physician, neurologist, or psychiatrist as appropriate.

Helpful Approaches

- *Remove from triggering place/event*—Give the individual time to cool down and forget incident; give more space; use a calm, reassuring voice and gently guide away.
- *Redirect*—Example: "I need your help watering my plant . . . walk with me. . . ."
- *Reassure*—Example: "I will keep you safe . . . I won't let anything bad happen to you . . . your family knows you are here. . . ."
- *Validate feelings*—Example: "You seem to be feeling frustrated and angry . . . let's go for a walk to-

gether. . . ."

- *Accept the behavior*—If the behavior does not threaten the safety of the older adult or others or does not interfere with essential care, consider ignoring or accepting it.
- *Distract*—Change the subject, talk about a favorite topic, involve the client in a favorite activity, offer favorite food, go for a walk, use music, massage, sing familiar song, quietly read to older adult, and so on.
- *Schedule activity alternating with rest or "down time"*
- *Assess the behavior systematically*—Use a behavior log or diary to assess triggers and evaluate the success of therapeutic approaches.

Stressors

Physical	Emotional
Poor vision	Depressed
Fatigue	Anxious
Dehydration	Afraid
Discomfort (constipation, pain, cold, hunger, foot soreness, etc.)	Hallucinating
Hidden illness (infection, electrolyte imbalance, thyroid disease, etc.)	Paranoid Delusional

Activities and Tasks

Too many activities	Unfamiliar
Too complicated	Uncomfortable
Results in failure	Too many choices
Too childlike or insulting	

Communication	Environment
Can't understand you	Room too large
Can't make self understood	Room too cluttered
Person is asked questions that require him to remember something	Too much noise
Scolded	Overstimulation
Confronted	Understimulation
Contradicted	Not enough structure
Caregiver is stressed	Change in routine
Caregiver is impatient	Change in caregiver
Caregiver is irritable	Nothing looks familiar
Caregiver is bossy	Not enough light or too much glare
	Others arguing nearby
	Physically restrained

SETTING-SPECIFIC ISSUES

Much of the care of demented older adults is delivered in long-term care settings either in specialty "dementia care" units or in more heterogeneous skilled nursing environments. There is also an emerging trend toward "assisted living" environments with a focus on dementia care. All caregivers working in such settings must be educated about the nature of dementia and appropriate care and therapeutic approaches. Caregivers should be taught to use behavior logs to identify patterns and triggers to difficult behaviors and to evaluate the effectiveness of interventions (see Fig. 3–3

Date	Time	Behavior or Inappropriate Response	Antecedants and Environmental Conditions	Caregivers Response to Behavior (Interventions)	Outcome

Figure 3–3. Behavior Log

for a sample behavior log). Readers are encouraged to consult Joanne Rader's book, *Individualized Dementia Care: Creative, Compassionate Approaches* (1995), as well as Robinson et al.'s book, *Understanding Difficult Behaviors: Some Practical Suggestions for Coping with Alzheimer's Disease and Related Illnesses* (1989) and Taft et al.'s article, "Dementia Care: Creating a Therapeutic Milieu" (1993). The goals of dementia care should include (1) accurate diagnosis, (2) early identification of excess disabilities, (3) maintenance of older adults's self-esteem, (4) matching abilities with demands, and (5) cueing and assistance with activities that require lost abilities.

While dementia patients are at higher risk of delirium in any setting, hospital nurses need to be particularly aware of the increased likelihood of delirium in older patients with preexisting brain disorders.

■ DELIRIUM

It has been estimated that 10% to 30% of all confusion is reversible (Levkoff et al., 1992). Acute confusion or delirium represents acute brain failure in response to underlying medical or mental illness that requires prompt diagnosis and treatment. Acute confusion or delirium carries with it serious consequences. Delirious older adults are more likely to suffer from falls and iatrogenic sequelae of physical and chemical restraints. Some studies have suggested that hospitalized patients with delirium are twice as likely to die as their nondelirious counterparts (Lipowski, 1983, Inouye et al., 1990).

PREVENTION

Acute confusion is often the first presenting sign of serious medical illness such as pneumonia, appendicitis, or myocardial infarction and as such, is not inherently preventable. However, acute confusion may also result from smaller cumulative insults such as sleep deprivation, pain, unfamiliar environments, overstimulation, new medicines, and mild fluid and electrolyte imbalances ("ICU psychosis" is a classic example). These insults are potentially preventable. Recognizing clients at risk for delirium and working with front-line caregivers to maximize nutrition, hydration, oxygenation, sleep, physical activity, mental activity and comfort will foster optimum mental function. The number of medications (prescription and over the counter [OTC]) should be minimized. Optimizing vision, hearing, lighting, and meaningful social interaction may also decrease the risk of delirium.

CLINICAL PRESENTATION

Delirium is characterized by disorientation to time, place, or person; disorganized thinking; memory impairment; and sleep–wake disturbances. Delirium, or acute confusion, is distinguished from dementia by its acute versus gradual onset. Delirium is also characterized by decreased alertness and impaired attention

or distractability. Mental status fluctuation is a common feature of delirium, with possible lucid intervals. The delirious older adult may also experience disturbances of perception such as hallucinations. Table 3–6 differentiates acute confusion, dementia, and depression. It is important to recognize that it is very common for older persons with dementia to suffer from a superimposed reversible delirium, which, if treated, can greatly improve function.

CLINICAL PEARL

Changes in mental status, behavior, or function in demented clients that are not consistent with their baseline or with their "stage" of the dementing illness should be evaluated for a coexistent delirium.

The agitated, disoriented, uncooperative older adult will be easily recognized as requiring further assessment, but the withdrawn, half-somnolent, quietly hallucinating elder may be entirely overlooked as a victim of delirium unless the clinician specifically tests for features such as impaired attention and fluctuating cognition. Physicians and nurses often fail to detect cases of delirium (Levkof et al., 1992).

The following clinical vignettes illustrate the presentation of acute confusion.

vignette

Mrs. Jones is an 80-year-old resident of an intermediate-care facility. She has lived there for 5 years and has been alert, oriented, and inde-

TABLE 3–6.   COMPARISON OF ACUTE CONFUSION, DEMENTIA, AND DEPRESSION

Clinical Feature	Acute Confusion	Dementia	Depression
Onset	Acute/subacute, depends on cause; often at twilight or in darkness	Chronic, generally insidious, depends on cause	Coincides with major life changes, often abrupt
Course	Short, diurnal fluctuations in symptoms, worse at night, in darkness, and on awakening	Long, no diurnal effects, symptoms progressive yet relatively stable over time	Diurnal effects, typically worse in the morning; situational fluctuations but less than with acute confusion
Progression	Abrupt	Slow but uneven	Variable, rapid or slow, but even
Duration	Hours to less than 1 month, seldom longer	Months to years	At least 2 weeks, can be several months to years (Note: *DSM-IV* guidelines specify at least 6 weeks in duration for diagnosis.)
Awareness	Reduced	Clear	Clear
Alertness	Fluctuates, lethargic or hypervigilant	Generally normal	Normal
Attention	Impaired, fluctuates	Generally normal	Minimal impairment but is distractable
Orientation	Generally impaired, severity varies	May be impaired	Selective disorientation
Memory	Recent and immediate impaired	Recent and remote impaired	Selective or patchy impairment, "islands" of intact memory
Thinking	Disorganized, distorted, fragmented; incoherent speech, either slow or accelerated	Difficulty with abstraction, thoughts impoverished, judgment impaired, words difficult to find	Intact but with themes of hopelessness, helplessness, or self-deprecation
Perception	Distorted, illusions, delusions, and hallucinations; difficulty distinguishing between reality and misperceptions	Misperceptions usually absent	Intact, delusions and hallucinations absent except in severe cases

(Continues)

TABLE 3–6.   COMPARISON OF ACUTE CONFUSION, DEMENTIA, AND DEPRESSION (CONT.)

Clinical Feature	Acute Confusion	Dementia	Depression
Psychomotor behavior	Variable, hypokinetic, hyperkinetic, and mixed	Normal, may have apraxia	Variable, psychomotor retardation or agitation
Sleep/wake cycle	Disturbed, cycle reversed	Fragmented	Disturbed, usually early morning awakening
Associated features	Variable affective changes, symptoms of autonomic hyperarousal, exaggeration of personality type, associated with acute physical illness	Affect tends to be superficial, inappropriate, and labile; attempts to conceal deficits in intellect; personality changes, aphasia, agnosia may be present; lacks insight	Affect depressed, dysphoric mood, exaggerated and detailed complaints, preoccupied with personal thoughts, insight present, verbal elaboration
Mental status testing	Distracted from task, numerous errors	Failings highlighted by family, frequent "near miss" answers, struggles with test, great effort to find an appropriate reply, frequent requests for feedback on performance	Failings highlighted by patient, frequent "don't know," little effort, frequently gives up, indifferent toward exam, doesn't care or attempt to find answer

Source: Reprinted with permission from Foreman, M., and Zane, D. (1996). Nursing strategies for acute confusion in elders. *AJN, 96*(4), 44–52.

pendent in all aspects of self-care. She was originally admitted with a diagnosis of recurrent depression and anxiety, and she attends a weekly mental health group. For the past 2 nights, Mrs. Jones has been wakeful and anxious, ringing the call bell and insisting it was time to get up. Her daytime behavior is normal. She received two doses of lorazepam for anxiety, with no beneficial effect. She had one episode of urinary incontinence and fell last night. The advanced practice nurse (APN) is consulted and finds that Mrs. Jones is cooperative but easily distracted. Her clothing is disheveled and her hair uncombed. A screening mental status

exam reveals problems with attention span and short-term memory. Her physical exam is within normal limits. A urine dipstick reveals nitrates, leukocytes, and blood. She is cultured and treated for a urinary tract infection (UTI), and her behavior and functional status return to baseline within 72 hours.

.... *vignette* ....

Mr. Goodman was brought to the clinic at 8 A.M. to be seen by the nurse practitioner after he was found to be wandering in the halls of his retirement home at 3 A.M., knocking on doors and yelling at other residents. He is a 78-year-old man known to the APN from prior visits and annual checkups. He has no past history of disorientation. His medical history includes diagnoses of prostate cancer with metastases to the ribs and spine, hypertension, and coronary artery disease. His medications include aldactizide, tenormin, and acetaminophen. Mr. Goodman is alert and smiling when seen in the clinic. He does not recall the events of last night and suggests that "those others made it up to get rid of me." His score on a screening mental status exam is unchanged since his last physical exam 4 months prior. His physical exam is unremarkable. His blood pressure is 100/60 and pulse 58 with occasional premature beats. After physician collaboration, lab work is ordered and Mr. Goodman is given a follow-up appointement. The next morning, he is brought back to the clinic for the same reason. He is once again alert and oriented but is now fatigued and short of breath. His pulse is 48 and an electrocardiogram (ECG) reveals severe heart block. After eventual pacemaker insertion, Mr. Goodman suffers no new incidents of disorientation.

These vignettes illustrate many of the diagnostic featues of delirium, including disrupted sleep pattern, fluctuating mental status with lucid intervals, acute onset, and decreased alertness and attention (distractibility). The vignettes also illustrate the complexity of diagnosis in the patient with concurrent symptoms of psychological disorders.

ASSESSMENT

The most effective means of recognizing delirium is to formally screen mental status and to maintain a high index of suspicion while searching for the characteristic features. A baseline mental status assessment is required during each annual physical, as well as an interim assessment during episodes of questionable impairment. Serial testing is often highly useful in revealing the fluctuant nature of the cognitive deficits related to delirium. One of the most widely used tools for this purpose is the MMSE (Appendix A).

CLINICAL PEARL

Prior to administering a mental status exam, explain to the client that physical illness in the older adult often causes subtle changes in memory, concentration, and thinking and that it is important to examine these functions so that any changes are recognized early.

As an adjunct to the mental status exam, the APN may use tests that specifically measure attention and concentration such as the digit span, serial subtraction, or listing the days of the week or months of the year in reverse order. Appendix E at the back of the book contains examples of these tools.

Figure 3–4 provides a mnemonic for the possible reversible causes of confusion. The history, physical examination, and diagnostic testing should be geared toward the discovery of any of these conditions. History should identify onset, timing and progression of symptoms, and any fluctuation over time. Older adults and/or caregivers should be questioned

Metabolic/biochemical abnormality
 I infection/impaction/inability to void/injury
Neoplasm/nutritional deficiency/normal pressure
  hydrocephalus
Drugs/drug withdrawal

Environmental toxins/environmental changes
Sleep deprivation/sensory overload/sensory
  deprivation
Cardiac/cerebrovascular/central nervous system
  disease
Alcohol/alcohol withdrawal/anemia
Pain
Emotional/mental illness

Figure 3–4. Mnemonic for Reversible Causes of Confusion. *Courtesy of Sheila L. Molony.*

about sleep pattern disturbances, changes in alertness or attention, misperceptions, and changes in sleep patterns. The past medical and psychiatric history should be sought. A recent history of psychosocial stress or illness is important to illuminate but should not be accepted as the proximate cause of a delirium without a thorough search for other factors. An assessment of nutrition and substance use should be carried out. A comprehensive review of systems is indicated. Medications, both prescription and OTC, should be scrutinized, as medication reactions comprise the most common cause of reversible confusion. Drug interactions, drug–alcohol interactions, and drug or alcohol withdrawal must also be considered.

Physical Examination

A comprehensive physical examination is required. Assess vision and hearing. Assess for signs of occult infection; malignancy; and neurologic, cardiac, or endocrine disease. Assess for urinary retention or fecal impaction.

Diagnostic Studies

The diagnostic studies are the same as those listed in the workup of dementia. Many clinicians would also include an ECG and chest x-ray. The workup progresses from least to most invasive or costly.

CLINICAL MANAGEMENT

The single most important principle in the management of delirium is to diagnose and treat the cause(s). Suspicious medications should be eliminated, infections treated, and electrolyte imbalances corrected. Often, the cause is multifactorial. The delirious older adult should be reassured; reoriented, if possible; and distracted from frightening stimuli. It is helpful to respond to the feelings of the delirious person rather than to the content of their speech. Using logic and reasoning or arguing with the client is usually ineffective. Time is an ally in delirium management due to the fluctuating nature of the impairment. An older adult who is agitated and belligerent one moment may be lethargic or withdrawn the next.

Small doses of antipsychotic medicines are sometimes helpful but should be used conservatively since they may worsen an existing delirium. They are most effective in managing psychotic symptoms such as delusions or hallucinations and are invaluable in managing clients experiencing extreme fear related to these perceptual disturbances. These medicines should be discontinued after the acute episode is managed. The behavioral strategies listed in Figure 3–2 may also be useful.

■ DEPRESSION

Depression is discussed more fully in Chapter 15, but is important to recognize as a contributor to cognitive dysfunction and as a dementia mimic. Depressed older adults may score poorly on screening mental status examinations, but the deficit is frequently one of decreased motivation or lack of effort in the cognitive attempt. They may answer "I don't know" or "I can't" on the mental status exam or may exaggerate their own cognitive deficits. Depression frequently coexists with dementia, and it is essential to any workup of cognitive impairment to screen for symptoms of depression. A screening instrument such as the Yesavage Geriatric Depression Scale (Appendix C) (Yesavage, 1988) may be used to further document depressive symptoms and to provide a baseline assessment against which to measure treatment-related improvements. Agitation, weight loss, and sleep disturbance may also be present in dementia, making the differential diagnosis difficult. Psychiatric consultation and/or an empiric trial of antidepressant therapy may be warranted in such cases. It is always important to weigh the impact of the depression on cognitive function against the potential delirium common with the use of antidepressants in demented persons. Although the cognitive gain may be temporary, it is often worth the risk if it improves quality of life. Newer antidepressant agents such as the selective serotonin reuptake inhibitors (SSRIs) may be better tolerated in these patients.

■ SLEEP DISORDERS

Sleep problems are a prevalent complaint among the older population. At least 50% of community-dwelling elders and up to 90% of institutional-dwelling elders experience sleep disturbance (National Commission on Sleep Disorders, 1993). These complaints include difficulty in falling asleep, in staying asleep, and in feeling rested in the morning (Newman et al., 1997). Sleep issues can be multifactorial, arising from age-related sleep changes, physical illness, emotional concerns, environmental conditions, medications, and bad habits. Inadequate sleep often leads to mood disorders, alcoholism, automobile accidents, and other outcomes that can adversely affect quality of life. Pollack et al. (1990) found sleep disturbances to increase the risk of institutionalization and death of older adults. This chapter will explore the assessment of these factors and discuss management strategies for sleep disturbances in the older adult.

AGE-RELATED CHANGES

It is believed that loss of neurons in the brain may be responsible for the following changes in the sleep cycle, which occur as a process of normal aging:

- A longer time to fall asleep
- Increased time spent in the lighter stages of sleep (stages 1 and 2)
- Decreased time spent in the deeper stages of sleep (stages 3 and 4) and in rapid eye movement (REM) sleep, which is necessary for feeling rested and for rejuvenating the body

- Increased and shorter repetitions of the sleep cycle, leading to more nighttime awakenings
- Altered circadian rhythm, specifically, an earlier falling asleep time (8 to 9 P.M.) and an earlier awakening time (2 to 4 A.M.) (total sleep time is unchanged)

CLINICAL PRESENTATION

Sleep disorders can be transitional, as in reaction to a situational event (illness, death of a loved one, retirement, relocation). Other disorders can be chronic and longstanding, often developing in early or middle adulthood and exacerbating when coupled with age-related sleep changes.

Sleep apnea is a serious and potentially life-threatening disorder, characterized by repeated cycles of airway obstruction and interrupted breathing. Loud snoring accompanied by multiple apnea–hypopnea events (usually reported by the bed partner) may lead to complaints of daytime hypersomnolence, fatigue, irritability, and decreased intellectual function (Dealberto et al., 1996).

Restless leg syndrome (RLS) (a creepy, crawly, painful feeling in the leg muscles) and nocturnal myoclonus (leg jerks) are both conditions that involve repetitive movements of the lower extremities during sleep, confirmed by the bed partner, which often disrupt the sleep pattern. The individual reports motor restlessness and difficulty falling asleep due to this feeling of needing to move the legs. These conditions may be related to iron-deficiency states, with or without anemia, uremia, and other chronic medical problems.

ASSESSMENT

History

A comprehensive history is essential to categorize the type and etiology of the sleep complaint. Gathering data from both the older adult and his or her bed partner is helpful. Asking the person to complete a sleep diary for several weeks can increase the accuracy of reporting (see Fig. 3–5).

Characterization of the Chief Complaint

Begin with a standard investigation of the onset, duration, severity, and consequences of the sleep issue. Characterizing the troublesome components of the sleep phase will assist the examiner in further questioning (falling asleep, staying asleep, early morning awakening, feelings of fatigue). It is essential to determine whether insomnia is related to another treatable symptom such as pain, depression, anxiety, or breathlessness. Asking the individual to describe the scenario surrounding the complaint can often expose the multifactorial causes and lead to more successful treatment.

Inquire into past sleep patterns to determine how sleep is now different. Some individuals mistake normal aging changes in sleep for pathology and expose themselves to futile measures to correct this. Individuals often alter their sleep habits following retirement from their jobs, which can cause sleep problems.

Explore sleep promotion and maintenance habits. This should include inquiring about time of retiring and time of arising; use of alcohol, nicotine, tobacco, and sleep aids; bedtime rituals; environmental barriers (noise, light, temperature); and total sleep time in a 24-hour period.

	Sunday	Monday	Tuesday	Wednesday	Thursday	Friday	Saturday
Date							
Time to bed							
Length of time to fall asleep							
Time got up in morning							
Number of nocturnal awakenings							
Time of daytime nap							
Duration of daytime nap							
Estimated time asleep in 24 hours							
Self-assessment of feeling rested							
Things done to enhance sleep							
Factors which hindered sleep							

Figure 3–5. Sleep Diary

Illness Profile

Cardiovascular (Hypertension, Angina, Congestive Heart Failure, Arrhythmias). Fletcher (1995) found that 50% of persons with sleep apnea had systolic hypertension (HTN). Stouts et al. (1996) found a similar correlation between HTN and sleep apnea. Guilleminault et al.

(1983) and Shepard et al. (1985) noted that many persons with sleep apnea experienced cardiac arrhythmias, both bradycardia and ventricular tachycardia.

Respiratory (Chronic Obstructive Pulmonary Disease, Lower Respiratory Infection). Fletcher et al. (1987) noted that persons with chronic obstructive pulmonary disease (COPD) often desaturate during sleep, disrupting their rest and leading to the risk of pulmonary HTN. Persons with acute respiratory illness often report that sleeping in a recliner chair leads to more restful sleep.

Pain. Pain (acute or chronic) can cause sleep disturbance. Musculoskeletal complaints are common among the elderly, often interfering with rest. Consider pain in hospitalized and postsurgical patients who complain of sleep disturbance.

Gastrointestinal Disorders (Gastroesophageal Reflux Disease, Ulcer Disease). Gastroesophogeal reflux on recumbency may disrupt sleep and cause nocturnal cough or asthmatic symptoms.

Endocrine Disorders (Diabetes Mellitus, Thyroid Disorders). Diabetes can disturb sleep if hypoglycemia or hyperglycemia occurs during the night and can contribute to restless legs. Urinary problems such as nocturia due to hyperglycemia or overflow incontinence due to diabetic neuropathy can also impact on sleep. Hypothyroid or hyperthyroid states can affect all phases of the sleep cycle.

Urinary Tract and Renal Disorders (Urinary Tract Infection, Benign Prostatic Hypertrophy, End-stage Renal Disease). Moore (1989) found persons with end-stage renal failure to report poor sleep patterns. Uremic states exacerbate RLS and nocturnal myoclonus. Urinary frequency and urgency associated with urinary tract infection (UTI) and benign prostatic hypertrophy (BPH) can contribute to frequent nighttime awakenings.

Cognitive Impairment (Alzheimer's Disease, Delirium). Hoch et al. (1987) and others have found a high incidence of sleep apnea among persons with Alzheimer's disease. Alzheimer's disease is also thought to alter circadian rhythms, leading to the frequent symptom of day–night reversal. Persons experiencing delirium often display a sleep disturbance, either excessive sleeping with an altered level of consciousness or a paucity of sleep.

Psychiatric Disorders (Depression, Anxiety, Mania). Inadequate amounts of sleep often accompany these illnesses, although depression can present with either excessive sleep or lack of sleep.

Medication Profile

Medications can affect sleep in a variety of ways. Diuretics may increase nighttime urgency and voiding, thus interrupting sleep patterns. Agents known to delay sleep onset and hinder deep sleep are antiparkinsonian medications, steroids, theophylline, cimetidine, phenytoin, thyroid preparations, and fluoxetine. Caffeine, nicotine, and alcohol have similar deleterious effects on the sleep cycle. Calcium channel blockers, lithium, and neuroleptics can exacerbate RLS and periodic leg movement syndrome (PLMS) during sleep.

Medications used for sleep can often lead to tolerance or side effects such as daytime hangover, urinary retention, and rebound insomnia, which often exacerbate the underlying sleep disorder (See Table 3–7).

Physical Examination

- General: Obesity, state of alertness.
- Mental status: Attentional testing to assess concentration; MMSE (initial

TABLE 3–7. PHARMACOLOGIC SLEEP AIDS

Drug Name	Half-Life (hr)	Dosage	Sleep Onset	Sleep Maintenance	Adverse Effects
Triazolam (Halcion)	1.6–5.4 hr	0.125 mg	x	x	Short-acting, may need to repeat; retrograde amnesia, rebound insomnia, hallucinations
Zolpidem (Ambien)	1.4–4.5 hr	5 mg	x		
Estazolam (Prosom)	10–24 hr	0.5–1 mg	x	x	Daytime sedation, retrograde amnesia
Restoril (Temazepam)	10–20 hr	7.5–15 mg	x	x	Daytime sedation, retrograde amnesia

Source: Adapted from Farney, R. & Walker, J. (1995) Office management of common sleep–wake disorders. *Med Clin North Am, 79*(2), 391–414; and Becker, P. and Jamieson, A. (1992). Common sleep disorders in the elderly: Diagnosis and treatment. *Geriatrics 47*(3), 41–52.

and periodic) to screen for cognitive decline.

- Emotional status: Geriatric Depression Scale (Appendix C) to screen for depression. Assess for anxiety, irritability, and other potential psychiatric components of a sleep disorder.
- Eyes, ears, nose, throat (EENT). Examine nose and throat for obstructive causes (tonsillitis, enlarged uvula, deviated septum, polyps, palate malformation). Note neck circumference (large neck associated with sleep apnea). Check palpebral conjunctiva for evidence of iron deficiency anemia.

- Respiratory: Assess for acute or chronic respiratory disease.
- Cardiovascular: Blood pressure, cardiac exam to identify arrhythmias or CHF.
- Neuromuscular: Deep tendon reflexes (DTRs), clonus, muscle strength, tremor, cogwheeling, paresthesias, or dysesthesias.
- Genitourinary: Prostate exam to rule out BPH, palpate bladder postvoid to rule out urinary retention.

Diagnostic Studies

The selection of diagnostic studies will be based on the history and physical exam findings. Testing may include CBC, electrolytes, BUN, creatinine, ionized calcium, magnesium, serum iron, ferritin, glucose, thyroid profile, liver profile, toxicology screen, arterial blood gases (ABGs), pulse oximetry, pulmonary function tests (PFTs), and ECG.

Polysomnography involves an overnight stay in a sleep laboratory. During this session, the examiner monitors sleep staging, airflow, ventilatory effort, arterial oxygen saturation, ECG, body positioning, and periodic limb movements. Portions of this testing can also be done in the home setting.

CLINICAL MANAGEMENT

Pharmacologic Measures

The treatment of sleep disturbance is a challenge for practitioners. Medications to treat age-related sleep complaints are ineffective and inappropriate. Persons aged 65 and older consume more than 40% of all prescription sleep medicines. Drugs for transient and chronic insomnia are not without adverse effects and should be prescribed thoughtfully according to National Institutes of Health (NIH) Task Force Hypnotic Treatment Guidelines (Table 3–8).

The practitioner chooses the best medication for the patient based on the characteristics of the sleep disturbance and its proposed etiology. When a medical cause is found, the illness is treated. For example, sedating antidepressants such as trazadone (Desyrel) 50 to 300 mg or doxepin (Sinequan, Adaptin) 10 to 150 mg may be helpful for sleep disturbances related to depression. However, doxepin has anticholinergic side effects, and trazadone may produce cardiac problems or priapism. Acetaminophen (Tylenol) or other analgesics may assist persons who are in pain from musculoskeletal disease. H2 antagonists or pro-

---

TABLE 3–8.   NIH TASK FORCE HYPNOTIC TREATMENT GUIDELINES

■ **SHORT-TERM INSOMNIA**

Review sleep hygiene and sleep routines.

If a hypnotic is needed, use a benzodiazepine with a short elimination half-life at the lowest effective dose.

Use intermittently; skip nightly dose after 1 or 2 good nights' sleep.

Use medication for no more than 3 weeks and discontinue gradually.

■ **LONG-TERM INSOMNIA**

Hypnotics should be used in conjunction with psychologic–behavioral therapy.

A benzodiazepine with a long elimination half-life may be preferable but should only be used intermittently (eg, every third night).

Sedating antidepressants may be effective.

Once treatment is successful, discontinue medication gradually after 3–4 months.

Consider referral to a psychiatrist or sleep laboratory for difficult cases.

Source: Adapted from National Institutes of Health Consensus Task Force, Consensus Development Conference (1984). Drugs and insomnias: The use of medication to promote sleep. *JAMA, 251,* 2410–2414.

ton pump inhibitors may relieve the symptoms of gastroesophageal reflux disease (GERD).

Insomnia is most commonly and effectively treated with benzodiazepines. Table 3–9 lists the most commonly used medications with their therapeutic and side effect profiles. The practitioner must follow the response to these medications very carefully to achieve the therapeutic effect. Limited amounts should be dispensed to assist with titration and eventual weaning.

Pharmacologic treatments for RLS and nocturnal myoclonus are listed in Table 3–9. All associated conditions should be identified and treated in order

CLINICAL PEARL

Persons with sleep apnea should avoid use of pharmacologic sleep aids, as they may reduce their body's ability to recover from apneic episodes.

to minimize these movements. Treatment is based on the severity of the condition and effect on sleep and daytime function.

Homeopathic remedies have been introduced as alternative or adjunctive

TABLE 3–9.   MEDICATIONS FOR RESTLESS LEG SYNDROME (RLS) AND PERIODIC LEG MOVEMENT SYNDROME (PLMS)

Timing/Severity of Symptoms	Medication	Dosage	
Mild or present only at night	Sinemet CR	1/2–1 tablet 50/200 mg at bedtime	
	OR		
	Clonazepam (Klonopin)	1/2–1 tablet 0.5 mg at bedtime	May be used in combination
	OR		
	Propoxyphen (Darvon)	1–2 65 mg capsules at bedtime	
Moderate to severe symptoms	Bromocriptine mesylate (Parlodel)	1/2–1 tablet 2.5 mg at bedtime	
	OR		
	Codeine	30–60 mg at bedtime	May be used in combination
	OR		
	Pergaloid (Permax)	0.5 mg at bedtime	

Source: Adapted from Becker, P., & Jamieson, A. (1992). Common sleep disorders in the elderly: Diagnosis and treatment. *Geriatrics 47*(13), 41–52; and Hening, W. (1997) Restless leg syndrome. *Hospital Medicine,* November, 54–75.

therapy for sleep disorders. Melatonin is thought to assist in sleep induction by helping the body to relax for sleep and to reset the body's internal clock. The brain produces melatonin in response to darkness. Its use as a sleeping aid is controversial, with few studies confirming its effectiveness or safety. Vitamin E, folic acid, B vitamins, and quinine are thought to help in calming periodic leg movements.

Nonpharmacologic Measures

Light Therapy. Many studies have been done investigating the effect of light therapy on sleep patterns in healthy older adults, with encouraging findings. (Campbell et al., 1993; Campbell et al., 1995; Dawson & Campbell, 1990; Lack & Wright, 1993). Sunlight, dim light, and bright light have all been tested as measures to help affect the circadian rhythm and temperature phases of sleep. It is thought that evening light exposure (sitting under a light for several hours before bedtime) lengthens the total sleep time and delays morning wake-up time.

Light therapy has also been tested on persons with dementia to help with day–night reversal. Castor et al. (1991) found that exposure to sunlight increased mean sleep hours, increased nighttime uninterrupted sleep, decreased the number of nighttime awakenings, and decreased daytime sleep episodes. Satlin et al. (1992) found that bright light pulses for 2 hours during the evening helped to alleviate day–night reversal by restoring daytime wakefulness and nighttime sleep.

Sleep Hygiene. Johnson (1988) found bed routines to enhance sleep patterns. Such routines include adhering to a consistent bedtime and wake-up time; avoiding daytime napping; and using the bedroom for sleep and not eating, reading, or TV viewing. Environmental strategies include a comfortable bedroom temperature, a diminished noise level, a darkened room, and comfortable sleepwear. The installation of locks and smoke alarms can increase feelings of safety and peace of mind. Engaging in regular exercise of moderate intensity in the morning or early afternoon has been found to improve sleep onset, duration, and quality (King et al., 1997). Leaving the bed promptly if unable to fall asleep after 15 minutes and returning when feeling drowsy can help to avoid frustration. Weight loss and proper head positioning (avoiding neck flexion) are helpful with obstructive sleep apnea. Avoiding large meals before bedtime and limiting or avoiding the use of alcohol, nicotine, caffeine, and foods that contain monosodium glutamate can minimize sleep disturbances. It is thought that foods containing tryptophan, such as milk, turkey, and lettuce, can help with sleep induction. Relaxation techniques such as meditation, music therapy, guided imagery, progressive muscle relaxation, and self-hypnosis have been found to enhance sleep onset, decrease the number of nighttime awakenings, and increase sleep satisfaction (Johnson, 1991).

CLIENT EDUCATION

Older adults should be educated about the sleep changes related to normal aging prior to their onset. This may decrease the use of pharmaceutical sleep aids and promote healthy sleep habits. In persons with transient or chronic sleep disturbances, a combination of behavioral (nonpharmacologic) and pharmacologic interventions is recommended. When prescribing a sleep aid, the practitioner must educate the client as to the plan of treatment. Assessment of the underlying cause and treatment of such is key, using sleeping medication as an adjunctive and temporary therapy, rather than lifelong treatment. Discussions of scheduled doses and weaning are important to discuss with the client to promote understanding of the plan and to improve compliance. Formulating realistic plans to gradually decrease the habitual use of substances and modify poor sleep habits with continual reinforcement and praise is crucial to success.

 ## CASE STUDY

Mr. Benson is an 88-year-old gentleman living in a congregate living center in the community. His medical history includes COPD, non–insulin-dependent diabetes mellitus (NIDDM), CHF, and osteoarthritis of the spine. He tells you that he has been feeling very tired lately, nearly falling asleep during meals and while driving. He has some trouble falling asleep (sleep onset time, 15 minutes) but finds himself waking up "every 15 minutes." He believes he sleeps better in his recliner than in his bed. He has been taking temazepam (Restoril) 15 mg every night for years, but has recently taken two each night since one does not seem to be helping.

QUESTIONS

1. How might you proceed to collect more assessment data about Mr. Benson's sleep complaint?

2. What physical exam and diagnostic studies might you pursue at this time?

3. Discuss potential differential diagnoses and your approach to their treatment and management.

ANSWERS

1. Asking Mr. Benson to complete a sleep diary can give you a more complete and objective assessment of his sleep problem. Also ask him to show you all of the prescription and OTC medications that he takes regularly and occasionally. Collect information about his sleep hygiene habits and rituals. Ask if he has had any recent stress in his life. Perform a complete review of systems, focusing on the respiratory, cardiac, and endocrine systems (considering his

past medical history). Assess his pain control related to his musculoskeletal problems. Inquire about nighttime urination as a potential disturbance.

2. Perform a comprehensive physical exam with focus on respiratory, cardiac, endocrine, musculoskeletal, and psychosocial systems. Administration of the Geriatric Depression Scale can help to identify a contributing mood disorder. An MMSE is useful to screen for depression or cognitive impairment, which often accompany sleep disturbance. Appropriate diagnostic studies would be determined based on physical exam findings. Potential studies in this client might be a CBC (rule out UTI, respiratory infection), electrolytes, BUN, creatinine (to detect imbalances or renal changes that can contribute to drug toxicity or other conditions), intermittent blood sugar levels (including during the night) to detect hypoglycemia or hyperglycemia, TSH to detect thyroid abnormalities (common with diabetes), UA to look for UTI, and pulse oximetry at different points in time (including during sleep, if possible) to detect hypoxia. An ECG can be helpful if angina (common in diabetes) is suspected. A chest x-ray may be indicated if acute respiratory conditions are suspected. A formal sleep study in a sleep lab is also an option, especially if sleep apnea or RLS/PLMS is suspected.

3. Mr. Benson has the potential for many contributing factors to be affecting his sleep. If he is experiencing an acute respiratory infection (common with COPD), appropriate antibiotic and adjunctive therapy would be warranted. Cardiac problems may require nitrate therapy (if anginal) or further workup may be necessary. Blood sugar abnormalities may require an adjustment in diet or hypoglycemic agent. Thyroid imbalance warrants further workup and probable pharmacotherapy. Urinary tract infections (common in diabetics) requires antibiotic therapy and increased fluids. Stress or depression may require counseling and possibly short-term pharmacotherapy. Poor sleep hygiene would warrant an assessment of Mr. Benson's understanding and motivation to change his habits and patterns to enhance sleep. A gradual weaning of temazepam may be indicated, especially if sleep apnea is suspected. Additional measures for improvement of sleep apnea would include weight loss (if overweight), proper head positioning during sleep (with a collar), continuous positive airway pressure, and surgery.

■ REFERENCES

Agostinelli, B., Demers, K., Garrigan, D., & Waszynski, C. (1994). Targeted interventions: Use of the Mini-Mental State Exam. *J Gerontol Nurs, 20*(8), 15–23.

American Psychiatric Association (1994). *Diagnostic and statistical manual of mental disorders (4th ed.)* (pp. 123–133). Washington, DC: Author.

Campbell S., Dawson, D., & Anderson, M. (1993). Alleviation of sleep maintenance insomnia with timed exposure to bright light. *J Am Geriatr Soc, 41*(8), 829–836.

Campbell, S., Terman, M., Lewy, A., et al. (1995). Light treatment of sleep disorders: Consenss report V. Age related disturbances. *J Biolog Rhythms, 10*(2), 151–154.

Castor, D., Woods, D., Pigott, K., et al. (1991). Effect of sunlight on sleep patterns of the elderly. *J Am Acad Phys Assist, 4,* 321–326.

Cohen, D., & Eisdorfer, C. (1986). Dementing disorders. In Calkins, E., Davis, P., & Ford, A. (Eds.). *The practice of geriatrics* (pp. 194–205). Philadelphia: W. B. Saunders.

Consensus Development Conference. (1984). Drugs and insomnia: The use of medication to promote sleep. *JAMA, 251,* 2410–2414.

Costa, P. T. Jr., Williams, T. F., Somerfield, M., et al. (1996) *Early identification of Alzheimer's disease and related dementias.* Clinical Practice Guideline Quick Reference Guide for Clinicians, No. 19. Rockville, MD: U.S. Department of Health and Human Services, Public Health Service, Agency for Health Care Policy and Research. AHCPR Publication No 97-0703, November.

Crum, R. M., Anthony, J. C., Bassett, S. S., et al. (1993) Population-based norms for the Mini-Mental State Examination by age and educational level. *JAMA, 269,* 2386–2391.

Dawson D., & Campbell, S. (1990). Bright light treatment: Are we keeping our subjects in the dark? *Sleep, 13*(3), 267–270.

Dealberto, M. J., Pajot, N., Courcon, D., et al. (1996). Breathing disorders during sleep and cognitive performance in an older community sample: the EVA study. *J Am Geriatr Soc, 44,* 1287–1294.

Fletcher, E. C., Miller, J., Divine, G. W., et al. (1987). Nocturnal oxyhemoglobin desaturation in COPD patients with arterial oxygen tensions above 60 mm Hg. *Chest, 92,* 604–608.

Fletcher, E. C. (1995). The relationship between systemic hypertension and obstructive sleep apnea: Facts and theory. *Am J Med, 98,* 118–128.

Folstein, M., Folstein, S., & McHugh, P. (1975). Mini-mental state. *J Psychiatr Res, 12,* 189–198.

Foreman, M. (1989). Confusion in the hospitalized elderly: Incidence, onset and associated factors. *Res Nurs Health, 12*(1): 21–29.

Guilleminault, C., Connolly, S. J., & Winkle, R. A. (1983). Cardiac arrthymia and conduction disturbances during sleep in 400 patients with sleep apnea syndrome. *Am J Cardiol, 52,* 490–494.

Hoch, C., Reynolds, C., & Houck, P. (1987). Sleep apnea in Alzheimer's patients and the healthy elderly. *Sch Inq Nurs Pract, 1,* 221–235.

Inouye, S. K., van Dyck, C. H., Alessi, C. A., et al. (1990). Clarifying confusion: the Confusion Assessment Method—a new method for detection of delirium. *Ann Intern Med, 113,* 941–948.

Johnson, J. (1988). Effect of benzodiazepines on older women. *JCHN, 5,* 119–127.

Johnson, J. (1991). Progressive relaxation and the sleep of older noninstitutionalized women. *Appl Nurs Res, 4,* 165–170.

Jorm, A., Korten, A., & Henderson, A. (1987). The prevalence of dementia: A quantitative integration of the literature. *ACTA Psychiatr Scand, 76,* 464–479.

Katzman, R., & Kawas, C. (1994). The epidemiology of dementia and Alzheimer disease. In Terry, R., Katzman, R., & Bick, K. (Eds.). *Alzheimer disease* (pp. 105–122). New York: Raven Press.

King, A. C., Oman, R. F., Brassington, M. A., Bliwise, D. L., & Haskell, W. L. (1997). Moderate-intensity exercise and self-rated quality of sleep in older adults: A randomized controlled trial. *JAMA, 277*(1), 32–37.

Lack, L., & Wright, H. (1993). The effect of evening bright light in delaying the circadian rhythms and lengthening the sleep of early morning awakening insomniacs. *Sleep, 16*(5), 436–443.

Lawton, M., & Brody, E. (1969). Assessment of older people: self-maintaining and instrumental activities of daily living. *Gerontologist, 9,* 179–186.

Levkoff, S. E., Evans, D. A., Liptzin, B., et al. (1992). Delirium: The occurrence and persistence of symptoms among elderly hospitalized patients. *Arch Intern Med, 152,* 334–340.

Lipowski, Z. (1983). Transient cognitive disorders in the elderly. *Am J Psych, 140*(11), 1426–1434.

Mangino, M. & Middlemiss, C. (1997). Alzheimer's disease: Preventing and recognizing a misdiagnosis. *Nurse Pract, 22*(10), 58–75.

Matteson, M. (1997). Age-related changes in the neurological system. In Matteson, M., McConnell, E., & Linton, A. (Eds.). *Gerontological nursing: Concepts and practice* (pp. 282–315). Philadelphia: W. B. Saunders.

Moore, M. N. (1989). Development of a sleep wake instrument for use in a chronic renal population. *ANNA J, 16,* 15–19.

National Commission on Sleep Disorders Research (1993). Wake up America, A National Sleep Alert. (Executive summary and executive report, submitted to the United States Congress and to the U.S. Department of Health and Human Services, January.)

Neelon, V., Champagne, M., & McCourd, E. (1987). Acute confusion in the hospitalized elderly: patterns and early diagnosis. Abstract published in *Nursing advances in health: Model, methods and applications, international nursing research conference abstracts* (p. 323). Kansas City, MO: American Nurses Association.

Newman, A. B., Enright, P. L., Manilio, T. A., et al. (1997). Sleep disturbance, psychosocial correlates and cardiovascular disease in 5201 older adults; The cardiovascular health study. *J Am Geriatr Soc, 45,* 1–7.

Pfeiffer, R., Kurosaki, T., Harrah, C., et al. (1982). Measurement of functional activities of older adults in the community. *J Gerontol, 37,* 323–339.

Pollack, C. P., Perlick, D., Linsner, J. P., Wenston, J., & Heish, F. (1990). Sleep problems in the community elderly as predictors of death and nursing home placement. *JCH, 15,* 123–134.

Bick, K. (Eds.), *Alzheimer disease* (pp. 231–261). New York: Raven Press.

Rader, J. (1995). In Tornquist, E. (Ed.), *Individualized dementia care: Creative, compassionate approaches.* New York: Springer-Verlag.

Robinson, A., Spencer, B., & White, L. (1989). *Understanding difficult behavior.* Ypsilanti, MI: Eastern Michigan University Press.

Satlin, A., Volicer, L., Ross, V., Herz, L., & Campbell, S. (1992). Bright light treatment of behavioral and sleep disturbances in patients with Alzheimer's disease. *Am J Psych, 149*(8), 1028–1032.

Shepard, J. W., Garrison, M. W., Grither, D. A., & Dolan, G. E. (1985). The relationship of ventricular ectopy to oxyhemoglobin desaturation in patients with obstructive sleep apnea. *Chest, 88,* 335–340.

Sloohs, R. A., Gingold, J., Cohrs, S., et al. (1996). Sleep-disordered breathing and systemic hypertension in the older male. *J Am Geriatr Soc, 44,* 1295–1300.

Small, G., Rabins, P., Barry, P., et al. (1997). Diagnosis and treatment of Alzheimer's disease and related disorders: Consensus statement of the American Association for Geriatric Psychiatry, the Alzheimer's Association and the American Geriatrics Society. *JAMA, 278*(16), 1363–1371.

Taft, L., Delaney, K., Seman, D., et al. (1993). Dementia care: Creating a therapeutic milieu. *J Gerontol Nurs, 19*(10), 30–39.

Tangalos, E., Smith, G., Ivnik, R., et al. (1996). The Mini-Mental State Examination in general medical practice: Clinical utility and acceptance. *Mayo Clin Proc, 71,* 829–837.

U.S. Department of Veterans Affairs and University Healthsystem Consortium. (1997). *Dementia identification and assessment: Guidelines for primary care practitioners.* Washington, DC: U.S. Department of Veterans Affairs 1363–1371.

Vermeersch, P. (1990). The clinical assessment of confusion. *Appl Nurs Res, 3,* 129–133.

Wolanin, M., & Phillips, L. (1981). *Confusion: Prevention and care.* St. Louis: C. V. Mosby.

Yesavage, J. A. (1988). Geriatric depression scale. *Psychopharmacol Bull,* 24, 709–711.

4

TOPICS IN EYE, EAR, HEAD, AND NECK CARE

Evelyn Woodman Godwin

■ INTRODUCTION

The eyes, ears, nose, mouth, and throat undergo major changes in the aging process that can have a major impact on quality of life. Older adults may need to make numerous adjustments both personally and in the environment to compensate for these changes. Aids such as glasses, hearing aids, and dentures may become an integral part of their life. The role of the advanced practice nurse (APN) is key in identifying these changes and assisting older adults to adapt to their changing needs in order to maintain their independence.

■ EYES

AGE-RELATED CHANGES

The human eye undergoes numerous physiologic changes with aging. Visual acuity diminishes slowly from age 40 to 70, and thereafter at a more rapid pace. Near vision declines as the lens loses its elasticity and therefore its ability to focus on near objects. Peripheral vision and color intensity also decrease. Color discrimination, specifically for shades of blue, green, and purple, becomes less acute. Night vision is impaired due to decreased accommodation. With diminished accommodation, it takes longer for the older adult to adjust to a change in lighting such as when coming indoors after being exposed to the sunlight. This can also be a problem when one is going from one room to the next, particularly at night when the light in a darkened room is abruptly turned on. Decreased tear production and viscosity lead to increased dryness, irritation, and a predisposition to infection. Altered depth perception occurs as a result of a decrease in contrast sensitivity, which affects one's ability to accurately predict gait adjustment on uneven surfaces such as stairs, curbs, and thresholds. Older adults also are extremely sensitive to glare from windows and polished floors. It is imperative for the clinician to recognize that in addition to the numerous age-related changes, visual function is also affected by medications and systemic illnesses.

COMMON EYE DISORDERS

Blepharitis

Blepharitis is an inflammation of the hair follicles and glands of the eyelid margins. Frequently, the condition is chronic with acute flare-ups, and on occasion can result in a coinciding infection. Conditions such as seborrheic dermatitis of the eyebrows or forehead, commonly found in clients with Parkinson's disease, can cause blepharitis.

Clinical Presentation. Typically, the eyelid margins are slightly edematous and hyperemic, with crusting and greasy, scaly deposits on the lids and eyelashes. This may be accompanied by erythematous and itchy eyes. On occasion, ulcerations of the margins may be noted.

Clinical Management. Lid scrubs three times a day for 7 days with a solution of 1/2-strength baby shampoo are recommended. In cases of coinciding infection, a 3- to 5-day course of antibiotic therapy with ophthalmic drops/ointment such as erythromycin, sulfonamide sulfacetamide Na 10% (Sulamyd), bacitracin, neomycin (Neosporin), or tobramycin is indicated. It is important to note that long-term use of Neosporin can result in neomycin allergy. With repeated episodes of blepharitis, a scheduled program of once or twice a day lid scrubs may be warranted. If steroid-containing agents are used, avoid long-term use to prevent complications.

Blepharochalasis

Blepharochalasis, sometimes referred to as "false ptosis," is a drooping of the skin over an eyelid due to loss of elasticity. The space between the eyelids (palpebral fissure) is diminished, resulting in a decrease in visual acuity.

Clinical Management. The client should be referred to an ophthalmologist for surgical correction of this condition.

Cataracts

Cataracts are formed when the normally transparent lens becomes opaque. This is a normal aging process that generally affects both eyes. It is the most common cause of decreased vision in the older adult. The three age-related cataracts are nuclear sclerotic, cortical (peripheral), and posterior subcapsular opacification.

Clinical Presentation. The client complains of increased glare and gradual visual loss due to clouding. Objects appear darker and less clear, with less vivid colors. Frequently, the client will claim to see near objects better without glasses. Upon fundoscopic exam, a peripheral opacity of the lens appears as dark spokes radiating toward the center of the lens. In contrast, the posterior subcapsular cataract is a 1- to 2-mm black spot located in the center of the lens. A nuclear sclerotic cataract presents as a central darkening of the red reflex.

Older adults with cataracts are often very aware of the deficits they cause. They frequently adjust their environment to fit these deficits (placement of lights, room design). Collecting the data and attempting to modify new environments (hospital/rehab setting) to meet clients' needs is essential to promote maximum function and safety.

The decision for cataract surgery is based on the effect on function and not age. Many older adults will consider surgery when they no longer are able to perform the activities they value and enjoy.

CLINICAL PEARL

Cataract surgery can be appropriate in older adults with dementia as a way to improve sensory input and maximize function.

Clinical Management. Surgical removal of the lens, followed by an intraocular lens implantation, generally restores vision to its precataract state. It is not uncommon to have clouding of the posterior capsule from 6 months to several years post–cataract surgery. Without correction, visual acuity is decreased. This is easily corrected with laser surgery.

Chalazion

Chalazion is caused by a chronic granulomatous inflammation of a meibomian gland.

Clinical Presentation. A small, hard, nontender nodule is found located deep within the lid near the conjunctival surface. The surrounding area is red.

Clinical Management. No treatment is necessary unless the nodule is pressing on the eyeball; surgical removal is then recommended. Treat infected, painful chalazions with warm, moist compresses four times a day.

Conjunctivitis

Conjunctivitis is an inflammation of the conjunctiva that can be of allergic, bacterial, or viral origin.

Clinical Presentation. The client will complain of a burning or itching sensation. Frequently, increased tearing and an exudate will be present. The client will complain of the eyelids sticking shut, especially when awakening in the morning. The eyelids may be swollen, and the conjunctiva red and possibly swollen. Visual acuity is not compromised.

CLINICAL PEARL

In clients with recurrent conjunctivitis, one should suspect blepharitis.

Allergic conjunctivitis is due to seasonal, chemical, or animal allergy. This condition is often associated with itchy, swollen conjunctiva and red, edematous eyelids. There is a white, ropy discharge from the eyes, rhinorrhea, and sneezing.

Clinical Management. Generally, this condition resolves once the offending allergen is removed. Artificial tears, topical vasoconstrictors, and systemic antihistamines, as well as cool moist compresses, may provide symptomatic relief. In severe cases, steroids may need to be used short term. For those clients who are highly sensitive, a referral to an allergist is indicated.

Bacterial conjunctivitis is caused by a bacterial infection. The conjunctiva is edematous and red with a thick, purulent discharge. The older adult may complain of sensation of a foreign body, burning, or itching.

Clinical Management. Instill ophthalmic drops/ointment such as Neosporin, Sulamyd, or erythromycin.

Viral conjunctivitis is a viral infection causing inflammation. Viral conjunctivitis is often preceded by fever, general myalgia, and pharyngitis. This form of conjunctivitis is highly contagious. Although initially it involves only one eye, the other eye frequently becomes infected as well. The conjunctivae are inflamed and the corneas may be steamy. The eyelids are red and edematous. The client may complain of blurred vision. A watery or mucoid discharge is present. Usually, the preauricular nodes are palpable (Speight and Cunha, 1995).

Clinical Management. Treat symptomatically with cool, moist compresses; artificial tears; vasoconstrictors; and antihistamines. Instruct the client to avoid touching the eyes, sharing towels, or shaking hands.

Diabetic Retinopathy

Diabetic retinopathy is a leading cause of blindness in the older adult with a long-standing history of diabetes mellitus. It is caused by microvascular degenerative changes such as mini-hemorrhages and aneurysms of the retina, as well as proliferative changes of neovascularization. Retinal detachment is a complication due to development of scar tissue and hemorrhages.

Clinical Presentation. The client complains of blurred and distorted vision, with blind spots or floaters.

Clinical Management. Proper management of diabetes must be adhered to. Disease progression of neovascularization changes can be slowed with laser photocoagulation.

Ectropion

Ectropion is an eversion of the eyelid, generally the lower lid. This causes continual exposure of the conjunctiva, which can result in thickening and keratinization. The eye is exposed to chronic irritation and tearing. Corneal dryness and decreased visual acuity can occur if untreated.

Clinical Management. Treat with artificial tears, securing the lid shut at night with a patch. If necessary, surgery can correct this, but it may recur.

Entropion

Entropion is the inversion of the eyelid, usually involving the lower eyelid. This causes the eyelashes to rub against and scratch the cornea. As a result of this constant trauma to the cornea, scarring and decreased visual acuity can occur.

Clinical Presentation. Clients with this condition complain of burning and a sensation of a foreign body in the eye. Increased lacrimation and photophobia are also present.

Clinical Management. The client should be referred to an ophthalmologist for surgical correction.

Glaucoma

Glaucoma is a common disease among older adults. Risk factors for developing glaucoma are black race, diabetes, hypertension, history of a head injury, and family history of glaucoma. Glaucoma can also be provoked by some drugs. Glaucoma may present unilaterally or bilaterally. It is characterized by an increase in intraocular pressure due to an accumulation of aqueous humor. Decreased elasticity of the sclera and increased rigidity of the eyeball combined with other aging changes can inhibit the normal drainage of aqueous fluid from the anterior chamber. This combined with increased production of aqueous fluid will elevate the intraocular pressure. If left untreated or in extreme cases, it can cause optic nerve atrophy and blindness. There are two forms of glaucoma: open-angle/chronic simple, which is the most common form, and acute angle-closure glaucoma, which is relatively uncommon. The use of anticholinergics, anticonvulsants, antidepressants, antihistamines, bronchodilators, central nervous system (CNS) stimulants, mydriatics, vasopressors, and vasodilators should be avoided or used cauiously in the older adult with glaucoma, as they increase intraocular pressure and can lead to acute angle-closure glaucoma.

Open-angle/chronic simple glaucoma is caused by increased intraocular pressure due to closure of the canal of Schlemm. It generally is insidious, affecting both eyes, and goes undetected for many years.

Clinical Presentation. The client may complain of seeing halos around lights, blurred vision, or decreased peripheral vision. He or she may complain of eye discomfort, chronic headache, or difficulty adjusting to the dark. Older adults with glaucoma often complain that their recently corrected eyeglass prescription is not helping their visual acuity. Fundoscopy shows cupping of the optic disc and atrophy of the optic nerve. Intraocular pressure is over 22 mm Hg.

Clinical Management. When glaucoma is suspected, the client should be referred to an ophthalmologist. If detected early, damage is frequently reversible. Topical and systemic medications can be used to decrease the production of aqueous humor or increase the drainage of aqueous humor from the anterior chamber. Use of long-acting beta blockers to decrease aqueous production such as timolol (Timoptic), betaxolol (Betoptic), and Levobunolol (Betagan) are very effective. Cholinergic agents such as pilocarpine 2% are used to cause pupillary constriction and decrease resistance to aqueous humor outflow. Corrective lenses with either prisms or reverse telescopic lenses are used to bring peripheral vision into the center. Glaucoma can also be treated with trabeculoplasty or laser if medical management is unsuccessful.

Acute angle-closure glaucoma is also seen with increasing age, but unlike open-angle/chronic simple glaucoma, it is relatively rare, unilateral, and more frequently seen in those who are farsighted and with a family history of glaucoma. It may be induced by mydriatic eyedrops or systemic anticholinergic medications. It is sometimes caused by a shallow anterior chamber that has a decreased filtration angle and thus decreased outflow.

Clinical Presentation. The client will have sudden, acute eye pain, headache, nausea/vomiting, and abdominal discomfort. A key finding is decreased vision, which can progress to severe and rapid visual loss over hours to days. The client may report seeing colored halos around lights due to corneal edema. The eye is firm and inflamed, with a steamy appearance of the iris and pupil. The pupil is unreactive and partially dilated. There is conjunctival and corneal edema, and the intraocular pressure is elevated. Cupping of the optic disc can be seen, as well as pallor and atrophy of the optic nerve. There are visual field deficits.

Clinical Management. This is a true medical emergency and requires immediate referral to an ophthalmologist. Treatment to reduce aqueous humor production and to decrease the outflow resistance can be accomplished with medications, laser, and/or surgery. Generally, medication is used first, often followed by surgery. Drugs of choice are long-acting beta blockers such as timolol to decrease aqueous production. A cholinomimetic (pilocarpine 2%) is used to cause pupillary constriction and decrease resistance to aqueous outflow. Oral carbonic anhydrase inhibitors (Diamox) decrease aqueous production. Laser iridotomy is the surgical treatment.

Keratoconjunctivitis

Keratoconjunctivitis, also known as "dry eye syndrome," is characterized by a burning or scratchy sensation. The conjunctiva and cornea are inflamed, and the normally glassy luster is absent. Vision is blurred, and occasionally excessive tearing is noted.

Clinical Management. Symptomatic relief can be obtained with the use of artificial tears. Review the client's drugs to see if any may be contributing to the problem, and, if possible, discontinue their use.

Macular Degeneration

Macular degeneration is commonly seen with increasing age and tends to be familial. There are three types of macular degeneration: dry form, wet form (subretinal neovascularization), and pigment epithelial detachment (blister formation on the macula).

Clinical Presentation. The client will complain of a gradual but occasionally rapid generalized decline in vision. This is characterized by a loss of central vision without a change in peripheral vision. With disease progression, whitish-yellow spots (Drusen spots) are noted around the macula. On Amsler grid, straight lines are perceived as bent or having a missing center section. Age-related macular degeneration progresses slowly, with minimal loss of visual acuity.

Clinical Management. The client should be referred to an ophthalmologist if macular degeneration is suspected. Clients with early age-related macular degeneration are given an Amsler grid to check their vision on a weekly basis to monitor the disease progression so that macular edema and subretinal neovascularization can be detected and managed early. Although there is no treatment for early age-related macular degeneration, subretinal neovascularization may respond to laser photocoagulation and thus prevention of further damage in the wet form. Some clients benefit from the use of magnifying glasses for close-up work and telescopic lenses for distance. Individuals can learn how to use their peripheral vision. Eventually, central vision blindness can occur.

Pinguecula

Pinguecula is a painless, triangular-shaped, yellowish thickening of bulbar conjunctiva found on the inner and outer margins of the cornea (Fig. 4–1).

Clinical Management. No treatment is needed. Ocular lubricants or artificial tears can be used in the presence of inflammation.

Pterygium

Pterygium is a triangular thickening of the bulbar conjunctiva that extends from the inner canthus to the border of the cornea. It is a painless, cloudy growth (Fig. 4–2).

Clinical Management. Treatment is not indicated unless it extends to the pupillary axis; then, surgical intervention is required. According to Soong, Johnston, and Sugar (1998), its formation may be due to actinic radiation, wind, drying, or dust.

Ptosis

Ptosis is a drooping of the upper eyelid. It generally is caused by weakness of the levator muscle but can be caused by injury to the third cranial nerve.

Clinical Management. Generally, no treatment is needed. In pronounced cases, surgery is indicated.

Presbyopia

Presbyopia (farsightedness) is diminished near vision as a result of decreased lens elasticity and decreased ability to focus. Reading material is held at arm's length to enhance focusing.

Clinical Management. Vision may be improved with the use of magnifying or corrective lenses.

Retinal Detachment

Retinal detachment may occur after trauma or cataract surgery, or spontaneously.

Clinical Presentation. The client will complain of a sudden onset of floaters or flashes of light peripherally, with decreased visual acuity. Partial loss of pe-

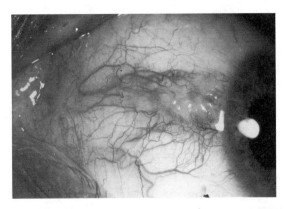

Figure 4–1. Pinguecula. (*Source: Vaughan, D., Asbury, T., & Riordan-Eva, P. [1999]. General Ophthalmology [15th ed.]. Stamford, CT: Appleton & Lange.)*

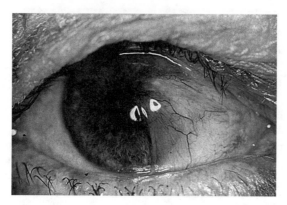

Figure 4–2. Pterygium encroaching on the cornea. (*Source: Vaughan, D., Asbury, T., & Riordan-Eva, P. [1999]. General Ophthalmology [15th ed.]. Stamford, CT: Appleton & Lange.)*

ripheral vision and distortion of images will be reported. The client may describe the visual loss as "like having a curtain come down across the field of vision." The retina is wavy and slightly gray or pale.

Clinical Management. The client should be referred immediately to an ophthalmologist. Surgery or laser treatment may be required.

Retinal Vein Occlusion

Retinal vein occlusion is seen in older adults with long-standing medical problems such as cardiovascular disease (arteriosclerosis), hypertension, and diabetes (Scimeca et al., 1989) (Fig. 4–3).

Clinical Presentation. The client will complain of a sudden onset of painless, unilateral loss of vision. Edema and hemorrhages are noted in the section of the retina with the affected vein. The surrounding venous system is darker in color, tortuous, dilated, and distended with blood. Frequently, retinal edema is present, and there is blurring of the disc margin. Occasionally, cotton-wool patches can be seen.

Clinical Management. Immediate referral to an ophthalmologist is indicated. It is felt that low-dose acetylsalicylic acid (ASA) is probably helpful in decreasing the incidence of thrombosis. In some cases, laser photocoagulation has been beneficial.

Sty

Sty is a bacterial (generally staphylococcal) infection of a sebaceous gland of the eyelid. External styes are superficial and on the rim of the eyelid. Internal styes are located under the eyelid and apt to progress to abscess formation.

Clinical Presentation. The sty is a small, painful, circumscribed swelling. The conjunctiva is injected, and ptosis may be present if the upper lid is involved. The eyelids may be edematous and erythematous.

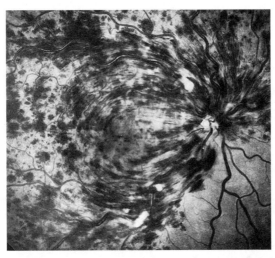

Figure 4–3. Central retinal vein occlusion with extensive superficial retinal hemorrhage obscuring macular and optic nerve detail. *(Source: Vaughan, D., Asbury, T., & Riordan-Eva, P. [1999]. General Ophthalmology [15th ed.]. Stamford, CT: Appleton & Lange.)*

Clinical Management. Application of warm, moist packs provides comfort. The infection is treated with topical antibiotics and corticosteriods. In some cases, it may be necessary to treat with systemic antibiotics (dicloxacillin 250 to 500 mg qid for 5 to 7 days).

Subconjunctival Hemorrhage

Subconjunctival hemorrhage is caused from a ruptured conjunctival vessel. It is unilateral and asymptomatic. A bright red area that is well demarcated appears on the bulbar conjunctiva. Frequently, the patient does not recall how it occurred. It is painless and reabsorbs in 1 to 3 weeks. No treatment is necessary.

Clinical Management. Preventive measures to consider with the aging eye include prophylactic use of artificial tears if the person is taking anticholinergic

agents, providing a means for proper closure of the eyelids, and adequate lighting to compensate for visual decline. Add contrasting colors to the bottom stair or in areas where the floor level may drop or incline. Glare can be eliminated with the use of soft lighting and avoidance of highly polished floors. Night-lights can prevent falls in unfamiliar, dark settings by avoiding extremes in lighting changes. Use of large print calendars/books/telephone dials helps clients with decreased vision. Discourage visual blood sugar monitoring (without monitor) due to inability to distinguish shades of blue and green. Be sure eyeglasses are clean and in use. Avoid disrupting the person's environmental cues which promote function (eg, location and order of pill bottles). Contact local resources for community services available to persons with visual impairment.

■ EARS

AGE-RELATED CHANGES

The aging ear undergoes a number of changes. The auricle (pinna) becomes elongated and broader. The cartilage is less elastic and thus less flexible. Tophi may appear on the pinna. The earlobes become longer and flatter. The hairs of the external ear canal become longer and more coarse. With age, the tympanic membrane becomes thicker, more fixed, less translucent, and loses its luster. Because of a decrease in the number of cerumen glands, the cerumen is thicker, drier, and consequently harder. As a result of this decreased lubrication, the skin of the ear canal is drier and more easily irritated. Atrophic changes of the skin result in thinner, dry, and itchy skin. In the cochlea, hair cells, neurons supporting cells, ganglion cells, and fibers are decreased; these changes, combined with diminished blood flow to the cochlea, can cause generalized deterioration of hearing (Winters, 1989), as well as problems with balance (equilibrium), including dizziness and lightheadedness. Aging changes can have a negative effect on the ability to discriminate speech, as well as a decreased sensitivity to sound.

COMMON EAR DISORDERS

Acoustic Neuroma

Acoustic neuroma (vestibular schwannoma) is a benign tumor along the eighth cranial nerve.

Clinical Presentation. This condition presents with varying degrees of unilateral sensorineural hearing loss and tinnitus. Occasionally, disequilibrium and facial hypesthesia are also present.

Clinical Management. A complete auditory exam (inner and outer ear evaluation, Weber and Rinne tests) should be followed by cranial nerve testing. Further testing would include the auditory brain response (ABR) and magnetic resonance imaging (MRI). Acoustic neuromas are surgically excised.

Cellulitis of the External Ear

Clinical Presentation. This condition generally presents as a painful, erythematous swelling of the auricle.

Clinical Management. Since the blood supply to this area is poor, intravenous (IV) antibiotics such as dicloxacillin, cephalosporin, or erythromycin may be beneficial if the client is running a high fever. In less severe cases, oral antibiotics are sufficient. Warm compresses should be applied four times a day for several days.

Cerumen Impaction

Cerumen impaction is a common problem of the older adult, and if left untreated can result in otitis externa. Hearing aids not only stimulate the production of cerumen but also impede its flow from the canal.

Clinical Presentation. Clients note a sensation of fullness, decreased hearing, pain, or itching. Upon examination, cerumen will be seen in the external canal. Depending on its age and consistency, the wax can appear yellow, tan, light or dark brown, maroon, or black. It can be mistaken for purulent drainage or dried blood.

Clinical Management. Prior to initiating treatment, a comprehensive history should be taken to confirm that the patient has not had inner ear surgery or a ruptured tympanic membrane.

CLINICAL PEARL

Cerumen removal should not be attempted with a curette or by irrigation without pretreatment with cerumen softener. The skin of the external ear canal is quite friable and bleeding is more likely to occur.

Instill cerumen-softening drops such as carbamide peroxide (Debrox) (5 drops twice a day for 4 days). Mineral oil, vegetable oil, liquid glycerine or liquid ducosate sodium may be substituted as an ear wax softener. Instruct the client to lie with the affected ear toward the ceiling and to maintain that position for at least 10 minutes following drop insertion to assure penetration and absorption. Remove wax by curette or lavage. A curette (cerumen loop) is preferable if cerumen is close to the opening of the canal. If irrigation is necessary, use of a 30-cc plastic syringe with a 1-inch intercath sheath can be less threatening and more manageable. A Waterpik or 50-cc metal irrigation syringe are other options. Irrigate gently with warm, sterile water or normal saline. Warming the solution to body temperature decreases the incidence of labyrinth stimulation, which may cause nausea, vomiting, or vertigo. To open and straighten the ear canal, pull the helix of the ear upward and outward. When performing ear irrigation, point the syringe tip superiorly

so that the cerumen is flushed away from the tympanic membrane. After irrigation, have the client turn to the affected side to promote drainage of the residual water left in the external canal to decrease the incidence of infection (Freeman, 1995).

Although it is common practice to irrigate with nonsterile water, if an undetected perforated tympanic membrane is irrigated, water and infectious agents can be introduced into the middle ear space, causing infection. A mixture of equal parts of hydrogen peroxide and sterile water or normal saline may also be used as an irrigant but the foaming action may decrease the clinician's ability to visualize the ear canal. It is common to have to repeat the course of eardrops and irrigation before the ear canal is sufficiently cleared. Occasionally, repeat irrigation is unsuccessful, and it is necessary to refer the client to an ear specialist for cerumen removal. To prevent hearing aid damage, instruct the older adult not to wear the hearing aid during the time frame that cerumen-softening agents are used or for at least 24 hours after ear irrigation.

CLINICAL PEARL

If cerumen is dislodging slowly, massage the trague of the ear to enhance loosening of the cerumen from the canal and promote cerumen removal.

CLINICAL PEARL

Do not attempt irrigation if a ruptured tympanic membrane is suspected.

Setting-specific Issues. Older adults who live independently should be cautioned not to use cotton swabs to clean their ear canals as they tend to push the wax up against the ear canal causing further impaction and potential injury to the tympanic membrane.

Hearing Impairment

Hearing impairment is an alteration in hearing that is classified as conductive, sensorineural, or mixed.

Clinical Presentation. In *conductive hearing loss,* the normal flow of sound vibration is obstructed by an abnormality of either the external ear canal, the tympanic membrane, or the middle ear ossicles. These abnormalities may include a foreign body, cerumen impaction, infection, or otosclerosis. The client usually talks in a normal voice and can hear better if others talk loudly. Hearing can be restored with removal of cerumen impaction on foreign body or by treatment of infection.

Sensorineural hearing loss (presbycusis) occurs when the brain stem, cortical auditory pathways, inner ear, or eighth cranial nerve are not functioning properly. Normal aging changes, cerebrovascular accident (CVA), ototoxic drugs (see Table 4–1), infection, intense or prolonged noise or trauma, can all cause sensorineural hearing loss. Diabetes mellitus, hyperlipidemia, hypothyroidism, renal failure, tumor, polyarteritis, lupus erythematosus, and radiation therapy are all less common causes of sensorineural hearing loss. The client with sensorineural hearing loss may talk in a loud voice since he cannot hear his own voice. Hearing may be improved with a hearing aid. *Mixed hearing loss* is a combination of both conductive and sensorineural hearing loss.

Age-related sensorineural hearing loss is the most common form of hearing loss in this country. It involves the slow but progressive loss of high tones bilaterally. Cochlear degeneration may cause decreased acuity for high-frequency tones, such as P, B, T, F, S, H, G, Z, TH, and SH sounds, resulting in difficulty with speech discrimination (Anderson et al., 1983). Although hearing itself is normal, the client is no longer able to distinguish certain sounds, and comprehension is impaired. This is all compounded by slowed central processing of auditory information (Morris & McManus, 1991). Noisy environments make it more difficult to understand speech. According to Fitzgerald (1985), most hearing loss in the older adult is both symmetric and bilateral.

Clinical Management. Some nonpharmacologic treatment modalities include hearing aids, assistive listening devices, telephone adapters, blinking lights to indicate a ringing phone/doorbell, and infrared or audio loop systems for TV, radio, church, theater, and lecture hall settings (Rupp, Vaughn, & Lightfoot, 1984).

Unilateral hearing loss is seldom related to presbycusis. Acute unilateral hearing loss can be associated with hypertension (HTN). If a hearing loss is sudden and only in one ear, it most likely is due to an embolic or thrombotic occlusion of the internal auditory artery. This may partially improve over several weeks to months. When unilateral hearing loss and tinnitus occur, acoustic neuroma should be a major consideration. Beside acoustic neuroma, peripheral disorders such as cholesteatoma, chronic infection, Ménière's disease, meningioma, otosclerosis, and trauma can cause unilateral hearing loss or tinnitus. Sudden hearing

TABLE 4–1. OTOTOXIC DRUGS

Alkylating agents	
Carboplatin	Paraplatin
Cisplatin	Platinol
Nitrogen mustard	Mustargen
Aminoglycoside antibiotics	
Amikacin sulfate	Amikin
Gentamicin sulfate	Garamycin, Gentafair, Jenamicin
Kanamycin sulfate	Kantrex, Klebcil
Neomycin sulfate	Mycifradin
Netilmicin sulfate	Netromycin
Streptomycin sulfate	
Tobramycin sulfate	Nebcin
Analgesics	
Salicylates	ASA, ASA Enseals, Ecotrin, Empirin, Trilisate, Arthropan, Extra-Strength Doan's, Mobidin, Original Doan's, Disalcid, Mono-Gesic, Salgesic, Uracel-5, Asproject
Anti-infectives	
Vancomycin hydrochloride	Vancocin
Antimalarials	
Chloroquine hydrochloride	Aralen HCL
Chloroquine phosphate	Aralen Phosphate
Hydroychloroquine sulfate	Plaquenil
Guinine sulfate	Legatrin, Quinamm, Quinidan
Loop diuretics	
Bumetanide	Bumex
Ethacrynate sulfate	Edecrin sodium
Ethacrynic acid	Edecrin
Furosemide	Lasix, Myrosemide
Nonsteroidal anti-inflammatory drugs	
Indomethacin	Indameth, Indocin
Oxyphenbutazone	
Phenylbutazone	Butazolidin

loss should be considered a medical emergency. Without treatment, permanent sensorineural hearing loss can occur. One such cause of sudden hearing loss is related to a perilymphatic fistula that occurs after a sudden rise in cerebral spinal pressure (Fitzgerald, 1985). This rise in pressure is conveyed to the inner ear fluid (perilymph), which results in a rupture of the oval/round window. The rupture causes a sudden hearing loss, as well as positional vertigo. This is treated with bedrest and surgical repair of the rupture if hearing does not return quickly.

Clinical Management. Vascular occlusion of the labyrinthine artery, a common cause of sudden hearing loss, often responds to

> ## CLINICAL PEARL
>
> Be sure to test the hearing of an older adult who gives incorrect or inappropriate responses to questions. These clients may be misdiagnosed with a cognitive impairment.

> ## CLINICAL PEARL
>
> It takes time to adjust to a hearing aid, and the older adult may be at risk for falls during this period.

vasodilators which may reverse the hearing deficit. If examination results are consistent with sudden, acute damage to the eighth cranial nerve, the patient should be referred immediately to a neurologist.

Setting-specific Issues

If the older adult wears a hearing aid, assess his knowledge with regard to proper insertion, battery replacement, operation, and proper care.

Hearing aids amplify background noise, as well as what the client wants amplified. The sound will be louder, but not clearer. Often clarity, not volume, is the issue.

Installation of blinking lights to indicate a ringing doorbell or telephone may be helpful, especially if the client refuses to wear a hearing aid.

Communication with the hearing impaired client who does not wear a hearing aid can be accomplished by writing or using an amplifier with headphones or ear piece.

Mastoiditis

Mastoiditis is an inflammation of the mastoid process that can develop as a result of untreated or chronic otitis media.

Clinical Presentation. The client may complain of tenderness of the mastoid process or ear pain. Drainage of pus or blood (if the tympanic membrane is ruptured) and fever and chills may be present. Sepsis can occur in severe cases.

Clinical Management. Depending upon the severity of the infection, IV antibiotics may be indicated. An otolaryngologic consultation should also be obtained.

Ototoxicity

Ototoxicity can be an unwarranted side effect of numerous prescription and over-the-counter (OTC) drugs and can result in permanent hearing loss or deafness. (See Table 4–1 for a listing of ototoxic drugs.) Clients with preexisting hearing deficits or renal insufficiency are at increased risk of this complication.

Clinical Management. If ototoxic drugs cannot be avoided, serial audiometry should be considered throughout the course of treatment.

Otitis Externa

Otitis externa is an inflammation of the pinna and external auditory canal. Causes can stem from swimming (frequently referred to as "swimmer's ear"), seborrheic dermatitis, heat and humidity, eczema, hearing aid use (including an allergic reaction to the hearing aid material itself) (Fields, 1991), narrow canal, excessive cerumen production, or trauma.

Clinical Presentation. The client may complain of a sensation of fullness, decreased hearing (due to edema), itching, and pain that is exacerbated with jaw movement. Manipulation of the outer ear or pressure placed on the tragus will also cause pain. Erythema, presence of moisture, and edema of the ear canal may be noted on otoscopic examination. The external ear canal may be filled with purulent exudate and blood. The tympanic membrane will be intact and possibly erythematous. Lymphadenopathy may be present toward the angle of the mandible or in the pretragal region. According to Curtis (1990), the most common organisms are *Pseudomonas aeruginosa, Bacillus proteus,* and *Staphylococcus aureus.*

Clinical Management. Use of broad-spectrum antibiotic otic drops is the accepted mode of therapy. If significant ear canal edema exists, the use of an ear wick (small sponge) may be necessary. A 5-day course of treatment with Cortisporin otic drops; chloramphenicol drops; or topical combinations of neomycin, polymyxin, and hydrocortisone are local treatments. If systemic antibiotics are required for severe infections or punctured tympanic membrane, a 7- to 10-day course of dicloxacillin, erythromycin, or cephalosporin is an effective treatment regime.

Otitis Interna
Otitis interna is an inflammation of the internal ear structures, which consist of the vestibule, three semicircular canals (which control balance), and the cochlea (affects hearing).

Clinical Presentation. The client may complain of vertigo, nausea and vomiting, or problems with balance.

Clinical Management. Prior to treatment, the cause of the inflammation must be determined.

Otitis Media
Otitis media is an inflammation of the middle ear, which is frequently precipitated by an upper respiratory infection (URI), sinusitis, or allergies.

Clinical Presentation. The client may complain of congestion and pain, with mild hearing loss. This may be compounded by tinnitus and vertigo. The eardrum may be retracted or bulging, dull or red, with diminished mobility and an alteration in the normal landmarks (Curtis, 1990). Sometimes, a fluid level can be seen on the tympanic membrane. (In cases of serous otitis media, the tympanic membrane is usually amber in color and may or may not have an air–fluid level.) If the tympanic membrane is ruptured, there may be bloody or purulent drainage in the canal. The client may complain of soreness of adjacent nodes. Without treatment, the tympanic membrane will rupture.

Clinical Management. Analgesics such as Tylenol (acetaminophen) or Tylenol with codeine are often needed for 3 to 5 days. The infection should be treated for 10 to 14 days with Augmentin (amoxicillin/clavulanate), Amoxil (amoxicillin), or Bactrim (trimethoprim–sulfamethoxazole). An oral decongestant is also prescribed for 3 to 5 days to promote drainage of fluid from the middle ear and sinuses.

Tinnitus
Tinnitus is frequently described as a loud or muted ringing noise heard inside the ear or head. The tinnitus related to presbycusis (presbycusis is almost always associated with tinnitus) is most likely caused by a deterioration of the hair cells in the

cochlea, as well as deterioration of the central auditory pathways in the brain. This deterioration is thought to create an imbalance between the oxcitatory and inhibitory influences on auditory nerve cells and thus result in tinnitus. When conductive hearing loss is also present, tinnitus is accentuated to the affected ear. The sound may be pulsatile if associated with the heartbeat, or low-pitched if associated with nasal respiration. Other causes of tinnitus are drug toxicity (see Table 4–1), Ménière's disease, multiple sclerosis, otitis media, and a perforated tympanic membrane.

Ciocon et al. (1995) describes two types of tinnitus: subjective and objective. *Subjective tinnitus* is described as either a constant or intermittent buzzing, humming, or ringing sound. Causes of subjective tinnitus include acoustic neuroma, cerumen, drug toxicity, fluid in the middle ear, hyperthyroidism, hypothyroidism, hypotension, infection, Ménière's disease, multiple sclerosis, otitis media, perforated tympanic membrane, stress, trauma, and zinc deficiency. *Objective tinnitus* is a noise that can also be heard by the clinician. It may be a blowing sound that corresponds with respirations, a pulsatile sound that coincides with the heartbeat, or a rapid clicking sound. Vascular disorders such as arteriovenous malformation, carotid artery stenosis, carotid body or glomus tumor, or valvular heart disease are common causes of objective tinnitus. Other causes include HTN, hypotension, and mechanical disorders such as temporomandibular joint (TMJ) dysfunction.

Clinical Presentation. Tinnitus can be described as a minor nuisance to an incapacitating noise. It may interfere with the client's normal activities and hearing, creating anxiety, depression, decreased concentration, and insomnia.

Clinical Management. Prior to initiation of treatment, the underlying cause must be determined. The workup for this should include a comprehensive history and physical (medication review including OTC drugs, stimulants such as caffeine and chocolate, diet, and noise exposure). Laboratory studies should include complete blood count (CBC), sedimentation rate, chemistry profile, and thyroid function studies. An audiologic examination should be performed and an MRI considered.

Treatment of tinnitus caused by middle and external ear problems is generally much more effective than that of CNS or inner ear origin. Depending on the cause of the tinnitus, the following interventions will be indicated: antibiotic therapy, removal of impacted cerumen, cessation of offending drugs, dietary changes, use of vasodilators, anticonvulsants (eg, carbamazepine), tranquilizers, amplification with hearing aids, tinnitus maskers, and biofeedback (Fitzgerald, 1985).

Tympanic Membrane Perforation

Tympanic membrane perforation is caused by otitis media or trauma. Ninety percent of perforations will heal spontaneously without residual hearing loss, generally within 3 to 6 weeks.

Clinical Presentation. The client will usually complain of sudden, severe earache that abruptly stops. He or she may notice purulent fluid or blood draining from the ear. There will be hearing loss immediately after the rupture.

Clinical Management. The area should be kept dry while open. The client should follow up with an otolaryngologist if healing does not occur within 6 weeks.

Tympanosclerosis

Tympanosclerosis is sclerotic changes of the tympanic membrane and middle ear mucosa from previous infections of the middle ear cleft.

Clinical Presentation. Chalky, white plaques are seen on the tympanic membrane, and there is frequently an associated hearing loss due to the involvement of the ossicular chain.

Clinical Management. The client should be referred to an otolaryngologist for surgical removal and reconstruction of the ossicle.

■ NOSE AND SINUSES

AGE-RELATED CHANGES

Several noticeable changes take place with aging. The nose becomes longer and narrower, with a more pronounced droop at the tip. The sense of smell is impaired. The nasal mucosa is thinner and less elastic. Decreased mucus production makes the mucosa dryer and more fragile, thus more vulnerable for epistaxis and nasal irritation. A common complaint among older clients is increased rhinorrhea or nasal dripping when eating, especially spicy or hot foods. This is thought to be due to improperly functioning parasympathetic vasomotor secretory fibers in the nose, and there is no treatment for this condition (Abrams et al., 1990).

COMMON NOSE AND SINUS DISORDERS

Allergic Rhinitis

Allergic rhinitis is common, usually familial, and frequently seasonal. It is uncommon for it to develop after age 50 (Griffith, 1994).

Clinical Presentation. The client may complain of itchiness of the membranes of the eyes, nose, and palate. Profuse intermittent rhinorrhea is watery and stringy. Rhinorrhea may be accompanied by nasal congestion, sneezing, postnasal drip, dry cough, wheezing, sinus tenderness, a sensation of fullness, and ear popping. The conjunctiva are watery and injected. A middle ear effusion may be present. The nasal mucosa are pale, swollen, boggy, and gray. In chronic allergic rhinitis, the following might be noted: a high palatine arch, palatal patechiae, malocclusion, geographic tongue, mouth breathing, edematous turbinates, and allergic shiners.

Clinical Management. Treatment involves avoiding exposure to the offending allergens and providing symptomatic relief with antihistamines, decongestants, and, occasionally, short-term use of corticosteroids. Antihistamines relieve the rhinorrhea, sneezing, and itching but have anticholinergic side effects that can cause drowsiness and dry mucous membranes. Use of antihistamines should be done cautiously in clients with narrow-angle glaucoma, epilepsy, stenosing peptic ulcer, and bladder neck obstruction. Patients should be monitored carefully if antihistamines are given in combination with monoamine oxidase inhibitors (MAOIs), tricyclic antidepressants (TCAs), alcohol, antiparkinsonian medications, barbiturates, narcotics, and tranquilizers.

Terfenadine (Seldane) and astemizole (Hismanal) are second-generation antihistamines that have minimal to no sedative or anticholinergic effects. However, Seldane and Hismanal have serious cardiac side effects if given simultaneously with erythromycin, ketoconazole, or itraconzole. Loratadine (Claritin), fexofenadine hydrochloride (Allegra) and cetirizine hydrochloride (Zyrtec) are long-acting antihistamines that can be given in conjunction with erythromycin, ketoconazole, or itraconzole. Usual dosing is as follows: Allegra 60 mg twice a day; Claritin 10 mg every day or every other day; Hismanal 10 mg every day; and Zyrtec 5 to 10 mg every day. Like Hismanal and Seldane, Claritin is an effective antihistamine that is particularly good in the geriatric population due to its minimal sedating and cholinergic effects.

The vasoconstrictive action of decongestants helps to decrease edema and congestion. Entex LA (phenylporparolamine) one tablet twice a day and Sudafed one tablet twice a day are effective decongestants that should be used with caution in the older adult due to their sympathomimetic action, which can cause HTN and tachycardia. Topical decongestants should be reserved for short-term use due to their rebound effect (Hoffman, 1995). Claritin-D is an effective antihistamine–decongestant that can be taken every 12 hours.

Epistaxis

Epistaxis is usually due to self-inflicted trauma to the anterior nasal septum. Since the mucosa is thin and fragile, nose picking can easily cause subsequent bleeding. It can also be caused by dry environment or HTN. Seldom is epistaxis due to abnormal bleeding states.

Clinical Management. The nares should be carefully inspected for lesions and ulcerations. Epistaxis usually resolves spontaneously or with application of pressure just beyond the bone. When epistaxis is caused by a dry environment, humidifiers with cool mist humidification or placement of containers of water around the room will increase the moisture. If HTN or abnormal bleeding states are the cause, a complete workup should be done.

Furuncles

Furuncles (boils) are painful, swollen pustules surrounding a hair follicle. The lesion is smooth, shiny, and tender. Keep in mind that manipulation may spread the infection. The organism is generally *Staphylococcus.*

Clinical Management. The pustules frequently either come to a head and rupture spontaneously or regress and eventually reabsorb. Moist heat is used to facilitate resolution, and may require incision and drainage. If the infected area is unusually large or the older adult is immunologically compromised or feverish, then systemic antibiotics such as dicloxacillin 500 mg every 6 hours should be given.

Polyps

Polyps are small, smooth, mobile, soft, gray, pedunculated nasal swellings that frequently develop in patients who are prone to allergic rhinitis. They may be highly vascular and protrude from the middle turbinate, causing a nasal obstruction.

Clinical Management. The client should be referred to a physician or otolaryngologist for surgical removal.

Sinusitis

Sinusitis is an inflammation of the mucous membranes of the paranasal sinuses. It frequently occurs after a cold. It may be bacterial (> 50%), viral (10% to 15%), or allergenic in nature. Obstructions due to septal deviation, polyps, and enlarged turbinates interfere with drainage and result in stasis and infection. Other contributing factors include chronic rhinitis, air pollutants, allergens, smoke, and debilitation. The maxillary sinuses are the most frequently infected in adults.

Clinical Presentation. The sinuses are edematous and irritated; congestion and purulent drainage are present. There is aching, tenderness, or a pressure sensation over the involved sinuses. The pain may shift from side to side with movement, especially when sleeping at night. Bending over creates an increased sensation of pressure and pain. Headache with facial and periorbital pain is frequently present on the affected side. Fever, malaise, and cough, which is worse at night resulting in increased sputum production upon awakening, often accompany it (Berczeller, 1991). Some individuals complain of pain with mastication. Keep in mind that rhinitis and URIs also have a similar presentation but would be treated differently. Purulent drainage from the middle meatus is a consistent finding with sinusitis. If the maxillary and frontal sinuses cannot be transilluminated, the likelihood of sinusitis is increased. Sinus films are considered the "gold standard" for diagnosing sinusitis, but they are expensive and should not be done routinely.

Clinical Management. Antibiotic therapy is indicated for a 2- to 3-week period.

The following antibiotics have been found to be equally effective:

- Ampicillin 500 mg q6h
- Amoxicillin 250 to 500 mg tid
- Doxycycline 200 mg initially and then 100 mg qd
- Bactrim-DS bid for 2 weeks

Analgesics and oral decongestants such as Claritin 10 mg daily, pseudoephedrine 30 mg every 4 hours for 3 days, or Entex LA one tablet twice a day may be needed. The side effect of tachycardia may be poorly tolerated by the older adult, especially with agents containing phenylpropanolamine (Entex). Application of local heat, high humidity via warm vaporizer, or showers may contribute to comfort. The client should be encouraged to push fluids if not otherwise contraindicated. Referral to an otolaryngologist should be made if the sinusitis is resistant to treatment or recurrent.

■ MOUTH

AGE-RELATED CHANGES

The lips are thin and pale. The tissue of the oral mucosa is thinner, paler, and less elastic. Small yellow sebaceous glands may be seen in the buccal mucosa and lips. The dorsum and margins of the tongue may have decreased number and size of papillae and may be coated with a thin white film. Increased fissures may be noted on the dorsal aspect of the tongue. The undersurface is smooth, with a bluish-purple hue from an increased number of varicosities. Taste buds atrophy, and the sense of taste likewise diminishes, especially for sweets and salt. The use of herbs and spices can enhance taste. The submaxillary, pituitary, and salivary glands atrophy, leaving the mouth much drier.

The gums are thinner and receded, making teeth loose and exposing roots. There is a tendency to have fewer surface cavities but an increase in root cavities. Tooth enamel is diminished, the tooth surface is softer, and there is an increase in pigmentation of the superficial layers. Dentin is not as well hydrated, and it becomes less translucent. Along with decreased dental pulp mass due to infringement of its space by dentin; there is a decrease in cell population of pulp, with diminished perfusion and sensitivity. Atrophy of alveolar bone mass may occur with partial or complete loss of dentition, which then impairs mastication. Although dentures solve some of the problems of poor mastication, they tend to alter taste and texture sensation. Increased lower facial and lip droop are due to diminished muscle tone, and decreased bone support is seen in the edentulous person. An inability to close the lips may result in drooling and spilled food.

Aphthous Ulcers
Aphthous ulcers (canker sores) are ulcerations of the oral mucosa that are thought to be due to a delayed hypersensitivity reaction. They are noncontagious, and may possibly be of autoimmune ethology (Bhaskan, 1990). They can recur intermittently and are frequently associated with foods such as chocolate, nuts, and fruit. In addition to these foods, stress, trauma, menstruation, and gastrointestinal (GI) ailments can be the cause.

Clinical Presentation. The client has one or more small, painful, white, oval ulcerations with erythematous borders. They are located on the mobile, nonkeratinized mucosa of the mouth. They usually disappear after 1 to 2 weeks.

Clinical Management. Generally, no treatment is needed. However, application of a topical anti-infective or anti-inflammatory agent such as Orajel and Orabase HCA increases comfort. Cleansing several times a day with toothpaste enhances healing. Depending on the severity, the ulceration may need to be debrided and treated with tetracycline rinses four times daily.

Black Tongue
Black tongue (hairy tongue, lingua nigra) is a condition in which there is an overgrowth of the papillae of the tongue. This is caused by an imbalance of the normal flora, which may be due to antibiotics and excessive use of mouthwash.

Clinical Presentation. The dorsum of the tongue has a black, furry appearance.

Clinical Management. Consider stopping antibiotic therapy.

Candidiasis
Candidiasis (moniliasis, thrush) is a fungal infection of the mucous membranes frequently seen in the immunocompromised client and in the client on long-term or high-dose antibiotic therapy. It is also common in clients with diabetes mellitus and lupus erythematosus, and those who are human immunodeficiency virus (HIV) positive. Be aware that beta blockers can cause xerostomia and increase the susceptibility for candidiasis.

Clinical Presentation. There are creamy white patches on erythematous mucous membranes. According to Bhaskar (1990), bleeding of the underlying tissue may occur if the patch is scraped. The tongue may be smooth, or papillae may be hypertrophic. Local lymph nodes may be enlarged and tender. The client may complain of a sore mouth, sore throat, and difficulty swallowing. If there is esophageal involvement, look for ulcerations. If the client has chronic candidiasis, test for acquired immunodeficiency syndrome (AIDS), as the condition is diagnostic for AIDS.

Clinical Management. Oral candidiasis responds well to clotrimazole troches (Mycelex) 10 mg dissolved slowly in the mouth five times a day for 14 days or nystatin suspension (Mycostatin) 100,000 U/mL 4to 6 mL swish and swallow four times a day for 14 days. If esophageal involvement is present, use a systemic antifungal agent such as fluconazole 200 mg on day 1, followed by 100 mg daily for 21 days. Clients using steroid inhalers should be instructed to rinse their mouth with water after each use to prevent candidiasis infections.

Geographic Tongue

Geographic tongue is a common condition that is generally asymptomatic. It is more commonly seen in the presence of systemic diseases, but it may also come and go without apparent cause.

Clinical Presentation. A map-like pattern of multiple denuded, pale red patches surrounded by white, raised borders is present on the doral surface of the tongue. Occasionally, the patient may complain of a sore tongue or burning sensation.

Clinical Management. Generally, there is no need for treatment, but Orajel or lidocaine may be indicated for pain relief.

Herpes Simplex

Herpes simplex (cold sore, fever blister) is a viral infection that comes in two forms. The primary form or first attack is usually seen in children and young adults. It commonly presents with an eruption of vesicles around the vermilion border of the lips or in the oral cavity and pharynx. Lesions can also be seen on the forehead, eyelids, cheek, and chin. Primary attacks can be severe, with stomatitis, local adenopathy, and URI, or mild, with presentation of a small cluster of vesicles.

The second type of herpes simplex involves the reactivation of the dormant virus with subsequent recurrence of the lesions in the same or adjacent sites as the first attack. This is primarily seen in older adults. The attacks are almost always triggered by a precipitating factor such as fever, stress, sun, illness, trauma, or immunodeficiency.

Clinical Presentation. There may be a sensation of burning or itching just prior to the eruption of vesicles. Typically, the vesicles are small, gradually enlarging and coalescing after they break. Lesions are often found on the lips, tongue, palate, floor of the mouth, buccal mucosa, gingivae, and oropharynx. They may be painful and can last for 1 to 2 weeks.

Clinical Management. Generally, the lesions crust over in several days and totally resolve in 1 to 2 weeks without any intervention. Preventive measures, such as avoiding direct sun exposure or wearing sunscreen preparations in cases of sun-induced herpes simplex, are more effective than treatment. Taking acyclovir 400 mg twice daily or lysine 1000 mg daily prophylactically will prevent recurrent attacks; however, once the drug is stopped, the virus will be reactivated and a more severe attack may result. Eating foods that are rich in lysine (eg, milk, fish, chicken, pork, and legumes) may help lessen the frequency or severity of attacks. Foods high in argimine (eg, nuts, chocolate, popcorn, gelatin, brown rice, and raisins) should be avoided. Taking acyclovir at the first sign of an attack may decrease the severity and length of the attack. Encourage increased fluids to prevent dehydration, especially if the lesions are causing oropharynx pain. Treat with analgesics. Apply acyclovir ointment to external lesions every 3 hours 6 times a day, or prescribe oral acyclovir 200 mg every 4 hours while awake (5 times a day) for 10 days.

Leukoplakias

Leukoplakias are thickened, white plaques that adhere to the oral mucosa and tongue. These lesions may be premalignant, especially if they present on the soft palate, floor of the mouth or tongue and if the individual is age 50 or more (Bhaskar, 1990).

Clinical Presentation. The plaques are shaggy, white, and thick. They are firm and do not wipe off when rubbed.

Clinical Management: Physician referral or an ear, nose, and throat (ENT) consult should be made with plan for biopsy.

Malignant Tumors

Malignant tumors are seen frequently in clients with a history of significant alcohol and tobacco use. Clients with poorly fitting dentures can develop chronic ulcerations that are precursors to malignant lesions.

Clinical Presentation. The majority of lesions occur on the lateral borders of the tongue. Lesions are also found on the floor of mouth, retromolar trigone, and the lateral areas of the soft palate. Hyperkeratotic changes with the presence of white patches and/or erythematous mucous membranes with dysplastic changes are signs of premalignancy. Lesions may have poorly defined borders with a velvety appearance, polypoid growths, or red or white ulcerations. The soft tissue may be indurated. Local lymph nodes may show signs of metastasis. Reports of bleeding, local soreness, or pain on chewing or swallowing are late symptoms of an oral carcinoma.

Clinical Management. A dental evaluation should be performed, with biopsies of all suspicious-looking lesions. Depending on the findings, a more extensive workup may be needed. If the client is to undergo treatment for cancer, dental caries and any gum disorders should be taken care of first to prevent infection.

Periodontal Disease

Periodontal disease is a slow, progressive disease that results from years of poor oral hygiene and plaque accumulation.

Clinical Presentation. Clients have tender, edematous gums that bleed without provocation. Eventually, destruction of bone and periodontal ligament leads to tooth loss. Decreased saliva production contributes to the disease progression.

Clinical Management. Good oral hygiene with frequent dental care should be encouraged. Rinsing with antiplaque agents and occasionally using toothpaste with chlorhexidine may be helpful. (Regular use can cause tooth staining.)

Sialadenitis

Sialadenitis is an inflammation of the parotid and submandibular glands. It occurs as a result of diminished salivary production and chronic dehydration. Most elderly persons are dehydrated because of medications and a decreased sensation of thirst.

Clinical Presentation. Pain, erythema, and swelling of the affected gland; purulent drainage (organism is usually *Staphylococcus aureus*), fever, and leukocytosis may also be present.

Clinical Management. Adequate rehydration and antibiotics are generally sufficient, but occasionally incision and drainage is needed.

Temporomandibular Joint Dysfunction

Temporomandibular joint dysfunction is characterized by unilateral facial pain with jaw movement. It can be caused by malocclusion, trauma, muscle spasm and fatigue, congenital abnormality, joint disease, tensing of muscles, or grinding and clenching of teeth.

Clinical Presentation. The pain is usually at the TMJ site, but it can be referred to the face or neck. Pain increases with jaw movement. There usually is tenderness with palpation of the masseter muscle. The client often complains of a clicking or popping sensation of the joint, as well as muscle spasms, slightly decreased range of motion, crunching tinnitus, headache, crepitus at the joint, and sometimes ear discomfort (Vallerand et al., 1989).

Clinical Management. This condition should be treated with the application of heat/cold, nonsteroidal anti-inflammatory drugs (NSAIDs), and muscle relaxants. A soft diet is better tolerated than a regular. Massage, exercise, ultrasound, and electric muscle stimulation all provide varying degrees of relief. If the client grinds or clenches his teeth, a bite splint will help to decrease the muscle spasms and fatigue that occur. If there is poor response after 3 to 6 months of conservative treatment, surgery should be considered. A dental or oral consult should be obtained initially as well as x-rays with transcranial or panographic views. In some cases, magnetic resonance imaging (MRI), arthrography, or tomography may also be indicated (Vallerand et al., 1989).

Xerostomia

Xerostomia (dry mouth) is common in the older adult. Several factors contribute to its cause: medication, diminished production of saliva, inadequate fluid intake, atrophy of oral mucosa, vitamin deficiencies, poor nutrition and hygiene.

Clinical Presentation. Clients may complain of difficulty swallowing dry food or difficulty speaking for long periods. They may have a sudden increase in tooth decay.

Clinical Management. Evaluate the salivary gland for patency. Perform a medication review to see if any drugs contributing to the problem can be discontinued. Diuretics and anticholinergics are the primary offenders. Encourage increased fluid intake. Instruct the client to drink liquids when swallowing. Treat with moisture or other artificial saliva products.

■ THROAT AND NECK

AGE-RELATED CHANGES

Decreased neck muscle tone occurs with aging, with subsequent weakening of head movement against resistance. Neck vessels are more prominent as a result of loss of muscle tone as well as diminished skin elasticity. Range of motion is diminished, and there is a tilting forward and shortening of the neck. Carotid bruits may be detected in patients with atherosclerotic disease. The gag reflex is often decreased. Muscle atrophy, loss of minor salivary tissue, diminished fibrous tissue support, decreased vibratory mass, and decreased moisture of the larynx occur and can cause an irritating tickle sensation in the throat, with constant clearing. A weak, trembly, high-pitched voice in men is due to decreased pulmonary volume and expiratory effort, as well as diminished elasticity and muscle mass, which has a bowing effect on the vocal cords. The clinician should not attribute changes in the voice to normal aging changes without first completing a thorough workup.

COMMON THROAT AND NECK DISORDERS

Dysphagia

Dysphagia is a decrease in the ability to swallow. The client may complain of a choking sensation or lump in the throat.

It is a common problem following stroke, and it is also seen with esophageal lesions, Parkinson's disease, traumatic head injury, and myasthenia gravis.

Clinical Presentation. Symptoms may include coughing, drooling, choking, clearing of the throat, or regurgitation. Initially, clients usually experience difficulty with swallowing solids and finally thin liquids.

Clinical Management. A thorough history and oropharyngeal exam should be done. A swallow evaluation by a speech therapist should follow with modified barium swallow if indicated. Once the cause is determined, it should be treated as indicated and appropriate diet consistency ordered. In some cases, swallowing exercises may be indicated.

Viral Laryngitis

Viral laryngitis is a common cause of hoarseness. It occurs more frequently in the winter.

Clinical Presentation. The onset is acute and often associated with rhinopharyngitis and cough.

Clinical Management. Provide increased humidity, hydration, and cough suppressants if needed. If the condition is not resolved in 10 days, an ENT evaluation should be obtained to rule out other common causes such as polyps, ulcerations, foreign bodies, and cancer.

Viral Pharyngitis

Viral pharyngitis is an inflammation of the pharynx, caused by a virus.

Clinical Presentation. The pharynx may be erythematous. The client will complain of a mild sore throat. The temperature is usually less than 101°F, and head cold symptoms and cough are frequently present.

Clinical Management. Treat with lozenges, gargling with warm saline solution, analgesics, and rest. If not contraindicated, push fluids to at least 2000 cc per day.

CASE STUDY #1

Mrs. Andrews is a community-dwelling 86-year-old woman with a history of schizophrenia, which is currently well controlled on haloperidol (Haldol) 1 mg bid. Several years ago she developed a severe eye infection during an exacerbation of her mental illness, which led to enucleation of her left eye. She is now experiencing visual changes in her right eye. She asks your advice on how to proceed.

QUESTIONS

1. What additional history would you obtain surrounding her chief complaint?
2. What risk factors would you consider when advising Mrs. Andrews?

ANSWERS

1. Additional history to collect would include the functional impact of the visual loss on Mrs. Andrews activities of daily living (ADL) and instrumental activities of daily living (IADL). This will help to identify the severity of the condition on her day-to-day life and will help to guide teratment decisions. The course of the visual loss (acute versus gradual) will determine the urgency of a referral to an ophthalmologist. Any acute visual change must be referred immediately to rule out acute-angle glaucoma, retinal detachment, or other optic emergencies. It would be important to review Mrs. Andrews medication regimen, looking for agents that could contribute to visual changes (digoxin, anticholinergics). Being aware of her living situation and support system would be helpful when considering the impact of this visual change and potential interventions. Ask Mrs. Andrews how she compensates for this visual change (environmental modifications, changes in routine). An examination of her right eye for visual acuity, peripheral vision, extraocular movements (EOMs), pupillary response, accommodation, and structural changes would be appropriate by the APN.

   You find that Mrs. Andrews has a ripe cataract in her right eye. She shares that she has stopped writing poetry, reading favorite books, and visiting friends for lunch at the church basement across the street due to her visual changes. She is quite distressed about these losses and is agreeable to a consultation with an ophthalmologist to discuss cataract removal and lens implantation to restore her function.

2. Risk factors to consider in Mrs. Andrews case are a bit unique due to her history of mental illness and enucleation of her left eye. She will have extremely limited vision for a short period of time following cataract surgery and will need close observation and monitoring. The consequences of a postsurgical infection could lead to total blindness. She may also be at risk for delirium due to the initial postoperative visual limitation. Since she lives alone with no strong social supports, a short stay in a rehabilitation facility or 24-hour home care may be indicated.

Mrs. Andrews has cataract removal with artificial lens implantation. She recuperates for 2 days in an extended-care facility and is discharged to home with close follow-up by in-home nursing services. Within 1 week, she has resumed her previous level of function and is once again enjoying her life.

 ## CASE STUDY #2

Mr. Reed resides in an extended-care facility. The nursing assistant comments to you that he has been more sleepy and less interactive in the past few weeks, often not responding to questions or requests. She wonders if he has had a stroke or is receiving too much medicine.

As you enter Mr. Reed's room, he is dozing in a chair. He does not respond as you call his name but is easily arousable to gentle touch. He smiles at you, but his answers to your simple questions do not make sense. He speaks in clear, full sentences, but the content is unrelated to your question.

QUESTIONS

1. How would you proceed in the workup of Mr. Reed?
2. What interventions would you implement to correct each of your most likely proposed diagnoses?

ANSWERS

1. In order to investigate Mr. Reed's change in status, an accurate baseline and change from baseline should be determined. Performing a Folstein Mini-Mental Status Exam (MMSE), at-

tentional testing, and a Geriatric Depression Scale and comparing it to previous performance can be invaluable in raising or ruling out dementia, delirium, and depression. A thorough medication review to look for drugs that may be interacting or causing adverse effects is necessary. A full physical exam with a focus on neurologic findings is indicated to rule out a physical cause for this change in behavior. Laboratory studies may include CBC, chemistry panel, and urinalysis to rule out common causes of lethargy.

You are keyed into checking Mr. Reed's hearing as you administer the cognitive tests and receive strange answers from this very attentive gentleman. He fails the whisper test. Upon exam, you find significant cerumen impaction bilaterally.

2. You order earwax-softening treatment for Mr. Reed, to be instilled by the nurses every night for 5 nights. You explain that the patient must lie on his right side for 10 minutes following the application of the drops in his left ear. This procedure is then reversed for the opposite ear. Eardrops often are ineffective if the patient does not lie in these positions to allow for penetration of the solution into the wax impaction. After 5 days, the APN returns and is able to scoop out a large amount of soft wax from each ear. Gentle irrigation with warm water and intermittent massage of the area anterior to the tragus of each ear allows for total removal of wax bilaterally

without trauma or discomfort to Mr. Reed.

Following cerumen removal, Mr. Reed's hearing is completely restored. He becomes appropriately conversant and returns to his baseline status of alert and participatory in daily activities.

■ REFERENCES

Abrams, W. B., Berkow, R., & Fletcher, A. J. (Eds.) (1990). *The Merck manual of geriatrics.* Rahway, NJ: Merck.

Anderson, R. G., Simpson, K., & Ross, R. (1983). Auditory dysfunction and rehabilitation. *Geriatrics, 38*(9), 101–112.

Berczeller, P. H. (1991). A fresh look at sinusitis and bronchitis. *Hospital Practice, 26*(6), 167–170.

Bhaskar, S. N., Lilly, G. E., & Pratt, L. W. (1990). A practical, high-yield mouth exam. *Patient Care, 24*(2), 53–74.

Ciocon, J. O., Amede, F., Lechtenberg, C., & Astor, A. (1995). Tinnitus: A stepwise workup to quite the noise within. *Geriatrics, 50*(2), 18–24. 1: Disorders of the ear. *Physician Assistant, 14*(9), 23–46.

Fields, S. D. (1991). Special considerations in the physical exam of older patients. *Geriatrics, 46*(8), 39–44.

Fitzgerald, D. C. (1985). The aging ear. *AFP, 31*(2), 225–232.

Freeman, R. B. (1995). Impacted cerumen: How to safely remove earwax in an office visit. *Geriatrics, 50*(6), 52–53.

Griffith, C. J. (1994). Allergic rhinitis: Practical guide to diagnosis and management. *Physician Assistant, 18*(7), 19–36.

Hoffman, B. (1995). Adrenoceptor-activating & other sympathomimetic drugs. In Katzung, B. E. (Ed.). Basic & clinical pharmacology, (6th ed.). Norwalk, CT: Appleton & Lange.

Morris, J. C., & McManus, D. Q. (1991). The neurology of aging: Normal versus pathologic change. *Geriatrics, 46*(8), 47–54.

Rupp, R. R., Vaughn, G. R., & Lightfoot, R. K. (1984). Nontraditional "aids" to hearing: Assistive listening devices. *Geriatrics, 39*(3), 55–73.

Scimeca, G. H., Magargal, L. E., Jaeger, E. A., & Robb-Doyle, E. (1989). An eye disorder caused by chronic cardiovascular disease. *Geriatrics, 44*(5), 98–102.

Soong, H. K., Johnston, M. E., & Sugar, A. (1988). Clinical significance of common eye changes in older patients. *Geriatrics, 43*(5), 49–55.

Speight, J. L., & Cunha, B. A. (1995). Spotting red eye. *IM, 16*(6), 33–37.

Vallerand, A. H., Russin, M. M., & Vallerand, W. P. (1989). Taking the bite out of TMJ syndrome. *AJN, 89*(5), 688–690.

Vaughan, D., Asbury, T., & Riordan-Eva, P. (1999). *General ophthalmology* (15th ed.). Stamford, CT: Appleton & Lange.

Winters, R. K. V. (1989). Adapting the environment to age-related sensory losses. *JAANP, 1*(4), 106–111.

5

TOPICS IN RESPIRATORY CARE

Mary Frances Rooney Lewis • Margaret Campbell Haggerty

■ INTRODUCTION

Changes in host defense mechanisms may make the elderly more susceptible to respiratory illness. Diminished immunologic response, decreased cough, decreased ciliary action, and decreased immunoglobulin A (IgA) in the nasal and respiratory surfaces alter the elderly's response to pathogens. Coupled with years of exposure to respiratory irritants such as tobacco smoke and pollutants, the elderly are at increased risk for life-threatening disorders. Respiratory disorders are considered to be the fourth leading cause of death in this population (Ebersole & Hess, 1990).

Respiratory diseases may be classified as acute or chronic, and further classified as those involving the upper airways or lower respiratory tract. They may also be classified by their affect on pulmonary function: obstructive lung diseases, restrictive lung diseases, and diffusion de-

fects as shown in Table 5–1. Obstructive lung diseases are those that cause resistance to expiratory airflow due to lumenal obstruction, intrinsic airway narrowing, or peribronchial obstruction. Emphysema, chronic bronchitis, asthma, bronchiectasis, and cystic fibrosis are the major chronic obstructive lung diseases. Acute bronchitis and bronchiolitis are the main acute obstructive disorders of the lower respiratory tract. Restrictive lung diseases include disorders that limit lung expansion and cause a decrease in total lung capacity. This chapter is limited to diseases of the lower respiratory tract, that is, involving the airways and lung tissue below the level of the carina.

Some respiratory disorders may have elements of both obstruction and restriction. Restrictive and obstructive diseases are distinguished primarily by history and pulmonary function tests. Diffusion defects include pulmonary vascular disease, and may coexist with obstructive and restrictive diseases.

TABLE 5–1.   CLASSIFICATION OF RESPIRATORY DISEASES

Restrictive Lung Diseases		Obstructive Lung Diseases		Diffusion Defects
Chronic	*Acute*	*Chronic*	*Acute*	
Pulmonary fibrosis	Atelectasis	Emphysema	Acute bronchitis	
Bony malformations	Congestive heart failure	Chronic bronchitis		Pulmonary vascular disease
Neurologic conditions	Pneumonia	Bronchiectasis	Bronchiolitis	
Sarcoidosis*		Sarcoidosis*		
		Asthma		

*Can present as restrictive or obstructive.

■ OBSTRUCTIVE LUNG DISEASES

CHRONIC OBSTRUCTIVE PULMONARY DISEASE

Incidence

Fifteen million people in the United States have chronic obstructive pulmonary disease (COPD). These diseases are the fourth most frequent cause of death in the elderly and are second only to heart disease as a cause of disability. Managing this disability directly and indirectly cost billions of dollars.

Emphysema is an anatomic diagnosis characterized by destruction of alveolar/capillary units and chest hyperinflation. A presumptive diagnosis can be made by pulmonary function tests on the basis of the irreversible expiratory airflow limitation and decreased diffusion capacity. A chest x-ray is sometimes helpful in diagnosing more advanced emphysema in that it can reveal hyperinflation of the chest, flattened diaphragms, and sometimes bullae.

Chronic bronchitis is a clinical rather than anatomic diagnosis and is defined as daily productive cough for at least 3 months each year for 2 consecutive years, which is not due to other conditions such as tuberculosis or bronchiectasis. Chronic bronchitis is further delineated as simple chronic bronchitis (ie, mucus hypersecretion without obstruction and chronic obstructive airflow limitation). Chronic obstructive pulmonary disease is a nonspecific term characterized by "persistent slowing of airflow during forced expiration" (American Thoracic Society, 1995). Because emphysema and chronic obstructive bronchitis often coexist, these disorders will be described together.

Etiology

The largest etiologic agent contributing to the development of COPD is cigarette smoking (80% to 90%). Occupational and community pollutants (eg, sulfur dioxide, coal dust, mineral quartz, cotton mill dust, toluence diiocyanate) may also contribute to the development of COPD. Repeated exposure to second-hand smoke and familial factors may play an additional role. A small percentage (1% to 2%) of cases of emphysema are linked to a genetic deficiency of alpha-1 antitrypsin. Alpha-1 antitrypsin levels can be measured in the blood.

Clinical Presentation

Assessment. History taking should focus on the onset and setting of dyspnea, which is frequently described by clients as shortness of breath, breathing difficulty, or an inability to get a deep breath or sufficient air. In COPD, dyspnea is usually insidious in onset, beginning with heavy exertion such as stair climbing and progressing to less strenuous activities such as activities of daily living (ADL). In the later stages of the disease, individuals may experience dyspnea with minimal exertion or at rest. Both pathophysiologic features and emotional factors, including anxiety and depression, are thought to contribute to the development of dyspnea in COPD (Sweer & Zwillich, 1990; Janson-Bjerklie, 1993).

A visual analogue scale can be a useful tool for quantifying the change in dyspnea for an individual patient. The patient is asked to mark a 100-mm line with one end labeled "no shortness of breath" and the other end labeled "the worst shortness of breath" (Fig. 5–1). A sudden change in the patient's usual amount of dyspnea may indicate an exacerbation of COPD or an additional problem. Cardiovascular disease, neuromuscular disease, anemia, metabolic acidosis, hypothyroidism, collagen vascular disease, and concomitant lung disease (eg,

bronchogenic cancer, interstitial lung disease, pulmonary embolism, pneumonia, pleural effusion, pneumothorax, pulmonary vascular disease, upper airway obstruction) should be considered in the differential diagnoses of the dyspneic client.

Paroxysmal nocturnal dyspnea (PND) may be cardiac in origin and should be investigated as such. If dyspnea is noted to be sudden or combined with chest pain, the cause may be a pneumothorax or a pulmonary emboli.

Cough is also a common chief complaint in the older adult with COPD. Generally, the cough begins as an early morning cough, productive of clear to white sputum. A variety of stimuli may trigger cough in the COPD client: postnasal drip, exposure to respiratory irritants, and retained secretions from an impaired mucociliary clearance system. Often, a cough is described as a "smoker's cough," which may begin upon arising in the morning and progress to a cough throughout the day.

Cough is typical in chronic bronchitis. In addition to bronchietasis, differential diagnosis for cough should include asthma, neoplasm, mitral stenosis, congestive heart failure (CHF), and infection. If cough produces more than 1 ounce of sputum, brochiectasis (chronic dilatation of the bronchi) should be suspected.

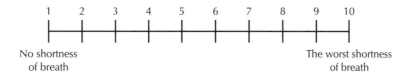

Figure 5–1. Visual Analog Scale for Dyspnea

CLINICAL PEARL

Clients with bronchiectasis typically develop many serious pulmonary infections and thereby warrant earlier treatment with antibiotics than a client with chronic bronchitis without accompanying bronchiectasis.

Review of Systems

- General: fatigue (may be a sign of pulmonary hypertension)
- Head, eyes, ears, nose, and throat (HEENT): early morning headache (may be indicative of nocturnal hypoxemia, sinusitis, or postnasal drip)
- Cardiac: ankle edema, palpitations (may be a sign of pulmonary hypertension)
- Lungs: PND (may be a sign of pulmonary hypertension)
- Neurologic: changes in mentation, insomnia, nocturnal headache, nightmares; personality changes at night may indicate nocturnal oxygen desaturation
- Activity: dyspnea with activities that are exertional; change in sexual function, work role, functioning around the home, hobbies, and social functioning
- Coping: associated anxiety, depression, or panic disorders
- Nutrition: weight gain (secondary to being sedentary) or weight loss (may be indicative of excess calories being utilized for breathing. Tuberculosis [TB] and cancer should also be considered.)

Physical Examination

- General: Tired, anxious (or depressed), ill-appearing, obese (or cachectic)
- Neck: Jugular venous distention (JVD) associated with cor pulmonale (right-sided heart failure)
- Cardiac: S3 to right of apex, S4 left parasternal, murmur of tricuspid regurgitation (may be heard in cor pulmonale)
- Lungs:
  1. Increased anterior–posterior diameter and costal angles > 90 degrees
  2. Respiratory rate > 20
  3. Accessory muscle use during inspiration
  4. Retractions due to increased work of breath
  5. Tripod position may be used spontaneously—back straight, leaning slightly forward, shoulders in a fixed position, with hands placed on either knees or a table
  6. Pursed lip breathing
  7. Decreased chest expansion and decreased fremitus
  8. Hyperresonance to percussion (particularly in the very thin)
  9. Flattened diaphragms with dullness to percussion noted lower on chest wall
  10. Decreased breath sounds upon auscultation/prolonged exhalation (> 2:1) throughout lung fields
  11. Adventitious sounds (coarse crackles, wheeze)
- Abdomen: hepatomegaly (in right ventricular hypertrophy)

Diagnostic Studies. Laboratory data for the initial workup is guided by the history and physical and may include a complete blood count (CBC) with differential, chemistry screen, thyroid function, and arterial blood gas and/or oxygen saturation by oximetry at rest and with exercise. The white blood count (WBC) may be elevated in the client taking corticosteroids or with an infection. Arterial blood gas analysis may show varying degrees of hypoxemia, hypercarbia, compensated or uncompensated respiratory acidosis, and normal or decreased oxygen saturation. Oxygen levels determined by arterial blood gases are more accurate than pulse oximetry. Blood gases are necessary when acid–base balance and PA_{CO_2} are needed.

Pulse oximetry may be useful in determining the client's response to sleep and/or exercise. If the client has any perfusion deficits or cardiac arrhythmias, the results may be less accurate because they are dependent on perfusion to the site where the probe is placed—the finger, earlobe, or forehead.

CLINICAL PEARL

Pulse oximetry results can also be skewed upward in a smoker because carbon monoxide found in cigarette smoke can cause a falsely elevated oxygen saturation (SaO_2).

An electrocardiogram (ECG) is useful in evaluating the client for right ventricular hypertrophy and cor pulmonale. Right axis deviation, tall pointed p waves in leads II and AVF, pointed V_1 and V_2,

and negative p wave in AVL are consistent with right ventricular hypertrophy.

Other laboratory tests that are occasionally useful include sputum for culture and sensitivity in cases of suspected infection, sleep studies in suspected concomitant sleep apnea, and exercise studies.

A chest x-ray may be useful to establish a client's baseline or diagnose an infiltrate or other cardiopulmonary abnormalities. Routine chest x-rays are not helpful in mild cases of COPD because chest films may appear normal. In later stages, however, flattened diaphragms, hyperinflated lungs, bullae, and a narrow cardiac silhouette may be detected.

Pulmonary function tests include spirometry, lung volumes, and diffusion capacity. Flow rates (FEV_1, FVC, and FEV_1/FVC) will be decreased, volumes (RV, TLC, and RV/TLC) will be increased, and diffusion capacity may be reduced. (For pulmonary function definitions, see Table 5–2.)

Clinical Management

Table 5–3 lists common problems of patients with COPD. The goals of management of COPD are to stabilize clients, reduce symptoms and the risk of exacerbation, promote maximal functional capacity, and prevent premature disability. Therapeutic considerations include smoking cessation, secretion clearance techniques, early identification and management of exacerbations, breathing retraining, client education and rehabilitation, psychologic support and management of depression and anxiety, nutritional support, and supplemental oxygen therapy (see Table 5–4).

Pharmocologic Measures. Pharmacologic management includes bronchodila-

TABLE 5–2.   PULMONARY FUNCTION INTERPRETATION

■ PULMONARY SPIROMETRY TESTS	■ DEFINITION
FVC Forced vital capacity	The volume of air expired forcefully and rapidly after maximal inspiration. Validity depends on client's best effort
FEV_1 Forced expiratory volume	The forced expired volume measured over a 1-second time interval
FEV_1/FVC ratio	The ratio of FEV_1 to FVC, expressed as the percentage of FVC that a given FEV_1 represents
■ LUNG VOLUME TEST	
RV Residual volume	The volume of air remaining in the lungs at the end of maximal expiration
■ LUNG CAPACITY TESTS	
TLC Total lung capacity	The volume of air contained in the lung at the end of a maximal inspiration
RV/TLC ratio	This ratio expresses the percentage of TLC that can be defined as RV

tor therapy, antibiotics for exacerbations caused by infection, corticosteroids in select individuals, and supplemental oxygen therapy in hypoxemic patients. Clients demonstrating a greater than 15% increase in FEV_1 may benefit from bronchodilator therapy, although those showing no objective improvement may report symptomatic relief. A clinical trial may therefore be useful.

The inhaled route (by hand-held metered-dose inhalers [MDIs] or electrically powered nebulizers) offers advantages over the systemic route for the administration of bronchodilators and corticosteroids. The drug reaches the target or-

TABLE 5–3.   COMMON PROBLEMS OF PATIENTS WITH COPD

1. Dyspnea, decreased exercise tolerance
2. Ineffective secretion clearance
3. Blood gas abnormalities: hypoxemia, hypercarbia, desaturation with exercise/sleep
4. Increased risk for infection and respiratory failure
5. Sleep disturbance
6. Nutritional problems
7. Anxiety, panic, depression
8. Right ventricular hypertrophy and failure
9. Family-related problems

TABLE 5–4.   CRITERIA FOR HOME OXYGEN PRESCRIPTION

Health conditions	COPD, diffuse interstitial lung disease, cystic fibrosis, bronchiectasis, pulmonary neoplasm, pulmonary hypertension, cor pulmonale, erythrocytosis, delirium, nocturnal restlessness, morning headache
Laboratory evidence	$PaO_2 < 55$ mm Hg or $SaO_2 < 88\%$ $PaO_2 = 56–59$ mm Hg or $SaO_2 = 89\%$ in cor pulmonale, erythrocythemia with hematocrit $< 56\%$, recurring edema related to right-sided CHF

gan directly, and less drug can be used to achieve the same therapeutic benefit. Proper technique for metered-dose inhaler use is critical to the success of inhalation therapy.

CLINICAL PEARL

Less than 30% of clients use their inhalers correctly. Less than 30% of health-care workers teach use of inhalers correctly.

Coordinating activation of the inhaler with inspiration can be particularly difficult for geriatric clients. Spacer devices for those unable to learn correct inhaler technique may increase drug delivery to the lungs (Reardon & Bragdon, 1993). Use of spacers should not be relied on totally, as clients may not carry them. Correct inhaler use should be taught and reinforced with and without spacers. Seven steps must be accomplished in approximately 15 seconds (Fig. 5–2).

Inhaler technique can take much practice and reinforcement over time. A useful technique for teaching correct inhaler use is to instruct clients to take a deep "drag" on the inhaler like they used to smoke a cigarette. Former smokers

can understand the desired technique almost immediately.

Bronchodilators fall into three broad categories: (1) anticholinergics, (2) sympathomimetics, and (3) theophylline.

- Sympathomimetics are administered orally or by the inhaled route (more commonly) and are useful for symptomatic relief. Frequently used sympathomimetic agents include albuterol, metaproterenol, pirbuterol, and terbutaline. Two puffs of a quick-acting sympathomimetic are often prescribed on an as-needed basis.
- Ipratropium bromide (Atrovent), an anticholinergic, is advocated as first-line therapy for the client with chronic symptoms (dyspnea every day). Three to six puffs of Atrovent four times a day may be needed to achieve effective bronchodilatation. Clients need to be taught to expect less dramatic results than with sympathomimetics, as the onset of action of Atrovent is 15 minutes. If the client is taught to use the anticholinergic inhalers properly with a routine dosing schedule, good relief of symptoms can be experienced with virtually no side effects.
- Theophylline, once a mainstay of treatment, is now considered third-line therapy. Its narrow therapeutic

Using a metered-dose inhaler is a good way to take asthma medicines. There are few side effects because the medicine goes right to the lungs and not to other parts of the body. It takes only 5 to 10 minutes for inhaled beta$_2$-agonists to have an effect compared to the liquid or pill form, which can take 15 minutes to 1 hour. Inhalers can be used by all asthma patients age 5 and older. A spacer or holding chamber attached to the inhaler can help make taking the medicine easier.

The inhaler must be cleaned often to prevent buildup that will clog it or reduce how well it works.

■ The guidelines that follow will help you use the inhaler the correct way.
■ Ask your doctor or nurse to show you how to use the inhaler.

Using the Inhaler

1. Remove the cap and hold the inhaler upright.
2. Shake the inhaler.
3. Tilt your head back slightly and breathe out.
4. Use the inhaler in any one of these ways. (A and B are the best ways. B is recommended for young children, older adults, and those taking inhaled steroids. C is okay if you are having trouble with A or B.)
   A. Open mouth with inhaler 1 to 2 inches away.
   B. Use spacer (ask for the handout on spacers).
   C. Put inhaler in mouth and seal lips around the mouthpiece.

5. Press down on the inhaler to release the medicine as you start to breathe in slowly.
6. Breathe in *slowly* for 3 to 5 seconds.
7. *Hold* your breath for 10 seconds to allow the medicine to reach deeply into your lungs.
8. Repeat puffs as prescribed. Waiting 1 minute between puffs may permit the second puff to go deeper into the lungs.

Note: Dry powder capsules are used differently. To use a dry powder inhaler, close your mouth tightly around the mouthpiece and inhale very fast.

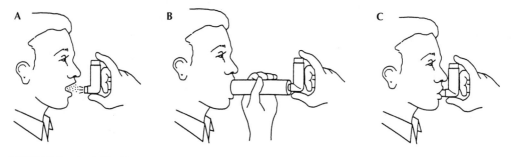

Figure 5–2. Your Metered-Dose Inhaler: How to Use It. *(Source: Nurses' Asthma Education Working Group. [1995] Nurses: Partners in Asthma Care.[NIH Publication No. 95-3308.])*

range and minor bronchodilator effect limit its usefulness. However, theophylline may improve mucociliary clearance, diaphragmatic muscle function, and central respiratory drive, and assist in reducing airway inflammation (Ferguson & Cherniak, 1993). Some clinicians prescribe theophylline at bedtime for

nocturnal symptoms not controlled by sympathomimetics and ipratropium.

• Corticosteroids are reserved for clients who remain symptomatic despite maximum bronchodilator therapy. A therapeutic trial may be useful to determine whether symptoms improve with the addition of corticosteroids. Careful monitoring for side effects is essential (Ferguson & Cherniak, 1993; Solheim, 1993). Consultation with a physician should be considered prior to initiating PO steroids.

- Other pharmacologic agents include annual influenza vaccination, pneumococcal vaccination, antibiotics for exacerbations, and cough preparations for symptom control. Augmentation therapy with Prolastin, an alpha$_1$ protease inhibitor, has been approved for use in clients with alpha-1 antitrypsin deficiency. Prolastin's long-term effects in slowing the course of emphysema are not known. Narcotics are occasionally prescribed for unremitting dyspnea in clients with advanced disease. Their use should be carefully monitored and reserved for clients not responding to the more traditional pharmacologic and nonpharmacologic approaches. (Sweer & Zwillich, 1990).

Supplemental oxygen therapy is prescribed to relieve hypoxia, decrease pulmonary hypertension, and improve neuropsychologic function (Nocturnal/Oxygen Therapy Trial Group, 1980; MRC, 1981). Specific criteria for prescribing long-term supplemental oxygen have been developed. Traditionally oxygen is delivered by nasal cannula or mask. Newer approaches include transtracheal oxygen and the addition of oxygen-conserving devices.

Nonpharmacologic Measures. The importance of smoking cessation should be stressed in all clients diagnosed with COPD. A nonjudgmental approach, as-

> ## CLINICAL PEARL
> Supplemental O$_2$, however, *may* or *may not* improve dyspnea, which is difficult for clients to understand. It is important for a client and caregivers to understand the concept that O$_2$ is administered to protect their heart and brain from hypoxemia.

sessment of readiness to quit, a determination of the need for nicotine replacement, and early relapse prevention strategies are keys to successfully aiding smokers to quit. A thorough review of smoking cessation techniques is not within the scope of this chapter, but excellent reviews exist (Nett and Obrigewitch, 1993). A promising new agent in assisting smokers to quit is Zyban (unpublished data from GlaxoWellcome, Inc.).

Rehabilitation. Pulmonary rehabilitation is a comprehensive approach to the symptomatic COPD client and includes assessment of the common problems, breathing retraining, secretion clearance techniques, physical reconditioning, energy conservation, education, strategies for coping with the psychologic effects, and providing support. Clients who have gone through pulmonary rehabilitation have been shown to have fewer hospitalizations and exacerbations. Since pulmonary rehabilitation ultimately saves money, insurance companies generally reimburse for a limited program.

Elderly clients with COPD respond well to rehabilitation. Simple dyspnea management techniques can be taught to alleviate an acute episode of dyspnea (Fig. 5–3).

Step 1: Position
  Find the most comfortable position to relieve your shortness of breath. For most people this is sitting with your back straight, leaning slightly forward or leaning over a table while standing or sitting. The idea is to rest most of your body and help your breathing muscles work better.

Step 2: Pursed Lip Breathing
  Begin to control your breathing. If you're very short of breath, breathe in through your mouth and out through pursed lips (slightly puckered). Try to breathe out at least twice as long as you breathe in. It may also be helpful to puff out your cheeks as you breathe out through pursed lips to avoid breathing out with too much force. Gradually slow down your breathing by breathing *out* longer and longer. As it gets easier, take a slow deep breath in through your nose and a longer breath out through pursed lips.

Step 3: Relaxation
  As your breathing gradually slows down, remind yourself to relax your neck and shoulders. Allow your arms to become relaxed and limp. Close your eyes if that helps you to relax.

Additional points
  Once your breathing is back in control, resume your previous activity but at a slower pace. Try to match your pace with your body's ability to breathe. Breathe out for the hardest part of the exertion (for example, while climbing stairs, picking up heavy objects, pushing things).
  Practice the method for catching your breath when you are not short of breath. You'll be less likely to panic if you practice ahead of time.
  If your shortness of breath continues or becomes worse than usual, call your nurse practitioner or doctor.

NOTE. Table may be photocopied for patient use.

Figure 5–3. Outpatient Management of an Acute Episode of Shortness of Breath. *(Source: Haggerty, M. C. [1993]. Outpatient management of common problems in the patient with COPD, Nurse Practitioner Forum 4, 19. Copyright © 1993 by W. B. Saunders. Reprinted with permission.)*

CLINICAL PEARL

Pursed lip breathing can be accomplished by instructing the client to:

1. Breathe in through the nose.
2. Imagine there is a candle about 6 inches in front of you. Don't blow hard enough to blow that candle out; try to flicker that flame. Gently exhale through slightly puckered lips.

Diaphragmatic breathing may be helpful, but it requires much practice and many times may not be worth the effort. Clients may find that keeping their shoulders relaxed, using pursed lip breathing, and coordinating their activities with breathing are more effective than hours of diaphragmatic training.

Additional important treatments include influenza and pneumococcal prophylactic immunizations. Early recognition and effective management of bronchopulmonary infections and CHF can help reduce acute exacerbations of respiratory failure. Support groups supplement rehabilitation and are useful adjuncts to care. Home-care programs for select clients may also be useful and have been shown to decrease hospitalizations and health-care costs (Haggerty et al., 1991).

Complications
Exacerbations are caused by infections of the upper and lower respiratory tract, a

progression of the disease, acute respiratory failure caused by infectious or noninfectious agents, and problems with oxygenation that may lead to organ failure such as right ventricular failure (cor pulmonale).

Coexisting disorders such as neoplasm, pulmonary edema, embolism, or other medical problems can complicate the picture. Clients who are difficult to diagnose, do not respond to outpatient management, show signs of rapid deterioration, or require special procedures or surgery should be referred to a pulmonary specialist (Pitman, Sherman, & Black-Shaffer, 1991). An iatrogenic problem of COPD clients can be osteoporosis secondary to chronic oral steroid use.

Skin breakdown can be an issue in that clients many times lean on their elbows and can develop irritation, soreness, and lesions, as well as infections in those lesions. Sores on the auricles of the ears from O_2 tubing is also common. Preventive use of pressure-relieving devices is recommended.

ASTHMA

Asthma is a chronic inflammatory disorder of the airways in which many cells and cellular elements play a role. In susceptible individuals, this inflammation causes recurrent episodes of wheezing, breathlessness, chest tightness, and cough, particularly at night and in the early morning (Second Expert Panel, 1997).

Asthma is manifested by increased airway responsiveness to a variety of stimuli, mucous hypersecretion, and generally reversible airway obstruction. Fourteen to sixteen million Americans are diagnosed with asthma. Severity can range from mild intermittent (with completely re-

versible pulmonary function tests), to severe persistent (with permanent, chronic obstructive airflow) (see Table 5–5). Asthma rates have increased 29% in the past decade. Deaths have increased by 31%. The cause of the increased prevalence is subject to debate: reporting variances versus actual increase.

While asthma is usually a disease that begins in early adulthood or childhood, there is a subpopulation of people who develop asthma in their later years. It tends to occur more frequently in women than in men in the older population.

Pathophysiology
Asthma has an early phase of bronchospasm, which is a mechanical reaction to an irritant. A sustained late-phase contraction of airway smooth muscle is induced by mast cell degranulation and release of mediators. Mediators from mast cells attract other inflammatory cells (eosinophils, neutrophils, basophils, lymphocytes) to the airway. Both allergic and viral antigens are important in this inflammatory chain of events. Individual asthmatics may show elements of early phase, late phase, or both.

Clinical Presentation
Asthmatics typically present with wheezing, coughing, chest tightness, and/or shortness of breath in response to an irritant. Nocturnal awakenings may signal worsening asthma. The common triggers of an asthma episode include those listed in Table 5–6.

Assessment

History. Explore the following seven attributes of cough, wheezing, chest tightness, and sputum:

TABLE 5–5.   ASTHMA SEVERITY

Classification of Severity: Clinical Features Before Treatment[a]

	Symptoms[b]	Nighttime Symptoms	Lung Function
STEP 4 **Severe persistent**	■ Continual symptoms ■ Limited physical activity ■ Frequent exacerbations	Frequent	■ FEV$_1$ or PEF ≤ 60% predicted ■ PEF variability > 30%
STEP 3 **Moderate persistent**	■ Daily symptoms ■ Daily use of inhaled short-acting beta$_2$-agonist ■ Exacerbations affect activity ■ Exacerbations ≥ 2 times a week; may last days	> 1 time a week	■ FEV$_1$ or PEF > 60% ≤ 80% predicted ■ PEF variability > 30%
STEP 2 **Mild persistent**	■ Symptoms > 2 times a week but < 1 time a day ■ Exacerbations may affect activity	> 2 times a month	■ FEV$_1$ or PEF ≥ 80% predicted ■ PEF variability 20–30%
STEP 1 **Mild intermittment**	■ Symptoms ≤ 2 times a week ■ Asymptomatic and normal PEF between exacerbations ■ Exacerbations brief (from a few hours to a few days); intensity may vary	≤ 2 times a month	■ FEV$_1$ or PEF ≥ 80% predicted ■ PEF variability < 20%

[a]The presence of one of the features of severity is sufficient to place a patient in that category. An individual should be assigned to the most severe grade in which any feature occurs. The characteristics noted in this figure are general and may overlap because asthma is highly variable. Furthermore, an individual's classification may change over time.
[b]Patients at any level of severity can have mild, moderate, or severe exacerbations. Some clients with intermittent asthma experience severe and life-threatening exacerbations separated by long periods of normal lung function and no symptoms.
Source: Adapted from Second Expert Panel on the Management of Asthma. (1997). *Guidelines for the diagnosis and management of asthma* (p. 29). (NIH Publication No. 97-4051A.)

TABLE 5–6.   ASTHMA TRIGGERS

Allergens (Immune System Reaction)	Irritants (Mechanical Reaction)
Pollens (tree, grass, ragweed)	Primary and second-hand smoke
Molds (indoor/outdoor)	Fumes/odors
Warm-blooded animals	Cold air
House dust mites	Exercise
Cockroaches	Viral infections
Certain foods (eg, peanuts, shellfish)	Pollutants (eg, sulfur dioxide, nitrous oxide)
	Rhinitis and sinusitis
	Gastroesophageal reflux
	Certain medications (eg, beta blockers)

1. What is the onset and pattern of symptoms? Is the pattern continuous or episodic? Could it be described as seasonal? What early warning signs precede bronchospasm? Common ones are itchy, watery eyes; scratchy throat; cough; stuffiness or rhinitis; and tightness in the chest. Many chronic asthmatic clients become desensitized to their early warning signs and ignore them.

2. To what was the client exposed?

3. When did the symptom occur? Particularly watch for nocturnal awakenings.

4. How severe is the symptom on a scale of 1 to 10?

5. How long did the symptom last?

6. In what setting does it occur?

7. What relieved the symptom or made it better?

Clinical Management

A national, multidisciplinary expert panel established by the U.S. Department of Health and Human Services, developed guidelines for asthma management. The guidelines include recommendations for the following:

- Measures of assessment and monitoring
- Control of factors contributing to asthma severity
- Pharmacologic therapy
- Education for a partnership in asthma care (Second Expert Panel, 1997)

Measures of Assessment and Monitoring. Several types of monitoring are recommended:

- Signs and symptoms
- Pulmonary function
- Quality of life/functional status
- History of asthma exacerbations
- Pharmacotherapy
- Client–provider communication
- Client satisfaction (Second Expert Panel, 1997)

Goals for asthma management and classification of asthma severity are listed in Table 5–7.

Monitoring Pulmonary Function. Maintenance of an asthma diary and use of a peak flowmeter are two effective ways of self-monitoring asthma. With an asthma diary, clients are asked to assess their

TABLE 5–7.   STEPWISE APPROACH FOR MANAGING ASTHMA IN ADULTS AND CHILDREN OVER 5 YEARS OLD

Goals of Asthma Treatment

- Prevent chronic and troublesome symptoms (eg, coughing or breathlessness in the night, in the early morning, or after exertion).
- Maintain (near) "normal" pulmonary function.
- Maintain normal activity levels (including exercise and other physical activity).
- Prevent recurrent exacerbations of asthma and minimize the need for emergency department visits or hospitalizations.
- Provide optimal pharmacotherapy with minimal or no adverse effects.
- Meet clients' and families' expectation of and satisfaction with asthma care.

Source: Adapted from Second Expert Panel on the Management of Asthma. (1997). *Guidelines for the diagnosis and management of asthma* (p. 29). (NIH Publication No. 97-4051A.)

ease of breathing, how much wheezing they are having, how often they need to use their reliever therapy, and how much their asthma is interfering with their life. Peak flowmeters are portable pulmonary function devices that monitor maximum expiratory airflow. Clients should be instructed to breathe to total lung capacity and exhale as quickly and forcefully as possible. (See Fig. 5–4 for peak flow instructions.) The best measure of three efforts is recorded. The highest number reached is recorded in L/min. There are predictive tables of peak flow for height, weight, gender, and age. Establishing the client's personal best when asthma is stable enables the clinician to evaluate asthma and predict exacerbations more easily. If the peak flow dips to less than 20% of one's personal best, more preventive therapy may be initiated. Partnership management can be initiated by teaching the client which peak flow trends necessitate changing therapy. It is useful to ask new clients to record their peak flows in the morning for two weeks to establish a baseline and reveal the variation of that individual's asthma. If exercise-induced

asthma is suspected, peak flow before and after exercise can be useful. A drop of greater than 20% indicates an element of exercise-induced bronchospasm. Peak flows are useful both in diagnosis and treatment. Peak flowmeters may be purchased for $25 each, but they can often be obtained as samples from respiratory drug companies.

Managing Triggers. Environmental triggers may often be underreported because clients may be embarassed to say that they live in a damp home, a dirty home, or a home with roaches. Use generic-type statements, such as "Some people have problems with roaches, and the recommendation is . . ." or "Some people live in older homes. There can sometimes be hidden sources of mold in such a home, and what can be done to control the mold is . . ." In this way, information can be passed on without making a value judgment regarding a particular lifestyle. See Table 5–8 for a listing of common environmental triggers, and strategies for minimizing them.

A peak flowmeter is a device that measures how well air moves out of your lungs. During an asthma episode, the airways of the lungs begin to narrow slowly. The peak flowmeter will tell you if there is narrowing in the airways days—even hours—before you have any symptoms of asthma.

By taking your medicine(s) early (before symptoms), you may be able to stop the episode quickly and avoid a severe episode of asthma. Peak flowmeters are used to check your asthma the way that blood pressure cuffs are used to check high blood pressure.

The peak flowmeter can also be used to help you and your doctor:

- Learn what makes your asthma worse.
- Decide if your medicine plan is working well.
- Decide when to add or stop medicine.
- Decide when to seek emergency care.

A peak flowmeter is most helpful for patients who must take asthma medicine daily. Patients age 5 and older are able to use a peak flowmeter. Ask your doctor or nurse to show you how to use a peak flowmeter.

How to Use Your Peak Flowmeter
- Do the following five steps with your peak flowmeter:
  1. Put the indicator at the bottom of the numbered scale.
  2. Stand up.
  3. Take a deep breath.
  4. Place the meter in your mouth and close your lips around the mouthpiece. Do not put your tongue inside the hole.
  5. Blow out as hard and fast as you can.
- Write down the number you get.
- Repeat steps 1 through 5 two more times and write down the numbers you get.
- Write down in "My Asthma Symptoms and Peak Flow Diary" the highest of the three numbers achieved.

Find Your Personal Best Peak Flow Number
Your personal best peak flow number is the highest peak flow number you can achieve over a 2-week period when your asthma is under good control. Good control is when you feel good and do not have any asthma symptoms.

Each client's asthma is different, and your best peak flow may be higher or lower than the peak flow of someone of your same height, weight, and sex. This means that it is important for you to find your own personal best peak flow number. Your medicine plan needs to be based on your own personal best peak flow number.

To find out your personal best peak flow number, take peak flow readings:
- Every day for 2 weeks
- Mornings and early afternoons or evenings (when you wake up and between 12:00 and 2:00 P.M.)

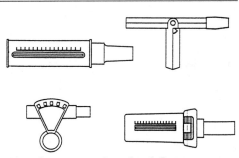

There are a variety of peak flowmeters.

- Before and after taking inhaled beta$_2$-agonist (*if* you take this medicine)
- As instructed by your doctor

Write down these readings in your peak flow diary.

Actions to Take When Peak Flow Numbers Change
- Peak expiratory flow rate (PEFR) goes more than 20% below your personal best (PEFR is in the yellow zone).
  ACTION: Take an inhaled short-acting bronchodilator as prescribed by your doctor.
- PEFR changes 20% or more between the morning and early afternoon or evening (measure your PEFR before taking medicine).
  or
- PEFR increases 20% or more when measured before and after taking an inhaled short-acting bronchodilator.
  ACTION: Talk to your doctor about adding more medicine to control your asthma better (for example, an anti-inflammatory medication).

Figure 5–4. How to Use Your Peak Flowmeter. *(Source: Adapted from National Asthma Education and Prevention Program, National Heart, Lung, and Blood Institute. [1995]. Nurses: Partners in Asthma Care. [NIH Publication No. 95-3308.])*

TABLE 5–8. CONTROL OF ENVIRONMENTAL FACTORS

House dust mites	Focus on the bedroom. Wash the bedding (pillowcases, mattress covers, sheets, blankets, spreads) weekly in hot (130°F) water in order to kill house dust mites. Remove carpeting from the bedroom. Encase mattress and pillows in allergen-impermeable covers.
Pollen	Abide by weather reports and ozone layer reports, which provide warning to asthmatics not to spend as muich time as usual outside and/or to use premedication more to reduce responsiveness to this allergen.
Exercise-induced asthma	Warm up and cool down slowly. Wear protection over the nose and mouth if the air is cool. Neck gators or rolled up turtlenecks warm inhaled air.
Animal dander	Rid house of warm-blooded animals. Keep animal out of the bedroom.

Smoking has not been shown to be a cause of asthma in adults, but exposure to second-hand smoke can be a major trigger for asthma. Asthmatics who smoke do not recover from their exacerbations as quickly. Teaching about smoking can be specific with asthmatics, relating smoking directly with symptoms. Family members sometimes need to be involved in an educational session, in that their second-hand smoke can precipitate an asthmatic attack.

Room air filters (high-efficiency particle air filters [HEPA] are the most effective) may be rented from a medical supply company for a month before purchasing (at a cost of $300). This trial can reveal whether it will make a significant difference in helping to control a client's asthma.

Upper respiratory infections (URIs) (postnasal drip, rhinitis) and gastroesophogeal reflux can aggravate asthma. If ordinary measures are not helping, such a client may need to see an asthma specialist.

Pharmacologic Measures. Pharmacologic management has undergone considerable change in the past 15 years and is based on current knowledge of pathophysiology.

Long-term–control medications and Quick-relief medications are key terms and concepts that asthma clients need to understand. Long-term–control medications are used to achieve and maintain control of persistent asthma. Quick-relief medications are used to treat acute symptoms and exacerbations. The stepwise approach to asthma therapy emphasizes initiating higher-level therapy at the onset to establish prompt control and then stepping down to the minimum dose required to maintain control, thus reducing potential side effects (Second Expert Panel, 1997).

Long-term–control Medications. Inhaled corticosteroids are the mainstay of long-term asthma control. They stabilize airways and therefore prevent asthma. Inhaled corticosteroids do not cause the devastating side effects of systemic corti-costeroids. Beclomethasone diproprion-ate (Vanceril, Beclovent), triamcinolone acetonide (Azmacort), flunisolide (Aero-bid), and fluticasone (Flovent) are the most commonly used inhaled steroids in the United States. Aerobid is more po-tent than other inhaled steroids. Flutica-sone, the newest agent, comes in three different doses.

Comparative daily dosages for inhaled corticosteroids are shown in Table 5–9. There are few side effects if used in ap-propriate doses. Inhaled steroids are not helpful during a moderate or severe asthma exacerbation. During a mild asthma attack, however, a double dose of inhaled steroids may reduce symptoms. Once daily doses of more than 1500 μg are administered, some systemic absorp-

TABLE 5–9.   ESTIMATED COMPARATIVE DAILY DOSAGES FOR INHALED CORTICOSTEROIDS

Adults			
Drug	*Low Dose*	*Medium Dose*	*High Dose*
Beclomethasone dipropionate	168–504 μg	504–840 μg	> 840 μg
42 μg/puff	(4–12 puffs—42 μg)	(12–20 puffs—42 μg)	(> 20 puffs—42 μg)
84 μg/puff	(2–6 puffs—84 μg)	(6–10 puffs—84 μg)	(> 10 puffs—84 μg)
Budesonide Turbuhaler	200–400 μg	400–600 μg	>600 μg
200 μg/dose	(1–2 inhalations)	(2–3 inhalations)	(> 3 inhalations)
Flunisolide	500–1000 μg	1000–2000 μg	> 2000 μg
250 μg/puff	(2–4 puffs)	(4–8 puffs)	(> 8 puffs)
Fluticasone	88–264 μg	264–660 μg	> 660 μg
MDI: 44, 110, 220 μg/puff	(2–6 puffs—44 μg) or (2 puffs—110 μg)	(2–6 puffs—110 g)	(> 6 puffs—110 μg) or (> 3 puffs—220 μg)
DPI: 50, 100, 250 μg/dose	(2–6 inhalations—50 μg)	(3–6 inhalations—100 μg)	(> 6 inhalations—100 μg) or (> 2 inhalations—250 μg)
Triamcinolone acetonide	400–1000 μg	1000–2000 μg	> 2000 μg
100 μg/puff	(4–10 puffs)	(10–20 puffs)	(> 20 puffs)

NOTES:
■ *The most important determinant of appropriate dosing is the clinician's judgment of the client's response to therapy.* The clinician must monitor the client's response on several clinical parameters and adjust the dose accordingly. The stepwise approach to therapy emphasizes that once control of asthma is achieved, the dose of medication should be carefully titrated to the minimum dose required to maintain control, thus reducing the potential for adverse effect.
■ Some dosages may be outside package labeling.
■ Metered-dose inhaler (MDI) dosages are expressed as the actuater dose (the amount of drug leaving the actuater and delivered to the client), which is the labeling required in the United States. This is different from the dosage expressed as the valve dose (the amount of drug leaving the valve, all of which is not available to the patient), which is used in many European countries and in some of the scientific literature. Dry powder inhaler (DPI) doses (eg, Turbuhaler) are expressed as the amount of drug in the inhaler following activation.
Source: Adapted from Second Expert Panel on the Management of Asthma. (1997). *Guidelines for the diagnosis and management of asthma* (p. 35). (NIH Publication No. 97-4051A.)

tion takes place. Inhaled steroids can affect oral flora with secondary yeast infections (thrush) resulting.

CLINICAL PEARL

Clients are advised to rinse their mouth and spit the fluid out after using inhaled steroids. Using a spacer also cuts down on the incidence of thrush.

There is no immediate relief of symptoms with inhaled corticosteroids. Clients need to be educated that inhaled steroids differ from sympathomimetics in that on a long-term basis they stabilize the airways. Therefore, compliance with inhaled steroids can be key to managing asthma effectively. Oral steroids can be critical and lifesaving in asthmatic clients. Oral steroids can be used in the short term for acute exacerbations of asthma. A common approach is to give 40 to 60 mg of prednisone to adults and taper the dose slowly over 5 to 10 days. Long-term use of corticosteroids is reserved for those with unremitting symptoms due to their side effects: hypertension (HTN), osteoporosis, hyperglycemia, and gastrointestinal (GI) irritation.

Theophylline was once the mainstay of asthma therapy. Its role has changed markedly in recent years. Low-dose, sustained-release theophylline is used as an adjunct to corticosteroids, especially for control of nocturnal symptoms. The long-acting sympathomimetic agent, Serevent, can also reduce nocturnal symptoms. Serevent is not quick-relief

therapy; it is long-term–control medication. After the recent introduction of Serevent, there was a rise in asthma-related deaths. This is thought to be due to the fact that clients were mistakenly using Serevent for treatment and rescue therapy. It must be stressed that a client is to use no more than the prescribed two puffs per day (one puff bid). There is some suspicion that Serevent has tachyphylaxis (a rapid production of immunity). After about 3 months of use, it ceases to work as well as it initially did. The short-acting bronchodilators, however, do not precipitate much tachyphylaxis.

The nonsteroidal anti-inflammatory drugs (NSAIDs) nedocromil sodium (Tilade) and cromolyn (Intal) are noted to be more useful in decreasing exercise-induced asthma in children than in adults.

It had been hoped that leukotriene inhibitors would revolutionize the field of asthma. People who need chronic systemic corticosteroids may benefit from the addition of leukotriene inhibitors in an attempt to decrease systemic steroid use. Leukotriene modifiers (Zafirlukast, Zileuton) are considered alternative therapy to low-dose inhaled corticosteroids. A clinical trial is needed to determine which clients may benefit from these agents.

Quick-relief Medications. Short-acting sympathomimetic (beta$_2$-agonist) bronchodilators may be used in the inhaled or oral form for symptom relief. The inhaled route is the preferred and the most commonly used route. Sympathomimetics may be delivered via hand-held nebulizer or MDI. There is no advantage to a nebulizer over an MDI if each is used correctly. Each client must be individually evaluated to see which method is best suited to him or her. The disadvantage of nebulizers is that infection can be more of an issue than with MDIs if they are not cleaned effectively.

The most widely used agents are albuterol (Ventolin, Proventil), pirbuterol (Maxair), metaproterenol (Alupent), and terbutaline (Brethair). Anticholinergics such as ipratropium bromide (Atrovent) provide additive benefit to inhaled beta$_2$-agonists in severe exacerbations in selected clients.

Systemic corticosteroids may be used to speed asthma exacerbation recovery. Oral steroids must be taken exactly as directed. Any forgotten doses need to be made up. Oral steroids must be tapered, especially if they are taken longer than 10 to 14 days. A switch to the inhaled form of corticosteroids should be accomplished as soon as possible (see Table 5–10).

Immunizations. The principle behind immunizations is to expose a person to a small amount of an allergen and eventually a resistance is developed to that particular allergen. Allergy immunizations are more standardized than they were previously. Selected clients may benefit from immunization therapy when specific allergies are identified. Cost and the necessity for long-term therapy may limit their use.

Client Education

The National Asthma Education Program promotes the concept of clients as partners—giving clients the knowledge and skills to enable them to co-manage their asthma with the health-

care provider. The goals of management include the following:

1. Prevent chronic and troublesome symptoms (eg, coughing or breathlessness in the night, in the early morning, or after exertion).
2. Maintain (near) "normal" pulmonary function rates.
3. Maintain normal activity levels (including exercise).
4. Prevent recurrent exacerbations of asthma, and minimize the need for emergency department visits or hospitalizations.
5. Avoid adverse effects from asthma medications.
6. Meet clients' and families' expectations of and satisfaction with asthma care (Second Expert Panel, 1997).

Specific components of the clinician's follow-up assessment can be found in Fig. 5–5. Helpful tools for teaching clients can be found in *Teach Your Patients About Asthma,* published by the National Asthma Education Program (1992).

Support groups are many times available through the American Lung Association and through some hospitals.

Exacerbations. Underrecognition of exacerbation is by far the greatest factor in asthma-related deaths. Some older adults fail to perceive inadequate response to treatment and repeatedly use beta agonists to blunt symptoms rather than seek evaluation. Increasing airway inflammation can be masked, which may result in sudden rapid deterioration (Janson-Bjerklie, 1993). Exacerbations may present as progressively worsening episodes of shortness of breath, cough, wheezing,

TABLE 5–10. QUICK-RELIEF ASTHMA MEDICATIONS

Medication	Dosage Form	Usual Dosages for Quick-relief Medications		Comments
		Adult Dose	Child Dose	
■ SHORT-ACTING INHALED BETA₂-Agonists				
	Metered Dose Inhalers (MDIs)			
Albuterol	■ 90 µg/puff, 200 puffs	■ 2 puffs 5 minutes prior to exercise	■ 1–2 puffs 5 minutes prior to exercise	■ An increasing use or lack of expected effect indicates diminished control of asthma.
Albuterol HFA	■ 90 µg/puff, 200 puffs	■ 2 puffs tid–qid	■ 2 puffs tid–qid	■ Not generally recommended for long-term treatment. Regular use on a daily basis indicates the need for additional long-term control therapy.
Bitolterol	■ 370 µg/puff, 300 puffs			■ Differences in potency exist so that all products are essentially equipotent on a per puff basis.
Pirbuterol	■ 200 µg/puff, 400 puffs			■ May double usual dose for mild exacerbations.
Terbutaline	■ 200 µg/puff, 300 puffs			■ Nonselective agents (ie, epinephrine, isoproterenol, metaproterenol) are not recommended due to their potential for excessive cardiac stimulation, especially at high doses.

Medication	Dosage Forms	Adult Dose	Child Dose	Comments
Dry Powder Inhalers (DPIs)				
Albuterol Rotahaler	■ 200 µg/capsule	■ 1–2 capsules q 4–6 hours as needed and prior to exercise	■ 1 capsule q 4–6 hours as needed and prior to exercise	■ May mix with cromolyn or ipratropium nebulizer solutions. May double dose for mild exacerbations.
	Nebulizer solution			
Albuterol	■ 5 mg/mL (0.5%)	■ 1.25–5 mg (0.25–1 cc) in 2–3 cc of saline q 4–8 hours	■ 0.05 mg/kg (min 1.25 mg, max 2.5 mg) in 2–3 cc of saline q 4–6 hours	■ May not mix with other nebulizer solutions.
Bitolterol	■ 2 mg/mL (0.2%)	■ 0.5–3.5 mg (0.25–1 cc) in 2–3 cc of saline q 4–8 hours	■ Not established	
■ ANTICHOLINERGICS				
	MDIs			
Ipratropium	■ 18 µg/puff, 200 puffs	■ 2–3 puffs q 6 hours	■ 1–2 puffs q 6 hours	■ Evidence is lacking for producing added benefit to beta$_2$-agonists in long-term asthma therapy.
	Nebulizer solution			
	■ 0.25 mg/mL (0.025%)	■ 0.25–0.5 mg q 6 hours	■ 0.25 mg q 6 hours	
■ SYSTEMIC CORTICOSTEROIDS				
Methylprednisolone	■ 2-, 4-, 8-, 16-, 32-mg tablets	■ Short course "burst": 40–60 mg/day as single or 2 divided doses for 3–10 days	■ Short course "burst": 1–2 mg/kg/day, maximum 60 mg/day, for 3–10 days	■ Short courses or "bursts" are effective for establishing control when initiating therapy or during a period of gradual deterioration.

(Continues)

TABLE 5–10. QUICK-RELIEF ASTHMA MEDICATIONS (CONT.)

Usual Dosages for Quick-Relief Medications

Medication	Dosage Form	Adult Dose	Child Dose	Comments
Prednisolone	■ 5-mg tabs, 5 mg/cc, 15 mg/cc			■ The burst should be continued until patient achieves 80% peak expiratory flow personal best or symptoms resolve. This usually requires 3–10 days but may require longer. There is no evidence that tapering the dose following improvement prevents relapse.
Prednisone	■ 1-, 2.5-, 5-, 10-, 20-, 25-mg tabs; 5 mg/cc solution			

Source: Adapted from Second Expert Panel on the Management of Asthma. (1997). *Guidelines for the diagnosis and management of asthma* (p. 38). (NIH Publication No. 97-4051A.)

Monitoring Signs and Symptoms of Asthma

(Global assessment) "Has your asthma been better or worse since your last visit?"

(Recent assessment) "In the past 2 weeks, how many days have you:

- Had problems with coughing, wheezing, shortness of breath, or chest tightness during the day?"
- Awakened at night from sleep because of coughing or other asthma symptoms?"
- Awakened in the morning with asthma symptoms that did not improve within 15 minutes of inhaling a short-acting inhaled beta$_2$-agonist?"
- Had symptoms while exercising or playing?"

Monitoring Pulmonary Function

Lung Function

"What is the highest and lowest your peak flow has been since your last visit?"

"Has your peak flow dropped below _____ L/min (80% of personal best) since your last visit?"

"What did you do when this occurred?"

Peak Flow Monitoring Technique

"Please show me how you measure your peak flow."

"When do you usually measure your peak flow?"

Monitoring Quality of Life/Functional Status

"Since your last visit, how many days has your asthma caused you to:

- Miss work or school?"
- Reduce your activities?"
- (For caregivers) Change your activity because of your child's asthma?"

"Have you had any unscheduled or emergency department visits or hospital stays?"

Monitoring Exacerbation History

"Since your last visit, have you had any episodes/times when your asthma symptoms were a lot worse than usual?"

If yes—"What do you think caused the symptoms to get worse?"

If yes—"What did you do to control the symptoms?"

Monitoring Pharmacotherapy

Medications

"What medications are you taking?"

"How often do you take each medication? How much do you take each time?"

"Have you missed or stopped taking any regular doses of your medications for any reason?"

"Have you had trouble filling your prescriptions?"

"How many puffs of your short-acting inhaled beta$_2$-agonist (quick-relief medicine) do you use per day?"

"How many _____ [name short-acting inhaled beta$_2$-agonist] inhalers [or pumps] have you been through in the past month?"

"Have you tried any other medicines or remedies?"

Monitoring Pharmacotherapy

Side Effects

"Has your asthma medicine caused you any problems?"

- Shakiness, nervousness, bad taste, sore throat, cough, upset stomach

Inhaler Technique

"Please show me how you use your inhaler."

Monitoring Client–Provider Communication and Client Satisfaction

"What questions have you had about your asthma daily self-management plan and action plan?"

"What problems have you had following your daily self-management plan? Your action plan?"

"Has anything prevented you from getting the treatment you need for your asthma from me or anyone else?"

"Have the costs of your asthma treatment interfered with your ability to get asthma care?"

"How can we improve your asthma care?"

"Let's review some important information:"

- "When should you increase your medications? Which medication(s)?"
- "When should you call me [your doctor or nurse practitioner]?" "Do you know the after-hours phone number?"
- "If you can't reach me, what emergency department would you go to?"

* These questions are examples and do not represent a standardized assessment instrument. The validity and reliability of these questions have not been assessed.

Figure 5–5. Components of the Clinician's Followup Assessment: Sample Routine Clinical Assessment Questions.* *(Source: Adapted from Second Expert Panel on the Management of Asthma. [1997]. Guidelines for the diagnosis and management of asthma [pp. 11–12]. [NIH Publication No. 97-4051A.])*

Assess Asthma Severity

Measure PEF: Value < 50% personal best or predicted suggests severe exacerbation.

Note signs and symptoms: Degrees of cough, breathlessness, wheeze, and chest tightness correlate imperfectly with severity of exacerbation. Accessory muscle use and suprasternal retractions suggest severe exacerbation.

↓

Initial Treatment

- Inhaled short-acting beta$_2$-agonist: up to three treatments of 2–4 puffs by MDI at 20-minute intervals or single nebulizer treatment.

Good Response

Mild Episode

PEF > 80% predicted or personal best

No wheezing or shortness of breath

Response to beta$_2$-agonist sustained for 4 hours

- May continue beta$_2$-agonist every 3–4 hours for 24–48 hours

- For clients on inhaled corticosteroids, double dose for 7–10 days

↓

- Contact clinician for followup instructions

Incomplete Response

Moderate Episode

PEF 50%-80% predicted or personal best

Persistent wheezing and shortness of breath

- Add oral corticosteriod

- Continue beta$_2$-agonist

↓

- Contact clinician urgently (this day) for instructions

Poor Response

Severe Episode

PEF < 50% predicted or personal best

Marked wheezing and shortness of breath

- Add oral corticosteriod

- Repeat beta$_2$-agonist immediately

- If distress is severe and nonresponsive, call your doctor and proceed to emergency department: consider calling ambulance or 9-1-1

↓

- Proceed to emergency department

Figure 5–6. Management of Asthma Exacerbations: Home Treatment. *(Source: Adapted from Second Expert Panel on the Management of Asthma. [1997]. Guidelines for the diagnosis and management of asthma [p. 41]. [NIH Publication No. 97-4051A.])*

chest tightness, and nocturnal awakenings with symptoms. The Second Expert Panel on the Diagnosis and Management of Asthma (1997) recommends initial therapy of up to three treatments of two to four puffs of an inhaled short-acting beta agonist by MDI at 20-minute intervals or a single nebulizer treatment (see Fig. 5–6 for full decision tree). In the elderly, recognition of irreversible obstruction and treatment of comorbid conditions is crucial. A client should be referred to a specialist when poor asthma control makes management difficult; a life-threatening acute asthma exacerbation has occurred; atypical signs and symptoms make the diagnosis doubtful; or sinusitis, nasal polyps, or gastroesophageal reflux complicate the management (Janson-Bjerklie, 1993).

■ ACUTE DISEASES

INFLUENZA

Influenza is a viral infection of the upper or lower respiratory tract. Influenza viruses are classified as A, B, or C. Much of the morbidity and mortality of viral influenza occurs in the elderly. A heavy smoker or an individual with preexisting lung disease is at risk to develop complications such as bronchitis, pneumonia, respiratory failure, or death. Pneumonia following flu is generally due to *Haemophilus influenzae* or *Streptococcus pneumoniae* but may be staphylococcal. Diagnosis is usually made based on clinical symptomatology, coupled with epidemiologic evidence of influenza in the community. Physical examination and x-ray findings are nonspecific unless the client is compromised. Specific diagnosis rests on culture from throat washings and or rise in serum titer with this virus.

Prevention

Epidemics of influenza occur mainly in the winter months and are influenced by the level of immunity of the population at risk. It is recommended that all persons over the age of 65, their caretakers, persons with chronic disease, and healthcare professionals who interact with older adults be vaccinated annually for influenza. Amantadine can be used prophylactically and in the first 48 hours after exposure to influenza A (but *not* influenza B). Amantadine is usually given in a reduced dosage of 100 mg/d orally in elderly persons. For some debilitated older adults, dosage may be titrated based on creatinine clearance (Calkins et al., 1992). See Chapter 1 for additional discussion of influenza vaccination.

Assessment

History includes rhinorrhea, headache, fever, malaise, and myalgias. Influenza is diagnosed empirically, the greatest risk being the secondary risk for developing pneumonia.

Clinical Management

Rest, fluids, and acetaminophen for fever, headache, and myalgias are the mainstays of treatment.

ACUTE BRONCHITIS

Bronchitis may be broadly defined as inflammation of the tracheobronchial tree that frequently accompanies an upper respiratory infection (URI). Clinically, bronchitis is "acute cough with sputum in the absence of pneumonia." Bronchitis may be classified as viral or bacterial. Most cases are viral, caused by influenza, rhinoviruses, adenoviruses, or *Mycoplasma pneumoniae,* and resolve spontaneously. Organisms commonly causing bacterial bronchitis include *S. pneumoniae* and *H. influenzae* (Biller, 1987).

Assessment

History	Recent URI for 1 to 2 weeks
	Cough (productive or nonproductive)
	Purulent sputum production in bacterial bronchitis
Physical exam	Coarse crackles
	Localized or diffuse wheezes/rhonchi
	Absence of pulmonary consolidation signs
Labs	Slightly elevated WBC, rarely more than 15,000
Chest x-ray	Negative for signs of consolidation or infiltrate

Pharmacologic Measures

Acute bronchitis may not require antibiotic treatment unless pulmonary illness lasts for 7 to 10 days without signs of improvement. Consider use of one of the following broad-spectrum antibiotics:

- Erythromycin 250 to 500 mg qid for 7 to 10 days
- Tetracycline 500 mg qid for 7 to 10 days
- Ampicillin 500 mg qid for 7 to 10 days
- Trimethoprim–sulfamethoxazole 160 to 800 mg bid for 7 to 10 days

Antipyretic analgessics such as aspirin or acetaminophen (Tylenol) may be used if the fever is higher than 101°F or the client is compromised in some way. Fluids liquefy secretions well for easy expectoration; in lieu of liquids, guaifenesin is helpful with sputum expectoration. Cough suppressants should be used only when significant interference with a client's rest occurs.

In clients with concomitant chronic bronchitis, consider antibiotics if two of the three cardinal symptoms are present: increased sputum volume, increased sputum purulence, and increased dyspnea. Antibiotic therapy is recommended against *S. pneumoniae, H. influenzae, Moraxella catarrhalis,* and possibly some atypical pathogens. Cefuroxime, azithromycin, and clarithromycin are often good choices. These drugs are more expensive than trimethoprim–sulfamethoxazole and tetracycline, but they have a broader antimicrobial spectrum (Davis et al., 1996). If a patient has had three or more acute exacerbations of bronchitis, a gram-negative organism deserves consideration. In this case, a trial of ciprofloxacin or ofloxacin may be effective.

CLINICAL PEARL

Antihistamines should be avoided because they dry out secretions.

Nonpharmacologic Measures

Smoking cessation, rest, well-balanced diet, increased oral fluids, and humidification are all important nonpharmacologic interventions in acute bronchitis.

If a client with acute bronchitis is not showing signs of improvement within 3 days, further measures may be required. A chest x-ray rules out pneumonia or a pulmonary mass. Consider sinusitis if the client has a persistent cough. A trial with a decongestant may be worthwhile if evidence of sinusitis exists. An antihistamine may help if there is an allergic component, but the possible side effects and drug interactions may restrict their use. Asthma should be considered when a client has a lingering (many times dry), refractory cough of 1 month or longer, following bronchitis. *Chlamydia pneumoniae* is often the responsible agent (Kauopnen et al., 1995), which may be treated with doxycycline 100 mg twice a day for 1 week or azithromycin 1000 mg once weekly for a mean of 4 weeks (Hahn, 1995). Gastroesophageal reflux disease (GERD) also needs to be considered, especially if symptoms occur almost exclusively when the client is in bed.

INFECTIOUS PNEUMONIA

Incidence
Pneumonia is the most common infectious cause of death in older adults and the most common infection requiring hospitalization. Older adults with other comorbid conditions, such as diabetes, cancer, stroke, CHF, dementia, and renal failure, often die of pneumonia. (Satin, 1994). Advanced age has become a well-recognized risk factor for death in clients with pneumonia. Combined with influenza, pneumonia is the fifth leading cause of death in the United States in older adults (Metlay et al., 1997).

There are 4 million cases of community-acquired pneumonia each year, with peak incidences in the winter and spring, and 15% to 20% of those cases require hospitalization. The mortality in outpatients is 1% to 5%, but in those who require hospitalization, it is as high as 25% (American Thoracic Society, 1993).

Pathophysiology
Pneumonia is consolidation and inflammation of the lung parenchyma, caused by an infectious agent, either viral or bacterial. Infection only rarely occurs by droplet nuclei directly into the lung. More commonly, the organism resides in the oropharynx, grows in number, and secondarily contaminates the lung through aspiration. This can happen more readily in an elderly person in whom the host defenses such as coughing, mucociliary clearance, and phagocytic action in the aveoli are depressed. Those elderly with chronic lung disease or immunosuppression are even more susceptible to pneumonia.

Pathogens among outpatients 60 years of age or older include *S. pneumoniae*, respiratory viruses, *H. influenzae*, aerobic gram-negative bacilli, *Staphylococcus aureus*, and miscellaneous pathogens such as *M. catarrhalis*, *Legionella* spp., *Mycobacterium tuberculosis*, and endemic fungi. Therapy is a second-generation cephalosporin, trimethoprim–sulfamethoxazole (Bactrim), or a beta-lactam/lactamase inhibitor plus possibly erythromycin or another macrolide. No single test is presently available that can identify all potential pathogens, and each diagnostic test has limitations (American Thoracic Society, 1993).

CLINICAL PEARL

Although early etiologic diagnosis is optimal, particularly in the aged, the responsible pathogen is unable to be identified in as many as 50% of clients.

Prevention

Prevention is best accomplished by reducing the risk of aspiration by avoiding sedating drugs, alcohol, and nasogastric tubes when possible. Immunization with pneumococcal vaccine is recommended every 10 years (Calkins et al., 1992). Some authorities recommend boosting patients in 5 years, but there are clear standards at this time. Influenza, which can predispose a patient to development of a subsequent pneumonia, can be prevented with an annual influenza immunization. See Chapter 1 for more information on prevention of pneumonia.

Clinical Presentation

Usual Presentation of Disease. A recent study verifies what is seen routinely: Older adults with community-acquired pneumonia report a significantly lower number of respiratory and nonrespiratory symptoms than younger clients. (Metlay et al., 1997). Signs of pneumonia are often blunted in older adults. Of those that are evident, the most commonly reported respiratory signs and symptoms are cough, dyspnea, and sputum production. Commonly reported nonrespiratory signs and symptoms are fatigue, fever, and chills.

Atypical Presentation of Disease. Pneumonia has a more subtle presentation in the older adult. Typical symptoms, such as a productive cough, fever, and pleuritic chest pain, are frequently absent. Subtle symptoms, such as delirium, alteration of sleep–wake cycles, a fall, increased CHF, anorexia, and failure to thrive are more common. Misdiagnosis and late diagnosis contribute to the high mortality of pneumonia (Satin, 1994).

CLINICAL PEARL

Cognitive changes and/or unexplained falls may be an early atypical presentation of physical illness such as community-acquired pneumonia.

Assessment

History. Perform a symptom analysis of complaints of cough, change in sputum from baseline, hemoptysis, sustained fever (> 102°F could indicate *S. pneumoniae* or *Legionella*), and diarrhea (could indicate *Legionella*). A URI 2 to 14 days prior will often be reported. Aggravating factors include concomitant illness.

Physical Examination. Check vital signs and mental status in addition to the respiratory exam. Note splinting, accessory muscle use, adventitious breath sounds, dullness to percussion, and other signs of consolidation (Bates, 1995).

Laboratory and Diagnostic Measures. The white blood count will be increased. Blood cultures may be helpful. Lab abnormalities associated with increased mortality are listed in Table 5–11.

TABLE 5–11. LAB ABNORMALTIES ASSOCIATED WITH INCREASED MORTALITY

Hematocrit	< 30%
Blood urea nitrogen (BUN)	> 30 mg/dL
Glucose	> 250 mg/dL
Na	< 130
PaO$_2$	< 60 mm Hg
Artrial pH	< 7.35

Source: Fine, M. J., Auble, T. E., Yealy, D. M., et al. (1997). A prediction rule to identify low-risk patients with community-acquired pneumonia. *N Engl J Med, 336*(4), 243–250.

Chest X-ray. A chest x-ray can reveal infiltrates that help differentiate pneumonia from acute bronchitis and help evaluate severity (multilobar involvement). A chest x-ray can also suggest specific etiologies (TB, lung abscess, *Pneumocystis carinii*, etc.) and coexisting conditions (bronchial obstruction, pleural effusion, etc.) (Fine et al., 1997).

CLINICAL PEARL

Rehydration of a dehydrated client may cause an infiltrate to "appear" where none could be seen on a chest x-ray.

Sputum for Gram Stain and Culture and Sensitivity. The single most important diagnostic test for determining initial antibiotic therapy is identification of the causative bacteria in a sputum sample (Satin, 1994). Fifty percent of the time, a pathogen is unable to be identified. Early morning is the best time to obtain a specimen.

CLINICAL PEARL

An adequate sputum specimen must contain < 5 epithelial cells from the oropharynx and at least 25 neutrophils.

Clinical Management

Pharmacologic Measures. Therapy is often empiric in that sputum specimens are difficult to obtain in a dehydrated and uncooperative elderly client. Pathogens among outpatients with coexisting disease and/or who are 60 years of age or older include *S. pneumoniae, H. influenzae,* aerobic gram-negative bacilli, and *S. aureus. M. catarrhalis, Legionella* spp., *Mycobacterium* spp., and endemic fungi are less common pathogens. Mortality in the outpatient setting is less than 5%, but 20% of patients initially treated may require hospitalization.

In nursing-home clients, the following pathogens are recognized more frequently than in clients with the same coexisting illnesses who are residing in the community: methicillin-resistant *S. aureus, M. tuberculosis,* and certain viral agents (eg, adenovirus, respiratory syncytial virus, and influenza). Adjustments can be made if sputum culture data becomes available (Calkins et al., 1992).

Treatment with a second-generation cephalosporin, trimethoprim–sulfamethoxazole, a beta-lactam/lactamase inhibitor, and/or a macrolide are recommended for outpatient management of the elderly (American Thoracic Society, 1993).

Nonpharmacologic Measures. Table 5–12 outlines other therapeutic interventions. A crucial part of the strategy is deciding whether the client can be treated as an outpatient by the advanced practice nurse (APN) and whether the client needs to be referred to an internist or a specialist and/or hospitalized. Research identifies age greater than 65 years as a risk factor for increased morbidity/mortality, which is a relative indication for inpatient care. Several other risk factors are associated with increased mortality:

- Male sex
- Tachypnea R > 30
- Hypotension < 90 systolic; < 60 diastolic
- Leukopenia
- Hypothermia < 95
- Multilobar radiographic pulmonary infiltrate
- Pleuritic chest pain
- Pleural effusion
- Bacteremia

Medical practitioners could use these prognostic factors to help determine the initial site of care (home versus hospital) and the intensity of initial empiric antibiotic therapy.

If outpatient treatment is indicated, contact with the client every 24 to 48 hours is important to ensure improvement. Clients may be referred to physicians if they have (1) inadequate response to therapy (fever lasting > 2 to 4 days after initiation of therapy, lack of improvement within 48 to 72 hours, or clinical deterioration); (2) physical findings that reveal a complicated course of recovery (respiratory rate > 30, tachycardia > 125, temp > 101°F or < 95°F, hypotension, delirium, evidence of extrapulmonary sites of disease); or (3) laboratory findings that predict increased morbidity. A prediction model for identifying the at-risk patient has been developed (Fig. 5–7).

CLINICAL PEARL

Develop a strategy for further diagnostic testing or therapeutic interventions considering the tempo and degree of illness.

TABLE 5–12. CLINICAL MANAGEMENT OF PNEUMONIA

Hydration

Frequent rest periods while preventing deconditioning

Breathing exercises and secretion clearance techniques such as coughing and deep breathing, incentive spirometry, stimulating a cough, and/or suctioning

Chest physical therapy and postural drainage if sputum > 1 oz./day and client is unable to cough

Aerosolized bronchodilator such as albuterol

Pain control

Cough control

Fever control

Management of concomitant disease

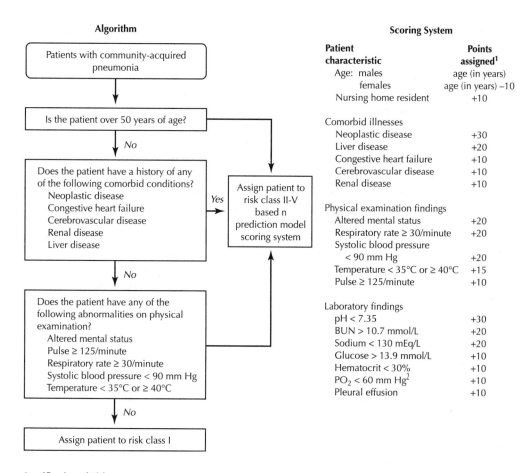

Algorithm

Patients with community-acquired pneumonia

Is the patient over 50 years of age?

No

Does the patient have a history of any of the following comorbid conditions?
Neoplastic disease
Congestive heart failure
Cerebrovascular disease
Renal disease
Liver disease

No

Does the patient have any of the following abnormalities on physical examination?
Altered mental status
Pulse ≥ 125/minute
Respiratory rate ≥ 30/minute
Systolic blood pressure < 90 mm Hg
Temperature < 35°C or ≥ 40°C

No

Assign patient to risk class I

Yes → Assign patient to risk class II-V based n prediction model scoring system

Scoring System

Patient characteristic	Points assigned[1]
Age: males	age (in years)
females	age (in years) −10
Nursing home resident	+10
Comorbid illnesses	
Neoplastic disease	+30
Liver disease	+20
Congestive heart failure	+10
Cerebrovascular disease	+10
Renal disease	+10
Physical examination findings	
Altered mental status	+20
Respiratory rate ≥ 30/minute	+20
Systolic blood pressure < 90 mm Hg	+20
Temperature < 35°C or ≥ 40°C	+15
Pulse ≥ 125/minute	+10
Laboratory findings	
pH < 7.35	+30
BUN > 10.7 mmol/L	+20
Sodium < 130 mEq/L	+20
Glucose > 13.9 mmol/L	+10
Hematocrit < 30%	+10
PO_2 < 60 mm Hg[2]	+10
Pleural effusion	+10

Stratification of Risk Score

Risk	Risk class	Based on
	I	Algorithm
Low	II	≤ 70 total points
	III	71–90 total points
Moderate	IV	91–130 total points
High	V	> 130 total points

[1] A risk score (total point score) for a given patient is obtained by summing the patient age in years (age −10 for females) and the points for each applicable patient characteristic.

[2] Oxygen saturation < 90% also was considered abnormal.

This prediction model for prognosis in patients with community-acquired pneumonia may be used to help guide the initial decision on site of care. However, its use may not be appropriate for all patients with this illness and therefore should be applied in conjunction with physician judgment.

Figure 5–7. Prediction Model for Identification of Patient Risk for Persons With Community-Acquired Pneumonia. *(Source: Adapted from Fine, M. J., Auble, T. E., Yealy, D. M., et. al. [1997]. A prediction rule to identify low-risk patients with community-acquired pneumonia. N Engl J Med. 336[4], 243–250.)*

Setting-specific Issues

In a hospital or nursing home setting, the following technique can assist in producing a cough in a client unable to follow commands: A cough may be spontaneously generated to clear the lungs by gently stimulating the trachea, using sterile technique and a size 10 French suction catheter and water-soluble lubricating gel. A nasal trumpet may be used if this procedure needs to be ongoing. This procedure could precipitate laryngospasm and hypoxemia, so pulse oximetry and emergency equipment should be available.

TUBERCULOSIS

Incidence

M. tuberculosis infection occurs more frequently and has higher mortality rates in the older population (Yoshikawa, 1990). Many geriatric clients have been exposed to TB (latent infection), and reactivation may occur. The reactivation rate is increased by alcoholism, malnutrition, diabetes, immunosuppression, neoplasia, and renal dialysis.

TB is spread by airborne transmission of droplet nuclei 1 to 5 microns in diameter. There are two stages in the TB disease process. In the infected (or latent) period, the client has been exposed to and harbors the *Mycobacterium* bacillus, without having any active signs or symptoms of the disease, and is not capable of transmitting the disease to others. In the second disease stage, the bacterium has become active. The patient experiences signs and symptoms of the disease and becomes capable of transmitting the disease through airborne droplet nuclei.

Pulmonary TB usually presents as an infiltrate in the apical and posterior segments of the upper lobes. The client may be asymptomatic or have nonspecific symptoms of a chronic respiratory infection: cough (productive or nonproductive), anorexia, weight loss, chronic fatigue, fever, night sweats, and hemoptysis. The chest x-ray may reveal a nondescript fluffy process in the upper lung fields but frequently shows cavity formation or fibrosis with volume loss or both. Routine lab studies in pulmonary TB are nonspecific. Hyponatremia (usually attributable to the syndrome of inappropriate antidiuretic hormone production) occurs in more than 10% of clients with pulmonary tuberculosis. A definitive diagnosis of pulmonary TB can be obtained only by culture of infected material. Smears alone will miss up to 60% of active TB cases. Cultures are essential (Bordow & Moser, 1994). One of the major limitations of the culture technique is that it takes 4 to 8 weeks to obtain results. When sputum is not available, bronchoscopy with brushings, transbronchial biopsy, or needle aspiration can provide material for diagnosis.

New laboratory diagnostic techniques could revolutionize the diagnosis of mycobacterial diseases. The BACTEC$_R$ system, a rapid radiometric culture technique, can detect mycobacterial growth in 5 to 8 days. Deoxyribonucleic acid (DNA) probe technology can detect mycobacteria in sputum within hours. Bordow and Moser (1996) predict genus-specific *Mycobacterium* probes may soon be available as an excellent screening test for TB in sputum.

Assessment

Physical exam is not particularly helpful. Rales and bronchial breath sounds (if there is consolidation) may be the only indicators of underlying disease. If there is cavitation, the breath sounds may resemble the noise made by blowing across the mouth of a bottle (Hopwell & Bloom, 1994). See Table 5–13 for assessment of the latent stage versus active disease stage.

Prevention

Good pulmonary hygiene, yearly TB screening, preventive therapy for those with a positive purified protein derivative (PPD) tuberculin test, and chemoprophylaxis for those with a positive chest x-ray helps decrease the spread of TB. A person who is infected may lose skin test reactivity over a period of years, thus producing a falsely negative single Mantoux which involves the intracutaneous injection of 5 tuberculin units (TU) of purified protein derivative (PPD). A second Mantoux tuberculin test given within 1 to 2 weeks would then elicit a positive or

"boosted" response. A reaction greater than 10 mm is considered positive. If a person is suspected of being human immunodeficiency virus (HIV) positive or otherwise immunosuppressed, has had recent close contact with a TB infectious person, or has a chest x-ray suggestive of TB, greater than 5 mm PPD induration is considered positive (Murray & Nadel, 1994).

Rather than presenting with the usual clinical picture, older adults may present atypically with only anorexia, weight loss, or fever. Instead of typical upper lobe infiltrate or cavitary disease, they may present with pulmonary nodules, pleural effusion, infiltrates in locations other than the upper lobes, and miliary spread (Schrier, 1982).

Clinical Management

Management of clients in the latent stage consists of educating the patient as to the

TABLE 5–13.   TUBERCULOSIS ASSESSMENT

Latent Stage	Active Disease Stage
■ **HISTORY**	
Exposure to TB infectious person	Cough
	Anorexia
	Weight loss
	Chronic fatigue
	Gradual decline in functional status
	Fever
	Night sweats
	Hemoptysis
■ **PHYSICAL EXAMINATION**	
Skin test: Positive purified protein derivative (PPD) (Mantoux)	Positive PPD (Mantoux)
Chest x-ray: Negative	Upper zone infiltrates with or without cavitation
Sputum culture: Negative	Positive for TB bacillus

signs and symptoms of the disease becoming active, the airborne route of transmission, and the advisability of receiving preventive pharmacologic therapy. Clients who have converted to the active stage of the disease should begin therapy immediately with four TB drugs (isoniazid [INH], rifampin, pyrazinamide, and ethambutol or streptomycin). Direct observation therapy (DOT) of medication ingestion is advisable for all clients when possible. Clients with active TB should be isolated until sputum smears convert to negative (three consecutive negative smears from specimens collected on different days). All suspected or confirmed cases of TB should be reported to local public health TB control programs for epidemiologic follow-up of close contacts of the client. Clients should be monitored monthly for drug reactions, infectious status, and clinical and bacteriologic response to therapy. A TB expert should be consulted if susceptibility results show resistance to any of the first-line drugs, if the client has side effects from the pharmocologic regimen or remains symptomatic, and/or if the smear or culture remain positive after 3 months.

Pharmacologic Measures. In the past decade, the standard regime for the treatment of TB has undergone considerable change. INH, rifampin, ethambutol, and pyrazinamide are the first line drugs for treatment of TB. Streptomycin, the first drug available for tuberculosis therapy, is still occasionally used as a first-line drug; its value is limited, however, by dose-related renal and eighth cranial nerve toxicity.

A multidrug-resistant TB epidemic has been rampant in the 1990s. Current recommendations for initial TB therapy therefore include (1) initial drug susceptibility studies for all positive cultures, (2) initial four-drug therapy for all patients (except in very low drug-resistance areas), and (3) initial DOT for most patients. If significant drug resistance is demonstrated, the therapeutic regimen should be altered to include at least two drugs to which the organism is sensitive and the ineffective drug(s) should be discontinued. Factors influencing the likelihood of drug resistance include history of previous antituberculous therapy, country of origin (especially Southeast Asia and Latin America), and duration of residence in North America (Bordow & Moser, 1996).

Initial treatment includes INH, rifampin, pyrazinamide, and ethambutol for 2 months. INH and rifampin are continued for an additional 7 to 10 months and at least 6 months beyond culture negativity. If INH or rifampin resistance is present, therapy should be continued for at least 18 months and 12 months, respectively, beyond culture negativity (Bordow & Moser, 1996).

INH hepatitis is a concern in the elderly, especially in those with active liver disease or impaired liver function. Rifampin, in combination with INH, increases the risk of further liver damage. Another side effect of INH is peripheral neuritis. Despite its risks, INH prophylaxis is recommended for those who have latent TB and who are at high risk for developing active disease (those who also have chronic debilitating diseases: chronic renal failure, COPD, gastric resection, diabetes, silicosis, and alcoholism). Prophylactic therapy should be continued for 12 months.

Streptomycin may be substituted for rifampin. Side effects of streptomycin include eighth-nerve damage and nephrotoxicity. Optic neuritis is a side effect of ethambutol. See the *Core Curriculum on Tuberculosis* (U.S. Department of Health and Human Services, 1994) for a summary of recommended drugs for the initial treatment of tuberculosis and second-line antitubercular drugs.

Nonpharmacologic Measures. If a client develops active TB with symptoms, pharmacologic treatment is started. Isolation in a negative pressure room is used to decrease the risk of spread of airborne pathogens. HEPA masks are recommended for use by personnel who come in contact with the client. Good pulmonary hygiene (coughing or sneezing into a tissue and discarding) is vital for the client. When three early morning sputa are negative for acid-fast bacillus, the client is considered noninfectious and can be removed from isolation.

Extrapulmonary Tuberculosis

Tuberculosis can be present not only in the lung, but in extrapulmonary sites. Upper airway, laryngeal, lymphatic, pleural, and pericardial TB can occur. Gastrointestinal TB, disseminated (miliary) TB, tuberculous meningitis, genitourinary TB, and bone and joint TB have all been identified.

CASE STUDY #1

Mrs. Warner is a 76-year-old black woman who presents with a 3-week history of cough and wheeze. She describes her symptoms as starting with a cold that went into her chest. Her chest symptoms persisted and have worsened over the past 2 days. She describes her chest symptoms as a feeling of restricted breathing and an inability to get the air in deeply enough. At times, it feels like a tightness in her chest. She awakens once or twice a night to cough and feels chest tightness. She denies allergies to animals, medications, environment, or foods, but remembers having problems with her breathing as a child when she had colds or exercised. She denies a smoking history. She describes a history of chest tightness in damp environments such as a cellar. She recalls nasal stuffiness, postnasal drip, and increased breathing difficulties in the fall.

She is on no prescribed medications but has been taking over-the-counter (OTC) cold remedies. Her friend told her to try a Primatene (epinephrine) inhaler, which makes her breathing feel somewhat better for 1 to 2 hours. She also feels somewhat better after a strong cup of coffee.

Physical examination reveals a thin woman who is periodically coughing nonproductively. Her vital signs are: temperature, 98.6°F; blood pressure,

120/82; pulse, 88; and respirations, 20. Physical exam is normal except for swollen nasal mucosa; postnasal drip; and a high-pitched, expiratory wheeze scattered thoughout the chest.

---

1. What diagnoses should be included in the differential?

   Acute reactive airways related to a viral respiratory infection, asthma, COPD, mechanical obstruction of the airways, CHF, pulmonary embolism, and pulmonary infiltration with eosinophilia are included in the differential diagnoses. Current findings support the diagnosis of asthma, with an acute exacerbation precipitated by a respiratory tract infection. The absence of a history of smoking makes COPD less likely.

2. What diagnostic tests should be performed?

   Spirometry before and after bronchodilator therapy establishes baseline severity and reversibility of airflow obstruction. Peak flow measures and home monitoring establish the measure of the client's pulmonary function over time and response to treatment. Peak flow readings help the patient detect early signs of asthma exacerbation. Other diagnostic tests (eg, chest x-ray, WBC) can be ordered if the suspicion of other diagnoses is high.

3. What are some of the initial therapeutic measures that should be started with this client?

   Bronchodilator therapy with a sympathomimetic as needed; oral or inhaled steroids regularly, depending on objective measurements and your evaluation of asthma severity (peak flow, spirometry); antibiotics (if bacterial infection is thought to be contributing); and measures to control nasal symptoms (nasal lavage, decongestants, nasal steroids) are some of the initial therapeutic measures that should be started with this client. You should discuss environmental control measures (particularly the control of indoor molds, house dust mites, and cockroaches), consider initiating twice-a-day home peak flow measurements to establish a pattern of asthma, and initiate the concept of asthma management as a partnership. Teach proper inhaler technique. Only 30% of clients who used their inhalers correctly once will do so on subsequent evaluations; reinforcement is the key. It is common for clients to confuse medications taken for disease control and those used for symptomatic relief.

4. How soon should you see Mrs. Warner in follow-up?

   If your previous evaluation indicates that she is stable, follow up in 1 to 2 weeks to review home peak flow monitoring and the use of monitoring to predict worsening asthma, to recheck inhaler technique, and to remeasure spirometry. Instruct her to call sooner for worsening symptoms, a dramatic drop in peak flow, a sharp increase in her inhaler use (sympathomimetic), and an increase in nocturnal awakenings.

5. What are indicators of good asthma control in Mrs. Warner?

Ability to participate in desired activities, uninterrupted sleep, absence of symptoms (using reliever medication only a few times per week), are goals to discuss with Mrs. Warner.

6. What should be explored if symptoms do not improve at subsequent visits?

Evaluate other possible environmental triggers (eg, warm-blooded animals, cockroaches, inability to control house dust mites, mold, second-hand smoke, aspirin sensitivity). Evaluate peak flow monitoring and adherence to prescribed regimen and reinforce goals of therapy.

Evaluate nasal signs and symptom, consider GERD as a contributing factor. Refer to a specialist if symptoms worsen or do not subside.

 ## CASE STUDY #2

Mr. Simon is a 75-year-old white male presenting to your clinic with a chief complaint of dyspnea. He describes his dyspnea as occurring on exertion, particularly upon stair climbing, showering, and working in his yard. He cannot quite remember when the dyspnea began but thinks it was gradual over the past several years. Past medical history is negative for a history of asthma, heart disease, TB, cancer, stroke, or diabetes. He has no allergies. He takes Robitussin occasionally.

1. What further information should you obtain from Mr. Simon?

Ask Mr. Simon if he has ever had pneumonia and/or bronchitis ("chest colds"). Also ask about personal habits, particularly smoking. Mr. Simon reports a history of frequent chest colds, occurring once or twice a year and lasting 1 to 2 weeks. He has a 75 pack-year history of cigarette smoking but quit 3 years ago after an episode of bronchitis. He drinks alcohol occasionally and takes no recreational drugs. His review of systems is significant for dyspnea, daily cough and sputum (1 to 2 teaspoons of white, thick sputum), and wheezing associated with sputum production. Otherwise, his review of systems is negative.

2. What diagnoses are on your differential list?

COPD is strongly suspected in this client. Other diagnoses to consider include infection, asthma, restrictive lung disease, neoplasm, and pulmonary emboli. Physical examination reveals a thin man in no acute distress. His vital signs are temperature, 98.8°F; blood pressure, 130/84; pulse, 88, respirations, 26. He weighs 140 lb, and height is 5'10". Mr. Simon is sitting up and leaning forward with his arms braced on his legs. His chest wall motion is decreased overall. You notice bilateral intercostal retractions at the postaxillary line at the tenth intercostal space. (Bilateral intercostal retractions at the lower part of the chest are often seen in the client with acute or chronic hyperinflation, consistent with obstructive lung disease.) Mr. Simon's chest is hyperresonant to percussion. The expiratory phase of his breath sounds is prolonged in all lung fields. He has a sonorous wheeze in the bases, which clears with cough.

3. Has your differential diagnosis changed? What diagnostic tests should be performed?

Tests to consider at the initial evaluation are pulmonary function tests (spirometry; possibly lung volumes and diffusion capacity), chest x-ray for suspected infections and/or to establish a baseline, pulse oximetry and/or arterial blood gas at rest and with exercise, and blood chemistry and CBC. Keep in mind that O_2 saturation by pulse oximetry can be falsely elevated in a smoker for approximately 1 to 2 hours after smoking because carbon monoxide found in cigarette smoke is indistinguishable from oxygen by this indirect O_2 saturation measurement method.

Mr. Simon's spirometry reveals an FEV_1 of 0.98 (37% predicted), and FEV_1/FVC of 44%. His flow volume loop shows significant coving (concavely curved), which is indicative of airway obstruction. The pulmonary function test is consistent with severe obstructive lung disease. His oxygen saturation at rest is 94%, which decreases to 91% after 6 minutes of walking at a moderate pace. His chest x-ray shows hyperinflation and flattened diaphragms. There is no evidence of infiltrate or masses. His blood chemistries and CBC are within normal limits.

4. What is your diagnostic impression?

The history, physical exam, and laboratory data support the diagnosis of COPD. You start treatment with ipratropium 3 puffs qid. You also teach Mr. Simon the importance of yearly influenza immunization and administer Pneumovax, a vaccine against pneumococcal pneumonia.

5. What other therapeutic options should be considered?

You may also prescribe an inhaled sympathomimetic to be used on an as-needed basis. It is essential to review the correct administration of drugs taken by metered-dose inhalers and to check technique at subsequent client visits. You may also recommend a pulmonary rehabilitation program for education, breathing retraining, physical reconditioning, and support for dealing with the chronic nature of lung disease. You need to teach Mr. Simon the signs and symptoms of infection/exacerbation and when to notify you. As you get to know Mr. Simon, discuss advance directives and his views on how aggressive therapy should be.

6. How often should Mr. Simon be followed-up?

A visit would optimally be rescheduled within 2 to 4 weeks to determine Mr. Simon's response to his bronchodilator therapy, reinforce inhaler technique, and consider other therapeutic options. For suboptimal response, consider increasing his ipratropium dose to as much as 6 puffs qid and/or adding theophylline and/or a therapeutic trial of oral corticosteroids (depending on the severity and persistence of symptoms). After symptoms are relieved, back off to the lowest dose possible. Visits may then be scheduled every 3 to 6 months, depending on his course. Yearly visits for very stable clients with less severe disease may be adequate.

7. What future problems might you anticipate in this patient?

Nutritional problems, particularly weight loss; progressive dyspnea; hypoxemia; right ventricular hypertrophy; and exacerbations are probable future problems in this man with severe lung disease. Loss of functional status and independence may lead to anxiety and depression. Future assessments should be directed at early identification of problems. Periodic evaluation of oxygen saturation at rest, with exercise, and during sleep should be made.

Refer Mr. Simon to a specialist for symptoms not responding to conventional therapy, suspicion of other lung problems, a rapidly progressive course, or for consideration for specialized procedures (eg, bronchoscopy, cardiopulmonary stress testing, or lung volume reduction surgery).

 ## CASE STUDY #3

Mr. Oliver is a 92-year-old retired businessman who has a history of insulin-dependent diabetes mellitus, atrial fibrillation, hypertension, coronary artery disease, CHF, peripherial vascular disease, and multi-infarct dementia. Mr. Oliver is living with his wife and a 24-hour live-in companion in a two-bedroom apartment in an "assisted living" facility. The live-in companion reports that Mr. Oliver has had a runny nose for the past 5 days. She also reports that Mr. Oliver has not been ordering his meals in the dining room as he had been doing previously. He has not been following commands as well as he had previously. Two-step commands need to be broken down into one-step commands and many times have to be repeated.

The client presented with eyeglasses askew and inappropriately dressed; otherwise, the physical examination was unremarkable.

1. What do you think might be going on with this patient?

    A change in baseline cognition often indicates a change in physical condition. The physical exam is negative, and the fingerstick is within normal range. A urinalysis would be helful in ruling out a possible urinary tract infection (UTI). Continue to monitor Mr. Oliver's physical and mental status. Checking his fingerstick twice a day would be advisable.

    The urinalysis was negative, but Mr. Oliver continued to exhibit cognitive changes during the next week. He is having difficulty finding his way back to his bed after getting up to go to the bathroom at night, and he fell last night. He had no injury but had to be directed back to his bed. His fingerstick ranged from 150 to 189, which was on the high side for him. A chest x-ray revealed an infiltrate consistent with right lower lobe pneumonia. Scant rales were detected in the right posterior base on day 10.

2. What would be the treatment plan for Mr. Oliver?

    A second-generation cephalosporin (eg, Ceftin 500 mg bid for 10 days) would be a good choice of an antibiotic for community-acquired pneumonia. An extra 2 mg of regular insulin may be needed to cover his hyperglycemia

if Mr. Oliver's fingerstick is greater than 150. Fluids should be encouraged to 1600 cc/24 hr. Mr. Oliver should be observed for signs of CHF, which could include a weight gain of more than 3 lb and/or lower-extremity edema. Mr. Oliver would best be reminded to cough and deep breathe every 2 to 4 hours. Having him attempt to blow up a balloon may be helpful in helping him achieve the desired aveolar ventilation). Repeating the Folstein Mini-Mental State Exam (MMSE) may help document the cognitive changes being observed. After the antibiotics are completed, another MMSE will hopefully have returned to Mr. Oliver's baseline.

■ REFERENCES

American Thoracic Society, Medical Section of the American Lung Association. (1993). Guidelines for the initial management of adults with community-acquired pneumonia: Diagnosis, assessment of severity, and initial antimicrobial therapy. *Am Rev Resp Dis, 148,* 1418–1426.

American Thoracic Society, Medical Section of the American Lung Association. (1995). Standards for the diagnosis and care of patients with chronic obstructive pulmonary disease (COPD) and asthma. *Am J Resp Crit Care Med, 152,* S77–S120.

Bates, B. (1995). *A guide to physical examination and history taking* (6th ed.). New York: J. B. Lippincott.

Biller, P. L. (1987) Diagnosis and management of acute bronchitis and pneumonia in the ambulatory setting. *Nurse Pract* 12 (10): 12–15, 18, 23 passim.

Bordow, R. A., & Moser, K. M. (1996). *Manual of clinical problems in pulmonary medicine.* Boston: Litttle, Brown.

Calkins, E., Ford, A., & Katz P. (1992). *The practice of geriatrics.* (p. 559). Philadelphia: W. B. Saunders.

Davis, A., Hahn, A., Niederman, M., & O'-Connell, E. (1996). When chronic bronchitis turns acute. *Patient Care,* January, 124–128.

Ebersole, P., & Hess, P. (1990). *Toward healthy aging: Human needs and nursing response.* (p. 161). Baltimore: C. V. Mosby.

Ferguson, G. T., Cherniack, R. M. (1993). Management of chronic obstructive pulmonary disease. *N Engl J Med. 328:* 1017–1022.

Fine, M. J. (1990). Pneumonia in the elderly: The hospital admission and discharge decisions. *Sem Resp Infect, 5*(4), 303–313.

Fine, M. J., Auble, T. E., Yealy, D. M., et al. (1997). A prediction rule to identify low-risk patients with community-acquired pneumonia. *N Eng J Med, 336*(4), 243–250.

Haggerty, M. C., Stockdale-Woolley, R., & Nair, S. (1991). Respi-Care: An innovative home care program for the patient with chronic obstructive pulmonary disease. *Chest, 100,* 607–612.

Hahn D. L. (1995). Treatment of *Chlamydia pneumoniae* infection in adult asthma: A before–after trial. *J Fam Prac, 441,* 350.

Hopwell, P. C., & Bloom, B. R. (1994). Tuberculosis and other myocobacterial diseases. In Murray, J. F., & Nadel, J. A. (Eds). *Textbook of respiratory medicine* (2nd ed.) (pp. 1094–1154). Philadelphia: W. B. Saunders.

Janson-Bjerklie, S. (1993). Assessment and management of adults with asthma: guidelines for nurse practitioners. *Nurse Pract Forum, 4*(1), 23–29.

Kalafer, M. E. (1996). Tuberculosis: epidemiology and prophylaxis. In Bordow, R. A., Moser, K. M. (Eds.), *Manual of clinical problems in pulmonary medicine* (pp. 133–147). Boston: Little, Brown.

Kauopnen, M. T., Herva, E., Kiyala, P., et al. (1995). The etiology of community acquired pneumonia among hospitalized patients during a *Chlamydia pneumoniae* epidemic in Finland. *J Infect Dis, 172,* 1333.

Metlay, J. P., Schulz, R., Li, Y. H., et al. (1997). Influence of age on symptoms at presentation in patients with community-acquired pneumonia. *Arch Intern Med 157,* 1453–1459.

Medical Research Council Working Party (1981). Longterm domiciliary oxygen therapy in chronic hypoxic cor pulmonale complicating chronic bronchitis and emphysema. *Lancet,* i:681–686.

National Asthma Education Program (1992). *Teach your patients about asthma* (NIH Publication No. 92-2737). Washington, DC: U.S. Government Printing Office.

National Asthma Education and Prevention Program Working Group Report (1996). *Considerations for diagnosing and managing asthma in the elderly* (NIH Publication No. 95-3675). Washington, DC: U.S. Government Printing Office.

Nett, L. M., & Obrigewitch, R. (1993). Nicotine dependency treatment: A role for the nurse practitioner. *Nurse Prac Forum, 4*(1), 37–42.

Nocturnal Oxygen Therapy Trial Group (1988). Continuous or nocturnal oxygen therapy in hypoxic chronic obstructive lung disease. *Ann Intern Med, 93*:391–398.

Nurses' Asthma Education Working Group (1995). *Nurses: Partners in asthma care* (NIH Publication No. 95-3308). Washington, DC: U.S. Government Printing Office.

Pitman, M. B., Sherman, M. E., and Black-Schaffer, W. S. (1991). The use of fine-needle aspiration in the diagnosis of metastatic pulmonary adenoid cystic carcinoma. *Otolaryngol Head and Neck Surg, 104*(4), 441–447.

Pomilla, P. V., & Brown, R. B. (1994). Outpatient treatment of community-acquired pneumonia in adults. *Arch Intern Med, 154,* 1793–1801.

Reardon, J. Z. & Bragdon, R. L. (1993). Optimizing the use of metered-dose inhalers in chronic obstructive lung disease and asthma. *Nurse Pract Forum,* 4(1):53–57.

Satin, D. (Ed.). (1994). *The clinical care of the aged person.* NY: Oxford University Press.

Second Expert Panel on the Diagnosis and Management of Asthma (1997). *Guidelines for the diagnosis and management of asthma* (NIH Publication No. 97-4051-A). Washington, DC: U.S. Government Printing Office.

Schrier, R. W. (1982). *Clinical internal medicine in the aged.* Philadelphia: W. B. Saunders.

Solheim, K. (Mar. 1993). Managing prednisone in clients with chronic obstructive pulmonary disease. *Nurse Pract Forum,* 4(1):43–48.

Sweer, L. & Zwillich, C. W. (Sept. 1990). *Clinic Chest Med, 11*(3):417–45.

U.S. Department of Health and Human Services (1994). *Core curriculum on tuberculosis* (3rd ed.). Atlanta, GA: Public Health Service.

Yoshikawa, T. T. (1990). Antimicrobial therapy for the elderly patient. *J Am Geriatr Soc, 38*(12), 1353–1372.

6

TOPICS IN CARDIOVASCULAR CARE

Michele A. Marek • Janine Alfano Wilcox • Ann E. Cocks

■ INTRODUCTION

Cardiovascular disease remains the leading cause of death in older adults, accounting for 50% of the nearly one-half million fatalities and more than 3.5 million hospital admissions of those aged 65 and older in the United States each year. Specifically, coronary heart disease (CHD) is the main cause of activity limitation for 11.5% of the population, ranking behind only orthopedic impairments and arthritis. It is the leading reason for Social Security disability, accounting for one fourth to one third of the $16 billion cost of this program (Sullivan et al., 1996). Despite improvements in disease diagnostics and treatments, this trend has persisted since the 1940s, and, as recently as 1991, 42% of all deaths were secondary to major cardiovascular disease. Major health objectives of the nation by the year 2000 are the reduction of CHD by 26% and reduction of average serum cholesterol by 6% to an average of 200 mg/dL (Reece, 1995). Given these statistics, along with projections of increased numbers of the population living longer, advanced practice nurses (APNs) must be well versed in recognition and modification of risk factors related to CHD, diagnosis related to its disease ramifications, and current management strategies.

■ CORONARY HEART DISEASE

AGE-RELATED CHANGES

Coronary heart disease is said to occur when there is decreased blood flow to the myocardium as a result of atherosclerotic plaque buildup on the cardiac vessels. There exists a high correlation between elevated cholesterol levels and the development of CHD over the life span, with the elderly experiencing a higher incidence and greater severity of CHD. Although controversy exists regarding the issue of treatment of hypercholes-

161

terolemia in the elderly, most research supports the relationship between high cholesterol levels and CHD. Specifically, low-density lipoprotein (LDL), is directly related to the incidence of CHD. Reductions in blood levels of this fatty, waxy substance are associated with reductions in CHD risk, and vessel wall plaques actually regress as part of this process (Atkins & Garber, 1996). Interest in addressing cholesterol levels and atherosclerotic risk in childhood early years is now increasing (Larosa, 1996).

Atherosclerosis begins within the artery wall as a lesion, eventually leading to narrowing of the arterial lumen, causing decreased myocardial perfusion in the basal state and limiting increases in perfusion in demand states. Generally, when a stenosis reduces the cross-sectional lumen by 75%, full-range increases in flow to meet demands are not possible. When luminal area is reduced by 80%, resting blood flow may be reduced, and any minor decreases can reduce coronary blood flow dramatically, causing ischemia (Selwyn & Brounwald, 1993). It is also demonstrated that cholesterol plaques lead to reactive endothelial injury of the vessels, causing release of thrombi, mediated through platelets and other members of the clotting system. Many episodes of acute coronary insufficiency and infarction are associated with thrombosis.

ASSESSMENT

History
Evaluation of the client with suspected CHD begins with careful evaluation of the client's complete medical history, including identification of risk factors such as the following:

- Male sex or postmenopausal female
- Advanced age
- Family history of CHD; myocardial infarction (MI) or angina in parent or sibling before age 55
- Smoking > 10 cigarettes per day
- Hypertension (HTN)
- LDL > 100; high-density lipoprotein (HDL) < 35 in male or < 45 in female
- Diabetes mellitus (DM)
- History of cerebrovascular or occlusive peripheral vascular disease (PVD)
- Obesity > 30% of desirable weight

Other essential components of the health interview should include information regarding personal history of MI, angina, dyspnea, syncope, leg pain, numbness, sexual dysfunction, HTN, DM, thyroid disorder, obesity, PVD, renal disease, and cerebrovascular disease. Family history, including current age and health status of members; diet history, including types of foods and patterns of ingestion; exercise patterns; and tobacco and alcohol usage need to be determined.

Physical Examination
The following components are essential in evaluation of CHD in the elderly patient:

- Blood pressure (BP)—both arms
- Cardiac auscultation
- Assessment for carotid and femoral bruits
- Palpation of the abdomen for aortic aneurysm
- Palpation of peripheral pulses
- Examination of the skin for xanthomas and xanthelasmus

• Examination of the retina for abnormalities such as nicking (Bates, 1995)

Diagnostic Studies

Baseline lab tests should include complete blood count (CBC), urinalysis, glucose, creatinine, thyroid function tests, and lipid profile. A chest x-ray to rule out heart failure (CHF), ventricular aneurysm, and cardiac enlargement is also recommended. There is general agreement that the information obtained from an electrocardiogram (ECG) is invaluable in the initial diagnostic workup of cardiac clients. The ideal frequency of ECG in the stable elderly population has not been established; yearly testing as well as testing for changes in condition is warranted (Sivaram et al., 1996). An echocardiogram is recommended to assess the client for left ventricular hypertrophy, valvular dysfunction, thrombus, ejection fraction, and so forth. When history, physical examination, or ECG findings suggest the presence of CHD, stress testing is usually the next step in the diagnostic workup. Contraindications include recent unstable angina and MI, as well as uncontrolled HTN, CHF, severe ventricular arrhythmia, and severe valvular disease. As primary-care providers, APNs are responsible for recognizing when a stress test is indicated and initiating consultation with appropriate physician colleagues.

The basis of stress testing is to note cardiac response to standarized incremental increase in external workload while ECG, symptoms, and BP are recorded. Using either a bicycle or treadmill, depending on client ability, workloads are gradually increased until the client reaches 80% to 90% of the maximal heart rate, predicted on the basis of age, or the client experiences symptoms of chest pain, shortness of breath, lightheadedness, claudication, a drop in BP of greater than 15 mm Hg, ventricular arrhythmias, or ST depression f 2 mm or greater. In general, a test is considered positive if ST depression of 1 mm occurs. If radioactive scanning is included, the client will receive the appropriate agent, such as thallium, at the time of maximal exercise, with cardiac scanning immediately, and then repeated scanning 3 hours later, comparing myocardial perfusion at maximal workload to perfusion at rest. In the case of an elderly or debilitated client for whom exercise is not tolerable, a dipyridamole–thallium test can be performed; dipyridamole-dilated coronary arteries and results of test are as meaningful as thallium stress testing. In an older client, a negative study may be clinically meaningful at a lesser workload if the workload approximates the client's normal daily activity. Older client do have a greater frequency of resting ECG abnormalities, higher prevalence of intraventricular conduction delays, and prior MIs that might interfere with interpretation of exercise-induced ST segment changes, therefore necessitating careful weighing of pros and cons when considering whether testing is indicated and which type testing will yield the most useful data (Vaitkevicius & Fleg, 1996; Goroll et al., 1995).

CLINICAL MANAGEMENT

According to the National Institutes of Health (NIH) Consensus Statement (1993), the following should serve as guidelines in the treatment of CHD:

- Management of clients with CHD is based on evaluation of the individual client with respect to life patterns, risk factors, control of symptoms, and prevention of damage to the myocardium. Life-style factors that aggravate hypertriglyceridemia and low HDL levels, such as obesity, smoking, and sedentary life style, should be targeted for change.
- Weight loss alone can significantly decrease plasma triglycerides and increase HDL by 10% to 20%.
- Alcohol should be eliminated in clients with very high triglyceride levels.
- Diets should emphasize complex carbohydrates as compared to simple sugars; complex carbohydrates have been shown to lower total and LDL cholesterol.
- Population studies indicate that diets high in fish are associated with decreased cholesterol. Omega-3 fatty acids in large amounts may reduce excessive triglyceride levels, but their safety is not yet proven; they may also increase LDL and impair blood clotting and control of DM.
- Exercise can increase HDL and decrease triglycerides. Intervention studies have shown dose–response relationships between HDL and amount of exercise. In general, there is a 10% to 20% increase HDL in response to exercise (see Rehabilitation section for a discussion on type of exercise).
- Cigarette smoking has been shown to decrease HDL, as does passive smoke exposure. Smoking cessation decreases the risk for CHD and increases HDL.

- Health professional services such as dietitians, nutritionists, exercise physiatrists, and health educators should be utilized as support personnel for the client with CHD. The American Heart Association (AHA) advocates a specific plan for risk reduction for patients with coronary and other vascular disease. While many of their recommendations closely parallel those of the NIH, they additionally recommend that all Americans eat a diet in which 30% or less of calories come from fat, with less than 10% of these calories coming from saturated fats (AHA, 1995).
- Aspirin 80 mg to 325 mg should be started daily (if not contraindicated); Warfarin (Coumadin) should be given to post-MI patients who cannot take aspirin, with a goal of international normalized ratio of 2 to 3.5.
- Beta blockers and angiotensin-converting enzyme (ACE) inhibitors should be used post-MI if not contraindicated.
- Estrogen replacement therapy should be considered in all postmenopausal women.
- BP should be controlled to less than 140/90.

Although the above guidelines were not developed specifically related to care of the elderly, they are generally applicable to this population. Successful management of the client with or at risk for CHD involves a team approach, utilizing client investment and support from significant others, teaching, community involvement, and ongoing assessment and interventions by the APN providing primary care. Clients whose CHD symptoms become unstable should be referred for medical evaluation and management.

Pharmacologic Measures

Pharmacologic issues in CHD revolve around the management of lipids. Sources and panels continue to differ regarding the issues of testing and treatment of hyperlipidemia in the elderly. Generally speaking, adults 20 to 70 years of age should have cholesterol levels checked every 5 years. There are no concrete guidelines to date on checking cholesterol levels over the age of 70; at this time, recommendations are to base tests on individual CHD risk profiles. Usually, total cholesterol levels less than 200 are desirable; levels greater than 200 should be retested, and, if still elevated, risk factor assessment for CHD and further evaluation are warranted (Baron, 1992).

The use of cholesterol-lowering medications would be expected to result in a higher rate of drug-to-drug interactions and side effects in the elderly, secondary to decreased metabolism and complicated medical regimens. Conversely, many elderly individuals might greatly benefit from treatment, especially in the setting of multiple cardiac risk factors or established CHD. In a recent meta-analysis of research regarding statins in the role of cardiovascular and stroke reduction, this class of drug was found to cause a significant decrease in cardiovascular disease mortality (Hebert, 1997). While few research studies have included the elderly as subjects, those that do support the finding that elevated LDL cholesterol levels are associated with higher morbidity (though not overall mortality), especially where concomitant disease was a factor. Controversy continues to exist re-

garding the management of hypercholesterolemia in the elderly in whom CHD is not an established diagnosis.

In terms of selection of cholesterol-lowering drugs, recent studies support hepatic hydroxymethylglutaryl coenzyme A (HMG CoA) reductase inhibitors such as lovastatin, which have been demonstrated to help reduce the progression of CHD. Results of the Scandinavian Simvastatin Survival Study (4S study) confirmed the benefits of HMG CoA reductase inhibitors in preventing CHD morbidity and mortality in clients with a history of MI or angina (Bittle et al., 1996).

Hormone replacement therapy (HRT) has been shown to significantly reduce the risk of CHD in large-scale studies of postmenopausal women. Estrogen increases HDLs and reduces LDLs by as much as 15%, resulting in a 44% reduction in the risk of CHD in the postmenopause period (Arnstein et al., 1996). In a recent study of 76 postmenopausal women aged 48 to 76, using either estrogen, pravastatin, or a combination of the two, it was found that adding pravastatin to estrogen does not improve HDL but does improve LDL. For a woman already taking pravastatin, starting estrogen replacement therapy raises HDL but does not improve LDL significantly (O'Brien, 1997). Table 6–1 illustrates some characteristics of the various cholesterol-lowering agents available.

Use of prophylactic aspirin and other platelet-inhibiting drugs such as ticlopidine in CHD has gained support due to their ability to enhance fibrinolysis, thereby diminishing the effect of tissue reactivity to thrombus formation in the pathogenesis of infarction. A 30- to 50-mg daily dose of aspirin produces ap-

TABLE 6–1. LIPID-LOWERING AGENTS

Category/Relative Cost	Main Effect	Potential Side Effects
Niacin; nicotinic acid $	↑HDL ↓LDL ↓Triglycerides	Flushing gout, rash ↑ LFTs worsening diabetic control
Bile acid resins, ie, colestipol cholestyramine $$	↑HDL ↓LDL Can be used in clients with liver disease	Bloating, heartburn, constipa- tion, drug interactions common, may ↑ triglycerides
Fibric acid derivatives, ie, gemfibrozil (Lopid) $$$	↓TG (triglycerides) ↑HDL	May ↑ LDL rash, nausea con- traindicated in clients with poor renal or hepatic functions and in cholelithi- asis may ↑ INR
HMG-CoA reductase inhibitors, ie, lovastatin, lipitor $$$$	↓ LDL, ↑ HDL usually avoided in liver disease ↓ Triglycerides	Myositis, ↑ LFT, nausea, headache, rash
Estrogen $$	↓ LDL ↑ HDL	Endometrial and breast cancer

proximately 95% inhibition of platelet aggregation for the 8- to 10-day life span of the platelet. Higher doses are found to increase gastrointestinal (GI) intolerance and blood loss. Ticlopidine also irreversibly inhibits platelet reactivity for the life of the platelet, but, unlike aspirin, the clearance of the drug is prolonged by multiple dosing. In the elderly, it may remain in the circulation for weeks after it is discontinued. Adverse side effects include GI upset to cholestatic hepatitis or neutropenia (Zeleznick, 1996).

Rehabilitation

In general, cardiac rehabilitation involves commitment to life-style modification such as a cholesterol-lowering diet, smoking cessation, weight loss, and exercise. Exercise has been shown to reduce CHD morbidity and mortality both di-

rectly and through reducing levels of cardiovascular risk factors such as obesity.

Exercise increases HDL, decreases LDL, enhances insulin sensitivity, and promotes fibrinolysis. It is not entirely clear whether these effects are the same in the elderly. Other positive effects of exercise include increasing functional capacity, increasing effect tolerance and work capacity, and an improved sense of well being, including less anxiety and depression (Siscovich, 1992). In a recent study examining whether walking reduced the risk of cardiovascular disease, hospitalization, and death in men and women 65 years of age and older, it was found that walking more than 4 hours a week was associated significantly with a reduced risk of cardiovascular disease–related hospitalization in both sexes, compared with walking less than 1 hour a week (LaCroix, 1996).

Client Education

Establishment of therapeutic relationships with clients and their significant others is the first step in being able to affect their health status in a positive way. Elderly clients usually have longstanding beliefs and opinions about their health practices, including diet, exercise, tobacco and alcohol usage, and the like, and have to be willing to listen to the recommendations of the NIH and AHA. In order for them to do this, they must have faith in their health-care provider.

CLINICAL PEARL

Address life-style modification and the issue of hypercholesterolemia with your elderly clients. Individualize your approach based on national guidelines as well as what is appropriate for your client. Be prepared to answer questions regarding diet and exercise; your local AHA will be happy to send you free pamphlets regarding their recommendations for you to review and to share with your clients: 1-800-AHA-USA1 (1-800-242-8721).

Setting-specific Issues

Decisions regarding intensiveness of cardiac workup and aggressiveness of interventions must be individualized for the client, depending on overall condition, ability to tolerate workup and interventions, and overall functional status and quality of life issues. For the chronically ill elder, maintaining the individual at functional baseline should be prioritized.

Whenever possible, families and significant others, as well as the client, should be part of the decision-making process.

■ ANGINA

CLINICAL PRESENTATION

Chronic, stable angina reflects transient myocardial ischemia and usually presents in a crescendo–decrescendo pattern of chest pain or heaviness, lasting 1 to 5 minutes and involving the substernal chest region; left shoulder and arm; ulnar surfaces of both forearms and hands; back, neck, or jaw; teeth; or epigastrium. It is usually caused by exertion or emotion and relieved by rest, but it may also occur at rest. Episodes of angina that last more than 15 minutes or that are increasing in frequency or severity and begin occurring at rest suggest transition to unstable angina, with increased risk for MI and complications. Angina in the elderly is less typically in the substernal location, often nonexertional, less severe in intensity, and not as responsive to nitroglycerin (NTG) as typically seen in the younger population (Arnstein et al., 1996).

Prinzmetal's angina refers to pain that occurs at rest or awakens the client from sleep. It is caused by focal spasm of the proximal epicardial coronary arteries; 75% of the time, atherosclerotic coronary artery obstruction is present, and vasospasm occurs near stenotic lesion. Angina decubitus refers to angina that occurs at night or while the client is lying down, due to the expansion to the intrathoracic blood volume that occurs with recumbency, causing increased cardiac size and myocardial demand. Listed in Table 6–2 are examples of the numerous noncardiac causes of chest

TABLE 6–2. NONCARDIAC CAUSES OF CHEST PAIN

■ **CERVICAL PATHOLOGY**
Arthritis
Spondylitis
Disc herniation
Metastases

■ **CHEST WALL CAUSES**
Herpes zoster
Pectoral myositis and spasm
Costochondritis
Thrombophlebitis

■ **PULMONARY CAUSES**
Pulmonary embolism
Pneumothorax
Pneumonia
Pleurisy

■ **GI-RELATED CAUSES**
Gallbladder disease
Esophageal spasm
Reflux
Pancreatitis
Gaseous distention

■ **VASCULATURE**
Dissecting abdominal aneurysm

■ **PSYCHOGENIC**
Anxiety
Depression

pain that can mimic angina. Cardiac conditions other than CHD, including left ventricular hypertrophy (LVH), aortic stenosis or regurgitation, hypertrophic cardiomyopathy, pericardial effusion, pericarditis, and myocarditis are also potential causes of chest pain.

While chest pressure is the classic symptom of angina in the elderly, there is an increased incidence of "silent ischemia" (SI) in this population. It is estimated that as many as 2 million asymptomatic middle-aged and older individuals have SI, and this increases dramatically with advancing age. Three forms of SI have been identified in the literature. The first type is seen in clients who do not experience angina or an "anginal equivalent" such as indigestion, malaise, fatigue, and so on, because of an abnormal warning system. These clients may even experience MI without prodromal symptoms. The second type of SI occurs in clients who are asymptomatic after MI but demonstrate ischemia during stress testing or ambulatory monitoring. The third type of SI occurs in patients with CHD who have typical chronic stable angina, who will have episodes of ischemic ST-segment changes on Holter monitor that are not accompanied by symptoms (Vaitkevicius & Fleg, 1996). Coexisting illness such as communication disorder or dementia also may limit the elderly client's ability to report anginal symptoms. Changes in behavior, including agitation or delirium, or altered vital signs such as tachycardia or blood pressure variations may be the only overt symptoms of ischemia, thus representing anginal "equivalents" for that client.

CLINICAL PEARL

Remember that atypical presentations of angina, such as agitation or delirium, are common in the elderly and may need to be part of the differential diagnosis, based on the clinical picture and assessment of CHD risk factors. "Silent ischemia," evidenced by ECG changes, must be addressed in order to avoid future MI.

ASSESSMENT

History

The assessment of angina is based upon consideration of symptoms including quality, severity, location, and precipitating factors for pain, as well as duration, alleviation, associated symptoms, self-treatment, and frequency. A comprehensive medical history, with emphasis on risk factors for CHD, is essential. Contributing conditions such as diabetes, HTN, thyroid disorder, anemia, and chronic obstructive pulmonary disease (COPD) should also be evaluated. Precipitating factors associated with angina such as stress, overeating, vigorous exercise, sexual relations, and so forth also need to be delineated for each individual.

Physical Examination

Physical examination signs of risk factors (in addition to examination previously discussed under CHD) include xanthelosoma and xanthomas, diabetic skin lesions, nicotine stains, thickened or absent peripheral pulses, nicking of the fundi, and displacement of the point of maximal impulse.

Diagnostic Studies

As discussed under CHD, stress testing should be considered in an elderly client with angina or history of MI, especially when there is a change in clinical status. Angiography should also be considered when determining suitability for revascularization of clients who have failed medical management, and for detection of left mainstem and severe triple vessel disease. It should be done only if the client is a candidate for revascularization. Minor complications include arterial thrombosis; bleeding from the site; tran-

sient impairment of renal function, which may be more pronounced in the elderly; allergies; arrhythmias; and hypotension. In general, there are greater risks in the elderly with poor left ventricle (LV) function and peripheral vascular disease (Bittle et al., 1996).

CLINICAL PEARL

Stress tests can be modified so as to accommodate possible limitations due to aging and provide helpful information toward guiding treatment decisions. Interpretation of results is best done in consultation with a cardiologist.

CLINICAL MANAGEMENT

Medical treatment of angina focuses on identification of precipitating factors and modification of behaviors leading to it; life-style modification with emphasis on exercise, stress reduction, and diet; and treatment of concomitant disease. According to the Multiple Risk Factor Intervention Trial, there was a significant reduction in coronary deaths among men with abnormal stress tests who underwent closely supervised risk factor modification. The provider and client also need to establish end points that will define the need to consider revascularization such as bypass surgery or angioplasty (Amsterdam et al., 1996).

While no revascularization procedure cures CHD, both percutaneous transluminal coronary angioplasty (PTCA) and coronary artery bypass graft (CABG) effectively reduce angina if successful.

Coronary artery bypass graft has the clearest impact on life expectancy in patients with triple vessel disease plus decreased ejection fraction (EF), and in clients with left mainstem stenosis greater than 50%. Coronary artery bypass graft is also preferred when the proximal portion of the left arterior descending artery is involved, and when additional surgery such as valve replacement is necessary. With the recent advances in utilization of the internal mammary artery for grafting, patency rates of greater than 15 years can occur for the individual who quits smoking and whose lipids are well controlled. Clients up to age 90 often do well during and after bypass surgery as long as they are good candidates for anesthesia, are well nourished, do not present in shock, and are not in the end stage of another disease. CABG-related mortality is 10% for octogenarians, compared to 2% for PTCA clients. Octogenarians who survive CABG have 5-year survival rates similar to those of 70 year olds post-CABG (Bittle, 1996).

The ideal candidate for PTCA is less than 65 years of age, leads an active lifestyle, and has frequent symptoms that are refractory to medical therapy. It is also the procedure of choice for clients with isolated circumflex disease, clients with directly accessible lesions of the right coronary artery (RCA), and those with two-vessel disease that has been refractory to medical treatment. Angioplasty may also be recommended for very old clients or those who are poor candidates for anesthesia. However, in the elderly, lesions may not respond as well to angioplasty because of increased vessel tortuosity and calcification. A recent study comparing PTCA outcomes in el-

derly clients who had the procedure between 1980 and 1989 with those who had it between 1990 and 1992 suggested that short-term complication rates have decreased probably secondary to advances in technology. Intermediate and long-term survival rates have not appreciably changed (Bittle et al., 1996).

Pharmacologic Measures

Medical management of angina involves the use of nitrates, beta blockers, and calcium channel blockers. Nitrates are first-line therapy for treatment of angina and control symptoms in many clients. They increase coronary artery blood flow and decrease myocardial oxygen demand by producing dilation of venous circulation, thereby decreasing preload and ventricular volume. This improves efficiency of the heart, which decreases wall tension and ultimately decreases myocardial oxygen demand. Nitrates also cause arterial dilation, thereby reducing resistance to ventricular ejection. Many different dosage forms exist for the administration of nitrates. Nitrate tolerance refers to loss of hemodynamic benefits associated with continuous nitrate use over prolonged periods, thereby necessitating an interruption, usually at night, in their administration (Goroll et al., 1995). Beta blockers decrease heart rate, contractility, and blood pressure. These effects decrease myocardial oxygen demand and help prevent the frequency and severity of angina. They often prevent arrhythmias as well as rapid ventricular rates in patients with atrial fibrillation (AF). They can be helpful in controlling premature ventricular contractions (PVCs), which may predispose to dangerous ventricular arrhythmias in times of ischemia. Beta blockers should not be used in second-

or third-degree atrioventricular (AV) block or severe aortic stenosis, and they should be cautiously used in COPD (cardioselective) and CHF, in which agents with intrinsic sympathetic activity (ISA) may be preferred (Goroll et al., 1995).

Calcium channel blockers can be very effective for clients with stable angina, especially if caused by vasospasm. In general, clients with sick sinus syndrome should not be started on diltiazem secondary to the risk of bradycardia, and verapamil is contraindicated in clients with heart failure and conduction system disease. All calcium channel blockers should be used with caution in clients with EFs less than 40%, because they are negative inotropes and could further suppress the myocardium (Goroll et al., 1995). However, new research on calcium channel blockers is constantly being presented and views regarding usage may change in the future.

Collaboration/Interdisciplinary Involvement

Recovery post-PTCA and -CABG involves specific cardiac rehabilitation programs and critical pathways that are individualized to meet the needs of the client. It is essential to emphasize that CHD is a chronic disease, requiring life-style modification postrevascularization to prevent recurrence of vessel occlusion.

Client Education

Helping to educate significant others and caregivers regarding indications that angina has reached the point at which revascularization studies are warranted is an important role of the APN. Reluctance to accept progression of disease and denial of symptoms are common and can be dissipated through development of a therapeutic relationship with the client and significant others.

■ MYOCARDIAL INFARCTION

ASSESSMENT

Only 15% to 25% of clients who seek medical attention to rule out MI are actually having an ischemic event (Amsterdam et al., 1996). Symptoms of MI are related to the area of myocardium that is experiencing injury and can include chest pain, nausea, lightheadedness, and syncope. Table 6–3 summarizes acute MI location and possible ECG changes. In general, ischemia to the myocardium is

---

TABLE 6–3. MYOCARDIAL INFARCTION LOCATION AND AFFECTED ELECTROCARDIOGRAM LEADS

Anterior wall: Occlusion of anterior descending branch of left circumflex artery (LCA). ST segment elevation or Q waves in V1–V6.

Lateral wall: Occlusion of circumflex branch of left coronary artery (LCA). ST elevation or Q waves in 1, AVL.

Inferior wall: Occlusion of either right or left circumflex artery. ST elevation or Q waves in 11, 111, or AVF.

Posterior wall: Occlusion of right coronary artery (RCA). Large R wave in V1 and V2, with ST depression.

evidenced by ST-segment depression or T-wave inversion in the affected leads, while actual myocardial injury is evidenced by ST elevation and the gradual appearance of Q waves on the ECG. As a complete discussion of ECG changes is beyond the scope of this test, the reader is referred to an appropriate medical text for review.

CLINICAL PEARL

When evaluating a client for angina and the possibility of MI, obtain a past ECG for comparison whenever possible; there are variants of ST and T waves that can resemble ischemia but may be chronic for the client.

When in doubt, call an ambulance. The sooner the client is evaluated in an ER, the better the chance for survival; both thrombolytic therapy and PTCA are potential options for the elderly.

In the elderly client with concomitant disease such as diabetes or dementia, symptoms of MI can often be atypical, with mental status changes or delirium as presenting characteristics. Basic assessment involves analysis of symptoms; past medical history; vital signs; lab data, including cardiac enzymes; and ECG findings, preferably with comparison to prior ECG. Depending on the index of suspicion, clinical presentation of the client, and advance directives of the client, transferal to the emergency room (ER) for evaluation of possible MI is appropriate when aggressive interventions are to

be pursued. In circumstances in which comfort of the client is the goal, assessment by the APN at the bedside, with collaboration with the physician regarding medical interventions, might be appropriate.

CLINICAL MANAGEMENT

Patients who are experiencing acute MI can usually be separated into three groups:

1. Candidates for thrombolytics or angioplasty. These clients typically have significant regional ST elevation (more than 1 mm in two adjacent leads), and when given intravenous (IV) NTG still have elevated ST segments. If ST segments decrease post-NTG, this suggests unstable angina due to transient thrombus or Prinzmetal's angina. If segments remain high or deviations are regional with reciprocal changes, there is a high probability for MI. Based on Global Utilization of Streptokinase and Tissue Plasminogen Activator for Occluded Coronary Artery Trial (GUSTO) Results, thrombolysis, as soon as possible, is recommended when there is no cardiac catheterization lab for PTCA available. Elderly clients have excellent results from thrombolytic therapy, although it may be underused due to fear of hemorrhage. While the incidence of intracranial hemorrhage is approximately 1% in the general population, it rises to approximately three times that in the over-65 age group (Smith, 1995). If PTCA is available, time is less crucial than with thrombolytics. Lower morbid-

ity and mortality are associated with angioplasty versus thrombolysis in young and elderly clients (Bell & Pinkowish, 1996).

2. Clients with angina and ST depression and T-wave inversion or a non–Q-wave infarct are not candidates for thrombolysis or PTCA but need medical therapy.

3. Clients with angina but minimal or absent ECG changes are at low risk for MI. If it does happen, it is non–Q wave with limited myocardial necrosis and a low complication rate. These clients may benefit from an early stress test.

Pharmacologic Measures

Sublingual (SL) NTG is generally used as a first-line agent for the client with angina secondary to its vasodilatory properties, which help dilate the coronary arteries as well as decrease preload and work of the heart. When NTG, repeated up to three times and given minutes apart, does not relieve anginal symptoms, the assumption that the client is experiencing unstable angina and possibly acute MI must be made and emergency measures instituted. Pharmacologic interventions usually include IV NTG, IV or intramuscular (IM) morphine, antiarrhythmics, thrombolytics, ACE inhibitors, beta blockers, and possibly calcium channel blockers (Goroll et al., 1995).

Acetylsalicylic acid (aspirin) 325 mg, chewed to enhance absorption, is generally indicated for its antiplatelet effect for clients experiencing severe anginal symptoms. It has also been shown to be helpful post-MI. In a study of 5490 elderly patients who were hospitalized and survived an MI between June 1992 and February 1993, mortality rates for patients prescribed aspirin was 8.4%, compared with 17% in the group without aspirin. According to this study, aspirin had the greatest benefit in older women with a history of MI or diabetes (Harpaz et al., 1996).

Post-MI beta blockers are considered protective for the heart unless the client develops CHF, bradycardia, hypotension, or heart block. In a recent study involving over 5332 New Jersey residents older than 65 who survived an MI between 1986 and 1990, 90 days post-MI only 21% received a prescription for a beta blocker. The adjusted mortality rate for those taking beta blockers was 43% lower than for those who did not (Soumerai et al., 1997).

ACE inhibitors are especially helpful in clients with EFs less than 40%; they decrease afterload and risk of CHF, recurrent ischemia, and death. The Fourth International Study of Infarct Survivors (ISIS-4) found that captopril twice a day reduced 5-week mortality post-MI by 7% compared to placebo (Amsterdam et al., 1996).

The role of calcium channel blockers post-MI is still controversial, especially if the EF is less than 40% (Amsterdam et al., 1996). Decisions regarding their use are best made in conjunction with a cardiologist.

Collaborative/Interdisciplinary Involvement

Knowledge of typical and atypical presentation of angina/ischemia is critical, and immediate referral to the ER for the client who will be aggressively treated is the standard of care, with administration of supportive care such as SL NTG, ASA, and oxygen while waiting for transport.

Communicating effectively with emergency services personnel is an important role for the APN, as providing a history and review of the current situation is vital. The sooner the client reaches the ER, the better the chance for a favorable outcome.

Cardiac rehabilitation post-MI should be considered for elderly clients. Low to moderate levels of exercise can be safe for elders and improve exercise capacity, weight control, glucose tolerance, and lipid levels much the same as for younger clients (Amsterdam et al., 1996). Programs are typically structured to include four phases: (1) during hospitalization—aimed at preventing deconditioning, offering education and psychological support; (2) discharge to 6 weeks post-MI—return to level of physical conditioning prior to MI (eg, walking, stationary bike); (3) post–6 weeks—increase level of physical conditioning using an exercise plan in conjunction with rehab specialist/beginning modification of risk factors; and (4) lifelong adherence to rehab, including 6- to 12-month follow-up (Goroll et al., 1995).

Client Education

Working with the family or caregiver of a client who has just had an MI requires support and information sharing on the part of the APN. Multiple questions related to function and independence will be raised. Instruction regarding medications, diet, risk factors, and other components of cardiac rehab will need to be addressed. Fears of losing independence after heart attack may be paramount in a previously healthy individual, especially if the MI was severe. For the chronically ill, further decline in global functioning is a possibility. Both groups are also at risk for depression, which often needs to be addressed by the family as a whole. Community resources, such as programs sponsored by the AHA for various types of support groups aimed at cardiac health, should be introduced to the interested client.

CLINICAL PEARL

Always address the issue of depression in your elderly post-MI patients; they are experiencing stress regarding possible loss of independence, and possibly helplessness and depression related to their illness.

■ ATRIAL FIBRILLATION

Atrial fibrillation affects more than 1 million Americans, more than half of whom are 75 years of age and older. It is associated with considerable cardiovascular morbidity or mortality, causing clinical symptoms such as palpitations, dyspnea, angina, and syncope, and is associated with heart failure as well as leading to cerebrovascular accident (CVA) in approximately 35% of people if left untreated (Futterman & Lemberg, 1996). Atrial fibrillation can have cardiac and noncardiac causes. Cardiac conditions such as CHD, cardiomyopathy, HTN, CHF, and the like can all predispose to AF, as well as noncardiac conditions such as chronic lung disease, diabetes, hyperthyroidism, cancer, pneumonia, postoperative complications, and pulmonary embolus. Occasionally, factors such as alcohol, cocaine, sympathomimetic drugs, excessive coffee intake, metabolic derangement, hypoxia, and emotional stress can potentiate it (Aronow, 1996).

ASSESSMENT

History
Diagnostic clues to the presence of AF include complaints of palpitations, lightheadedness or syncope, fatigue, cough, poor exercise tolerance, and chest pain. Other clients may not have any symptoms, and AF is discovered while assessing vital signs, auscultating the heart, or obtaining a routine ECG.

Physical Examination
Determination of whether the client is in any distress is the first step in the assessment of AF. Rapid AF can be a medical emergency when cardiac output is reduced, possibly leading to angina, CHF, and pulmonary edema. Is mental status clear or at baseline? Is the client delirious or is his or her level of consciousness impaired? Is there obvious pulmonary compromise? If the client appears stable, further assessment is then undergone. The client's heart should be auscultated for rate, rhythm, and quality. Blood pressure and peripheral pulses should be assessed for determination of perfusion. Lung sounds should be checked for appearance of rales, which might indicate CHF.

Diagnostic Studies
A 12-lead ECG is the first step in diagnosis of AF. A Holter monitor can be used to confirm AF and to monitor rates in AF, or if paroxysmal AF is suspected. Echocardiogram is also recommended in the evaluation of AF, especially if cardioversion is being considered.

CLINICAL PEARL
AF cannot be diagnosed by auscultation of the heart; a rhythm may sound like it is AF but be something completely different; an ECG or rhythm strip is needed to document (and possibly a Holter monitor) if it is paroxysmal.

CLINICAL MANAGEMENT
Transfer to the ER, with preparation for cardioversion, is the treatment of choice for the client with unstable AF (presence of hypotension, syncope, angina, or CHF), or a very fast ventricular rate. Older clients with a fast rate (eg, 140 and above) but without symptoms might be managed in a hospital setting with medications such as beta blockers, calcium channel blockers, and digoxin. Occasionally, antiarrhythmics such as amiodarone are necessary. If AF is not rapid, elders should not be given drugs that depress AV node conduction. Prevention of embolism becomes the focus of treatment.

Radiofrequency catheter ablation or surgical ablation of the accessory pathway is sometimes necessary if the ventricular rate cannot be slowed with medications. Occasionally, complete ablation and placement of a pacemaker is necessary to control AF (Aronow, 1996).

Whenever possible, treatment of the underlying cause of the AF should be attempted. Conditions such as pneumonia, hyperthyroidism, hypoglycemia, hypoxia, or infection all can contribute to AF, especially if the client is a frail elder whose general health is compromised.

Pharmacologic Measures

Treatment of stable AF revolves around the issues of rate control and anticoagulation. There is not so much of a push to convert stable AF to sinus rhythm by the use of antiarrhthymics, such as quinidine, mainly because of their side effect profile. There are some newer antiarrhythmic drugs that may be promising, such as amiodarone, and consultation with a cardiologist regarding their usage is appropriate.

Rate control in AF is often accomplished with the use of digoxin, which increases the responsiveness of AV nodal tissue to vagal stimuli. It is especially helpful in systolic dysfunction by enhancing contraction. Based on weight and renal function, clients are generally given a loading dose of digoxin over a 24-hour period, usually followed by a daily dose. Levels should be checked at least every 2 weeks until stabilized. As it is a highly protein-bound drug, its serum level may be lower than the actual free drug level that is circulating, and toxicity can occur at levels within the therapeutic guidelines of 0.6 to 2.0. Digoxin is not as effective in controlling heart rate when vagal tone is low and adrenergic stimulation is high, such as with exercise. In this case, another category of drug, such as a calcium channel blocker or beta blocker, should be considered. Because of the higher incidence of AV node dysfunction in the elderly, their usage should be carefully contemplated (Futterman & Lemberg, 1996; Goroll et al., 1995). Unless contraindicated by a history of recent hemorrhagic CVA, frequent falls, blood dyscrasia, or severe GI bleeding, anticoagulation with Coumadin is now an integral component of the pharmacologic management of AF. Over the last 5 years,

several studies have investigated the safety of oral anticoagulation for stroke prevention in clients with AF. Conclusions documented an approximately 70% reduction in stroke risk and very low complication rate. The Stroke Prevention in Atrial Fibrillation (SPAF) study concluded that Coumadin was more effective than aspirin for stroke reduction, especially in clients older than 75. SPAF 2 indicated that there was a higher risk of intracranial bleed in the elderly who had an international normalized ratio (INR) greater than three (Albers, 1994). For patients over age 75 who have AF without any concomitant heart disease (lone AF), aspirin, instead of Coumadin, is recommended (Futterman & Lemberg, 1996).

If the decision to use Coumadin is made, clients usually are given a high initial dose of 5 to 10 mg for 1 to 3 days. It generally takes approximately 3 days for levels to stabilize, but in the beginning week of therapy prothrombin time/INR should be checked daily. In the frail or high-risk elderly, low doses of 1 to 2 mg per day may be appropriate. After stabi-

CLINICAL PEARL

Coumadin levels can be profoundly altered by many other medications, including most classes of antibiotics, nonsteroidal anti-inflammatory drugs (NSAIDs), and barbiturates, to name only a few. It is prudent to measure PT/INR levels at least one time within 1 to 2 weeks after the initiation of any new medication.

lization on the drug, or if side effects develop, such as GI bleeding, levels are checked every 1 to 3 months. Generally, the greatest reduction in stroke occurrence is found when the INR is kept between 2 and 3. However, the target range must be individualized based upon concurrent illness and the risk of bleeding or falling.

Collaborative/Interdisciplinary Involvement

The commitment to treatment of AF is based on the premise of decreasing risk factors for stroke. For every client, the question of whether to anticoagulate or how to aggressively address rate control is asked, and sometimes is best answered with the help of the client's significant others and the input of a cardiologist.

■ HYPERTENSION

One of the leading health-care problems treated by practitioners each day is HTN. The Joint National Committee Fifth Report (JNC V) on Detection, Evaluation, and Treatment of High Blood Pressure states that nearly 50 million Americans live with this disease. Hypertension brings with it the risk of CHD and CVAs. Those at greatest risk for HTN are the elderly, women over 65 years of age, blacks, and lower socioeconomic groups (JNC V).

Hypertension is a circulatory disease characterized by a sustained elevation of systemic arterial pressure. There are two types of hypertension: primary and secondary. Primary HTN, also known as essential or idiopathic HTN, accounts for 90% of the cases. The sustained systemic

arterial pressure of primary HTN is not clearly understood and is often asymptomatic. Primary HTN leads to CHD, ventricular hypertrophy, CHF, PVD, decreased kidney function from decreased renal blood flow, and decreased cerebral artery blood flow and stroke. Secondary HTN accounts for 10% of cases and is associated with other disease such as renal artery disease, pheochromocytoma, hyperaldosteronism, extravascular compression caused by tumors, and thyroid disease, to name a few (JNC V, 1993).

Hypertension is defined as systolic blood pressure (SBP) greater than 140 mm Hg and/or diastolic blood pressure (DBP) greater than 90 mm Hg, found two or more times, on two or more separate occasions (JNC V, 1993). (See Table 1–3 for classification of HTN.) Decreasing diastolic pressure by as much as 6 mm Hg reduced overall mortality from vascular disease by 21%, fatal and nonfatal stroke by 42%, and fatal and nonfatal CHD by 14% (Hahn, 1995). The JNC V also describes the increased morbidity and mortality in the older adult associated with isolated systolic hypertension (ISH), defined as elevated SBP and normal DBP. Isolated systolic hypertension accounts for the majority of HTN in advancing age, and its cause is unknown. Isolated systolic hypertension must be treated. Nearly 4 million older adults have ISH. Of this aged population, women have a greater incidence of ISH than men (Bergman-Evans, 1996). These statistics illustrate the challenge that practitioners face when caring for the older adult. The goal must be to effectively treat this disease and prevent further complications of stroke and/or coronary disease. Treating ISH resulted in a 36% reduction in stroke and a 25% reduction in CHD (Hahn, 1995).

AGE-RELATED CHANGES

Increased peripheral vascular resistance with aging leads to a greater risk of HTN. Loss of blood vessel elasticity, also common with aging, causes a slight rise in SBP. The older adult is at increased risk for orthostatic hypotension due to a decline in baroreceptor activity with age. This risk, although only about 6% in healthy older adults, increases often due to the side effects of many antihypertensive medications (Calkins et al., 1992). Orthostatic hypotension is defined as a drop in SBP of greater than or equal to 20 mm Hg or a drop in DBP of greater than or equal to 10 mm Hg with position change.

Heart rate is also measured to look for a compensatory response to position change. Look for an increase of 5 to 10 beats per minute.

This change in heart rate does not always occur, indicating an impaired response. An increase in heart rate of greater than 10 beats per minute above baseline with position change may indicate an overcompensation, which can also be problematic. Evaluation of orthostatic hypotension should be done in the *lying, sitting,* and *standing positions.*

CLINICAL PRESENTATION

Usual Presentation of Disease

The presentation of HTN is usually not obvious unless target organ damage occurs. Hypertension is usually discovered during routine office visits. It is never diagnosed from one blood pressure reading. As stated by the JNC V, two elevated readings on two separate occasions over one to several weeks are needed to diagnose HTN.

A pulse deficit can occur when measuring blood pressures in a person with

CLINICAL PEARL

Orthostatic readings do not always occur immediately upon standing, but may appear 1 to 2 minutes after standing. Some clients fall shortly after getting up. Waiting 1 to 2 minutes also allows for the normally slowed baroreceptor response in the older adult. Therefore, the APN should adopt a standard practice of measuring blood pressure and heart rate in the lying, sitting, immediate standing positions and after the client has remained standing for 2 minutes when assessing for positional vital sign changes.

aortic insufficiency. In this condition, there is a wide range between the symbolic and diastolic blood pressures.

Atypical Presentation of Disease

"White coat" HTN has been described as elevated BPs detected only in the presence of a health-care provider. It usually requires several BP follow-ups in the community to accurately identify this condition. "Pseudohypertension" is a falsely high BP that is not caused by true hypertensive disease. Pseudohypertension is more common in the older adult and should be suspected when grossly disparate readings are found when comparing BPs in each arm. The falsely high reading is due to arteriosclerosis of the brachial artery, which becomes so rigid that the cuff cannot compress it. On examination, the radial artery is often palpable despite cuff inflation above the systolic pressure. Atherosclerosis can also cause the diastolic to register at or near zero. Another cause of disparate blood pressure readings between arms is coarctation of the aorta. The location of the aortic structure will determine if the blood pressures vary.

ASSESSMENT

Blood pressures should be checked on all initial and routine examinations. When the diagnosis of HTN has been made, all secondary causes should be initially ruled out. Physical findings that may indicate secondary causes are abdominal or renal masses associated with polycystic kidneys, abdominal bruits of renovascular disease, absent or delayed femoral pulses of aortic coarctation, tachycardia, orthostasis, tremor, and pallor associated with pheochromocytoma. (JNC V, 1993).

History

A thorough history is essential to identify actual and potential contributors to HTN. Medical history should include family and client history of high BP, coronary artery disease, diabetes, hyperlipidemia, and stroke (JNC V, 1993). Other contributing factors that need to be identified are obesity; smoking; excessive alcohol use; stress; lack of regular physical exercise; and dietary consumption of sodium, cholesterol, and fats.

Physical Examination

The physical exam of the hypertensive client has been outlined by the JNC V.

1. Two or more BPs separated by 2 minutes in both a sitting or lying position and then standing

2. Height and weight
3. Fundoscopic exam (hemorrhages or arteriovenous nicking, indicating secondary damage)
4. Heart exam for rate, rhythm, murmurs, S3, S4, size (signs of ventricular hypertrophy, heart failure)
5. Abdominal exam (masses, bruits)
6. Peripheral exam (absent or diminished pulses, edema)
7. Neurologic exam (evidence of stroke or transient ischemic attacks [TIAs]
8. Neck exam (carotid bruits)

Diagnostic Studies

Diagnostic tests should include chest x-ray and ECG to determine heart size and function. Lab work should include CBC, potassium, fasting blood sugar, calcium, creatinine, uric acid, cholesterol, and urinalysis.

CLINICAL MANAGEMENT

The ultimate goal of treating HTN is to reduce the morbidity and mortality associated with this disease by reducing SBP to 140 or less and DBP to 90 or less. The APN should always start with determining contributing factors of the disease process. When planning treatment, the following factors should be noted: (1) life style, (2) ability and willingness to understand and comply with prescribed treatment, and (3) concomitant disease.

The JNC V treatment guidelines use the stepped-care approach, beginning with nonpharmacologic, life-style changes and leading to pharmacologic interventions.

I. Life-style changes: Weight reduction, increased physical activity, moderation of sodium and alcohol intake, and smoking cessation (see Chap. 1).

If there is no success in reducing BP to less than 140 mm Hg systolic or less than 90 mm Hg diastolic within 3 to 6 months, or if BPs initially are greater than 160 mm/Hg systolic, pharmacologic intervention should begin.

- II. Pharmacologic intervention:
  - Continue life-style modification
- Step 2:
  - Initiate diuretic or beta blocker
  - *No response* within 1 to 3 months:
  - Increase dose of first durg
  - *No response:*
- Step 3:
  - Substitute another drug from another class (calcium channel blocker, ACE inhibitor, or vasodilator)
  - *OR*
- Step 4:
  - Add second agent from a different class
  - *OR*
- Step 5:
  - May add second or third agent or diuretic if not already prescribed

Follow-up should be in 1 to 2 months after initial drug treatment or any modification in the initial regime. Once stable, BP follow-up can be every 3 to 6 months.

Pharmacologic Measures

The goals of pharmacologic intervention are to lower BP with minimal adverse effects. The physiologic benefits that can be achieved with the use of antihypertensive medications are as follows:

- Reduction of sodium and water in the vessels

- Reduction of total peripheral resistance
- Improved blood flow to the heart, brain, and kidneys
- Improved structure and function of the heart (compensating for ventricular hypertrophy)
- Avoidance of decreasing cardiac output
- Inhibition of the renin–angiotensin–aldosterone system

Hypertension can be treated with the stepped-care approach. When choosing medications, consider the effect you are anticipating from the medications and other concomitant diseases that can also be treated with this medication regimen. The Systolic Hypertension in the Elderly Program (SHEP) looked at persons aged 60 and older with ISH and treated them using stepped-care treatment with a low-dose diuretic (chlorthalidone). This step-one medication reduced the incidence of total stroke by 36% and of major cardiovascular events, including CHF, by 32% (SHEP Cooperative Research Group, 1997).

Table 6–4 outlines medications used in the pharmacologic treatment of HTN. As always, when medicating the older adult, *"start low and go slow."* The decrease in kidney and liver function with aging requires a reduction in medication dosage and slow titration. Most antihypertensive medications should not be adjusted within 2 weeks of a change.

Collaboration/Interdisciplinary Involvement

As an APN, collaboration with a physician on a client's HTN therapy will depend upon the collaborative practice agreement and protocols you have de-

TABLE 6–4. PHARMACOLOGIC MANAGEMENT OF HYPERTENSION

Drug	Action	Side Effect	Special Considerations
Diuretics Thiazides	First line for uncomplicated hypertension	Hypokalemia; glucose intolerance; hypercholesterolemia	Not to be used in clients with renal failure or creatinine > 2.5
Loop	↑ Na+ excretion causes excessive loss of K+ and water	Hyperuricemia hypotension; electrolyte imbalance	Used with concomitant renal insufficiency or CHF
Adrenergic inhibiting agents	Interfere with sympathetic nervous system on a central and peripheral level (brain and nerve endings); compete with epinephrine for beta receptor sites inhibiting beta stimulation; ↓ cardiac output, force of contraction, rate	Fatigue, insomnia, depression, ↓ glucose tolerance, bradycardia, dry mouth, bronchospasm, confusion, hypotension	Beta blockers that are noncardioselective should not be used in clients with asthma, COPD, diabetes mellitus Diuretics and beta blockers used in combination ↓ cardiac morbidity and mortality. Hold for SBP < 90 or heart rate < 55; avoid use with pacemakers; avoid highly lipid-soluble agents (eg, propranolol, methyldopa)—may cause central nervous system side effects such as delirium and depression
Calcium channel blockers	Act peripherally and centrally to ↓ BP and myocardial contractility; forces Ca+ to leave cells, causing negative intropic effect; ↓ PVR	Flushing, edema, headache, constipation, bradycardia	Good choice for concomitant angina or arrhythmia
ACE inhibitors	Prevent conversion of angiotensin I to angiotensin II, ↓ vascular tone; ↑ renal blood flow	Neutropenia, proteinuria, rash, dry cough, hypotension, hyperkalemia	Avoid use with K+ sparing diuretics or renal artery stenosis or compromised renal function; good choice for diabetics due to ↑ renal blood flow
Nitrates	Reduce preload and afterload; dilate	Syncope, hypotension, headaches, flushing	Should be used in combination with diuretic and beta blocker to counteract fluid retention and reflex tachycardia

signed. The stepped-care approach allows for a methodologic and measurable plan for treatment of HTN. Poor response to treatment or medication side effects are an indication for consultation. Physician involvement will also be necessary when secondary causes of HTN are suspected.

Collaboration with nutritionists is helpful when dealing with issues regarding weight control and dietary modifications, specifically sodium and fat/cholesterol. Physical therapists or those who treat exercise tolerance are good resources when establishing exercise programs.

Client Education

It is necessary that families and caregivers understand the importance of BP control and its treatment. Awareness of potential medication side effects is extremely important when dealing with the older adult due to issues of polypharmacy. All clients should be instructed to make their care provider aware of any medications they are on. Teach clients to bring in all medications to review each visit. Instruct clients to avoid antihypertensive medications within one hour before or after a meal to prevent hypotension related to digestive blood shunting.

Older adults who live alone need to be instructed on diet. Those who cook for themselves rely on processed foods that are often high in sodium and are unaware of its implications.

SETTING-SPECIFIC ISSUES

Determine potential side effects when prescribing treatments for older adults. For example, the use of captopril (an ACE inhibitor) should not be initiated in an unsupervised setting because of its potential for rapid hypotensive effects. More aggressive treatment can be prescribed when one has access to skilled caregivers and laboratory monitoring. Structured settings (hospitals, nursing homes) increase medication compliance and allow for closer BP monitoring.

vignette

Mr. Allen, an 86-year-old man in a long-term care facility with a diagnosis of Alzheimer's-type dementia and peptic ulcer, presented with blood pressures of 168–198/80–90 over the course of 3 weeks. This was first identified by a routine monthly BP check that prompted more frequent follow-up. The client was on no medications and was asymptomatic from elevated BPs. A phone call was made to the physician, and Mr. Allen was placed on metoprolol 25 mg twice a day.

Two weeks following initiation of treatment, the client began to show signs of increased confusion, agitation, and weepiness. His BP was moderately controlled at 150–160/80. He was evaluated by the APN, and the metoprolol was changed to hydrochorothiazide (HCTZ) 25 mg/d. Within the next 2 weeks, Mr. Allen began to return to baseline behavior, with BPs ranging 140–150/80.

Evaluating mental status changes always includes ruling out secondary causes, such as infection and medications reactions. Beta blockers have the potential side effects of delirium and depression. The initiation of a diuretic as a first-step approach offered better BP control and less side effects for this individual.

■ CONGESTIVE HEART FAILURE

Congestive heart failure is prevalent in nearly 3 million Americans and is the leading cause of hospitalization in the older adult. The risk of CHF increases with age unrelated to any specific disease because of the decreased ventricular function of the heart associated with aging. Congestive heart failure can become a chronic condition associated with disease such as hypertension, coronary artery disease, valvular heart disease, cardiomyopathy, and abnormal systolic and diastolic dysfunction. Congestive heart failure can also be an acute condition and develop suddenly as a result of MI. Other precipitating factors include hepatic or renal disease, anemia, fever, infection, thyrotoxicosis, pregnancy, arrhythmias, cardiac amyloidosis, or use of NSAIDs (Bales & Sorrentino, 1997).

It is important to understand that CHF is not a disease but rather a condition of impaired cardiac function. Impaired cardiac function is the result of an underlying problem or disease, and this impaired cardiac performance is responsible for CHF (Miller, 1997).

AGE-RELATED CHANGES

Myocardial collagen increases with age and the heart becomes stiffer, causing diastolic filling pressures to increase. Left ventricular function decreases, leading to a decrease in stroke volume and cardiac output. Peripheral vascular resistance increases, causing 66% of older adults to have an increased risk of systolic and diastolic hypertension and LVH, which can be an underlying contributor to CHF (Ebersole & Hess, 1990).

A suggested comprehensive cardiac review of the heart can be found in the book *Geriatric Cardiology* (Berman, 1982).

CLINICAL PRESENTATION

Usual Presentation of Disease

The presentation of CHF will depend on whether it is a chronic or an acute condition. The choice for treatment is based on the underlying etiology of systolic or diastolic dysfunction.

Systolic Dysfunction
- A contraction or "output" problem
- Inability to pump blood out of the heart
- Weak pumping action causes backflow into venous system

Diastolic Dysfunction
- A relaxation or "input" problem
- Inability to allow proper ventricular filling secondary to weak, thickened muscles
- Typically, the same signs and symptoms as those with systolic dysfunction

Diastolic dysfunction is more common in elderly since they are susceptible to ventricular stiffness from HTN, ischemia, and tachycardia (Spencer & Lang, 1997).

The effects of systolic or diastolic dysfunction on the body can become very apparent as the weak muscle and poor pumping action lead to the following cascade of events:

- Decreased cardiac output
- Poor organ perfusion and oxygenation
- Kidneys retain water and sodium
- Peripheral edema

- Weight gain
- Hypoxia

Signs and symptoms of heart failure include the following:

- Chronic CHF: anorexia, nocturia, peripheral edema, hyperpigmentation of lower extremeties, weakness, hepatomegaly, ascites, dyspnea with exertion, exercise intolerance, dusky skin, S3 heart sound or murmurs, bibasilar rales
- Acute CHF: anxiety, restlessness, weight gain, shortness of breath (SOB), dyspnea, orthopnea, cough, hemoptysis, coarse crackles throughout lungs, bronchial wheezes, fatigue, cyanosis, S3 heart sound or murmurs, weak or nonpalpable peripheral pulses as blood is shunted to vital organs, tachycardia, decreased urine output, increased systemic vasculature resistance, jugular vein distention

Atypical Presentation of Disease

The onset or presentation of acute CHF in the older adult may present atypically. Delirium or acute confusion may be an early sign. The elderly may also present with compliants of dizziness or syncope. The presentation may be subtle, with the client demonstrating a slightly decreased functional ability in activities of daily living (ADL) or instrumental activities of daily living (IADL) from baseline.

ASSESSMENT

History

The client may report fatigue, weakness, general malaise, lethargy, dyspnea with exertion, a lingering cold or cough, orthopnea, paroxysmal nocturnal dyspnea, weight gain, pedal edema, or memory impairment.

The history should also include known cardiac disease, HTN, coronary artery disease, valvular disease, and cardiomyopathy.

Physical Examination

- Heart: rate, rhythm, murmurs, S3, palpate for displaced PMI
- Lungs: rales, cough, wheeze, hemoptysis, oxygen saturation, use of accessory muscles
- Neck: jugular vein distention
- Abdomen: hepatomegaly, ascites
- Extremeties: edema, cyanosis, skin temperature, weight

Worsening CHF can be determined by a one-pound-per-day weight gain for 3 consecutive days (Yontz, 1994).

Diagnostic Studies

Diagnostic tests should include a chest x-ray. Eighty-seven percent of those in chronic CHF will show cardiomegaly on their chest x-ray. Right-sided or bilateral pleural effusions are also seen in this group (Miller, 1997). In the acute client, the lower pulmonary vessels constrict and the upper vessels become better perfused. Effusions, as well as interlobular septal swelling, may also occur with acute CHF.

Look for sinus tachycardia, ischemia, infarction, or atrial fibrillation on ECG, all of which may be a clue for the cause of CHF. Possible signs to look for on echocardiogram include weak or stiff ventricular wall motion, ventricular hypertrophy, diseased or dysfunctional valves, aneurysm, or intracardiac shunting.

CLINICAL PEARL

All clients with the diagnosis or suspected diagnosis of CHF should have an echocardiogram to determine whether systolic or diastolic failure is present. Treatment of CHF is influenced by the type of failure.

CLINICAL MANAGEMENT

Prompt recognition of the onset of CHF is vital for effective management. Strategies for treating CHF depend on whether it is a chronic or an acute problem and whether there is systolic or diastolic dysfunction. It is also important to determine the underlying cause of failure and to treat that as well as the symptoms (Miller, 1997).

Pharmacologic Measures

The goal of pharmacologic treatment is to reduce afterload and preload of the heart. Identifying whether one has systolic or diastolic failure is necessary to guide treatment. Table 6–5 is a glossary of terms that APNs must know.

The following drugs are considered the treatment of choice for managing acute and chronic CHF.

First-line drugs are usually diuretics. They reduce afterload, which is associated with systolic dysfunction, and relieve pulmonary congestion, which is associated with diastolic dysfunction.

- Thiazide diuretics (mild CHF)
- Loop diuretics (more effective than thiazides)
- Thiazide-related diuretics (eg, metolazone) (often used in combination with loop diuretics to increase fluid loss)
- K+-sparing diuretics

Second-line drugs to use with diuretics include ACE inhibitors, which are effective preload and afterload reducers (help increase cardiac output, decrease workload).

Traditionally, these drugs have been contraindicated in diastolic dysfunction because of potent afterload reduction, but their effects on reducing myocardial fibrosis and reversing left ventricular hypertrophy may be of benefit (Spencer & Lang, 1997).

- Digoxin: Drug of choice in rapid atrial fibrillation or systolic failure

TABLE 6–5.   GLOSSARY OF TERMS

Afterload: The force the ventricular muscle must generate at systole to overcome the pressure in the aorta to push blood through.

Preload: The passive stretching of the ventricular muscle at end diastole that allows blood to enter it. The more the ventricle is stretched, the greater its force is to release blood volume.

Inotropic state: + increase contractiility
                    – decrease contractility

Chronotropic state: + increase heart rate
                       – decrease heart rate

(works to increase contractility, decrease heart rate). It is *not* to be used with diastolic failure in which ventricular compliance for relaxation and filling is needed.

- Hydralazine: Reduces afterload (used for systolic dysfunction)
- Isosorbide dinitrate: Reduces preload and afterload for systolic dysfunction (Agency for Health Care Policy and Research, 1994). Potent vasodilators must be avoided with diastolic dysfunction (Spencer & Lang, 1997).
- Calcium channel blocker: This drug is effective for diastolic failure; it allows for ventricular relaxation and filling (should not be used with severe CHF because of its negative inotropic effects).
- Beta blocker: Although previously contraindicated because it depresses myocardial response, it is thought to be of benefit for the long-term effects that sympathetic nervous stimulation can have on the myocardium. Use with caution and consideration (Miller, 1997). It is thought to be of benefit in diastolic dysfunction by decreasing heart rate, preventing myocardial ischemia, and decreasing blood pressure and left ventricular hypertrophy (Spencer & Lang, 1997).

Nonpharmacologic Measures

Chronic CHF
- O_2 for room air saturations 85% or less or for complaints of dyspnea
- Dietary sodium restriction (less than 4 g/d)
- Discontinue medications with exacerbating effects such as NSAID

(whose prostaglandin effect on renal function can cause sodium and water retention) or cardiac meds such as digoxin if diastolic dysfunction is determined to be the underlying cause of CHF
- Consider fluid restriction (approximately 1200 to 1500 cc) if known to exacerbate client
- Regular exercise to tolerance
- Home health services
- Discuss advanced directives

Acute CHF (usually requires hospitalization)
- O_2 or mechanical ventilation
- Fluid restriction (less than 1.5 L/day for hyponatremia, or volume overload)
- Interventions used for chronic CHF

Collaboration/Interdisciplinary Involvement

As an APN, collaboration with a physician for managing CHF will depend on your collaborative practice agreement and protocols. Poor response to treatment or medication side effects are an indication for consultation. An acute exacerbation of CHF often requires hospitalization.

Client Education

Education of clients, families, and caregivers is vital for successful management of CHF. Understanding the illness and its treatment helps to promote compliance. A teaching plan focused on monitoring of daily weights, sodium intake, and exercise tolerance can often prevent exacerbations of CHF. Nutritionists can assist the older adult in choosing the appropriate diet. Physical therapists can work with individuals on activity tolerance and energy conservation.

SETTING-SPECIFIC ISSUES

Caring for the community client with CHF poses a challenge because the ability to involve supervision by trained individuals is compromised. Be aware that community clients are at a greater risk of making uninformed decisions regarding their care. Their lack of knowledge surrounding diet, activity tolerance, medications, and symptomatology can delay prompt treatment of exacerbations and promote complications.

In the long-term care setting, the challenge is educating staff to perform accurate and consistent weight monitoring and to report subtle changes in activity tolerance, mentation, and hydration status. These parameters are frequently dismissed as unimportant or as expected aging changes, and may not become apparent until the client becomes quite ill. This delayed recognition leads to poor outcomes.

·········· *vignette* ··········

Mrs. Ryan is an 86-year-old woman with moderate Alzheimer's disease, osteoporosis, and paroxysmal atrial tachycardia. She visits the office for her 3-month primary-care visit. Since her last visit, she has lost 8 lb. When asked how she is feeling, Mrs. Ryan announces that she is pregnant. The client's daughter has noticed a decline in her mother's appetite over the past 2 months. When asked, the daughter reports that her mother has been talking about having a baby for approximately 6 weeks. She is attributing this delusion to her mother's progressive dementia.

The APN reviews Mrs. Ryan's medication regimen. She is taking digoxin 0.125 mg daily

for paroxysmal atrial tachycardia (PAT), calcitonin (Miacalcin) nasal spray daily for osteoporosis, and aspirin 325 mg daily for CVA prevention. The patient's last digoxin level was 0.6 approximately 9 months ago.

On examination, Mrs. Ryan is at her baseline physically and cognitively. The APN is suspicious that Mrs. Ryan may be feeling nauseated from digoxin toxicity or from the Miacalcin and has mistaken this for pregnancy. The client's dementia limits her ability to be specific about her chief complaint.

The APN checks her digoxin level, which is found to be 1.2. The APN decreases the digoxin to 0.125 mg every other day. Upon return to the clinic in 1 month, the client no longer states that she is pregnant and she has regained 5 of the 8 lb she had originally lost. Her cardiac status remains stable.

Individuals with dementia are often unable to be specific about their chief complaint. They may relate their symptoms to past experiences. Caregivers often miss subtle cues to reversible illness, attributing them to a progressive dementia. A "therapeutic level" of a drug may cause toxic side effects.

·········· *vignette* ··········

Mr. Sloan is a 79-year-old white man with history of HTN, coronary artery disease, CABG, Alzheimer's-type dementia, Parkinson's disease, benign prostatic hypertrophy (BPH); atrial fibrillation, and non–insulin-dependent diabetes mellitus (NIDDM). He was admitted from the hospital to a skilled nursing facility status post left CVA, urinary tract infection (UTI), aspiration pneumonia, percutaneous gastrostomy tube (PEG) placement, and CHF (systolic dysfunction).

Medications
- *Metoprolol 25 mg bid*
- *Captopril 37.5 mm qd*
- *Isosorbide 20 mg tid*
- *Lasix 20 mg qd*
- *Coumadin 5 mg qd*
- *Glyburide 2.5 mg qd*

Two weeks after admission, Mr. Sloan had a heart rate of 150 beats/min, respiratory rate 30, and BP of 122/90 (increase from 104/78).

On examination, the client's lungs have bibasilar crackles L > R, with trace edema, and an irregular heartbeat (rate 150s), jugular venous distention (JVBD) is absent.

Assessment
- *Tachycardia and possible atrial fibrillation*
- *Infection*
- *Hypoxia*
- *CHF*
- *MI*

Plan
- *CXR*
- *O_2 saturation*
- *ECG*
- *Labs: CBC, chem panel*

Findings
- *ECG: supraventricular tachycardia (SVT), left bundle branch block (LBBB), atrial fibrillation (rate 130s)*
- *Labs: blood urea nitrogen (BUN) 57, creatinine 0.8, electrolytes within normal limits (WNI), CBC WNL*
- *Chest x-ray: Bilateral pleural effusions consistent with CHF*

Conclusion
- *Tachycardia secondary to CHF*

Plan
- *O_2 2L*
- *Lasix 80 mg today, 40 mg tomorrow, then 20 mg qd*
- *Digoxin 0.5 mg today, 0.25 mg tomorrow, 0.125 mg thereafter*
- *Labs: Lytes, BUN, CRT, digoxin level in 3 days*
- *Weights qd for 5 days*

Assessment after 1 week was as follows: regular heart rate 76; Lungs, clear; BUN 47; Lytes WNL; digoxin level 0.4.

Diuretics are the first choice to treat CHF. Monitoring labs is important with preexisting renal insufficiency. A beta blocker could also have been increased to treat tachycardia, but given a history of atrial fibrillation and DM, adding digoxin seemed a better choice. The ACE inhibitor was already at maximum dose and was therefore not increased.

■ PERIPHERAL VASCULAR DISEASE

Peripheral vascular disease is characterized by decreased tissue perfusion to the extremities, resulting from partial or total occlusion of the arteries and/or veins of the peripheral circulation. The lower extremities are frequently more affected than the upper extremities. Clients with PVD may experience activity intolerance, pain, impaired skin integrity and increased risk for infection.

PERIPHERAL ATHEROSCLEROSIS

Chronically altered blood flow often results in atherosclerosis. Atherosclerotic plaques (atheroma) form on the intimal surface of the artery, causing partial or total occlusion of blood flow to the affected extremity. Risk factors include cigarette smoking, DM, obesity, HTN, hyperlipidemia, positive family history, and advanced age. The development of atherosclerosis occurs insidiously over the course of decades, and symptoms commonly do not appear until over 70% of the artery is occluded (Abrams et al., 1995).

Age-related Changes

Peripheral arterial disease in the elderly, especially those who are sedentary, may be asymptomatic. The characteristic pain of intermittent claudication may be absent, with the client reporting only numbness, coolness, or skin color changes in the legs. These clients typically present to primary-care providers later in the course of the disease process with more serious symptoms such as rest pain or gangrene.

Clinical Presentation

In the client accustomed to walking, intermittent claudication, or pain on ambulation, is the most common complaint associated with chronic arterial occlusion. Pain occurs in the portion of the extremity distal to the occlusion. Occlusion of the femoropopliteal artery causes calf pain; iliofemoral occlusion causes thigh and calf pain, while occlusion of the aortoiliac artery causes pain in the hips and buttocks. Clients may describe a burning, squeezing, or dull ache that forces them to stop walking due to pain or loss of muscle function. Claudication occurs only during ambulation, is relieved by rest without position change, and is reproducible.

An important diagnostic feature to note is that the walk–pain–rest cycle remains constant. However, external factors such as cold and windy weather, walking rapidly, or walking up an incline may shorten the distance a client can ambulate before claudication occurs.

Rest pain is an ominous sign that signals progression of the disease. The pain is most frequently nocturnal and is described as a severe aching pain in the forefoot. The pain is aggravated by elevation of the leg and is relieved when the limb is placed in a dependent position such as hanging over the side of the bed.

Assessment

History. Assess for risk factors associated with arterial disease such as smoking, HTN, DM, hypercholesterolemia, and family history. Assess for pain with ambulation, noting the location, quality, quantity, timing, and setting in which the pain occurs. Assess for aggravating factors and most importantly for techniques the client uses to alleviate the pain.

Physical Examination. In the presence of arterial disease, the central focus of the physical examination should be on the status of the peripheral pulses. The presence or absence of pulses assists in determining the location of the occlusive lesion. Palpate the femoral, popliteal, posterior tibial, and dorsalis pedis arteries, comparing one leg with the other. Auscultate the abdominal aorta, iliac, and femoral arteries to assess for the presence of bruits. Inspect the extremities, comparing size and symmetry. Inspect the skin for changes in color, texture, hair distribution, edema, and the location of any ulcerations. Expect to find thin, dry, shiny skin; diminished hair growth; and thick, brittle toenails on the affected extremity. Elevation of the affected extremity will result in pallor, while dependency of the extremity will result in a deep red color, or rubor. Assess for temperature and capillary refill. The affected extremity will be cooler to the touch and show decreased capillary refill time than the unaffected extremity.

Inspect the feet, especially between the toes, for any ulcerations or necrosis. Ulcerations most commonly develop on distal portions of the foot such as the heels, metatarsal heads, and other bony prominences. The location, size, and depth of the ulcer should be noted, as well as the color of the base and any drainage. The ulcers are exquisitely painful, the with a dry, pale wound bed and absent granulation tissue. Most ulcers result from trauma to the foot by ill-fitting footwear or injuring the foot when walking barefoot.

Diagnostic Studies. When disease is suspected, a Doppler ultrasound examination is recommended to determine the extent of the decrease in blood flow to the lower extremities, to determine the severity of the disease, and to establish a baseline for future reference. Brachial systolic pressures taken in the thigh, upper calf, and ankle also provide useful diagnostic information (Fahey, 1994).

Clinical Management

Interventions are based on the presence or absence of symptoms that limit normal ADL or IADL, as well as the presence of rest pain. Surgical bypass of the occluded segment of the artery is a common and successful treatment option in clients with severe rest pain, persistent ulcerations, and gangrene. In clients considered to be poor surgical candidates,

percutaneous angioplasty is often used, with excellent results.

Medical management of arterial disease must focus on the diagnosis and treatment of underlying conditions such as DM, HTN, and hypercholesterolemia, as these illnesses greatly influence the development and progression of arterial disease. The clinician must also address issues of smoking habits and obesity.

The use of vasodilators has not been proven to be effective in the treatment of arterial disease. Pentoxifylline (Trental), a hemorrheologic agent, may be of some use as it increases oxygen delivery to ischemic areas by improving the flexibility of blood vessels (Kelley, 1994).

DEEP VENOUS THROMBOSIS

Acute thrombus formation can occur at any site within the venous system but most commonly occurs within the deep veins of the lower extremities. Characteristic but not always consistent signs of deep venous thrombosis (DVT) include unilateral swelling of the portion of the leg distal to the occlusion, erythema, and pain.

Clinical Presentation

Rapid onset of unilateral leg swelling with dependent edema is the hallmark of DVT (Abrams et al., 1995). Prerequisites for the development of thrombus formation are venous stasis, trauma to the endothelial lining of the vein wall, and the presence of a hypercoagulable state. Risk factors include prolonged bedrest, obesity, heart failure, history of past DVT, malignant tumors, and estrogen use. Most thrombi form distally and travel to proximal locations within the body such as the pulmonary artery.

Signs suggestive of DVT in the upper leg or thigh include warmth, tenderness, and swelling of the calf. Pain on dorsiflexion of the foot (Homan's sign) may or may not be present. In sedentary individuals such as the elderly, calf vein thrombosis is common without swelling and should be strongly considered in any nonambulating individual. In cases of a small thrombus or when collateral circulation is adequate, physical signs may be absent. The inconsistency of signs and symptoms among clients makes diagnosis difficult.

Assessment

History. Assess for risk factors for DVT. These include previous history of DVT, trauma, surgery, bedrest, and estrogen use.

Physical Examination. Inspect the leg for unilateral calf swelling, warmth, erythema, tenderness, and Homan's sign. Note that signs and symptoms may vary, depending on thrombus size, development of collateral circulation, and location of the affected vein.

Diagnostic Studies. Noninvasive testing for DVT includes combined Doppler and ultrasound imaging, duplex scanning, contrast venography, and impedance plethysmography. Contrast venography is the most reliable diagnostic tool for detection of DVT but has been replaced by noninvasive methods such as Doppler imaging. Laboratory data including a coagulation profile should be obtained along with diagnostic testing.

Clinical Management

In high-risk clients, preventative measures such as administration of low-dose heparin, combined with external compression via elastic stocking or pneumatic compression devices should be used as warranted. In clients with diagnosed DVT, bedrest to prevent the clot from being dislodged is paramount. Systemic heparinization should be initiated and continued for 1 week while simultaneously administering oral anticoagulation with warfarin. Anticoagulation should continue for 3 to 4 months, with close monitoring of the standardized INR. For treatment of DVT, an INR of 2.0 to 3.0 should be maintained (Fahey, 1994). Enoxaparin (Lovenox), a low-molecular-weight heparin (LMWH), can be used an alternative to standard heparin therapy. The advantages of LMWHs include home administration, more predictable dosing among clients, and decreased incidence of bleeding (Hillis, 1997).

 ## CASE STUDY #1

Mr. Cox is a 68-year-old black man with a past medical history of blindness secondary to macular degeneration, NIDDM, mild dementia, and cervical stenosis. He has been a nursing home resident for several years and is well known to the staff. You receive a phone call from the charge nurse on his unit telling you that somthing is not "right" with him. He is diaphoretic, somewhat agitated, and refusing to eat his breakfast.

1. What instructions would you give to the nurse?

   Obtain a full set of vital signs (VS) and oxygen saturation (if available), check his blood sugar, and bring oxygen to the bedside.

You are at Mr. Cox's bedside within 5 minutes. His respiratory rate is 26; he is in no apparent distress. He is slightly diaphoretic, with a temperature of 98.8°F. Oximetry on room air is 94%, his BP is 130/80, and his heart rate is 100 and slightly irregular. His blood glucose is 97. He is able to answer questions and states that he has had a "bad feeling" in his chest, which has come and gone since this morning.

2. What information should you seek through your iinterview and physical examination?

   You should focus on a detailed description of the chest discomfort: what brought it on, where it is located, any associated symptoms, what makes it better, what makes it worse, and whether it radiates. Ask Mr. Cox to describe the type of feeling in more detail. It is intermittent or constant? Has he ever had it before? Has he ever been diagnosed with angina or heart disease? It is usually helpful to ask the client to quantitate the degree of pain by using a scale of 1 to 10, in which 1 is the least bothersome pain and 10 is the most severe. In the case of a dementia client, it may be difficult to obtain answers to questions, and reliance on more objective data might be necessary.

Other information to gather from Mr. Cox's chart would be any diagnosis of CHD or angina, his medical diagnoses in general, medications, baseline ECG, risk factors for CHD, usual state of health, and advanced directives.

A physical exam should note any disturbance in neurologic status: Is it intact? Are there any focal changes? Is his mental status at baseline? Is his respiratory status labored or effort increased? Are his lungs clear, or are there adventitious sounds such as rales? Is his skin color normal, or is there cyanosis? Are heart sounds normal, or is there a new murmur or S3? Is his heart rate abnormally fast or slow? Are there changes in the ECG (if available)? The examination at this point should be focused, as decision making regarding the next treatment step is paramout.

Mr. Cox states that he has never had this type of feeling before; he is very nauseous and feels as though there is a heaviness across his shoulders. He says it has come and gone since before breakfast, and the Tylenol the nurse gave him did not help. He rates the pain a 6 on the pain scale. The pain does not radiate; it appears to be associated with nausea and diaphoresis. His past medical history is significant for pneumonia and DM; the physical exam is noncontributory, and ECG is not available. At this point, Mr. Cox is having the "bad feeling." You give him a 1/150 SL NTG and stay at his bedside.

3. What other supportive treatment might be appropriate at this time?

Administration of low flow oxygen 1 to 2 L.

Mr. Cox states that the feeling is a little better. His BP is 110/60; you give him a second NTG. The feeling is unchanged, and his BP is 100/60 in 5 minutes.

4. What would be your next step?

Repeat NTG for the third and final time. Ask the nursing staff to begin to prepare the paperwork for transfer to the ER, and call the physician. Give the client ASA 325 mg tab to be chewed, and explain that you are calling his doctor and advising that he be sent to the hospital for evaluation.

The physician agrees with your assessment of possible unstable angina with a risk factor of elderly male diabetic. You call triage in the ER to give them a report. When Mr. Cox arrives there an ECG shows a new left bundle branch block; cardiac enzymes and isoenzymes are drawn. He is treated with IV morphine and topical nitrates for pain and admitted to a monitored bed. His cardiac enzymes are normal. He is seen by a cardiologist, who makes the diagnosis of unstable angina but not MI.

5. What medication is he most likely to start on a regular basis?

Probably a PO nitrate as a first-line drug in the treatment of angina. Other possibilities include calcium channel blockers and beta blockers, depending on underlying conditions.

The cardiologist orders an echocardiogram, which shows some mitral regurgitation and an EF of 45%. He also recommends that a stress test be done on the client as an outpatient.

6. In terms of assessing CHD risk factors, what lab work needs to be checked on Mr. Cox?

Cholesterol profile, triglyceride levels, and glycosylated hemoglobin must be checked. Results are as follows:
- Total cholesterol: 230
- LDL: 156
- HDL: 24
- Triglycerides: 359
- Glycosylated hemoglobin: 10.6

Mr. Cox is on a regular diet with no added sweets secondary to his SM.

7. What information do you need to obtain as you begin to plan dietary modifications?

Determine his eating habits: Does he have trouble chewing? Does he eat only what is provided by the home, or does he have food brought in? Have there been recent fluctuations in his weight?

You find that Mr. Cox eats the food that the institution gives him; you speak with him regarding changing his diet to low cholesterol and he agrees to try.

8. What other life-style modifications need to be addressed?

Tobacco and alcohol usage, and exercise patterns.

Mr. Cox does not smoke tobacco or drink alcohol, nor does he have a history of either. Because of his sensory deficits, he leads a very sedentary life. He tells you he is most comfortable sitting in his room because he is afraid of falling.

9. What type interventions might you suggest?

Walking around the various floors in the facility for approximately 20 minutes three times a week, with the help of the recreation staff as well as participating in either weight lifting or an aerobic exercise in which he could be essentially stationary.

Mr. Cox agrees to the exercise and dietary changes.

10. When would be an appropriate time to recheck cholesterol level?

Approximately 6 weeks to 3 months.

 ## CASE STUDY #2

Mrs. Martin is a 75-year-old woman with a 10-year history of HTN and angina. She was recently diagnosed with breast cancer and is undergoing chemotherapy. Medications include diltiazem (Cardizem CD) 240 mg/d and ASA 325 mg/d. Approximately 10 days after her chemotherapy, she presents to your clinic complaining of cough productive of yellow sputum and a "racing heart." Her temperature is 98°F orally, respiratory rate is 32, BP is 100/54, and heart rate is irregular at approximately 136 beats/min. She appears to be in mild respiratory distress, with audible wheezing throughout, and states that she feels short of breath. On examination, the nasopharynx is clear; the lungs are auscultated for high-pitched inspiratory and expiratory wheezes, with decreased breath sounds at the bases; and the heartbeat is irregular, with 3/6 systolic murmur and no S3 gallop. The abdominal exam is benign; the extremities are cool, with 1+ pitting edema on the right; pulses throughout are equal.

1. What further actions would you take?

    a. Obtain O_2 saturation and/or arterial blood gases; apply oxygen

    b. Obtain stat chest x-ray to rule out infiltrate and CHF.

    c. Obtain stat ECG to rule out arrhythmia and ischemia.

Chest x-ray confirms a new left lower lobe infiltrate, with no change in chronic bilateral pleural effusions, right greater than left. An ECG demonstrates AF with a ventricular response of 130 to 140 and LVH. A CBC shows an absolute neutrophil count of 500. You call Mrs. Martin's oncologist with this update and he advises you to directly admit her to the intensive care unit (ICU) for rapid AF and pneumonia. As you are waiting for transport, she begins to complain of pain in her left arm and a feeling of nauseousness.

2. What interventions would be apppropriate?

    Recheck apical rate and BP; recheck EKG; draw a full set of labs, including cardiac enzymes; and administer SL NTG, noting any effect on pain.

Mrs. Martin feels better, but she still feels weak. She is transferred to the ICU for monitoring, treatment for pneumonia, and control of heart rate. She is loaded with IV digoxin over 24 hours to help reduce her heart rate, and started on metoprolol tartrate (Lopressor). The cardiologist orders a transesophageal echocardiogram.

3. What information can this test relay and what are potential reasons for his ordering this test?

    It provides information regarding valvular function, kinetics of wall movement, EF, whether any thrombi exist in the heart, and so forth. The cardiologist may be contemplating whether cardioversion might be an option in trying to convert the client out of AF to sinus rhythm and needs to determine risk of embolization from a thrombus..

Mrs. Martin's condition improves. Her neutropenia resolves, the pneumonia is responding to the antibiotics and respiratory treatments, and she has had no further chest pain. Electrocardiographic findings and cardiac enzymes are negative for MI. The cardiologist does recommend that Mrs. Martin be started on Coumadin, as AF is a major risk factor for stroke if the client is not anticoagulated. She discusses this with her oncologist, and they decide to go along with the anticoagulation. She is given a 5-mg dose on day 1, then reduced to 2 mg/d.

4. What blood tests are used to monitor the response to anticoagulation and what should be the target range?

    The client should have close monitoring of PT/INR, usually daily for approximately 4 to 5 days (takes approximately 3 days to reach steady state), then every 3 days minimally while having the dose adjusted. Because of the bleeding risks associated with chemotherapy, the desired range of anticoagulation for AF in this client is an INR of 1.5 to 2.5. An elderly client, in otherwise good health who is not a fall risk could be carefully maintained at an INR between 2 and 3 for optimal prophylaxis against stroke.

Mrs. Martin comes in for her follow-up clinic visit. She is taking a "break" from chemotherapy and is feeling much better. Her main concern is that the new medications are making her feel lightheaded and making it difficult to help care for her husband, who is wheelchair bound. You also suspect that she may be concerned about the cost of the additional medications.

5. How might you approach this situation?

Ask her directly if she believes the medicine is making her worse, and explain to her that the medications will help control her heart rate and reduce her chance of stroke. Ask her if she is having trouble coping with the care of her husband or with financial issues and if she would like to speak with a social worker or a representative from her community regarding resources that might be available for the elderly.

■ REFERENCES

Abrams, W. B., Beers, M. H., and Berkow, R. (Eds.). *The Merck manual of geriatrics.* (2nd ed.). (1995). Whitehouse Station, NJ: Merck.

Agency for Health Care Policy and Research. (1994) *Heart failure: Management of patients with left ventricular systolic dysfunction.* Rockville, MD: Author. Publication #94-0613.

AHA. (1995) American Heart Association consensus panel statement: Preventing heart attack and death in patients with coronary disease. *Circulation, 92,* 2–4.

Amsterdam, E. A., Lakier, J. B., & Wharton, T. P. (1996). Managing MI in the community hospital. *Patient Care, 30,* 26–33.

Albers, G. W. (1994). Atrial fibrillation and stroke. *Arch Intern Med, 154,* 1443–1448.

Arnstein, P. M., Buselli, E. F., & Rankin, S. H. (1996). Women and heart attacks: Prevention, diagnosis and care. *Nurs Pract, 21,* (5), 57–68.

Aronow, W. S. (1996) Management of Atrial Fibrillation in Older Nursing Home Residents. *Nur Home Med, 4*(11), 332–339.

Atkins, D., & Garber, A. When experts disagree: The cholesterol standoff. *Pat Care, 30*(20), 62–91.

Bales, A. C., & Sorrentino, M. J. (1997) Causes of congestive heart failure: Prompt diagnosis may affect prognosis. *Postgrad Med, 101*(1), 44–56.

Baron, R. B. (1992). High blood cholesterol: Screening and interventions. In Dornbrand, L., Hooke, A. J., & Pickard, G. (Eds.), *Manual of clinical problems in adult ambulatory care* (pp. 619–626). Boston: Little, Brown and Company.

Bates, B. (1995). A guide to physical examination and history taking. Philadelphia: J. B. Lippincott.

Bell, R. T., & Pinkowish, M. D. (1996). Primary angioplasty for community hospitals? *Pat Care, 29*(2), 22–25.

Bergman-Evans, B. (1996). Hypertension in older adults. *Adv Nurse Pract, 52,* 23–25.

Berman, N. D. (1982). *Geriatric cardiology* (pp. 11–20). Lexington, KY: The Callamore Press.

Bittle, J. A., Craver, J. M., Mills, N., Ryan, T. J.,

& Weintraub, W. (1996). Bypass or angioplasty: Which one when? *Pat Care, 30*(6), 18–31.

Calkins, E., Ford, A. B., & Katz, P. R. (1992). *Practice of geriatrics.* Philadelphia: W. B. Saunders.

Davidson, M. U., Testolin, L. M., Maki, K. C., von Dwillard, S., & Drennan, K. B. (1997). A comparison of estrogen replacement, pravastatin, and combined treatment for the management of hypercholesterolemia in postmenopausal women. *Arch Intern Med, 157*(11), 1186–1192.

Ebersole, P., & Hess, P. (1990). *Toward healthy aging: Human needs and nursing response* (3rd ed.). St. Louis: C. V. Mosby.

Fahey, V. A. (1994). Venous thromboembolism. In Fahey, V. A. (Ed.). *Vascular nursing.* (pp. 405–431). Philadelphia: W. B. Saunders.

Futterman, L. G., & Lemberg, L. (1996). Atrial fibrillation: An increasingly common and provocative arrhythmia. *Am J Crit Care, 5*(5), 379–387.

Goroll, A. H., May, L. A., & Mulley, A. G. (Eds). (1995). *Primary care medicine* (3rd ed.). Philadelphia: J. B. Lippincott.

Hahn, M. S. (1995). Matters of the heart. *Adv Nurse Pract,* 42, 13–19.

Harpaz, D., Benderly, M., Goldbourt, U. (1996). Effect of aspirin on mortality in women with symptomatic or silent myocardial ischemia. *Am J Cardiol, 78,* 1215–1219.

Hebert, P. R., Gaziano J. M., Chan, K. S., & Kennehan, C. H. (1997). Cholesterol lowering with itrial drop, risk of stroke, and mortality. *JAMA, 278*(4): 313–321.

Hillis, L. B. (1997). Low molecular weight heparins. A pharmacologic overview. *Adv for Nurse Pract, 5,* 53–56.

Joint National Committee on Detection, Evaluation, and Treatment of High Blood Pressure. (1993). The Fifth Report of the Joint National Committee on Detection, Evaluation, and Treatment of High Blood Pressure. National Institutes of Health, National Heart, Lung, and Blood Institute. NIH Publication No. 93-1088.

Kelley, W. N. (Ed.). (1994). *Essentials of internal medicine.* (pp. 49–52). Philadelphia: J. B. Lippincott.

La Croix, A. Z., Leweille, S. G. Hecht, J. A., Grothan, L. C., & Wagner, E. U. (1996). Does walking decrease the risk of cardiovascular disease hospitalizations and death in older adults? *J Am Geriatr Soc, 44,* 113–120.

Larosa, J. C. (1996). Does reducing cholesterol improve CAD survival? *Patient Care, 30*(5), 61–74.

Miller, S. K. (1997). Congestive heart failure: Clinical assessment and pharmacological management. *Ad for Nurse Pract, 5* (6), 17–26.

National Institutes of Health Consensus Statement. (1993). Coronary heart disease. *JAMA, 269*(4). 1186–1192.

Pennachio, D. (1996). When experts disagree: The cholesterol standoff. *Patient Care, 30*(20), 62–66.

Reece, S. M. (1995). Toward the prevention of coronary heart disease: Screening of children and adolescents for high blood cholesterol. *Nurs Pract, 20*(2), 22–35.

Selwyn, A. P., & Brownwald, E. (1993). Ischemic heart disease. In Iwelbacher, K. J., Brownworld, E., Wilson, J. D., Marhn, J. B., Fauci, A. S., & Ikospo, D. L. (Eds.). *Harrison's principles of internal medicine* (pp. 1077–1084). McGraw-Hill, Inc. (3rd ed.) New York.

SHEP Cooperative Research Group. (1997). Prevention of stroke by antihypertensive drug treatment in older persons with isolated systolic hypertension. *JAMA 278*(3), 212–216.

Siscovich, D. S. (1992). Exercise. In Dornbrand, L., Hoole, A. J., & Pickard, C. G. (Eds.), *Manual of clinical problems in adult ambulatory care* (pp. 626–629). Boston: Little, Brown.

Sivaram, C. A., Ahmed, N., & Lestina, J. R. (1996). Electrocardiogram in the ambulatory clinic in older patients with cardiac disease: An assessment of the contribution to management. *JAGS, 44,* 452–455.

Smith, S. C. (1995). Consensus panel statement: Preventing heart attack and death in patients with coronary disease. *Circulation, 92,* 2–4.

Soumerai, S. B., McLaughlin, T. J., & Speigelman, D. (1997). Adverse outcomes of underuse of β-blockers in elderly survivors of acute MI. *JAMA, 277,* 115–21.

Spencer, K. T., & Lang, R. M. (1997). Diastolic heart failure: What primary care physicians need to know. *Postgrad Med, 101*(1), 63–78.

Sullivan, M., Lacroix, A., Baum, C., et al. (1996). Coronary disease severity and functional impairment: How strong is the relation. *J Am Geriatr Soc, 44,* 1461–1465.

Vaitkevicius, P. V., & Fleg, J. L. (1996). An abnormal exercise treadmill test in an asymptomatic older patient. *J Am Geriatr Soc, 44,* 83–88.

Yontz, L. L. (1994). Congestive heart failure: Early recognition of congestive heart failure in the primary care setting. *J Am Acad Nurse Pract, 6*(6), 273–278.

Zeleznik, J., & Jacobs, L. G. (1996). Anticoagulation for prevention of stroke in long term care residents. *Long Term Care Forum, 6*(1), 1–15.

7

TOPICS IN GASTROINTESTINAL CARE

Courtney H. Lyder • Sheila L. Molony

■ INTRODUCTION

Gastrointestinal (GI) complaints in the elderly are common and potentially deceptive. Loss of appetite, vague abdominal discomfort, and changes in bowel habits may represent benign conditions such as gastroenteritis or irritable bowel syndrome, or may be the only clues to life-threatening emergencies such as mesenteric artery thrombosis or ruptured diverticulum.

Colorectal cancer, diverticulitis, gastritis, and peptic ulcer disease (PUD) may each present with silent blood loss as the earliest or only symptom. Older adults may not seek out a clinician to report symptoms of dyspepsia, bloating, weight loss, or constipation, viewing these as misfortunes of old age that must be tolerated. The advanced practice nurse (APN) needs to use case-finding strategies such as symptom review, weight screening, dietary recall, and testing stool for occult blood to improve detec-

tion and treatment outcomes. Chapters 1 and 2 in this text review prevention, case finding, and wellness care. The emphasis in this chapter is on commonly encountered conditions and nuances of disease presentation and management in the elderly.

■ ANOREXIA

Anorexia in the elderly is a frequent nonspecific symptom of underlying systemic disease. Its presence, particularly in conjunction with overall functional decline, warrants comprehensive assessment.

AGE-RELATED CHANGES

A decrease in the sense of taste and smell frequently accompanies aging and may impact appetite and food enjoyment. Poor dental health, poor-fitting dentures, and decreased saliva production may also adversely affect food intake. A significant change in appetite or intake, especially in conjunction with weight loss, warrants further assessment and should not be attributed to normal aging.

ASSESSMENT

History
Review oral health and cardiac, respiratory, GI, and urinary systems. Assess personal and family history of cancer, tuberculosis (TB), and thyroid disease. Assess dietary intake, prior eating patterns, food preferences, and weight history. Review alcohol and cigarette usage and medication history, including all over-the-counter (OTC) medicines. Take a careful history of bowel habits and use of laxatives or enemas. Assess history of bereavement, losses, life changes, and stressors. Assess for history of dementia or symptoms of memory loss or changes in cognition or mood. Determine functional abilities and degree of social isolation.

Physical Examination
Check weight and vital signs. Assess integumentary system, thyroid, heart, lungs, and abdomen. Perform oral, breast, prostate, and rectal exams and check stool for occult blood. Screen mental status and assess for depression.

Diagnostic Studies
Check glucose, electrolytes, blood urea nitrogen (BUN), creatinine, and B_{12} level. Perform a complete blood count (CBC), liver function tests (LFTs), thyroid studies, and urinalysis (UA). Check drug levels of any medicines with potential for toxicity. Obtain a chest x-ray if congestive heart failure (CHF) or pneumonia is suspected.

CLINICAL MANAGEMENT

Treatment of anorexia is dependent on identification and treatment of the specific cause (see Table 7–1). General measures to stimulate appetite such as attractive presentation of food; use of small portions; and a relaxed, social dining atmosphere are always useful. Food preferences should be honored whenever possible.

SETTING-SPECIFIC ISSUES

Elders living alone require assessment of food shopping and preparation abilities. It may be undesirable to dine alone or prepare a meal for one. Community resources such as grocery delivery, Meals on Wheels, congregate dining, and homemakers may be employed to improve nutritional intake. In the hospital or long-term care facility, special attention must be paid to the appearance, taste, temperature, and amount of food. Honoring client preferences and allowing home-cooked meals if available may improve appetite. Dietary restrictions should be critically examined for benefits and risks. Adequate feeding time and appropriate functional assistance are important interventions for clients dependent on a caregiver for nutrition. A relaxed, social, odor-free dining atmosphere may be difficult to achieve but will improve appetite.

COLLABORATION AND REFERRAL

Clients with persistent anorexia or significant weight loss should be referred to the physician. Follow-up to ensure adequate symptom resolution and prevention of weight loss and dehydration is es-

TABLE 7–1. POTENTIAL CAUSES OF ANOREXIA IN THE ELDERLY

Cancer	**Psychiatric disorders**
Tumor	Dementia
Radiation	Delirium
Chemotherapy	Paranoia
Pain	Mania
	Eating disorder
Depression/bereavement	
	Drugs
	Alcohol
GI tract disorders	Medication toxicity
Peptic ulcer	Medication side effect
Abdominal ischemia	
Esophageal candidiasis	**Metabolic disease**
Hepatitis	Thyroid disease
Gastritis	Pituitary disease
Loss of taste	Renal failure
Poor dentition/denture fit	Liver failure
Constipation/impaction	Diabetes
Mouth lesions	Pernicious anemia
	Ketoacidosis
Infection	Hypercalcemia
UTI	Hypokalemia
Pneumonia	
Appendicitis	**Other**
TB	New food or environment
AIDS	Social isolation
Repeated minor infections	Poverty
	Functional impairment
	Feeding problems
	Severe CHF

GI, gastrointestinal; UTI, urinary tract infection; TB, tuberculosis; AIDS, acquired immune deficiency syndrome; CHF, congestive heart failure.

sential. The registered dietitian is an invaluable resource in nutritional assessment and intervention. An occupational therapist may suggest feeding aids or strategies to improve functional independence in eating. A speech therapist may be consulted for symptoms of dysphagia. Psychiatric follow-up is indicated for clients with depression or symptoms suggestive of an eating disorder.

.... *vignette* ....

Mrs. Crane is a long-term care resident with a past history of cerebrovascular accident (CVA) with left-sided hemiparesis and global aphasia. She was seen in consultation by the APN for symptoms of poor appetite, poor oral intake, and progressive weight loss. Mrs. Crane was usually seen in bed, occasionally in a wheel-

chair, appearing apathetic and sad. Assessment first required determination of her ability to understand verbal communication and to respond to questions. An aphasia assessment was conducted, and it was determined that Mrs. Crane's receptive communication skills were intact and she could answer yes/no questions using eye blinks. History taking suggested severe depression with suicidal ideation but no plan. Physical examination revealed a painful oral abscess, probably caused by food pocketing. Lab studies revealed undiagnosed diabetes mellitus. Pharmacologic treatment for diabetes, abscess, depression, dental consultation, and supportive psychosocial measures were implemented. Nurses were educated in communication strategies, and a speech therapist was consulted. Mrs. Crane's weight and intake stabilized and her mood improved. She began smiling for the first time since her stroke and engaged in reading newspapers and listening to books and music on tape.

■ GASTROESOPHAGEAL REFLUX DISEASE

Approximately 36% of adults report heartburn at least once a month, while 7% reported daily symptoms (Goroll, May, & Mulley, 1995). An estimated 30% to 40% of these clients will have mucosal injury (esophagitis). Severe or chronic reflux may lead to esophageal ulcers, strictures, Barrett's esophagus, asthma, and chronic cough. Reflux occurs as a result of inappropriate relaxation of the lower esophageal sphincter (LES) or a decrease in LES tone. Increased intra-abdominal pressure and delayed gastric emptying (a common aging change) may

contribute to this problem. The presence of a hiatal hernia does not necessarily correlate with reflux and is not considered a primary factor in treatment of gastroesophageal reflux disease (GERD).

AGE-RELATED CHANGES

A decline in gastric motility and emptying has been noted with advancing age (Lonergan, 1996). These changes may contribute to reflux in the older population.

CLINICAL PRESENTATION

The typical symptoms of reflux include heartburn and regurgitation within 30 to 60 minutes of eating. Symptoms are aggravated by bending over or lying down and may be relieved with antacids. Some clients present with chest pain, heaviness, or pressure that mimics angina. Less typical presentations include recurrent pneumonia, bronchospasm, and chronic cough, which may be the result of nocturnal aspiration of gastric acid and enzymes. Excess saliva or "water brash," hoarseness, sore throat, and feeling a "lump in the throat" may also stem from GERD. Dental erosion has also been noted as an atypical presentation of disease (Schroeder et al., 1995). The disease does not present differently in the elderly but does require more detailed investigation since cardiac disease, cholelithiasis, PUD, and gastric carcinoma need to be considered in the differential diagnosis.

ASSESSMENT

History
Assess symptom onset, character, location, radiation, quality, and timing, including relation to meals, smoking, caf-

feine, or spicy foods. Review cardiopulmonary and GI systems. Medication history and dietary intake assessment should be performed. Aggravating and relieving factors and any associated symptoms such as dysphagia, nausea, bloating, fullness, belching, weight loss, and fatigue should be assessed.

Physical Examination

Assess heart, lungs, thorax, and abdomen and check stools for occult blood.

Diagnostic Studies

While younger clients with uncomplicated symptoms of reflux may be treated empirically, older adults should be referred to the physician or gastroenterologist for specific tests to confirm diagnosis and rule out gastric malignancy or ulceration. Studies may include 24-hour ambulatory esophageal pH monitoring, barium studies, or endoscopy. Electrocardiogram (ECG) and cardiac enzymes are indicated if the clinician suspects cardiac disease.

CLINICAL MANAGEMENT

Gastroesophageal reflux disease is a chronic condition requiring lifelong treatment. Relapse rates are high. Client education is crucial to symptom management. Nonpharmacologic measures form the cornerstone of any treatment plan. Clients should be instructed to avoid smoking, alcohol, spicy foods, caffeine, peppermint, and spearmint. They should avoid large meals and eating within 2 to 3 hours of bedtime or before lying down. A low-fat diet and maintenance of ideal body weight is helpful, as is elevating the head of the bed on 6- to 8-inch blocks.

Medications that lower esophageal sphincter pressure should be avoided if possible. These include theophylline, calcium channel blockers, anticholinergics, and benzodiazepines.

If nonpharmacologic measures fail to resolve the problem, medication therapy is initiated in stepwise fashion (see Table 7–2). Histamine (H_2-receptor) antagonists block parietal cell acid secretion and are the first and primary agents used in the management of GERD. Cimetidine has been reported to cause side effects in the elderly, such as confusion and dizziness, and poses significant drug interactions. H_2 blockers should be given twice a day (unlike ulcer therapy), and some clients require high-dose therapy for symptom relief. Approximately 50% of clients will have recurrent esophagitis despite high-dose H_2-blocker therapy (Sullivan & Samuelson, 1996).

The next step in GERD management would be to add a proton pump inhibitor, such as omeprazole or lansoprazole, which causes marked acid suppression. Omeprazole alone or in combination with cisapride has been shown to produce an 80% to 89% remission rate in clients with refractory disease (Vignieri et al., 1995). Klinkenberg-Knol et al. (1994) treated 86 patients with omeprazole for 5 years and found increases in gastrin levels and a progression toward atrophic gastritis. Further studies are needed to demonstrate long-term outcomes.

Prokinetic agents such as metoclopramide and cisapride increase LES pressure and enhance gastric emptying. They are useful particularly for nocturnal symptoms and for clients with gastroparesis. Metoclopramide may cause side effects in older adults, such as confusion, drowsiness, agitation, depression, and ex-

TABLE 7–2.   ACID SUPPRESSIVE AND PROMOTILITY MEDICATIONS

	Standard-dose Therapy	Cost for 30-Day Supply	High-dose Therapy	Cost for 30-Day Supply
Histamine H$_2$-Receptor Antagonists				
Cimetidine[a] (Tagamet[b])	800 mg qhs	$42.80 (generic) $81.80	800 mg bid	$80.60 (generic) $158.65
Famotidine (Pepcid**)	20 mg bid	$91.30	40 mg bid	$171.75
Nizatidine (Axid)	150 mg bid 300 mg qhs	$91.40 $88.60		
Ranitidine (Zantac)	150 mg bid	$94.30	300 mg bid	$167.20
Proton Pump Inhibitors				
Lansoprazole (Prevacid)	15 mg qd	$97.15	30 mg qd	$98.90
Omeprazole (Prilosec)	20 mg qd	$103.00	40 mg qd	$201.00
Prokinetic Agents				
Bethanechol (Urecholine)	25 mg qid[c]	$12.00		
Cisapride (Propulsid)	10 mg qid	$75.65		
Metoclopramide[a] (Reglan)	10 mg qid	$23.00 (generic) $98.00		

[a] Generic.
[b] Available in OTC strength.
[c] Contraindicated in asthma patients.

Source: Adapted from Sullivan, C. & Samuelson, W. (1996). Acid suppressive and promotility medications, *Nurse Practitioner, 21* (11):94. Used with permission from the November 1990 issue of *Nurse Practitioner.* © Springhouse Corporation.

trapyramidal symptoms, and should be used with caution. Cisapride is better tolerated in the elderly, but recent concerns about drug interactions warrant further study. Bethanechol is sometimes used to enhance LES pressure and increase amplitude of contractions in the GI tract. It does not result in an increase in coordinated contractions, and its use is contraindicated in asthma.

Clients with severe or relapsing disease should be referred for further evaluation and management.

■ PEPTIC ULCER DISEASE

Approximately 10% of Americans will have peptic ulcer disease at some time in their life (Heslin, 1997). Morbidity and mortality due to PUD rises rapidly with advancing age. Upper GI bleeding and perforation occur with increased frequency and are often subtle or silent in their presentation. The frequent use of nonsteroidal anti-inflammatory drugs (NSAIDs) in the older population increases ulcer risk. (Smalley and Griffin, 1996).

AGE-RELATED CHANGES

Stomach acid production may decrease slightly with age. There is an increase in achlorhydria, atrophic gastritis, and pernicious anemia. Mucosal defenses remain intact in the absence of NSAID therapy, *Helicobacter pylori* infection, or serious illness. Approximately 80% of the current population of older adults is infected with *H. pylori,* an important correlate of PUD.

CLINICAL PRESENTATION

Duodenal ulcers typically present with burning, gnawing epigastric pain that is relieved by food. Gastric ulcers may be aggravated by food intake. (Shaw, 1996). Both types of ulcers may be accompanied by nausea, vomiting, anorexia, and complaints of bloating or belching.

The older adult may experience little or no epigastric discomfort in the presence of severe ulcer disease. Significant anemia and bleeding may be the first indicators of pathology. Even in the presence of perforation with peritonitis, the usual indices such as pain, fever, and rebound tenderness may be absent. Involuntary guarding, mental confusion, and modest leukocytosis may be the only signs of inflammation.

ASSESSMENT

History

Review cardiac and GI symptoms, history of tobacco and alcohol usage, medication history, and psychosocial assessment. Assess the relationship between symptoms and food or antacid intake. Obtain past history of gallbladder disease or surgery, cardiac disease, gastritis, or ulcer disease.

Physical Examination

Abdominal, cardiac, and respiratory examination and stool guaiac are indicated.

Diagnostic Studies

A CBC will help detect leukocytosis and anemia. Check serum amylase and bilirubin. Liver function tests and abdominal ultrasound may be useful if gallbladder or pancreatic disease is suspected. Clients with burning or gnawing epigastric pain should be tested for *H. pylori* infection. Serologic and breath tests are available, but the consulting physician or gastroenterologist may wish to pursue *H. pylori* testing in conjunction with endoscopy.

CLINICAL MANAGEMENT

While empiric therapy is often initiated in the younger client, physician referral for endoscopy or other upper GI evaluation is indicated due to the higher incidence of gastric malignancies, gastritis, and bleeding ulcers. The cost effectiveness of this approach is currently being studied (Fendrick et al., 1996). Confirmation of ulcer disease with or without *H. pylori* infection warrants treatment.

Pharmacologic Measures

Eradication of *H. pylori* in affected individuals results in ulcer healing and dramatically decreases the recurrence rate. Many drug regimens have been recommended for this purpose. Combination therapy is indicated due to frequent drug resistance. Bismuth subsalicylate, metronidazole, and tetracycline or ampicillin is the most common regimen. Cost, client compliance, history of adverse drug reactions, and prior drug exposure will determine which regime is selected. Table 7–3 outlines cost and dosing schedules for several treatment regimes which result in healing in 83% to 94% of cases (*Medical Letter,* 1997). H_2 blockers are prescribed as part of or in addition to antibiotic therapy to improve healing. Maintenance H_2-blocker therapy is often prescribed for at least 6 months.

TABLE 7–3.   SOME DRUG REGIMENS FOR *H. PYLORI*

Drugs	Daily Dose	Duration	Cost[a]
*Bismuth subsalicylate (generic)	2 tablets (525 mg) qid	2 weeks	$10.38
+ Metronidazole (generic)	250 mg qid	2 weeks	1.85
+ Tetracycline (generic)	500 mg qid	2 weeks	3.49
+ Ranitidine (*Zantac*)[b]	150 mg bid	2 weeks	44.64
			$60.36
Helidac Therapy[c]		2 weeks	77.70
+ Ranitidine (*Zantac*)[b]	150 mg bid	2 weeks	44.64
			$122.34
*Clarithromycin (*Biaxin*)	500 mg tid	2 weeks	$136.91
+ Omeprazole (*Prilosec*)	40 mg once	2 weeks	101.64
followed by omeprazole	20 mg once	2 weeks	50.82
			$289.37
Clarithromycin	500 mg bid	10 days	65.20
+ Omeprazole	20 mg bid	10 days	72.60
OR lansoprazole (*Prevacid*)	15 mg bid	10 days	67.17
+ Metronidazole	500 mg bid	10 days	1.37
OR amoxicillin (generic)	1 gram bid	10 days	9.18
			$133.741–146.98
*Ranitidine bismuth citrate (*Tritec*)[d]	400 mg bid	2 weeks	$48.72
+ Clarithromycin	500 mg tid	2 weeks	136.91
followed by ranitidine bismuth citrate	400 mg bid	2 weeks	48.72
			$234.35

* FDA-approved regimens.
[a] Cost to pharmacist based on wholesale price (AWP or HCFA) listings in *Drug Topics Red Book* 1996 and December *Update*.
[b] Or any other H_2-receptor antagonist.
[c] *Helidac Therapy* is supplied as 14 blister cards, each containing eight 262.4-mg bismuth subsalicylate tablets, four 250-mg metronidazole tablets, and four 500-mg tetracycline tablets.
[d] Equivalent to 162 mg of ranitidine, 128 mg of trivalent bismuth, and 110 mg of citrate.
Source: Adapted from "Some drug regimens for *H. pylori*." (1997). *The Medical Letter, 39*(991), 2.

Irrespective of *H. pylori* infection, peptic ulcers may be treated pharmacologically using histamine blockers, sucralfate, or proton pump inhibitors. A single daily dose of ranitidine, famotidine, or nizatidine at bedtime is given for 8 to 12 weeks until healing occurs, followed by maintenance doses. Sucralfate is believed to form a protective coating on the ulcer base and is also effective in healing. It may cause constipation. Proton pump inhibitors (omeprazole and lansoprazole) profoundly decrease acid secretion and are recommended for Zollinger–Ellison syndrome and refractory GERD. Proton pump inhibitors are effective in ulcer healing even in the presence of NSAID therapy.

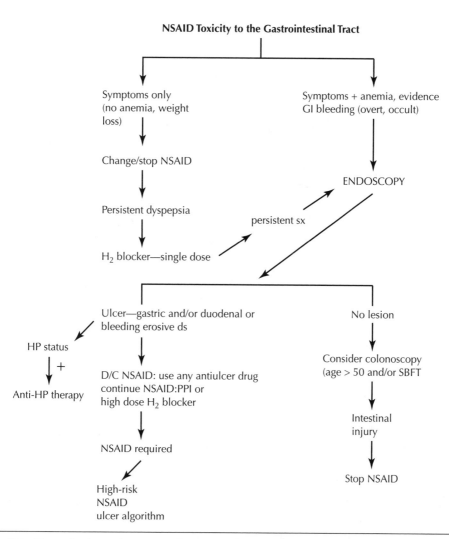

NSAID Toxicity to the Gastrointestinal Tract

Symptoms only (no anemia, weight loss)

Symptoms + anemia, evidence GI bleeding (overt, occult)

Change/stop NSAID

ENDOSCOPY

Persistent dyspepsia

persistent sx

H_2 blocker—single dose

Ulcer—gastric and/or duodenal or bleeding erosive ds

No lesion

HP status

+

Anti-HP therapy

D/C NSAID: use any antiulcer drug continue NSAID:PPI or high dose H_2 blocker

Consider colonoscopy (age > 50 and/or SBFT

NSAID required

Intestinal injury

High-risk NSAID ulcer algorithm

Stop NSAID

Figure 7–1.   The evaluation and treatment of patients with gastrointestinal side effects. *(Source: Adapted from Scheiman, J. (1996). NSAIDs, gastrointestinal injury, and cytoprotection.* Gastroenterol Clin North Am, *25(2), 292. Philadelphia: W. B. Saunders. Used with permission.)*
SBFT, small bowel follow through; HP, *Helicobacter pylori;* PPI, proton pump inhibitor; D/C, discontinue.

NSAIDs should be avoided if at all possible in clients with a history of gastritis or ulcer disease (Fay & Jaffe, 1996). Scheiman's article (1996) provides an excellent review of the use of NSAIDs in relation to GI toxicity. Agents such as salicyclic acid, nabutome, or etodolac have a lower risk profile for GI toxicity if an NSAID is required. Prophylaxis with misoprostol, omeprazole, lansoprazole, or a high-dose H_2 blocker may also decrease the risk of GI complications (Figs. 7–1 and 7–2).

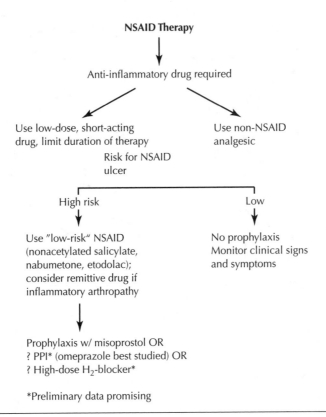

NSAID Therapy

↓

Anti-inflammatory drug required

Use low-dose, short-acting
drug, limit duration of therapy

Use non-NSAID
analgesic

Risk for NSAID
ulcer

High risk   Low

Use "low-risk" NSAID
(nonacetylated salicylate,
nabumetone, etodolac);
consider remittive drug if
inflammatory arthropathy

No prophylaxis
Monitor clinical signs
and symptoms

Prophylaxis w/ misoprostol OR
? PPI* (omeprazole best studied) OR
? High-dose H_2-blocker*

*Preliminary data promising

Figure 7–2. Preventing NSAID-induced injury. *(Source: Adapted from Scheiman, J. (1996). NSAIDs, gastrointestinal injury, and cytoprotection. Gastroenterol Clin North Am, 25(2), 292. Philadelphia: W. B. Saunders. Used with permission.)*
SBFT, small bowel follow through; HP, *Helicobacter pylori*; PPI, proton pump inhibitor; D/C, discontinue.

Nonpharmacologic Measures

Bland diets and milk should be discouraged as they are without therapeutic value and may worsen symptoms by increasing gastrin levels (Lonergan, 1995). The client should avoid tobacco, alcohol, and caffeine and take measures to reduce stress.

■ GASTRITIS

Gastritis is the inflammation of gastric mucosa. Acute gastritis may be caused by alcohol intake or aspirin or NSAID therapy, or

may be a correlate of any severe, life-threatening disease. Acute gastritis may result in erosions and upper GI bleeding.

The majority of cases of chronic gastritis are type B and are strongly correlated with *H. pylori* infection. Eradication of *H. pylori* results in disappearance of inflammatory changes (NIH Consensus Conference, 1994). A less common form of chronic gastritis, type A, is believed to be autoimmune in nature and is frequently associated with pernicious anemia.

Chronic inflammation from any cause begins as a superficial gastritis and progresses through glandular atrophy to gastric atrophy and achlorhydria. Approximately 10% of patients with gastric atrophy will develop gastric carcinoma. Gastric ulcer disease and gastric cancer share a similar etiologic mechanism (Hansson et al., 1996).

CLINICAL MANAGEMENT

Clients should be counseled about the effects of alcohol, aspirin, and NSAIDs on gastric mucosa, and these agents should be avoided if possible. *H. pylori* eradication therapy may benefit patients with type B gastritis. Some authors recommend serial endoscopic follow-up to detect gastric carcinoma in clients with gastric atrophy and pernicious anemia. The cost effectiveness of this approach has not yet been established.

■ GALLBLADDER DISEASE

Cholelithiasis is common in older age, and complications such as empyema, perforation, and choledocholithiasis are more likely in persons over 65 and in diabetics.

CLINICAL PRESENTATION

Right upper quadrant or epigastric pain radiating to the right shoulder or scapula is characteristic of biliary colic. Nausea and vomiting may also be present, and pain may be aggravated by deep inspiration. Jaundice or elevated bilirubin suggests common bile duct stones.

In the older adult, serious complications, such as gangrenous perforation of the gallbladder, may occur without significant fever or rebound tenderness. Anorexia, mental confusion, and low-grade fever may prevail.

ASSESSMENT

History

Obtain a description of pain type, location, radiation, severity, and progression. Determine association with meals and any aggravating factors (such as deep inspiration), relieving factors, and associated symptoms (fever, nausea). Assess past history of abdominal surgery, ulcer disease, cardiac disease, biliary colic, or stones.

Physical Examination

Assess vital signs, mental status, and abdominal exam. Check for Murphy's sign (right upper quadrant tenderness on palpation that increases with inspiration).

Diagnostic Studies

Check CBC with differential, LFTs, bilirubin, and amylase. Consult physician regarding abdominal ultrasound.

CLINICAL MANAGEMENT

Asymptomatic clients do not require intervention but should be educated to notify the health-care professional if symptoms of biliary colic do occur. Symptomatic clients should be referred to the physician or surgeon for follow-up studies and management. Laparoscopic cholecystectomy is associated with low morbidity when performed by an experienced surgeon. Medical therapy and extracorporeal shockwave lithotripsy (ESWL) are used when surgery is contraindicated or undesired. Endoscopic retrograde cholangiopancreatography (ERCP) with sphincterotomy is used in high-risk clients with common duct stones (Kowdly, 1996). Estrogen and thiazide diuretics should be reduced or discontinued if possible since they increase the risk of stone formation. Reducing fat and cholesterol intake offers no proven therapeutic benefit. Fasting or starvation diets should be avoided since they increase stone formation.

■ ABDOMINAL PAIN

Acute abdominal pain poses a diagnostic challenge in the elderly. Causes of acute abdominal pain include perforation or rupture (ulcer, spleen, diverticulum, abdominal aortic aneurysm, gallbladder, abscess, or hematoma), obstruction (bowel, biliary, or ureteral), vascular (aortic, hepatic, or splenic aneurysm; mesenteric artery infarct; myocardial infarct; or pelvic deep vein thrombosis), or inflammation (peritonitis, appendicitis, cholecystitis, pancreatitis, diverticulitis, pneumonia) (Burkhart, 1992; Lederle, 1990; Richter, 1995; Stone, 1996).

Clinical guidelines for the assessment of acute abdominal pain are found in Fig. 7–3 and Tables 7–4 and 7–5. Clinical management of pneumonia, myocardial infarction, cholecystitis, diverticulitis, and PUD are reviewed in this text. Acute conditions warrant physician referral. Atypical presentations are common. Peritonitis may be present in the absence of high fever, leukocytosis, severe pain or guarding. Confusion and functional decline are common harbingers of serious illness. Older adults with vague abdominal symptoms should be followed closely to promote early recognition of emergent or atypical presentations.

■ CONSTIPATION

Constipation is a frequent complaint of the elderly. The incidence and preva-

lence rates of constipation has not been established. However, it has been reported that approximately 30% of community-dwelling elders and 50% of nursing home residents suffer from constipation (Stewart et al., 1992; Whitehead et al., 1989). Moreover, approximately 19% to 50% of elders use laxatives regularly, contributing a large percentage of the $400 million dollars spent annually on laxatives in the United States (Cheskin et al, 1995; Harari et al., 1993).

AGE-RELATED CHANGES

Constipation is not a disease but rather a symptom with an underlying cause. Colonic motility whereby stool is delivered through the colon and subsequently evacuated through the rectum does not decline with age. Although many older adults may complain of constipation, it is not normal to the aging process. Thus, the underlying cause should be evaluated.

CLINICAL PRESENTATION

There is no definitive definition for constipation in the health literature. Three clinical definitions usually appear in the literature: (1) symptomatic—two or fewer bowel movements a week, of which 25% involve straining; (2) clinical—fecal retention in the rectal ampulla on digital examination, excessive fecal retention in the colon as evidence by abdominal radiograph, or both; and (3) subjective—self-reported constipation in the absence of symptomatic or clinical constipation (Minaker & Harari, 1995). Most APNs, however, tend to define constipation in the elderly as no more than two bowel movements every week and/or difficulty with defecation.

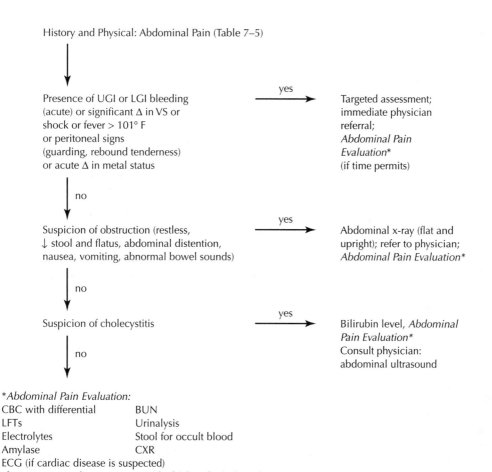

History and Physical: Abdominal Pain (Table 7–5)

Presence of UGI or LGI bleeding
(acute) or significant Δ in VS or
shock or fever > 101° F
or peritoneal signs
(guarding, rebound tenderness)
or acute Δ in metal status

→ yes → Targeted assessment;
immediate physician
referral;
*Abdominal Pain
Evaluation**
(if time permits)

no

Suspicion of obstruction (restless,
↓ stool and flatus, abdominal distention,
nausea, vomiting, abnormal bowel sounds)

→ yes → Abdominal x-ray (flat and
upright); refer to physician;
*Abdominal Pain Evaluation**

no

Suspicion of cholecystitis

→ yes → Bilirubin level, *Abdominal
Pain Evaluation**
Consult physician:
abdominal ultrasound

no

Abdominal Pain Evaluation:
CBC with differential   BUN
LFTs   Urinalysis
Electrolytes   Stool for occult blood
Amylase   CXR
ECG (if cardiac disease is suspected)
The more acute the symptoms or the higher the index of suspicion, the sooner the physician should be contacted.

Figure 7–3. Guidelines for Evaluation of Acute Abdominal Pain.
UGI, upper gastrointestinal; LGI, lower gastrointestinal; CBC, complete blood count; BUN, blood urea nitrogen; LFTs, liver function tests; CXR, chest x-ray; ECG, electrocardiogram.

History

Assess symptom onset, prior bowel pattern, frequency of bowel motion, characteristics of stool, incontinence (urinary and fecal), association of rectal pain to defecation, and laxative use. Assess for underlying illnesses (eg, non–insulin-dependent diabetes mellitus [NIDDM], depression, Parkinson's disease, stroke), history of hemorrhoids or anorectal disease, and mobility problems. Review prescription and OTC medications, dietary fiber history, and fluids. It is important to note that fiber can exacerbate constipation in elders with chronic constipation.

TABLE 7–4.   HISTORY AND PHYSICAL: ACUTE ABDOMINAL PAIN

* **Chief complaint:**
- Location/radiation
- Character/quality/severity
- Progression and onset (associated with meals, trauma, stress, movement, getting better or worse; interferes with sleep)
- Frequency and duration
- Aggravating factors (food, stress, position, cough, exertion, bowel movement)
  - Relieving factors (food, antacids, position, bowel movement)
  - Associated symptoms (change in bowel habits, heartburn, nausea, vomiting, fever, chills, food intolerance, bloating, urinary symptoms, tarry stools, anorexia, weight loss, decreased flatus, belching, cardiac symptoms, pulmonary symptoms)
- Past history (similar pain, cardiac disease, lung disease, ulcer disease, gallbladder disease, abominal surgery, diverticulosis, aneurysm, liver disease, pancreatitis, iritable bowel disease, kidney disease, diabetes, prostate disease, atrial fibrillation, varicella, presence of ovaries), travel history (? dysentery)
- Impact on life (social, recreational, functional status, significant others, fears, concerns, expectations, meaning of symptom)

* **Diet/nutritional assessment:** 24-hr recall, weight pattern

* **Meds**

- Anticholinergics
- Narcotics
- Steroids (may mask peritonitis)
- Anticoagulants (intra-abdominal bleed)
- Laxatives
- Antiacids or H_2 blockers
- Aspirin or NSAIDs
- Alcohol or drug use

* **Psychosocial assessment:** history of loss conflict, depression anxiety, stress

* **Review of systems:**

Cardiac	Respiratory	Genitourinary
Chest pain_____	Dyspnea/SOB_____	History of kidney stones_____
History of CAD/MI_____	Cough_____	Change in color/odor of urine_____
Orthopnea/PND_____	Sputum_____	Flank pain_____
Palpitations_____	Hemoptysis_____	Frequency/urgency_____
Edema_____	Wheezing_____	Hesitancy_____
Circulation probs_____	History of pneumonia_____	Incontinence_____
Last ECG_____	History of COPD_____	Nocturia_____
		Vaginal discharge_____
		Bleeding_____
		Prostate problems_____
		Scrotal mass_____
		Last pelvic exam_____

* **Physical exam:**

General: assess movement and positioning (tense and still in peritonitis; restless in bowel obstruction and biliary colic); change in mental status (peritonitis)

Skin: assess for jaundice or cirrhotic skin changes (hepatobiliary disease) pallor (anemia related to upper or lower GI bleed or aneurysm), diaphoresis (shock related to acute perforation or sepsis), mottling or cyanosis of lower extremities (ruptured AAA), herpes zoster lesions, turgor and mucous membranes for dehydration

TABLE 7–4.   HISTORY AND PHYSICAL: ACUTE ABDOMINAL PAIN (CONT.)

* Physical exam: (cont.)

Vital signs: fever, tachycardia, postural blood pressure (assess for shock, infection, hypovolemia related to bleeding)

Cardiac: complete exam; also assess for abdominal bruit, check pulses below the waist

Pulmonary: splinting, dullness, hemoptysis, decreased breath sounds, friction rub (pulmonary infarct or pneumonia)

Abdomen: complete exam, inspect for scars, distention, ascites pulsation, bruit (renal, epigastric, flank), bowel sounds, masses, tenderness, rebound, guarding, scars, sit-up maneuver, Murphy's sign, cough tenderness (peritonitis), hepatosplenomegaly, iliopsoas and obdurator signs

Rectal/genitourinary: check prostate, impaction, guaiac, masses, inguinal or femoral hernia; check for tenderness (appendicitis or diverticulitis) testicular torsion

Pelvic exam: if pain is in lower quadrants (assess for ovarian or retroperitoneal mass)

Other: check for CVA tenderness, perform mental status exam if indicated

NSAIDs, nonsteroidal anti-inflammatory drugs; SOB, shortness of breath; CAD, coronary artery disease; MI, myocardial infarction; PND, paroxysmal nocturnal dyspnea; ECG, electrocardiogram; COPD, chronic obstructive pulmonary disease; GI, gastrointestinal; AAA, abdominal aortic aneurysm; CVA, cardiovascular accident.

TABLE 7–5A.   POTENTIAL CAUSES OF ABDOMINAL PAIN

■ **CARDIOVASCULAR**
Myocardial infarction
Abdominal aortic aneurysm
Mesenteric artery ischemia
Mesenteric artery infarction
Pelvic deep vein thrombosis

■ **PULMONARY**
Pleurisy
Pneumonia

■ **OBSTRUCTION**
Small bowel obstruction
Large bowel obstruction
Biliary obstruction
Ureteral obstruction

■ **GENITOURINARY/GYNECOLOGIC**
Ovarian cyst
Ovarian torsion
Incarcerated inguinal hernia disorder
Renal calculi
Testicular torsion

■ **PERFORATION**
Perforated ulcer
Splenic rupture
Perforated gallbladder
Perforated colon

■ **INFLAMMATION/INFECTION**
Esophagitis
Gastritis
Pancreatitis
Cholecystitis
Appendicitis
Hepatitis
Diverticulitis
Regional enteritis
Ulcerative colitis

■ **OTHER**
Colon cancer
Gastroesophageal reflux
Irritable bowel syndrome

TABLE 7–5B.   DIAGNOSTIC TESTS USED IN EVALUATION OF ABDOMINAL PAIN

Complete blood count with differential	Flat plate and upright x-ray
Urinalysis	Abdominal ultrasound
Electrolytes	Electrocardiogram (ECG)
Liver enzymes	Stool for occult blood
Amylase	Endoscopy
Lipase	Sigmoidoscopy
Chest x-ray	Blood urea nitrogen
Serum creatinine	

TABLE 7–5C.   CLUES IN ABDOMINAL PAIN EVALUATION

Cholecystitis[a]	Right upper quandrant (RUQ) or epigastric pain radiating to right shoulder or scapula; may have history of gallbladder disease, jaundice, elevated *bilirubin,* elevated *white blood cell count (WBC) with left shift; abdominal ultrasound* shows dilatation and stones in biliary tree; *alkaline phosphatase* and *amylase* may be elevated; positive Murphy's sign
Appendicitis[b]	Diffuse pain which eventually localizes in right lower quadrant (RLQ); anorexia, nausea, vomiting; increased *WBC* with left shift; guarding, rebound tenderness, positive iliopsoas test, positive obdurator test
Bowel obstruction[c]	Bowel sounds abnormal (decreased or absent below obstruction, hyperactive before obstruction early in course); restlessness, distention, decreased stool, flatus, nausea, vomiting, *abdominal flat and upright x-ray* shows obstruction
Ulcer disease[d]	Recurrent upper abdominal pain; burning, gnawing, timing associated with food; nausea, vomiting, epigastric pain on palpation; *hemoccult + stool;* may have history of alcohol abuse, smoking, aspirin use, NSAID use; may test + for *Helicobacter pylori*
Inflammatory bowel disease[e]	Umbilical or RLQ pain; diarrhea alternating with constipation; low grade fever, fatigue, anorexia, weight loss, *anemia, hemoccult + for blood*
Diverticulitis	Left lower quadrant tenderness (LLQ), nausea, low grade fever, constipation, increased pain with bowel movements, increased *WBC,* guarding, mass in LLQ, *hemoccult + stool*
Pancreatitis	Left upper quadrant (LUQ) pain radiating to back; fever, elevated *WBC,* elevated *amylase*
Acute gastroenteritis	Nausea, vomiting, diarrhea, fever, flatulence, headache, myalgias
Acute mesenteric artery ischemia	History of vascular disease; postprandial abdominal pain, diarrhea, *hemoccult + stool,* acute confusion, new onset atrial fibrillation
Abdominal aortic aneurysm	Epigastric pain radiating to back or groin; abdominal bruit, pulsatile mass, history of vascular disease, decreased pulses below the waist, shock; *abdominal ultrasound* + for aneurysm

[a] Increased risk of abcess, perforation, pancreatitis in elders.
[b] Increased mortality in elders.
[c] Consider possible causes of obstruction: adhesions, tumor, hernia, volvulus, diverticulitis.
[d] Endoscopy is needed in older adults to rule out malignancy.
[e] Hemoccult + stool warrants workup for colorectal cancer.

Physical Examination

Assess abdomen, rectum, and sigmoid colon. In some elders, the transverse and descending colon can be assessed. *Note:* The absence of stool does not rule out constipation in the proximal colon.

Diagnostic Studies

Lab work is routinely not ordered if stool is felt in the rectum or sigmoid colon. Labs such as UA, BUN/creatinine, and CBC may be ordered to identify underlying infections. In conjunction with the digital examination, stool is tested for occult blood, and, if present, the older adult may be referred to a physician or gastroenterologist for a barium enema and/or endoscopy test to identify the origin of occult blood. An abdominal x-ray or ultrasound can also be ordered by the physician to identify fecal impaction within the colon.

CLINICAL MANAGEMENT

The goal in the management of constipation is to identify and treat the underlying etiology. The restoration of normal bowel patterns usually takes time, so older adults may become discouraged. The APN must dispel any preconceived myths surrounding "normal" bowel patterns. A normal bowel pattern ranges from three times per day to three times per week. Therefore, the APN must educate the older adult to the great variance in "normal" bowel patterns.

The first step in management of constipation is to educate the older adult

---

TABLE 7–6.   BOWEL TRAINING PROGRAM

1. Obtain bowel history and patterns.
2. Educate older adult about constipation and dispel any preconceived ideas about "normal" bowel movements (eg, one bowel movement per day).
3. Establish a "realistic" bowel regime that is achievable and meets older adults' schedules.
    (a) Commit to a regular time to have a bowel movement (10–15 minutes variance of regular schedule time is okay).
    (b) Commit to bowel evacuation 20–40 minutes after a regularly scheduled meal (breakfast is ideal due to the gastrocolic reflex).
    (c) Stimulate gastrocolic reflex, which is usually stimulated by ingestion of hot fluids/food during the first meal of the day. This reflex may also be stimulated by massaging the abdomen around the colon.
    (d) Stimulate anorectal reflex (either digital stimulation or glycerin suppository).
    (e) Instruct to sit on toilet seat or commode (if bedbound, then place bed at a 45-degree angle as tolerated). Placing feet on a stool and slightly leaning forward approximates the physiologic position for defecation.
    (f) Instruct to bear down and contract abdominal muscles when defecating. This maneuver increases intra-abdominal pressure which helps in defecation.
    (g) Encourage older adult to exercise or perform activities that may increase peristalsis prior to meal. If the older adult is bedbound, then range-of-motion exercises and abdominal massaging can be done prior to meal.
    (h) Instruct to drink six to eight 8-oz glasses of fluid per day (if not contraindicated) and educate about foods rich in fiber (eg, bran) and natural laxative foods (eg, raw fruits, whole grains, and vegetables).

about normal bowel habits and avoidance of laxatives (until diagnostic confirmation of constipation), as well as the need to be patient. A comprehensive bowel training program should consists of four elements: (1) diet, (2) activity, (3) toileting, and (4) medication.

Diet considerations are important in any bowel program. The diet plan should include increases in dietary fiber with bran cereal (10 g to 20 g), raw fruits and vegetables, and whole wheat breads. The older adult should be cautioned that bran may produce bloating, gas, and cramping; however, this will usually subside within 1 to 2 weeks. Fluids should be increased to 1.5 to 2.0 L/d.

If the general dietary measures do not work, then a bulk-forming agent (ie, hydrophilic muccoloid) should be tried. This should be coupled with increase of fluids (1.5 to 2.0 L) per day. Bulk-forming agents must be used on a regular basis and can be used long term. (Tedesco, 1978). Nonabsorbable sugar lactulose (15 mL to 30 mL/d) may also be used to manage constipation long term. Stool softeners (eg, docusate sodium) can be used for short-term treatment of constipation. In extremely constipated older adults (absence of bowel movement in 3 days), a glycerin suppository or tap water enema may be used. Irritant laxatives should always be avoided.

Bowel training (see Table 7–6) is another important component to any bowel program. Older adults should be instructed to attempt to move their bowels 10 to 15 minutes after each meal. They should remain sitting on the commode for at least 10 to 15 minutes. If a bowel movement is not forthcoming, then they they should increase their physical activity and attempt to move their bowels in 1 hour. Physical activity/exercise should also be encouraged since this may increase colonic peristalsis.

■ DIARRHEA

Diarrhea is the abnormal frequency and/or liquidity of stool compared to a person's normal stools. Diarrhea is not a frequent complaint of older adults. Diarrhea is divided into two types, acute and chronic, with different etiologies. Acute diarrhea in the older adult is usually caused by contaminated foods, medications (ie, antibiotics, laxatives), and infections. Chronic diarrhea in the older adult is usually caused by malabsorption problems (rare), fecal impaction, and irritable bowel syndrome (rare).

AGE-RELATED CHANGES

Diarrhea is a symptom of an underlying problem. It is not normal to the aging process.

CLINICAL PRESENTATION

The majority of diarrhea cases are acute in nature, lasting 1 to 2 days and resolving spontaneously without sequelae. Chronic diarrhea usually lasts approximately 2 to 3 weeks and occurs less frequently. Depending on the cause of the diarrhea, the older adult may complain of the onset of diarrhea after the start of a new medication, abdominal (cramping) pain, malodorous or foul-smelling stools, light-colored stools, large stools, liquid ("water") stools, blood-tinged stool, weight loss over a period of weeks, vomiting with abrupt onset, diarrhea with alternating constipation, malaise, and fever.

History

Assess onset of diarrhea, frequency, consistency, volume, and presence of blood and/or mucus. Obtain medication regimen, paying close attention to any new medications, especially the addition of antibiotics and overuse of laxatives. Obtain diet history, paying close attention to the addition of new foods or foods that may have been undercooked. Assess for fevers, malaise, or environmental stress, which may be related to irritable bowel syndrome.

Physical Examination

Examine abdomen for tenderness, rigidity, abnormal tympany, bowel sounds, and liver/spleen tenderness. Examine rectum for tenderness and masses, and stool for occult blood. Assess hydration status (ie, mucous membranes), rectal tenderness, decreased skin turgor, tachycardia, oliguria, and fever.

Diagnostic Studies

If the diarrhea lasts for 1 to 2 days and the older adult is asymptomatic, then no lab work is required. If the diarrhea lasts more than 2 days and the older adult is symptomatic (ie, fever, blood-tinged stools, wet prep indicates white blood cells [WBCs]), then obtain CBC for electrolyte imbalance, guaiac for occult blood, and ova and parasites (O&P) for enteric pathogens.

CLINICAL MANAGEMENT

The management of acute diarrhea caused by the ingestion of food requires only supportive therapy to prevent dehydration and antidiarrheal medications (eg, loperamide hydrochloride) for comfort and relief of symptoms. Diarrhea caused by toxigenic strains of *Escherichia coli* can be managed by large dosages of bismuth subsalicylate (Pepto-Bismol) given in dosages of 30 mL to 60 mL every 4 to 6 hours. Diarrhea caused by antibi-

otics will usually subside once the antibiotic is discontinued. If the antibiotic cannot be withdrawn, then treatment with vancomycin is usually helpful in decreasing the diarrhea by decreasing colonic motility. The disadvantage of vancomycin is related to its expense, and it may have adverse side effects in the elderly.

The management of chronic diarrhea should be referred to a physician or gastroenterologist for evaluation. The causes of chronic diarrhea (ie, malabsorption problems, irritable bowel syndrome, and constipation) usually require invasive diagnostic procedures (ie, barium studies and sigmoidoscopy) before effective treatment can be undertaken.

■ FECAL INCONTINENCE

Fecal incontinence, the involuntary loss of stool, can be both physically and psychologically devastating to the older adult. It may be acute or chronic in nature. Approximately 25% of older adults living in long-term care suffer with this problem. The exact incidence and prevalence for community-dwelling older adults has not been established; however, it is believed to be quite rare.

AGE-RELATED CHANGES

Fecal incontinence is not normal to the aging process. However, due to the aging process, some older adults may lose tonicity of the external sphincter, resulting in loss of stool during flatulence.

CLINICAL PRESENTATION

The majority of older adults with fecal incontinence will present with complaints of losing stool while having a flatulent episode. They may also complain of "soiling" their clothes, beds, chair, and floor.

History

There are many causes of fecal incontinence; therefore, an extensive history is needed to determine the etiology. Obtain bowel history (ie, frequency, consistency) and beliefs, dietary habits (ie, fiber and fluid intake), medications (especially use of laxatives, suppositories, and enemas), and activity level. Assess past medical and surgical abdominal history, anorectal disease, or disorienting disorders (dementia, depression, etc.).

Physical Examination

Assess abdomen for bowel sounds, tenderness, and masses; perform a rectal examination for impaction, external/internal hemorrhoids, and tonicity.

Diagnostic Studies

Obtain guaiac for occult blood. Refer to a physician for flexible sigmoidoscopy to rule out anterior rectal ulcers, inflammatory bowel disease, cancer, or infection.

CLINICAL MANAGEMENT

The goal is to treat the underlying cause of fecal incontinence. Establish a routine toilet schedule. Stop any laxatives that are currently being used, and increase bulk and fluids. If the older adult has diarrhea or constipation, then refer to the preceding sections for appropriate management. The perineum should be kept dry as possible, using a moisture barrier (petroleum-based cream or Desitin) to prevent skin ulcerations. Perineal dermatitis can occur within 48 hours in the presence of liquid diarrhea (Lyder et al., 1992). Provide emotional support.

■ DIVERTICULITIS

Diverticulitis, an inflammation of the colon, is a chronic disease that increases with age. The major cause of diverticular disease is absence of dietary fiber. The incidence of diverticulitis has been reported to be approximately 10% to 25% of all patients with diverticulosis (40% of older adults age 80 and older). Diverticulitis usually occurs in the sigmoid portion of the colon; however, it may occur throughout the colon. If undertreated, it may lead to abscesses, fistulas, perforations, and obstructions.

AGE-RELATED CHANGES

The intestines may also be affected by the aging process. They may atrophy, with fibrotic tissue replacing the normal parenchyma. This aging change may lead to malabsorption of nutrients.

CLINICAL PRESENTATION

The classic symptoms of diverticulitis in the elderly include abdominal pain (usually in the left lower quadrant), abdominal tenderness, diarrhea, constipation, or alternating diarrhea and constipation. Fever, malaise, anorexia, nausea and vomiting, and rectal bleeding may also be present in severe cases.

History

Assess for acute onset of abdominal pain and tenderness, and duration and intensity of discomfort. Obtain diet history to assess for fiber. Obtain stool history for consistency and painful defecation.

Physical Examination

Assess abdomen for bowel sounds, distention, rebound tenderness, and localized muscle spasms. Acute lower left quadrant abdominal pain is classic during physical examination. Low-grade fever may also be present during the physical examination.

Diagnostic Studies

Obtain guaiac and CBC (observe for elevated WBC with shift to the left). Refer to a physician or gastroenterologist to obtain x-ray, barium studies, flexible colonoscopy, and sigmoidoscopy.

CLINICAL MANAGEMENT

The older adult should be treated in consultation with a physician and/or gastroenterologist. The conservative management of diverticulitis consist of an increase in dietary fiber with added bran or bulking agent, antispasmodics (for colicky pain), and oral antibiotics such as gentamicin or ampicillin. If a conservative approach does not work within 1 week, the physician or gastroenterologist may recommend surgery.

 ## CASE STUDY

Mr. Drake, a 66-year-old type II diabetic on oral hypoglycemics, presented in the emergency room with a 3-day history of epigastric abdominal pain which is intermittent but progressively worsening and described as "gripping." An ECG is done and is within normal limits.

QUESTIONS

1. Describe the history, physical, and laboratory parameters to be assessed in this case.

2. What diagnose(s) should be considered in the differential?

ANSWERS

1. Mr. Drake's WBC is 15,000. A gallbladder ultrasound reveals several stones. He is sent home with pain meds and instructions to follow up with his primary physician. One week later, Mr. Drake begins hallucinating, has a temperature of 104.1°F, severe pain in upper quadrants, and hyperglycemia (fingerstick blood sugar of 382). His abdomen is distended, firm, and tender with guarding.

2. Mr. Drake was admitted to the hospital with a diagnosis of perforated gallbladder with hepatic abscess and sepsis.

▪ REFERENCES

Burkhart, C. (1992). Guidelines for rapid assessment of abdominal pain indicative of acute surgical abdomen. *Nurs Pract, 17*(6), 41–49.

Cheskin, L., Kamal, N., Crowell, M., et al. (1995). Mechanisms of constipation in older persons and effects of fiber compared with placebo. *J Am Geriatr Soc, 43*, 666–669.

Fay, M., & Jaffe, P. (1996). Diagnostic and treatment guidelines for *Helicobacter pylori*. *Nurse Pract., 21*(7), 28–35.

Fendrick, A., Chernew, M., Hirth, R., & Bloom, B. (1995). Alternative management strategies for patients with suspected peptic ulcer disease. *Am Coll Phys, 123*(4), 260–268.

Goroll, A., May, L., & Mulley, A. Jr. (1995).

Primary care medicine (3rd ed.) Philadelphia: J. B. Lippincott.

Hansson, L., Nyren, O., Hsing, A. W., et al. (1996). The risk of stomach cancer in patients with gastric or duodenal ulcer disease. *New Engl J Med, 335*(4):242–280.

Harari, D., Gurwitz, J., & Minaker, K. (1993). Constipation in the elderly. *J Am Geriatr Soc, 41,* 1130–1140.

Heslin, J. (1997). Peptic ulcer disease: Making a case against the prime suspect. *Nursing 97,* June, 34–39.

Klinkenberg-Knol, E., et al. (1994). Longterm treatment with omeprazole for refractory reflux esophagitis: efficacy and safety. *Ann Intern Med, 121*(3), 161–167.

Kowdley, K. (1996). Update on therapy for hepatobiliary diseases. *Nurs Pract, 21*(7), 78–88.

Lederle, F. (1990). Management of small abdominal aortic aneurysms. *Ann Intern Med, 113*(10), 731.

Lonergan, E. T. (Ed.). (1996). *Geriatrics: A Lange Clinical Manual.* Stamford, CT: Appleton & Lange.

Lyder, C., Clemes-Lorence, C., Davis, A., et al. (1992). A structured skin care regimen to prevent perineal dermatitis in the elderly. *J ET Nurs, 19*(1), 12–16.

The Medical Letter on Drugs and Therapeutics (1997). Drugs for treatment of peptic ulcers. 39(991) 1–4. New Rochelle, NY: The Medical Letter, Inc.

Minaker, K., & Harari, D. (1995). Constipation in the elderly. *Hospital Practice, 30*(5), 67–70.

NIH Consensus Conference 1994. *Helicobacter pylori* in peptic ulcer disease. *JAMA, 272*(1):65–69.

Scheiman, J. (1996). NSAIDS, gastrointestinal injury and cytoprotection. *Gastroenterol Clin North Am, 25*(2), 279–298.

Shaw, B. (1996). Primary care for women: management and treatment of gastrointestinal disorders. *J Nurse Midwife, 41*(2), 155–172.

Schroeder, P., Filler, S., Ramirez, B., et al. (1995). Dental erosion and reflux disease. *Ann Intern Med, 122,* 809–815.

Smalley, W., & Griffin, M. (1996). The risks and costs of upper gastrointestinal disease attributable to NSAIDs. *Gastroenterol Clin North Am 25*(2), 373–396.

Stewart, R., Moore, M., Marks, R., & Hale, W. (1992). Correlates of constipation in an ambulatory elderly population. *Am J Gastroenterol, 87,* 859–864.

Stone, R. (1996). Primary care diagnosis of acute abdominal pain. *Nurse Prac 21*(12), 19–39.

Sullivan, C., & Samuelson, W. (1996). Gastroesophageal reflux: A common exacerbating factor in adult asthma. *Nurs Pract, 21*(11), 82–96.

Tedesco, F. (1978). American College of Gastroenterology Committee on FDA related matters, laxative use in constipation. *Am J Gastroenterol, 80,* 303–309.

Vigneri, S., Termini, R., Leandro, G., et al. (1995). A comparison of five maintenance therapies for reflux esophagitis. *N Engl J Med, 333*(17): 1106–10.

Whitehead, W., Drinkwater, D., Cheskin, L., et al. (1989). Constipation in the elderly living at home: Definition, prevalence and relationship to lifestyle and health status. *J Am Geriatr Soc, 36,* 423–429.

8

NUTRITIONAL ISSUES

Mary Grace Kinahan

■ INTRODUCTION

It is well documented that nutrition affects all subgroups of older adults in all settings. The better nourished an individual is, the better he or she will thrive functionally, combat chronic long-term disease, and heal after a major assault from acute illness, trauma, or surgery. Promotion of adequate nutrition begins in the community setting with nutritional health education as the key. The Nutrition Screening Initiative (1992) (see Table 2–2) has developed valuable nutritional screening tools specific for the care of older Americans.

The effects of obesity are also of concern in the elderly population. Obesity is defined as an excess of body fat and is cited as one of the leading public health issues of this century and the next. It is linked to hypertension (HTN), type II diabetes, and hyperlipidemia. Of the seven leading causes of death in this country, four of them have been associated with

obesity: cardiovascular illness, cancer, stroke, and diabetes.

See Mitchell and Chernoff (1991) for in-depth information regarding nutrition in the elderly.

■ NUTRITION MANAGEMENT

AGE-RELATED CHANGES

Chernoff (1987) states that nutrition is a factor to human aging: "Normal aging changes, including changes in body composition, physical performance, organ function and condition, will occur to all individuals if they live long enough and this process will occur at different rates in different people." This depends on the specific dietary intake and where the individual's status is on the continuum of health.

Body composition represents the structure of the body. It is inevitable that, as the body ages, changes occur in body composition. These changes include a loss of lean body mass, bone density, and decrease in total body water with an increase in total body fat.

Physical endurance is maintained by proper intake of nutrients to preserve lean body mass. As the body ages, there is a slowing of metabolism, accompanied by a loss of protein mass. Decreasing calorie intake, providing adequate protein, and enhancing physical activity will preserve lean body mass and maintain endurance of the aging body.

Maintaining the function of the body is a dynamic process related to the condition of the internal vital organs. Research shows that as the body ages, there are changes in the reserve capacity or the organ's ability to deal with stress (Chernoff, 1987). Malnutrition may present rapidly in older clients who are stressed from acute disease states.

Other age-related changes occur with dentition, hearing, sight, smell, and taste. Potential impairment in gastrointestinal (GI) function includes decreased GI motility, decreased absorptive surface secondary to villous atrophy and achlorhydria, lactose intolerance, and constipation.

ASSESSMENT

History
Use the screening tools shown in Fig. 8–1 (Nutrition Screening Initiative, 1992), to screen older adults for nutrition-related problems. These tools will identify those individuals who should be further evaluated, determining who is at risk based on body weight, body mass index (BMI), eating habits, living environment, laboratory data, and functional and mental status.

Commonly used medications by the elderly can influence nutritional states because of the many drug–nutrient interactions and side effects from those medications (see Table 8–1).

A detailed history should include data on weight loss or gain, anorexia, substance abuse, tolerance to prescribed diet, food allergies, dentition, economic factors, and mental status. In the past medical history, assess for inflammatory bowel diseases, diabetes, HTN, osteoporosis or surgeries, and traumas of the GI tract. Consider past treatments with radiation, chemotherapy, and other medications. Psychosocial factors play a significant role in determining nutritional risk. Look for previous eating disorders. Assess mental status, emotional health, functional ability, cultural norms, and changes in life style.

Physical Examination
Review all systems with a focus on the GI system. Assess for underweight and overweight status by the BMI. Look for signs and symptoms of malnutrition (see Table 8–2). Recommended daily allowances (RDA) reflect the amount of nutrient adequate for healthy individuals. These values do not reflect amounts that may be needed to correct deficiencies.

An unintentional weight loss or gain greater than 10% of ideal body weight (IBW) in 3 to 6 months should be further investigated.

BMI = Body weight in kg divided by
height squared in meters

Refer to nomogram for body mass index on Level I or II screening tools to calculate BMI (Fig. 8–1).

Underweight = BMI less than 23
Obesity = BMI greater than 27

Level II Screen

Complete the following screen by interviewing the patient directly and/or by referring to the patient chart. If you do not routinely perform all of the described tests or ask all of the listed questions, please consider including them but do not be concerned if the entire screen is not completed. Please try to conduct a minimal screen on as many older patients as possible, and please try to collect serial measurements, which are extremely valuable in monitoring nutritional status. Please refer to the manual for additional information.

Anthropometrics

Measure height to the nearest inch and weight to the nearest pound. Record the values below and mark them on the Body Mass Index (BMI) scale to the right. Then use a straight edge (paper, ruler) to connect the two points and circle the spot where this straight line crosses the centerline (body mass index). Record the number below; healthy older adults should have a BMI between 24 and 27; check the appropriate box to flag an abnormally high or low value.

Height (in):_____
Weight (lbs):_____
Body Mass Index
(weight/height²):_____

Please place a check by any statement regarding BMI and recent weight loss that is true for the patient.

☐ Body mass index < 24
☐ Body mass index > 27
☐ Has lost or gained 10 pounds (or more) of body weight in the past 6 months

Record the measurement of mid-arm circumference to the nearest 0.1 centimeter and of triceps skinfold to the nearest 2 millimeters.

Mid-Arm Circumference (cm):_____
Triceps Skinfold (mm):_____
Mid-Arm Muscle Circumference (cm):_____

Refer to the table and check any abnormal values:

☐ Mid-arm muscle circumference < 10th percentile

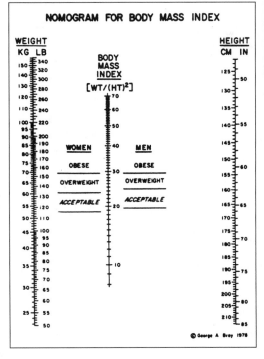

☐ Triceps skinfold < 10th percentile
☐ Triceps skinfold > 95th percentile

Note: mid-arm circumference (cm)-{0.314 x triceps skinfold (mm)}=mid-arm muscle circumference (cm)

For the remaining sections, please place a check by any statements that are true for the patient.

Laboratory Data
☐ Serum albumin below 3.5 g/dl
☐ Serum cholesterol below 160 mg/dl
☐ Serum cholesterol above 240 mg/dl

Drug Use
☐ Three or more prescription drugs OTC medications, and/or vitamin/mineral supplements daily

Clinical Features
Presence of (check each that apply):

☐ Problems with mouth, teeth, or gums
☐ Difficulty chewing
☐ Difficulty swallowing

Figure 8–1. Nutritional Screening Tool for Older Adults: Level II Screen (Continues)

□ Angular stomatitis
□ Glossitis
□ History of bone pain
□ History of bone fractures
□ Skin changes (dry, loose, nonspecific lesions, edema)

Eating Habits

□ Does not have enough food to eat each day
□ Usually eats alone
□ Does not eat anything on one or more days each month
□ Has poor appetite
□ Is on a special diet
□ Eats vegetables two or fewer times daily
□ Eats milk or milk products once or not at all daily
□ Eats fruit or drinks fruit juice once or not at all daily
□ Eats breads, cereals, pasta, rice or other grains five or fewer times daily
□ Has more than one alcoholic drink per day (if woman); more than two drinks per day (if man)

Living Environment

□ Lives on an income of less than $6,000 per year (per individual in the household)
□ Lives alone
□ Is housebound
□ Is concerned about home security
□ Lives in a home with inadequate heating or cooling
□ Does not have a stove and/or refrigerator
□ Is unable or prefers not to spend money on food (< $25-30 per person spent on food each week)

Functional Status

Usually or always needs assistance with (check each that apply):

□ Bathing
□ Dressing
□ Grooming

	Men		Women	
Percentile	55–65 y	65–75 y	55–65 y	65–75 y
Arm circumfrence (cm)				
10th	27.3	26.3	25.7	25.2
50th	31.7	30.7	30.3	29.9
95th	36.9	35.5	38.5	37.3
Arm muscle circumfrence (cm)				
10th	24.5	23.5	19.6	19.5
50th	27.8	26.8	22.5	22.5
95th	32.0	30.6	28.0	27.9
Triceps skinfold (mm)				
10th	6	6	16	14
50th	11	11	25	24
95th	22	22	38	36

From: Frisancho AR. New norms of upper limb fat and muscle areas for assessment of nutritional status. Am J Clin Nutr 1981; 34:2540–2545. 1981 © American Society for Clinical Nutrition.

□ Toileting
□ Eating
□ Walking or moving about
□ Traveling (outside the home)
□ Preparing food
□ Shopping for food or other necessities

Mental/Cognitive Status

□ Clinical evidence of impairment, e.g., Folstein < 26
□ Clinical evidence of depressive illness, e.g., Beck Depression Inventory > 15, Geriatric Depression Scale > 5

Patients in whom you have identified one or more major indicator (see pg 2) of poor nutritional status require immediate medical attention; if minor indicators are found, ensure that they are known to a health professional or to the patient's own physician. Patients who display risk factors (see pg 2) of poor nutritional status should be referred to the appropriate health care or social service professional (dietician, nurse, dentist, case manager, etc.).

Figure 8–1. Nutritional Screening Tool for Older Adults: Level II Screen (cont.) *(Source: Reprinted with permission by the Nutrition Screening Initiative, a project of the American Academy of Family Physicians, the American Dietetic Association, and the National Council on Aging, Inc., and funded in part by a grant from Ross Products Division, Abbott Laboratories.)*

TABLE 8–1. POTENTIAL DRUG–NUTRIENT INTERACTIONS FOR SOME COMMONLY USED DRUGS

Drug	Nutrient	Potential Side Effect
Alcohol	Thiamin	Deficiency
	Vitamin B$_6$	Deficiency
	Folate	Deficiency
	Zinc	Deficiency
	Calcium	Deficiency
	Magnesium	Deficiency
Aluminum hydroxide	Phosphorus	Binding
	Calcium	Deficiency
Antacids	Thiamin	Decreased absorption due to altered gastrointestinal pH
	Calcium	
	Iron	
Anticoagulants	Vitamin K	Deficiency
Antihistamines		Weight gain
Amphetamines		Appetite suppression
		Weight loss
Aspirin	Iron	Anemia
Cathartics	Calcium	Impaired gastrointestinal motility
	Potassium	Impaired gastrointestinal motility
Cholestyramine	Vitamins A, D, E, K	Deficiencies
Cimetidine	Vitamin B$_{12}$	Deficiency
Clofibrate	Carbohydrate	Enzume inactivation
	Vitamin B$_{12}$	Decreased absorption
	Carotene	
	Iron	
Colchicine	Vitamin B$_{12}$	Decreased absorption due to damaged intestinal mucosa
	Carotene	
	Magnesium	
Corticosteroids	Zinc	Damage to intestinal mucosa
	Calcium	
	Potassium	Gastrointestinal loss
Ethacrynic acid	Sodium	Depletion
Furosemide	Calcium	Diuretic effect
	Potassium	Depletion
	Sodium	
Gentamicin	Potassium	Depletion
	Sodium	
Levodopa	Protein	Competition for absorption

(Continues)

225

TABLE 8–1.   POTENTIAL DRUG–NUTRIENT INTERACTIONS FOR SOME COMMONLY USED DRUGS (CONT.)

Drug	Nutrient	Potential Side Effect
Neomycin	Fat Protein Sodium Potassium Calcium Iron Vitamin B_{12}	Decreases pancreatic lipase and binds bile salts and interferes with absorption
Penicillamine	Zinc Vitamin B_6 Sodium	Altered nutrient excretion
Phenobarbital	Vitamin D Folate	Impaired metabolism and utilization
Phenytoin	Vitamin D Folate	Impaired metabolism and utilization
Tetraacycline	Protein Iron	Imparied uptake and utilization General malabsorption
Tricyclic antidepressants		Weight gain due to appetite stimulation

Source: Chernoff, R. (1989). *Nutrition Today,* March/April, 4–11. Used with permission of Waverly, Williams & Wilkins, Baltimore, MD.

Nutritional History

Use the food pyramid (see Chapter 2, Fig. 2–1) to obtain information concerning the types and amounts of foods consumed by the client. Twenty-four-hour dietary recall information can be compared to the appropriate food selections, and inferences can be drawn concerning deficit and overindulgences. Look for food allergies and intolerance. Accurate information is essential.

Functional Exam

Assess oral health, use and fit of dentures, diseases of gums, tongue, oral lesions, and sense of taste and smell.

Assess for the patient's degree of independence with procuring food, and the ability to meet activities of daily living (ADL). See Fig. 8–1 for questions pertaining to functional ability.

Also assess for the ability to begin an exercise program to maintain physical condition. If the goal is weight loss, calorie counting and activities that provide maximum calorie burning should be promoted.

Diagnostic Studies

Albumin is an appropriate diagnostic study used in determining protein calorie malnutrition risk. Its value can determine the severity of depletion.

Mild depletion	2.8–3.5 g/dL
Moderate depletion	2.1–2.7 g/dL
Severe depletion	< 2.1 g/dL

TABLE 8–2. CLINICAL SIGNS OF NUTRITIONAL DEFICIENCIES WITH RECOMMENDED DAILY ALLOWANCES FOR PERSONS AGED 51 YEARS AND OLDER

Nutrient RDAs	Clinical Deficiency Symptoms
Vitamin A Males, 1000 μg Females, 800 μg	Eyes: Bitot's spots*, conjunctival and corneal xerosis (dryness), keratomalacia Skin: follicular hyperkeratosis, xerosis Hair: coiled, keratinized
Vitamin D Males, 5.0 μg Females, 5.0 μg	Bone: bowlegs, beading of ribs, pain, epiphyseal deformities
Vitamin E Males, 10 mg Females, 8 mg	Possible anemia
Vitamin K Males, 80 μg Females, 65 μg	Skin: subcutaneous hemorrhage, ecchymosis (bruises easily)
Thiamine (vitamin B_1) Males, 1.2 mg Females, 1.0 mg	Neurologic: mental confusion, irritability, sensory losses, weakness, parethesias, anorexia Eyes: ophthalmoplegia Cardiac: tachycardia, cardiomegaly, congestive heart failure Other: constipation, sudden death
Riboflavin (vitamin B_2) Males, 1.4 mg Females, 1.3 mg	Skin: nasolabial dermatitis, fissuring and redness around eyes and mouth, magenta tongue, genital dermatosis Eyes: corneal vascularization
Niacin (vitamin B_3) Males, 15 mg Females, 13 mg	Skin: nasolabial seborrhea, fissuring eyelid corners, angular fissures around mouth, papillary atrophy, pellagrous dermatitis Neurologic: mental confusion Other: diarrhea
Panthothenic acid (vitamin B_5 No RDA, recommend 4–7 mg	Headache, fatigue, apathy, nausea, sleep disturbances
Pyridoxine (vitamin B_6) Males, 2.0 mg Females, 1.6 mg	Skin: nasolabial seborrhea, glossitis Neurologic: paresthesia, peripheral neuropathy Other: anemia
Cobalamin (vitamin B_{12}) Males and females, 2 μg	Skin: glossitis, skin hyperpigmentation, pallor Neurologic: ataxia, optic neuritis, paresthesias, mental disorders Other: anemia, anorexia, diarrhea
Folic acid Males, 200 μg Females, 180 μg	Skin: glossitis, hyperpigmentation of tongue, pallor Neurologic: depression Other: diarrhea, anemia

(Continues)

TABLE 8–2.   CLINICAL SIGNS OF NUTRITIONAL DEFICIENCIES WITH RECOMMENDED DAILY ALLOWANCES FOR PERSONS AGED 51 YEARS AND OLDER (CONT.)

Nutrient RDAs	Clinical Deficiency Symptoms
Ascorbic acid (vitamin C) Males and females, 60 mg	Skin: petechiae, purpura, swollen, bleeding gums Other: bone pain, dental caries, depression, anorexia, delayed wound healing Smokers, 100 mg
Biotin No RDA, recommend 30–100 μg	Skin: pluckable, sparse hair, pallor, seborrheic dermatitis Neurologic: depression Other: anemia, fatigue
Iron Males and females, 10 mg	Skin: pallor, angular fissures, glossitis, spoon nails, pale conjunctiva Other: enlarged spleen
Zinc Males, 15 mg Females, 12 mg	Skin: seborrheic dermatitis, poor wound healing Eyes: photophobia Other: dysgeusia (altered sense of taste)
Iodine Males and females, 150 μg	Large, swollen tongue, goiter
Protein Males, 60 g Females, 50 g	Skin: dull, dry, easily pluckable hair; "flaky paint" dermatitis; edema
Protein energy No RDA Total energy: Males, 2300 kcal Females, 1900 kcal	Skin: loss of subcutaneous fat; dull, dry, easily pluckable hair; decubitus ulcers; muscle wasting
Water No RDA, recommend 2 quarts	Skin: mucosal xerosis, swollen tongue, sunken eyeballs Neurologic: mental confusion Renal: electrolyte disturbances, decreased urine output, acute renal failure Other: elevated temperature, constipation, nausea and vomiting, decreased blood pressure, altered drug effects

* White or gray triangular deposits on the bulbar conjunctiva adjacent to the lateral margin of the cornea.

Source: Adapted with permission from Mitchell, C. O., & Chernoff, R. (1991). Nutritional assessment in the elderly. In Chernoff, R. (Ed.) *Geriatric nutrition: The health professional's handbook* (pp. 365–366). Gaithersburg, MD: Aspen Publishers.

Albumin is an appropriate screening tool because it is widely available and inexpensive. Other diagnostic parameters appropriate for determining nutrition-related problems will be discussed in detail in the following section.

CLINICAL MANAGEMENT

Management of nutritional status in the community involves education on prevention and maintenance. The food pyramid serves as a widely used standard on which to base educational efforts. Knowledge of the food pyramid should provide adequate information on portion size and variety (see Chapter 2, Fig. 2–1). Management of obesity involves an appropriate eating plan, exercise regime, and behavior modification.

CLINICAL PEARL

Treatment goals should include strategies that promote burning as many calories as consumed. Although this concept seems like common sense, it is often overlooked.

There are many weight loss programs available in the community. This author advocates those programs that focus on balanced diets, home-prepared foods, exercise programs, behavior modification, and client support.

Many older adults are on specialized diets due to chronic disease states. Maintenance of proper nutrition with specialized diets is essential and can be achieved with education. Table 8–3 outlines common disease states and dietary recommendations.

Pharmacologic Measures

Polypharmacy is common with the elderly. Older adults are also known to have decreased drug tolerance and are more likely to suffer with GI tract adverse reactions to medications. Drugs may affect the efficient absorption and utilization of nutrients. Monitor drug profiles closely (see Table 8–4).

Micronutrient supplementation should be examined. Increasing numbers of older Americans are using vitamin, min-

eral, or herbal supplementation. Often, individuals will select supplements based on what they think they need versus sound research-based information. Nutrients must be provided in adequate combinations of amounts. Some nutrients, such as fat-soluble vitamins, in doses too large can be toxic. These should be considered in the drug profile. The RDAs may not reflect doses being used as antioxidants; therefore, recommendations for supplementation must come from the appropriate health-care professional. If deficiency or excess is suspected, specific nutrient profiles may be obtained but are not done routinely because of the expense.

Pharmacologic treatment of obesity was thought to be helpful when diet, exercise, and behavior modification had not produced the results intended. Care must be taken, because a pill alone is not the answer. Prior to September 1997, phentermine–fenfluramine combinations and dexfenfluramine were being used but were taken off the market suddenly because of studies linking them to valvular diseases of the heart. New pharmacologic treatments are being developed and emerging on the market.

COLLABORATION AND REFERRAL

Often, the advanced practice nurse (APN) is first to detect nutritional deficits. Orchestration of nutritional information requires input from many health-care professionals (registered nurses, registered dietitians, occupational/physical therapists, speech therapists, social workers, and psychologists) as well as from the client and significant others. As the client shifts from one

TABLE 8–3. COMMON DISEASE STATES AND NUTRITIONAL MANAGEMENT

Disease	Nutritional Presentation	Nutritional Management
Alcoholism	Varying degrees of liver function	Provide adequate protein; too much will add to liver dysfunction
	Protein and calorie deficiency	Encourage nutrient-dense choices; assess for infection comorbidity
	GI distress	Anorexia: small frequent feedings; limit caffeine and other stimulants; supplements may be useful, fortify food
		Nausea/vomiting and gastritis: nothing by mouth with nausea and vomiting, then provide sips of fluid if tolerated clear liquids. Advance as tolerated. Avoid spicy or fatty foods, alcohol, caffeine, nicotine. Don't lie down after meals
		Diarrhea/constipation: decrease fatty foods in diarrhea, fiber by diet and over-the-counter bulking agents; include adequate fluid. Look for malabsorption
	Vitamin B complex deficiency (especially thiamine, folic acid, and magnesium)	Good sources
		Thiamine: pork, liver, other meats, whole grains, legumes, nuts
		Folic acid: leafy vegetables, legumes, nuts, liver, oranges
		Magnesium: green vegetables; avocados; bananas; chocolate; whole, unprocessed grains; legumes, nuts, including peanut butter and seeds
		Supplement with multivitamin with RDA of thiamine, folic acid, and magnesium
	Fluid and electrolytes	Enhance maintenance fluid requirements to meet losses via GI tract and inadequate intake. Alcohol acts as a diuretic; monitor and replace potassium
Diabetes	Initially presents with excessive thirst, nocturia, polyuria, polydypsia, excessive craving for sweets	Diet should be well balanced of all nutrients of pyramid in controlled portions. Diet should consist of 50%–60% carbohydrate, 15%–20% protein and 20%–25% fat. Limit simple sugars or replace with a carbohydrate. Avoid excessive carbohydrates
	Presents with HTN, often obesity, hyperlipidemia	
		Encourage fiber-rich foods. Good sources: rice, beans, vegetables, barley, oat bran. Include potassium (bananas, cantaloupe, orange juice, baked potatoes, low-fat yogurt) and chromium (yeast, meat, mushrooms, nuts, potatoes, unpeeled apples). Provide adequate amounts of vitamins A, C, and E. Excess vitamin C can cause false-positive urine glucose

TABLE 8–3.   COMMON DISEASE STATES AND NUTRITIONAL MANAGEMENT (CONT.)

Disease	Nutritional Presentation	Nutritional Management
Diabetes (cont.)		Encourage eating same amounts and frequency every day; limit simple sugars
		Look for complications of diabetes that affect nutrient intake: gastroparesis, blindness, renal impairment
Heart disease	Hyperlipidemia: cholesterol and triglycerides	There are no plant sources of cholesterol. Encourage diet that limits all fat, not just cholesterol; encourage meatless meals
	HTN	No-added-salt diet (4 g/d). Avoid high-salt snacks, prepared processed foods, some condiments; rinse canned foods
	Angina	2-g salt diet with ischemia
	CHF	Encourage client to read labels to check sodium and cholesterol contents. Discuss spices and seasoning; Salt substitutes often have potassium chloride. Use with caution with ACE inhibitors and potassium-sparing diuretics
		Limit coffee and other caffeinated foods and beverages
Asthma and COPD	Respiratory distress and fatigue at mealtime	Control obesity, which will lessen the workload
		Provide small, frequent meals to prevent abdominal distention; correct malnutrition to provide maximum energy; improve ventilation prior to mealtime; avoid foods that are hot or cold, which may induce coughing
	Allergy	Identify and avoid allergens. Common foods to omit are milk, eggs, seafood, sulfites
	Decreased resistance to disease	Correct protein/calorie malnutrition to boost immune system. Provide foods rich in vitamins A, C, and B_6 and zinc
	Dehydration, tenacious sputum, constipation	Tenacious mucus interferes with intake; provide 1 mL/cal; encourage more fluid in dehydration. It will also help with constipation; encourage fiber in the form of bran, fruits, and vegetables
	Anorexia, malnutrition	Provide adequate calories and protein. Carbohydrate metabolism produces more CO_2 than fat; therefore, maximize calorie intake with fats. Encourage concentration of calories and protein in foods (eg, adding powdered milk, butter, sour cream, yogurt, peanut butter, etc. to foods)
	GI distress	Assess for slowed peristalsis, due to inadequate oxygenation; limit gas-producing foods if not tolerated; assess for gastric ulceration and avoid caffeine and alcohol

(Continues)

TABLE 8–3.   COMMON DISEASE STATES AND NUTRITIONAL MANAGEMENT (CONT.)

Disease	Nutritional Presentation	Nutritional Management
Renal failure	Uremia	Provision of protein dependent on degree of wasting and whether client is receiving dialysis. As little as 0.3 g/kg used to avoid dialysis, 1.0–1.2 g/kg with dialysis. Encourage eggs and milk instead of meat, which produces more nitrogen waste
	Hyperkalemia and hyper-phosphatemia	Encourage restriction of potassium (bananas, cantaloupe, orange juice, baked potatoes, yogurt) and phosphorus (high-protein foods, oatmeal, brown rice); monitor regularly; supplement vitamin D
	Osteomalacia	Encourage calcium foods without adding phosphorus (good sources: all diary products except butter; dried peas and beans; most dark, leafy greens except spinach and Swiss chard); may need to use supplements (1000–1500 mg/d) but avoid calcium phosphate
	Anemia (usually iron or protein deficiency anemia)	Iron supplement or recombinant human erythropoietin may be needed
		Provide protein in adequate amounts that are tolerated
	Muscle wasting	Encourage adequate calories (25–35 kcal/kg of body weight); use calorie supplementation if necessary
	Carbohydrate intolerance	Fructose, galactose, and sorbitol are well tolerated
	Edema	Fluid intake should be equal to output plus 500–1000 cc for insensible loss; monitor regularly, as compliance is difficult. Restrict sodium to 1.5–2.0 g; watch use of salt substitutes, as they contain potassium. Have client weigh self daily.
Gastrointestinal GERD GI ulcer	Heartburn, pain, GI bleeding, gastritis, cough, chest pain	Treat symptoms to promote intake. Little evidence that bland foods aid in healing. Encourage foods that are tolerated; avoid gastric stimulants such as alcohol, black pepper, garlic, cloves, chili powder, and caffeine. Use fewer saturated fats to avoid slowing of gastric motility. Avoid milk products to decrease production of acid. Eat small meals to avoid distention. Do not lie down for at least 1 hour after eating

TABLE 8–3. COMMON DISEASE STATES AND NUTRITIONAL MANAGEMENT (CONT.)

Disease	Nutritional Presentation	Nutritional Management
Irritable bowel syndrome	Belching, flatulence, heartburn, mucus in stool, cramplike pain usually in lower quadrant, constipation alternating with diarrhea, nausea	Encourage regular eating and defecation habits Monitor for lactose and gluten intolerance Use bland or soft foods, provide adequate fluids, and gradually add fiber; avoid constipation with high-fiber diet and bulking agents; omit gas-forming foods such as beans, barley, brussels sprouts, cabbage, nuts, and soybeans; alleviate pain with antispasmodic meds; encourage regular eating and bowel habits. Teach stress reduction or coping techniques, as stress can precipitate acute attacks. Look for symptoms of lactose or gluten intolerance and other food allergies
Diverticular disease	Diverticulosis— constipation, LLQ pain	Avoid constipation; increase stool caliber and volume by high-fiber diet and high fluid intake; add fiber gradually. Good dietary sources: whole grains, stewed or dried fruit, potato skins, raw carrots, celery. If diet is inadequate, begin with 1 tsp of bran daily and increase to 2 tsp/d
	Diverticulitis—distention, nausea, vomiting, constipation or diarrhea, fever, chills	Encourage complete bowel rest in acute attacks to prevent perforation; then clear liquids followed by soft, bland foods. Avoid seeds, nuts, and fibrous vegetables in inflamed states. Avoid laxative effect of excess fiber by adding fiber gradually. Treat promptly to prevent peritonitis and abscess. Monitor nutritional side effects of anticholingerics, stool softeners, and antibiotics
Osteoporosis	Pain (can be severe), kyphosis, height loss, proneness to fractures	Encourage weight loss in obese. Decrease precipitating factors such as anticonvulsants, corticosteroids, lactase deficiency, low calcium intake, calcium malabsorption, and sedentary life style. Calcium intake should be at least 800–1000 mg/d before menopause and 1500 mg/d after menopause (1 quart of milk per day). If dairy products are not well tolerated of if dietary calcium is inadequate, a calcium supplement is essential. Adequate amounts of vitamin D are required for absorption of calcium, at least 400 µg/d and maybe up to twice the RDA. Ensure control of gastric acidity to enhance absorption of calcium; encourage adequate fluid intake to prevent calcium stone formation or hypercalcemia.

(Continues)

TABLE 8–3. COMMON DISEASE STATES AND NUTRITIONAL MANAGEMENT (CONT.)

Disease	Nutritional Presentation	Nutritional Management
Osteoporosis (cont.)		Discourage alcohol, cigarette, and caffeine consumption. Explain that efficiency of calcium absorption declines with age
		Good sources of calcium: all dairy products except butter; dried peas and beans; most dark, leafy greens except spinach or Swiss chard; soft bones of canned fish
		Good sources of vitamin D: sunshine, cod-liver oil, fortified milk and other dairy products, butter, margarine, eggs, liver, oily fish such as salmon
Anemia	Iron deficiency—weakness, fatigue, vertigo, headache, irritability, heartburn, dysphagia, flatulence, vague abdominal pains, anorexia, pica, glossitis	Encourage diet adequate in iron as well as supplementation especially heme iron. Good sources of iron: liver, eggs, kidney, beef, dried fruit, whole-grain cereals, molasses. Good sources of heme iron: beef, pork, lamb. Increase intake of vitamin C, as an acid medium increases absorption of iron. Good sources: oranges, grapefruit, tomatoes, broccoli, cabbage, baked potatoes, strawberries. Avoid coffee and tea during meal to enhance absorption
	Stomatitis, pale skin, ankle edema, tingling extremities, palpitations	Detect pica behaviors. Foods chosen are often crunchy or brittle. After cure, clients often develop a revulsion to the craving. Common food cravings are ice, clay, starch, plaster, lettuce, celery, chips, chocolate
		Large doses of iron do not help alleviate anemia, as the body can synthesize only 5–10 mg of hemoglobin per day
		Check for malabsorption. Most iron is absorbed in small intestines. Look for surgical procedures that may have altered this anatomy
		Check for GI bleeding with stools for occult blood, colonoscopy; refer to gastroenterologist for GI bleeding. Eliminate culprits such as NSAIDs and ASA
	Folic acid deficiency— weight loss; anorexia; malnutrition; smooth, red tongue; cold extremities	Encourage diet high in folic acid as well as supplementation. Good sources: fresh fruits or vegetables, fish, legumes, whole grains, leafy greens, broccoli, grapefruits, meat; avoid overcooking
		Soft, bland, or liquid foods may be tolerated with sore tongue; 6–8 small feedings may be helpful
		Promote intake of vitamin C, which improves absorption. Avoid alcoholic beverages, which interfere with folate metabolism and

TABLE 8–3.   COMMON DISEASE STATES AND NUTRITIONAL MANAGEMENT (CONT.)

Disease	Nutritional Presentation	Nutritional Management
Anemia (cont.)		absorption. Large intakes of folate (≥ 1 mg/d) can cure anemia but may mask vitamin B_{12} deficiency; monitor carefully. Check blood levels after initiation of therapy
	Pernicious anemia— fatigue; flatulence; nausea/vomiting; diarrhea; constipation; anorexia; weight loss; pale, waxy skin; lemon yellow pallor; tachycardia; cardiomegaly; achlorhydria; glossitis	Provide foods rich in vitamin B_{12}. Good sources: meats, liver, fish, poultry, dairy products, eggs
		Provide foods that won't hurt sore mouth; average daily intake should be 2–30 µg
		Injections of vitamin B_{12} are lifelong. After deficient states are corrected, monthly injections are often employed; avoid megadosing. Usual dosage is 100 µg
		Look for concurrent hypothyroidism and vitamin B_6 or iron deficient anemias, which decrease absorption of vitamin B_{12}. Supplement diet with vitamin C, iron, and other B vitamins
		Monitor levels as needed at least once per year

GI, gastrointestinal; RDA, recommended daily allowance; HTN, hypertension; CHF, congestive heart failure; ACE, angiotensin-converting enzyme; COPD, chronic obstructive pulmonary disease; GERD, gastroesophageal reflux disease; LLQ, left lower quadrant; NSAIDs, nonsteroidal anti-inflammatory drugs; ASA, acetylsalicylic acid.

Source: Adapted from information from Escott-Stump, S. (1992). *Nutrition and diagnosis-related care* (3rd ed.). Philadelphia: Lea & Febiger.

health-care setting to another, nutritional profiles must be communicated.

Home delivery meals are offered in most communities through senior citizen centers or nursing associations. These are excellent options for homebound elders who are unable to prepare their own meals.

For the overweight, there are many weight loss programs available. Encourage clients to get involved with those that promote healthy weight loss and use the team approach, with support from many disciplines.

■ MALNUTRITION

As adults age, the risk of developing chronic disease rises. Many chronic diseases are associated with diet. Less than optimal nutrition puts the client at risk when acute events occur. Malnutrition is defined as the excessive or deficient intake of nutrients. It involves biochemical processes that are influenced by the proper balance of nutrients. In studies of marasmus (energy-deficiency malnutrition) in adults over age 75, there is a greater incidence of being underweight (Master et al., 1960). People with marasmus are particularly susceptible to progressing to protein calorie malnutrition secondary to their decreased reserve capacity.

Protein calorie malnutrition usually presents in hospitalized elderly. It is secondary to a primary disease state that caused or is caused by a nutrient imbalance.

TABLE 8–4. COMMON DRUGS IN THE ELDERLY THAT CAN NEGATIVELY INFLUENCE NUTRITION

Drug	Nutrition-related Side Effects
Alcohol	Anorexia, altered consciousness, amnesia, dizziness, headache, lethargy, paresthesias, vitamin/mineral deficiencies, weakness
Analgesics	
Aspirin	Anemia, GI hemorrhage
Antibiotics	Anorexia, diarrhea, nausea, vomiting
Anti-inflammatory agents	
Corticosteroids	Anorexia, appetite stimulation, edema, hyperglycemia, osteoporosis, weight gain
Nonsteroidal anti-inflammatory agents (NSAIDs)	Anemia, GI hemorrhage, edema, weight gain
Cardiovascular agents	
Antiarrhythmics	Anorexia, nausea, vomiting
ACE inhibitors	Anorexia, dry mouth, gastritis, hypoalbuminemia, hyperkalemia, loss of taste, nausea, weight loss
Beta blockers (lipid soluble)	Constipation, cramping, diarrhea, epigastric distress, nausea, vomiting, worsening of diabetic glucose control
Calcium channel blockers	Anorexia, constipation, diarrhea, dry mouth, dysgeusia, edema, nausea, vomiting
Diuretics	Anorexia, constipation, cramping, dehydration, diarrhea, fluid/electrolyte imbalance, gastric irritation, hyperglycemia, hyperlipidemia, hyperuricemia, nausea, vomiting
Cardiac glycosides	Anorexia, drug interactions, nausea, loss of taste, weight loss
Potassium supplements	Anorexia, gastric irritation, hyperkalemia
CNS agents	
Anticonvulsants	Anemia, antivitamin effects, hyperglycemia, oral health problems, nausea, osteoporosis, vomiting
Antidepressants	Anorexia, appetite stimulation, constipation, drowsiness, dry mouth, weight gain
Antipsychotics	Appetite stimulation, constipation, dry mouth, fluid retention, weight gain
Endocrine/metabolic agents	
Oral hypoglycemic agents	Appetite stimulation, dizziness, hypoglycemia
Gastrointestinal agents	
Antacids	Drug/nutrient binding, malabsorption, reduced iron absorption
Laxatives	Dehydration, diarrhea, malabsorption, weight loss
H_2-receptor antagonists	Confusion, diarrhea, dizziness, somnolence

Source: Modified from White, J. V. Risk factors associated with poor nutritional status in older Americans, Washington, DC, 1991, Nutrition Screening Initiative, a project of the American Academy of Family Physicians, the American Dietetic Association, and the National Council on Aging, Inc. and funded in part by a grant from Ross Products Division, Abbott Laboratories.
From White, J. V., & Ham, R. J. (1997). Nutrition.

The most serious consequence of malnutrition is the effect it has on the immune system. Nosocomial infections, which are prevalent in hospitalized or institutionalized elderly, further decrease the individual's reserves.

AGE-RELATED CHANGES

Energy
Healthy older adults have decreased energy needs. However, older adults who are acutely or chronically ill have increased needs due to stress, healing, and fighting infection. Individual assessment is essential to determine the energy requirements.

Protein
Protein requirements are not significantly affected by aging but are impacted by poor health. Immobility alone can cause negative nitrogen balance. It is imperative to individualize assessment and treatment.

Fat
Fat in the diet provides energy, essential fatty acids, and fat-soluble vitamins. Very little fat is required for essential fatty acids and vitamins stores. Therefore, as the energy requirement of the elderly decreases, so should the intake of fat to maintain calorie balance.

Carbohydrates
Carbohydrate metabolism declines with advancing age. Tolerance to glucose is altered. Lactose intolerance is also prevalent in the elderly. Energy needs of older adults are best met with a diet rich in complex carbohydrates, as they also serve as a valuable source for other nutrients.

Vitamins and Minerals
There is much speculation over the requirements of vitamins and minerals of older adults. Published recommended daily requirements for people over 51 years old encompass a large cross-section of populations. More research is needed to assess the specific micronutrient needs of older adults. Table 8–5 shows those micronutrients most affected by aging and associated consequences.

Water
Water is a nutrient that is often overlooked in the elderly. Symptoms associated with dehydration are hypotension, elevated temperature, constipation, nausea, vomiting, dry mucous membranes, decreased urinary output, and mental confusion.

CLINICAL PRESENTATION

Malnutrition or nutritional deficit often accompanies other illnesses such as malignancy, renal insufficiency, or major infection. Its presentation is often insidious, usually occurring as a comorbidity of a serious illness. Older adults who barely maintain their nutritional status when healthy can become malnourished when their reserve capacity is stressed with disease. These malnourished individuals often present with fatigue, anorexia, and frequent GI complaints. Unintentional weight loss, often difficult to document, is the common presenting symptom of malnutrition. Clients may or may not recognize anorexia as a concurrent symptom. This weight loss may be due to a myriad of physiologic, psychologic, or pathologic conditions, or they may occur in isolation. Rapid weight loss of greater than 10% in 3 to 6 months is cause for concern and warrants further investigation (Mansouri et al., 1994).

TABLE 8–5.   NUTRIENTS MOST OFTEN DEFICIENT IN THE ELDERLY

Micronutrient	Age-related Changes	Associated Conditions
Calcium, magnesium	Decreased intake	Osteoporosis
Zinc	Decreased intake	Poor wound healing, pressure sore development
Sodium	Decreased need	Excess intake associated with hypertension; deficiency associated with excessive use of laxatives or diuretics
Vitamin D	Decreased absorption—inadequate exposure to sunlight in homebound or institutionalized populations; possibly decreases in kidney function	Delayed wound healing, psoriasis, actinic keratoses, hyperproliferative disorders of cancer
Vitamin C	Associated with alcoholism	Fatigue, delayed wound healing, capillary hemorrhage, purpura, cataracts
Vitamin K	Deficiencies related to the use of sulfa or anticoagulation medications	Bleeding tendency
Vitamin B_{12}	Loss of intrinsic factor	Pernicious anemia
Folic acid	Alcohol related	Anemia
Thiamine (vitamin B_1)	Alcohol related	Depression, irritability, attention deficit, muscular weakness; in severe deficiency, it causes beriberi (edema, paralysis, and heart failure)
Iron	Deficiency state usually from blood loss	Iron deficiency anemia

Source: Adapted from Chernoff, R. (1990). Physiologic Aging and Nutritional Status. Nutrition in Clinical Practice, 5, 8–13.

CLINICAL PEARL

Do not assume that individuals who are over their ideal body weight cannot be malnourished or that they can live off the fat stores in their bodies.

Weight gain can be due to edema and is often a sign of hypoalbuminemia. This condition allows the oncotic pressure of the vascular system to rise and permits fluid to leak and accumulate in the dependent tissues. Obese individuals may be malnourished of protein and other micronutrients, which puts them at risk for infections, poor wound healing, and chronic states such as anemia and osteoporosis. Some elderly are chronically malnourished due to economic and social reasons. These individuals often present with osteoporosis, delayed wound healing, or chronic infections.

Institutionalized elderly are at great risk for malnutrition. Immobility and exposure to nosocomial infection add to the problem. It is well documented that 30% to 50% of hospitalized clients of many ages are malnourished. Diagnostic testing and surgical interventions only add to its severity.

ASSESSMENT

Elements of a complete nutritional history and physical are illustrated in Table 8–6.

History
Additional history may include current diagnoses that add to malnutrition (reason for hospitalizations), history of pressure ulcers or other skin lesions (draining wounds, etc.), mental status changes, malignancy, and therapies. Review current and past medications, looking for drug–nutrient interactions (see Table 8–1).

Physical Examination
Review all systems with a focus on signs and symptoms of malnutrition, giving special attention to those deficits common in the elderly. Assess for hypothyroidism or malignancy with rapid unintentional weight loss. Assess hydration status.

Assess height and weight. Always measure and record actual data because elderly adults are often not aware of their current height or weight. Then compare the measures to usual height/weight charts. The Metropolitan Life Insurance

CLINICAL PEARL

Hydration status is difficult to assess in the elderly by physical exam. Skin turgor and mucous membrane appearance are unreliable measures of fluid balance due to normal daily changes. Laboratory values may be somewhat helpful (electrolytes, blood urea nitrogen [BUN], creatinine) if baseline comparison is available.

scales are the most common. Assess IBW as follows:

Females: First 5 ft = 100 lb + 5 lb for each additional inch

Males: First 5 ft = 106 lb + 6 lb for each additional inch

Assess functional status. Clients who are immobile, bedbound, or nonambulatory may develop protein malnutrition secondary to a negative nitrogen balance.

Nutritional Assessment
A dietary history includes the current diet, the consistency of foods tolerated, food preferences, restrictions, allergies, and methods and assistance with food procurement. Daily food intake should be assessed in terms of meals, kinds of foods, and amounts. Obtain the assistance of a registered dietitian to provide information on calorie, protein, fat, and other nutrients from the dietary recall. In hospitalized clients, nutritional assessment should be completed in 3 to 5 days. In those with suspected malnutrition, nu-

TABLE 8–6.   COMPONENTS OF THE HISTORY AND PHYSICAL THAT ASSESS NUTRITIONAL STATUS

History	
Identifying data	Age, sex, ethnic origin, religious preference, marital status
Medical component	Chief complaint (especially if diet related)
	Presence of chronic disease or allergy
	Recent major illness or surgery
	Family history (diet-related disease)
	Usual weight and recent involuntary weight change
	Dental history
	Cognitive/emotional status
	Medications
	Exercise and sleep patterns
Psychosocial component	Occupation, income level
	Participation in economic assistance programs
	Living arrangements
	Transportation
	Shopping patterns
	Educational and reading level and learning style
	Motivation and compliance
Nutrition component	Changes in sensory perception
	Appetite
	Current meal and snack pattern
	Food intake over the last 24 hours
	Food preferences and tolerances
	Major food group intake
	Current and previous dietary modifications (duration, compliance, results)
	Use of supplements (purpose, content, frequency)
Physical	General appearance
	Measured height, weight, vital signs
	Other anthropometric parameters as indicated
	Physical signs and symptoms of nutrient deficiency or toxicity
	Oral cavity examination
	Vision and hearing status
Laboratory	Serum albumin (especially if hospitalized or institutionalized)
	Serum cholesterol (periodic monitoring: modify diet if elevated; check additional parameters if low)
	Blood glucose (especially postprandial)
	Hemoglobin/hematocrit, CBC
	Vitamin B_{12} (especially vegan diets or GI pathology)
	Individual nutrients (eg, K, Mg, Na—signs, symptoms, or chronic drug use dictates choice)

Source: Adapted from White, J., & Ham, R. (1997). Nutrition. In Ham, R., & Sloane, P. (Eds.). *Primary care geriatrics: A case-based approach* (3rd ed.) (p. 114). St. Louis: Mosby–Year Book.

tritional assessment should be completed in 24 hours.

Assessment of the nutritional requirements in the malnourished client is an essential part of the overall assessment. Requirement of nutrients is based on the client's basal requirements, current nutritional state, and the degree of stress or activity.

To assess calorie requirements, use the following Harris Benedict equation. It is based on the height, weight, sex, and age of the client and equals the client's basal energy expenditure (BEE).

For males 66.4 + 13.7 (weight in kg) + 5 (height in cm) − 6.8 (age in years)

For females 65.5 + 9.7 (weight in kg.) + 1.8 (height in cm.) − 4.7 (age in years)

To convert lb into kg = lb ÷ 2.2

To convert inches into cm = 2.54 × inches

To this number multiply a stress and/or activity factor.

Activity Factors

		Stress Factors	
Confined to		Minor surgery	1.2
bed	1.2	Skeletal	
Out of bed	1.3	trauma	1.3
		Major sepsis	1.6
		Severe burn	2.1

CLINICAL PEARL

More is not better. Overfeeding with calories only adds to increases in fat stores and should be avoided.

Some hospitals have available indirect calorimetry (which is currently not covered by Medicare) to determine the amount of calories being burned in a resting state. This reflects the measured energy expenditure. It is based on the oxygen consumed and the carbon dioxide produced and is a reflection of intercellular metabolism.

Calories are provided by carbohydrates, protein, and fats. If the client is in a catabolic state, adequate calories are provided by carbohydrates and fats to spare the protein for the building of anabolism. The ratio of fat calories to the total caloric intake should not succeed 30% to 40% depending on comorbities.

Protein requirements are also determined by stress factors. Stress levels must be quantified to assess the protein requirements.

No stress	0.5–0.8 g/kg/d
Mild stress	0.8–1.0 g/kg/d
Moderate stress	1.0–1.5 g/kg/d
Severe stress	1.5–2.0 g/kg/d

Very few clients need more than 1.3 to 1.5 g/kg/d.

Other micronutrients, including vitamins, minerals, trace elements, and electrolytes, are required at various amounts based initially on RDAs.

Diagnostic Studies

To determine the source of weight loss, assess complete blood count (CBC), creatinine, glucose, calcium, thyroid function studies, liver function studies, urinalysis, stool for occult blood, and chest x-ray.

Serum Proteins. The visceral protein status reflects the client's nutritional status and is assessed by serum albumin, transferrin, and prealbumin.

Albumin is the most abundant visceral protein. It has a half-life of 21 days and therefore is not the most sensitive nutritional marker. It is, however, a good screening tool because it is widely available and inexpensive. Serum albumin levels may be altered with edema, the administration of albumin, and fluid rehydration. This marker responds slowly to nutritional therapy.

Transferrin is a carrier protein for iron and is inversely proportionate to the serum iron. It has a half-life of 8 days and therefore is a more sensitive measurement.

Prealbumin is also a carrier protein for thyroxine that has a half-life of approximately 2 days. With nutritional therapy, the levels rise at a daily rate, making it one of the most sensitive parameters of protein depletion and repletion. Many believe that prealbumin is the best indicator and should be used in the assessment of nutritional support because of its sensitivity.

Measurement of these markers can indicate the severity of the protein depletion. Levels vary with the laboratory used.

Plasma Protein	Normal	Moderate Depletion	Severe Depletion
Albumin (mg/dL)	3.5–5.0	2.4–3.4	< 2.4
Transferrin (mg/dL)	155–355	100–150	< 100
Prealbumin (mg/dL)	10–40	5–10	< 5

Immunologic Measures. Immunologic measures may not be the best representation of nutritional deficiency in the elderly because of the decreased efficiency of the elder immune system. It is therefore wise to carefully consider immunologic data when assessing the older adult's nutritional status.

The total lymphocyte count (TLC) can be calculated to reflect protein depletion. Lymphocytes are produced by proteins and are an indication of an individual's ability to fight infection. This value can be influenced by diseases that affect the immune system and by immunosuppressive drugs. It is calculated as

$$TLC = \% \text{ lymphocytes} \times \frac{\text{white blood cells}}{100}$$

Cellular immune response by intradermal testing of the recall antigen has been used to identify protein depletion. The immunocompetent client will exhibit a response within 48 hours, with induration of at least 5 mm. With protein depletion, there is a decreased reproduction to antibody formation, leading to a diminished response to the antigen. However, the same result can be seen in normal elders making it difficult to assess this population.

CLINICAL MANAGEMENT

Clinical management of malnutrition is multifaceted, as nutrition is based on the client's physical, physiologic, social, psychologic, cultural, and spiritual self. Various factors play a role in its complete treatment. Recognition of acute malnutrition, assessment of risk, provision of proper requirements, monitoring of progress, and patient/caregiver education are the goals of management.

Pharmacologic Measures

Pharmacologic therapies for the treatment of malnutrition in the elderly have been based on symptom relief of GI tract distress and most often prove to be adequate. Antacids; H$_2$ blockers; proton pump inhibitors for heartburn; antiemetics for nausea and vomiting; prokinetic agents for enhancing gastric emptying; and antispasmodics for intestinal cramping, bloating, and flatulence are just a few that can provide relief. See Chapter 7 for more information.

There are pharmacologic options to enhance appetite and decrease anorexia, which are most often used in cachexia associated with cancer and acquired immune deficiency syndrome (AIDS). These agents (corticosteroids, anabolic steroids, appetite stimulants, progestational agents, metabolic inhibitors, and anticytokine) do not have a role in the treatment of age-related malnutrition other than that related to cancer and AIDS.

The nutritional rehabilitation of clients is slow. Weight gain of greater than 0.5 to 1 lb per week is usually a gain in fat or water, not lean mass.

CLINICAL PEARL

More is not better. Overfeeding without exercise will produce adipose tissue. The goal is to increase lean body or muscle mass.

Nonpharmacologic Measures

Nonpharmacologic measures include providing nutritious, appealing, appropriate meals and monitoring the intake. Alleviating isolation during meals may prove to be of some benefit. Older institutionalized adults sometimes increase their intake when meals are provided in a dining room atmosphere rather than isolated in their rooms.

There are many supplements on the market designed for specific disease entities such as renal failure and pulmonary compromise. Medicare does not reimburse for supplementation that is consumed by mouth, so the payment source must be considered for older populations at home. Most supplements provide 1 calorie per cc and the RDAs for all essential vitamins and minerals in 1000 cc of supplement. Protein contents can vary. Some supplements provide dietary fiber, which can be useful in elderly populations to prevent diarrhea and constipation. Some supplements are calorie and protein dense, providing 1.5 to 2.0 cal/cc and therefore supply less fluid. When using these supplements, monitor serum sodium levels and be cognizant of fluid needs, as dehydration may ensure, especially in older populations.

COLLABORATION AND REFERRAL

All malnourished older adults would benefit from the expertise of a registered dietitian. Prompt referral and frequent communication to the dietitian is essential for nutritional support therapy. Many acute-care institutions have nutritional support teams made up of physicians, nurses, pharmacists, and dietitians who are accountable for the nutritional support of the client. Collaboration with this group can prove invaluable.

■ EATING DISORDERS

Eating disorders are those in which the intake of nutrients is interrupted before they enter the body. These disorders may have neurologic, psychologic, or mechanical bases.

DEMENTIA

One of the most common neurologic disorders affecting nutritional intake is dementia. Dementia may be related to cerebrovascular accident (CVA), alcohol, vitamin B_{12} or folate deficiencies, or Alzheimer's disease. See Chapter 3 for more information related to dementia. Whatever the cause, memory loss will affect the nutritional status.

Clinical Presentation

Weight change (gain or loss) is common with dementia, as the client does not remember or is inattentive to food consumption. Vitamin and mineral deficiencies may ensue if these patterns are not recognized.

At stages of mild confusion, the client may exhibit changes in food behavior such as a tendency to overeat or leave meals. Supervision will be required as clients become unable to procure food and prepare meals independently. As dementia progresses, unusual food behaviors may develop such as excessive eating, forgetting to finish a meal, poorly coordinated feeding ability, loss of the desire to eat, bizarre food cravings, or eating foods in a particular fashion.

Assessment

A complete nutritional assessment, as outlined in previous sections, is important to calculate a balanced diet based on sex, age, and activity requirements.

In addition, knowledge of the type of dementia involved is essential to guide interventions. For example, management of a dementia secondary to vitamin deficiency will include replacement of vitamin B_{12} and folic acid, and nutritional interventions for alcoholic dementia will include avoidance of alcohol and the provision of proper nutrition (which may contribute to partial reversibility). Clinical features of the dementia will also influence the nutritional plan. Wanderers will require more nutrients than sedentary individuals.

Clinical Management

As dementia progresses, clients may require more supervision from the healthcare provider to maintain adequate nutrition. It is important that the intake of protein, calories, and other nutrients be maintained in advanced disease, as these clients are at risk for pressure ulcer formation and aspiration pneumonia secondary to their incontinence, immobility, and difficulty swallowing.

Tolerance of food consistency differs among clients with dementia and should be adapted to the individual. Some are more tolerant of liquids, whereas others do better with thicker consistencies. Smooth and sweet foods generally are more acceptable. Cooked cereal mixed with pudding, sweetened apple sauce, or eggnog is often a preferred choice.

Mealtime must be lengthened for clients with dementia, as it takes them longer to ingest, chew, and swallow food. Some may forget this process of eating and need constant reminders with both verbal and physical cues. Effective body positioning is useful to minimize losses from dribbling and prevent aspiration for clients with poor swallowing reflexes.

Creative interventions and diversions should be employed with combative or resistive clients. Hand holding, reassuring touches, coaxing, cheerful conversation, and singing softly have been known to be effective. It is often useful for the caregiver to join the client during mealtime, which provides initative cues as well as a sense of intimacy. Finger foods, high-lipped bowls and gripped utensils in colors which contrast with the tablecloth can promote self-feeding.

Persons with dementia often consume more at breakfast or lunch than at the eveining meal. This coincides with the "sundowning" phenomenon seen at the end of the day, which is displayed as restlessness, insecurity, and agitation. These behaviors will affect intake and should be recognized by caregivers. The goal is to provide support for maximum intake during the earlier meals if agitation is anticipated.

PSYCHOLOGIC DISORDERS

Depression is the most psychologically based explanation for nutritional problems. Weight loss or gain is often the symptom that takes the client to the primary-care provider. (See Chaps. 3 and 15 for more information on depression.) Assessment must be complete to rule out any physiologic causes of malnutrition. Depression often accompanies physical illness, which may add to nutritional deficits.

Anorexia nervosa and bulimia are most commonly found in adolescent populations. It is rate that psychologically based eating disorders present in elderly clients. They are most frequently a result of years of symptoms that have been battled or were subclinical and re-

mained undiagnosed. These behaviors may reappear during times of stress such as death of a spouse or loss of a home.

Clinical Presentation

Signs and symptoms of depression include anorexia or increases in appetite as well as weight change, poor sleep pattern, decreases in usual activity, loss of interest, fatigue, and diminished concentration, all of which can affect nutrient intake.

Anorexia nervosa is a condition that is related to severe rejection of food to the point of extreme weight loss and exhaustion, electrolyte imbalance, and metabolic disturbances. Bulimia is bingeing and purging of food by episodes of overeating, followed by laxative abuse or induced vomiting to expel food.

Assessment

In addition to the assessment parameters described in previous sections, special attention must be paid to eating habits. Assess whether the client's pattern tends toward overeating or undereating. Monitor weight weekly to assess progress. Loneliness, difficulties with ADL, boredom, inattention, and poor sleep can all play a role in nutrition-related problems. For eating disorders, assess for an intense preoccupation with body weight. Look for GI complaints that may be associated with bingeing and purging. Check for a physiologic cause. If none exists, look for misperceptions of body image, loneliness, passivity, sadness, chemical dependence, or suicidal behavior. Electrolyte imbalances are common.

Clinical Management

Management always includes a balanced diet. Emotional stress depletes the body of nitrogen and calcium, and therefore diets must be rich in these nutrients to prevent vitamin B deficiencies. Clinical depression is effectively treated by a combination of psychotherapy and medication. Some of the medications used have nutrient-related interactions, such as monoamine oxidase inhibitors (MAOIs), tricyclic antidepressants (TCAs), lithium carbonate, and nortriptyline (see Table 8–4).

Management of anorexia nervosa is extremely difficult, as the client is often very knowledgeable about food and may exaggerate on food amounts and frequency of meals. Never force the client to eat. Promote self-control in normal eating behaviors. Help the client identify nutritional hunger and strategies to satisfy it with nutritionally balanced food choices.

DYSPHAGIA

Dysphagia is a mechanical interruption of eating. It may be caused by a CVA, head trauma, obstructive tumor, or other neuromuscular disorders that affect the smooth muscle of the nasopharynx and esophagus. A disruption of swallowing can result in aspiration. The swallowing process can be interruted at many levels.

Age-Related Changes

Dysphagia is not a normal age-related change. It can be a result of age-related changes in dentition, mastication, and transport (slowing) of food through the esophagus. Swallowing time does decrease with age, which is consistent with the overall slowing of the central nervous system, but there are no significant increases in aspiration tendencies.

Clinical Presentation

There are three types of dysphagia. Mechanical dysphagia involves the inability to move food or liquids from the front to the back of the mouth, where it can be swallowed. This is usually associated with tumor. Dysphagia paralytica is a result of disease or trauma to the brain stem or cranial nerves associated with swallowing. Pseudobulbar dysphagia is commonly caused by stroke that has affected the upper part of the brain and cortex, which results in the inability to coordinate chewing, swallowing, and breathing.

Assessment

History. Assess for presence of diseases that are associated with dysphagia. Dietary history should include questions about types of foods with which the client is having difficulties. Some clients tolerate liquids and others tolerate semisolid foods. Some clients experience coughing and choking and others do not.

CLINICAL PEARL

Not all clients with dysphagia cough or choke while eating. Some are silent aspirators. Chronic congestion without fever or leukocytosis may be an indication of aspiration.

Clients often change their diets to accommodate their limitations without realizing it. Aspiration can be ongoing or intermittent.

Physical Examination. Look for significant weight loss. Assess level of consciousness. Look for temperature spikes, congestion after a meal, coughing, choking, drooling, difficulty initiating the swallowing process, poor head control, or poor lip closure. Look for a delay in the swallowing reflex or pocketing of food in the oropharynx. Assess both liquids and solids.

CLINICAL PEARL

Do not confuse behavioral eating problems such as clamping down, spitting out, refusal to eat when food is offered, or refusal to chew with true dysphagia.

Diagnostic Studies. If aspiration is suspected, check CBC with differential and chest x-ray. There is no widely accepted test for dysphagia. Current testing of dysphagia is bedside evaluation and observation, secretion monitors such as dyes and glucose, videofluoroscopy, and videoendoscopy. Bedside evaluation and observation should be done by speech therapists, as the trained individual will be able to accurately assess the more difficult cases of aspiration. Secretion monitoring has not proven to be a reliable assessment tool for dysphagia. Bedside evaluation alone will often underestimate the frequency and extent of aspiration. The most common study of dysphagia is the videofluoroscopy or barium swallow test. This technique not only allows for direct observation of swallowing but can also provide information on the causes of aspiration. Videoendoscopy allows direct visualization of the oropharyngeal structures, their function, and the swallowing maneuver. Frequent, on-going monitoring is recommended to watch for progress or decline.

Clinical Management

Management of dysphagia requires input from all team members (ie, speech therapists, nurses, dietitians, occupational therapists, and clinical practitioners). Based on data obtained in the assessment, dietary changes are made. Often, diets with semisolid consistencies are ordered. In this case, strict adherence to the diet is essential to reduce the risk of aspiration. Products are available to thicken the consistencies of liquids to an applesauce, thick nectar, or pudding consistency. These products are made from modified food starches.

Proper positioning during eating should be maintained. The client should sit up if at all possible. When the client is ready to swallow, he should tip his head slightly forward and hold his breath. Other body/head position techniques may be recommended by the physical or speech therapist.

Food should not be washed down by liquids. Some foods cause more difficulties than others. Milk-based products produce phlegm. Sticky foods such as mashed potatoes, bananas, and bread may be difficult to swallow. Dry foods should be moistened with gravy or other thick sauces. Temperature of food will affect the stimulation necessary for swallowing. Foods served at room temperature are most difficult to swallow. Foods served either hot or cold stimulate the swallowing reflex. The caregiver must be educated in order to continue this regime in the home setting. An understanding of the food consistency, body position, and special equipment required is essential.

Many clients become dehydrated because of the limitation of liquids in the diet. Some clients may not be able to maintain a balanced diet and become malnourished. Modules and supplements should then be employed. Modules contain single nutrients such as protein or carbohydrates that enhance nutrient concentrations of the diet. Supplements are meal replacement formulas. Each can augment diets to boost nutritional intakes. Timely assessment is imperative to prevent malnutrition and dehydration. If these modalities fail, enteral nutrition must be considered.

■ ENTERAL NUTRITION

ENTERAL ACCESS

Enteral nutrition is delivered by nasogastric/jejunostomy tubes, gastrostomy tubes (either surgically placed or percutaneously placed), or jejunostomy tubes (direct intubation or transgastrostomy jejunal intubation). Nasogastric/jejunostomy tubes are not to be used in long-term enteral feedings because of the multiple complications associated with them. Jejunostomy tubes are used when feeding into the stomach is unsuccessful, as with gastroparesis, and requires an x-ray to check for placement. Placement as

CLINICAL PEARL

Always be aware of what part of the GI tract the distal end of the tube occupies. This will determine delivery system and reasons for potential intolerance.

close as possible to the ligament of Treitz is ideal. Gastrostomy tubes are the most common access for enteral nutrition; they are easiest to care for and are associated with fewer complications.

ENTERAL PRESCRIPTIONS

There are a multitude of commercially available formulas with different nutrient concentrations. Some are higher in protein, some are concentrated delivering greater nutrients in smaller volumes, and some are "designer" products specific to disease states. Most are lactose free. Some include dietary fiber. Seek out the dietitian for recommendations of appropriate formulas and volumes. Generally, most standard formulas provide 1 cal/mL of volume and varying amounts of protein. The volume required to meet 100% of the RDA of vitamins varies between 1180 and 2000 cc.

Volume requirements are based on the calculated nutritional needs of the client minus the intake by mouth. Tube feeding must be initiated slowly and monitored for tolerance. It is not usually necessary to start with one-fourth-strength formula, as most formulas are isotonic. Start at 40 cc/hr full strength and increase to goal slowly, based on tolerance. It should be initiated over 24 hours until tolerance is established and then may be changed to a nighttime feeding if the client is able to take food by mouth. (Jejunostomy feedings require continuous delivery.) Stopping the tube feeding during the day may enhance PO feeding. However, some clients are NPO, and some are unable to tolerate feedings at fast rates. Other delivery methods are bolus feeding and intermittent pump feedings. Some feel that feeding intermittently is more physiologic and may be preferred for clients at home because it accommodates life styles.

Tolerance of tube feeding is based on the absence of nausea/vomiting, cramping, bloating, and/or diarrhea. If the client is able to verbalize, always remember that he or she is the best judge of tolerance. Residuals are to be checked at least every 4 hours upon initiation. There are many opinions as to what is an acceptable residual volume. Often, tube feedings are stopped or slowed because of "high" residuals adding to inadequate nutritional intake. An empty stomach has 100 cc of stomach contents. Residual consistency as well as volume must be considered. If the pump is delivering 100 cc/hr, there may be at least a 100-cc residual. The residual should be assessed over time, as the stomach does not constantly empty. If the residual is as large as the previous delivered volume after checking twice within a few minutes, the feeding should be held and resumed as soon as possible. There is no residual in a jejunostomy feeding, as the jejunum is not a reservoir.

Most enteral formulas deliver about 75% to 85% of fluid requirements, and therefore extra fluid must be provided, usually as a flushing volume. Free water deficit is apparent when hypernatremia occurs. Flushing the tube also helps prevent tube occlusion.

COMPLICATIONS

There are many potential complications associated with enteral nutrition. Some of the most distressing are aspiration, tube displacement, tube occlusion, and refeeding syndrome.

Aspiration is a serious complication of enteral nutrition and usually occurs with regurgitation of the enteral formula. It can be a result of improper positioning of the feeding tube or a delay in gastric emptying. Prevention can be enhanced by checking placement of the feeding tube and checking residuals. If gastric emptying is delayed, drugs such as cisapride can be used to improve the peristaltic action of the stomach. The risk of aspiration may also be prevented by raising the head of the bed whenever possible. This concept is based on the use of gravity when there is a potential for a delay in gastric emptying.

Tube displacement encompasses migration of tubes or complete disintubation. Gastrostomy or jejunostomy tubes can migrate up or down the GI tract. When a gastrostomy tube migrates further into the stoma, it may migrate to the pyloric sphincter, causing outlet obstruction, or up through the esophagus, causing a higher risk for aspiration. This will present with abrupt high residuals or vomiting. Prevention is based on keeping traction on the tube at the skin surface. A gastrostomy tube can be replaced (using a new tube) if the stoma tract is well formed and done in a timely fashion. Closure of the stoma may begin within hours, depending on how old the stoma is, so delays may make replacement difficult. A jejunal tube can also migrate. These tubes should be replaced by fluoroscopy or checked by x-ray to ensure a proper position.

Tubes that leak onto the surface of the skin will cause excoriation and eventual erosion. Prevention is the best defense against this complication. Keeping the tube in traction will prevent the stomach contents from leaking. If this does occur and excoriation ensues, protection of the skin surface with barrier creams or stoma devices can help.

TABLE 8–7. COMPLICATIONS, PREDISPOSING FACTORS, PREVENTION, AND THERAPY RELATED TO REFEEDING

Complication	Predisposing Factors	Prevention	Therapy
Hyperglycemia[a]	Rapid glucose infusion Diabetes Age > 60 years Steroid therapy Metabolic stress	Enteral rather than parenteral route if possible Initiate feedings slowly Daily monitoring of blood glucose initially Avoid excessive carbohydrate infusion	Decrease infusion rate Change to a lower-carbohydrate/higher-fat regimen Oral hypoglycemics or insulin therapy
Rebound hypoglycemia	Abrupt cessation of glucose infusion	Taper feedings Continuous administration schedules Daily monitoring of serum glucose	Supplemental IV or oral carbohydrate Glucagon therapy for severe hypoglycemia
Hypokalemia	Insulin therapy Diuretic therapy Diarrhea Vomiting Rapid glucose infusion Metabolic alkalosis	Daily monitoring of serum K^+ levels Initiate feedings slowly Adjust K^+ intake based on serum levels Close monitoring of high carbohydrate regimens	Supplemental K^+ administration (either IV or enteral)
Hyperkalemia	Metabolic acidosis Renal dysfunction Respiratory acidosis Hypoxia	Daily monitoring of serum K^+ Adjust K^+ intake based on serum levels	Potassium exchange resin enemas Glucose and insulin infusions Potassium wasting diuretics If acidotic, bicarbonate supplements Decrease K^+ content of IV feeding Change to an enteral formula containing less K^+ (ex: modular formulas)
Hypophosphatemia	Alcoholism Chronic antacid use Insulin therapy Malabsorption Hemodialysis Diabetic ketoacidosis	Biweekly monitoring of serum phosphorus Initiate feedings slowly Close monitoring of high-carbohydrate regimens Adjust phosphorus intake based on serum levels	Temporarily stop feeding Supplemental phosphorus

Complication	Predisposing Factors	Prevention	Therapy
Hypomagnesemia	Alcoholism Malabsorption Chronic diuretic therapy Ketoacidosis	Biweekly monitoring of serum magnesium Adjust magnesium intake based on serum levels	Supplemental magnesium
Hypocalcemia	Hypomagnesemia Hypoalbuminemia Hyperphosphatemia Hypoparathyroidism	Biweekly monitoring of serum calcium	If hypomagnesemic, supplemental magnesium will correct calcium If hypoalbuminemic, obtain ionized calcium; if normal, no supplementation is required If ionized calcium is low, supplement calcium
Refeeding edema	Low-sodium, low-carbohydrate diet Cardiac dysfunction Hypoalbuminemia	Avoid high-carbohydrate regimens Avoid high-sodium regimens Initiate feedings slowly	Mild edema usually resolves spontaneously Restrict Na$^+$ intake
Diarrhea	Malabsorption Hypoalbuminemia Antibiotic therapy Lactose intolerance Numerous medications[b]	Lactose-free enteral formulas Initiate enteral feedings slowly	Decrease tube-feeding infusion rate Increase fiber intake Change to a lower-fat enteral formula Antidiarrheal medications Peptide containing formula Discontinue medication causing diarrhea (if possible)
		Clostridium	If patient is receiving antibiotics: 1. Culture stool for Clostridium difficile 2. If culture is negative, restore normal gut flora with commercial lactobacillus acidophilus preparation

(Continues)

**TABLE 8–7.   COMPLICATIONS, PREDISPOSING FACTORS, PREVENTION, AND THERAPY
RELATED TO REFEEDING (CONT.)**

Complication	Predisposing Factors	Prevention	Therapy
Diarrhea (cont.)			3. If culture is *C. difficile* positive, the implicated antibiotic should be discontinued
Nausea and vomiting	Diabetes (gastroparesis) Poor gastrointestinal motility Obtunded patient Lactose intolerance	Avoid high-fat enteral regimens Initiate enteral feedings slowly Continuous administration schedules for tube feedings Avoid high osmolality enteral formulas Lactose-free enteral formulas	Decrease tube feeding infusion rate and/or concentration Change to a lower-fat enteral formula Antiemetic medication Elevate head of bed Place feeding tube distal to the pylorus
Cardiopulmonary failure	Cardiac dysfunction Pulmonary dysfunction Renal dysfunction	Low-sodium regimen Monitor cardiac dimensions and function Avoid overfeeding Avoid high carbohydrate intake Initiate feedings slowly	Dependent on severity and type of cardiopulmonary failure

[a] May lead to hyperglycemic, hyperosmolar, nonketotic coma.
[b] Magnesium-containing antacids, quinidine, digitalis, lactulose, aminophylline, propranolol, potassium, and phosphorus supplements.
Source: Adapted from Havala, T., & Shronts, E. (1990). Managing the complications associated with refeeding. *NCP, 5,* 25–26.

Tube occlusion can be prevented. Flushing of the feeding tube with at least 20 cc of water every 8 hours should clear the tube of residue. Not flushing the tube after stopping a continuous feeding will cause clogging. Improper medication administration through the tube may also cause gelatinous formations that will occlude the tube. Prudent medication administration includes giving each medication separately followed by 5 to 10 cc of water. If tube occlusion occurs, never use a syringe smaller than 10 cc to forcefully apply pressure in an attempt to dislodge the clot. The smaller the syringe, the greater the force. Manufacturers' recommendations of tubes clearly state that too great a force can puncture a tube, which can cause formula to be administered into the lungs. Studies done on irrigants such as cola, cranberry juice, and meat tenderizer mixed in water found that colas decreased the incidence of clogs better than acidic juices because of the carbonation's effervescent nature.

Refeeding the malnourished patient disrupts the adaptive state of semistarrvation (Hasvala & Shronts, 1990). See Table 8–7 for complications associated with refeeding, predisposing factors, prevention, and therapy. Close monitoring of the client's clinical and metabolic status and slow progression of enteral nutrition will decrease the incidence of refeeding complications.

 ## CASE STUDY #1

Mrs. Thomas is a 72-year-old woman with a long-standing history of nutritional problems. She presents with a gastrostomy tube, which is infusing Jevity at 40 cc/hr for 5 hours at night. She is not tolerating this amount and often needs to turn it off because of diarrhea, bloating, and cramping. Her past medical history includes a salivary gland cancer with metastasis to the lung, diagnosed 12 years ago, for which she underwent excision of the tumor and a left penumonectomy. She also had chemotherapy and radiation to the neck and thorax. She was hospitalized 2 months ago with staphylococcal pneumonia and congestive heart failure (CHF). She was ventilated with an oral endotracheal tube for 1 month and spent 2 weeks in a rehabilitation facility for intensive speech therapy to learn swallowing techniques and education on the care of her tube feeding. She is permitted foods by mouth as tolerated but wonders why she is not progressing to a full diet.

Significant findings during the initital visit include the following:

- History/Physical: malnutrition, CHF, tube-feeding intolerance, dysphagia secondary to surgery and decreased salivary production
- Medications: digoxin (Lanoxin) 0.125 mg qd, medroxyprogesterone acetate (Provera) 5 mg cyclically, estradiol (Estrace) 1 mg cyclically, captopril (Capotin) 25 mg tid, furosemide (Lasix) 20 md qd, sucralfate (Carafate) 1 g bid, simethicone 80 g qid
- Abnormal labs: albumin, 2.3; potassium, 3.1
- Nutritional assessment: height, 5'2" (157 cm); weight 85 lb (38.6 kg); lean body weight, 109 lb (49.6 kg)

QUESTIONS

1. What is your initial impression of Mrs. Thomas' condition? What factors can you identify that add to her nutritional condition? What is your plan?
2. What will you focus on in your history and physical exam? What additional

workup will you do?

3. What is her BMI? Is she malnourished? How severe?

Barium swallow at the rehabilitation facility 3 months ago was negative. She is still experiencing coughing when she eats.

4. What action would you take with this dysphagia symptom?

She is able to tolerate only 40 cc/hr of Jevity over 5 hours, which provides 208 calories and 8 g of protein. Her PO intake is minimal. The gastrostomy feeding tube intermittently migrates into the stoma causing pyloric obstruction.

5. What action would you take?

ANSWERS

1. Ms. Thomas' nutritional status is poor for several reasons. Radiation therapy and surgery have altered the structure and function of her upper GI tract. Her age also influences her ability to gain in nutritional status. Potential age-related deficiencies may include calcium; magnesium; sodium; zinc; vitamins D, C, K, and B_{12}; folic acid; thiamine; and iron. She is at risk for CHF, and therefore fluid volume needs to be considered. The initial plan is to determine why she is not tolerating the full volume of tube feeding and possibly rectify it to provide adequate nutritional support.

2. Look for clinical signs of specific nutrient deficiencies. Assess nutrient requirements and obtain data on diet intake and tolerance. Look for signs and symptoms of dysphagia. Assess for drug–nutrient interactions. Obtain prealbumin, accurate height and weight, and CBC.

3. Her BMI of 16 is well below what is considered underweight, and her albumin of 2.3 is considered severely protein malnourished.

4. Repeat barium swallow and bedside evaluation by a speech therapist. Swallowing training should be repeated and reinforced.

5. Anchor the feeding tube to the skin surface. Educate the client on techniques to prevent further migration episodes such as instructing her to check the length of her feeding tube when sudden nausea and vomiting occur. If the tube has migrated, gently pull the tube until resistance is met and anchor the tube. Obtain 24-hour dietary recall. Explore with the client foods that are well tolerated, and encourage her to progress to these foods and add them to her diet. Educate the client to the procedure of tube-feeding advancement. Begin with a volume of 40 cc/hr. If she is tolerating the feeding (ie, absence of cramping, bloating, nausea, vomiting, or diarrhea) after 2 to 4 hours, increase 20 to 40 cc/hr. Repeat this procedure until the client reaches the prescribed tube-feeding goal. Provide encouragement

to try new foods. Help the client identify barriers to progression. Monitor electrolytes and serum glucose during

progression. Monitor tolerance of tube feeding and suggest symptom-control methods.

 ## CASE STUDY #2

Mrs. Oatley is a 91-year-old woman who presents with a gradual weight loss of 50 lb over 1 year. She presents with her daughter, who states that she seems depressed. It was assumed that the weight loss was from depression, and bupropion hydrochloride (Wellbutrin) was initiated. She has a history of myocardial infarction (MI) 4 years ago, CHF, HTN, and diverticulosis. She lives alone and is a widow. Her mother had a history of Alzheimer's-type dementia, and her father died of kidney failure.

QUESTIONS

1. What are the possible factors related to Mrs. Oatley's weight loss?

2. What other course of action is prudent in assessing weight loss in this client?

The following lab values were obtained: BUN, 72; creatinine, 5.3. Mrs. Oatley was diagnosed with renal failure that was irreversible. The client refused dialysis, requested a DNR (do not resuscitate) status, and eventually expired.

3. How should Mrs. Oatley's diet be modified to meet her unique nutritional requirements?

ANSWERS

1. Depression can cause weight loss, especially in the elderly because their re-serves may already be compromised. However, depression can be a symptom of a more grave physiologic finding. The obvious should not be assumed. In this case, family history of renal failure is significant and should not be overlooked. Psychosocial issues with which Mrs. Oatley presents may have an effect on her nutritional intake because she is alone, elderly, and may not have the full support of her daughter with meal preparation. Unstable CHF may influence the client's ability to eat secondary to dyspnea. Diverticular disease causes pain with eating and may alter intake. With a family history, dementia should not be overlooked. All these factors may play a role in her weight loss.

2. A complete history and physical, including nutritional assessment and laboratory tests, are prudent in the as-

sessment of this client. History and physical should focus on signs and symptoms of nutritional deficit, with a detailed look at causes of weight loss other than depression. Assessment of cardiopulmonary status focusing on the incidence of CHF, assessment of mental status with the Folstein Mini-Mental State Exam or other mental status exams and assessment of the gastrointestinal tract would all rule out causes for weight loss. Laboratory data should include a complete pro-

file: Chem 24, CBC, thyroid profile studies, and nutritional parameters.

4. Protein should be limited to 0.5 g/kg of body weight until dialysis is initiated. Monitoring renal function and adjustment of protein intake is crucial. Provide at least 25 cal/kg of body weight because of muscle wasting. Restrict potassium and phosphorus. Assess for need of iron, and supplement as needed. Supplement calcium without adding phosphorus and vitamin D.

CASE STUDY #3

Mrs. Greenberg is an 84-year-old woman with a 10-lb weight loss over 8 months, which represents a 12% loss from her usual body weight of 80 lb. After probing for her history from her family, it was found that she has refused to eat over the last 8 months despite her husband's and family's encouragement. She has always been thin but not to this extreme. She has often been fixated on weight con-

trol and has been very demanding most of her adult life. All diagnostic tests for physiologic causes of weight loss were negative. Cognitive and emotional screening tests do not suggest dementia, delirium, or depression. After psychiatric consultation was obtained, a diagnosis of anorexia nervosa was made. Elements of this problem may have been present for years.

QUESTIONS

1. What diagnostic tests will be included in this workup for weight loss?
2. What questions should be explored if a psychologic component is suspected?

3. What strategies should be employed to enhance nutritional intake?

ANSWERS

1. The following diagnostic tests should be included: CBC, Chem 24, thyroid

profiles, swallowing study if indicated, and malignancy workup.

2. Assess for an intense preoccupation with body weight. Look for GI complaints that may be associated with bingeing and purging. Explore the use of laxatives, diuretics, and self-induced vomiting. Look for chemical dependence. Assess drug profiles.

3. Instruct the family to help the client maintain individual self-control over eating. Families often want to force feed. Encourage them to provide balanced diets at regular meals. Monitor electrolyte and nutritional parameters to assess progression.

■ REFERENCES

Chernoff, R. (19897). Aging and nutrition. *Nutrition Today, 22,* March/April, 4–11.

Hasvala, T., & Shronts, E. (1990). Managing the complications associated with refeeding. *NCP, 5,* 25–26.

Mansouri, A., Marton, K., & Verdery, R. (1994). Pinpointing the cause of unexplained weight loss. *Patient Care,* March 30, 43–46.

Master, A. M., Lasser, R. P., & Beckman, G. (1960). Tables of average weight and height of Americans aged 65 to 94 years. *JAMA, 172,* 658–662.

Mitchell, C. O., & Chernoff, R. (1991). Nutritional assessment of the elderly. In Chernoff, R. (Ed.). *Geriatric nutrition: The health professional's handbook* (pp. 365–366). Gaithersburg, MD: Aspen Publishers.

Nutrition Screening Initiative (1992). Nutritional problems related to medication use. In Greer, Margolis, Mitchell, Grunwald & Associates (Ed.). *Nutritional interventions manual for professionals caring for older adults* (p. 29). Washington, DC.

9

TOPICS IN GENITOURINARY CARE

Catherine Canivan

■ INTRODUCTION

The urinary system can be separated into upper and lower tracts. The upper tract consists of the kidneys, renal pelvis, and ureters. Basic structures of the lower tract are the urinary bladder and urethra. The upper tract's primary functional focus is urine production, whereas urine storage and elimination are the functional tasks of the lower tract. Other structures such as the uterus, vaginal vault, prostate gland, rectal vault, and pelvic floor muscles can also have a significant influence on genitourinary health. Body systems change over time in both anatomic structure and physiologic function, and the genitourinary (GU) system is no exception. Several subtle progressive alterations in functional tasks in both the upper and lower tracts accompany normal aging. The gradual nature of these changes usually allows the body to make adaptations. Commonly, the age-related functional alterations

within this system do not in themselves cause health problems but do create a more vulnerable environment. This chapter will be primarily concerned with problems of the lower tract and older adults.

■ AGE-RELATED CHANGES

Changes occur within the GU system after our twenties and are noticeable in most adults by age 60 to 70. These changes are both normal and subtle. The bladder (detrusor muscle) decreases in capacity, and the glomerular filtration rate in the kidneys loses efficiency with age. Changes in the cardiovascular system result in decreased blood flow to major organs such as the kidney, necessitating drugs such as diuretics, which can lead to increased frequency of urination. With improved blood perfusion of the kidneys while in a recumbent position (secondary to decreased gravity pressures on blood vessels to kidneys), increased filtration will result in larger volumes of urine stressing a bladder with reduced capacity and may also increase uninhibited bladder contraction and first urge to void at a higher urine volume.

Hormonal changes in women (menopause) can lead to a decrease in elasticity and moisture to the vaginal area. If severe enough, atrophic vaginitis occurs, which can precipitate urinary incontinence. Muscle strength and mass decline somewhat also, and for women this creates a problem. Many women have never learned how to strengthen their pelvic muscle floor and with the aging process easily develop poor pelvic floor muscle tone, putting them at high risk for stress incontinence.

In men, the normal enlargement of the prostate gland (benign prostatic hypertrophy [BPH]) may cause pressure on the urethra leading to overflow incontinence or urinary retention.

CLINICAL PEARL

When interpreting findings from a prostate exam, a normal exam from the rectal side does not rule out a potential enlargement on the urethral side, which may be the cause of retention or overflow incontinence.

The bowel slows with normal aging, making constipation a common problem. Constipation with resultant fecal impaction can cause sufficient pressure from the rectal vault to change the angle of the urethra, resulting in incomplete bladder emptying (may lead to retention, incontinence, or urinary tract infections [UTI]).

CLINICAL PEARL

If an older adult has a problem with nighttime incontinence, encourage the individual to lie down midday for at least 1 hour to increase kidney perfusion. Plan toileting prior to and at least one hour after lying down to help restore bladder control.

If constipation is a problem, instruct in using the "squat position" to defecate on a regular timed basis (20 to 60 minutes after meal usually coincides with the gastrocolic reflex). By using the squat position on a toilet (knees higher than hips), the body is in a more anatomically correct position to evacuate stool, which may decrease voiding problems. A pillow on the floor or a small footstool may help the individual to assume the squat position.

■ PATHOPHYSIOLOGY PROBLEMS

Older individuals may experience problems with their urinary systems that can vary from mild to severe. These problems can include increased urinary frequency, urinary incontinence, and UTIs.

URINARY FREQUENCY

Urinary frequency can result from a disease process such as polyuria secondary to hyperglycemia or hypercalcemia, a

UTI, or an obstruction in the lower urinary tract that prevents adequate bladder emptying. It may also be the result of reduced bladder capacity that accompanies normal aging. A thorough assessment of this symptom is essential to rule out pathology.

If no pathology is found, management techniques can include planned voiding times based on the individuals' voiding patterns; looking at the volume of oral fluids taken daily and the time of these fluids (the amount of fluids taken should be spread out over time, not taken in bolus amounts); using the recumbent position to help improve filtration and bladder emptying; or decreasing the amount of irritating fluids to the bladder such as cafffeinated drinks (coffee, tea, colas) and acidic fruit drinks, especially before nighttime sleep hours.

URINARY INCONTINENCE

Urinary incontinence (UI) is defined as an involuntary loss of urine that is sufficient to be a problem. Urinary incontinence is a symptom, not a disease, and not a normal part of aging. It can be an acute or chronic condition. It affects approximately 13 million people in the United States, according to the Agency for Health Care Policy and Research's Clinical Practice Guidelines (Fantl et al., 1996).

There are several types of UI such as stress, urge, overflow, and functional (see Table 9–1), which affect approximately 35% of adults in the United States and at least half of the nursing home population. The cost has been estimated at more than $15 billion annually (1995), with most of this expense being in nonmedical costs such as caretaking, pads, and laundry.

Acute or transient incontinence can be related to one or several factors. Older adults are especially at risk for this type of incontinence, as it often accompanies other conditions causing abrupt decline in physical, cognitive, and functional status. It is critical that acute incontinence be recognized and treated so that it does not become chronic or accepted as an individual's state of health. The factors associated with acute or transient incontinence are shown in Table 9–2. To remember easily, think of the mnemonic DIAPPERS (Resnick, 1986).

D **Delirium.** Acute confusion, or delirium, may cause a temporary functional leakage.

I **Infection.** Symptomatic UTI can increase the irritability of the bladder wall leading to unstable detrusor contraction. The older female is at greater risk for this development secondary to the length of the urethra (short) and probable previous infection in her younger years.

A **Atrophic vaginitis.** Atrophic vaginitis results from the dryness of the vaginal vault tissue secondary to decreased hormonal levels (menopause). This often leads to increased urinary frequency and may cause previous stress or urge incontinence to worsen.

P **Pharmacology.** Drugs such as sedatives, narcotics, or sleeping pills increase the risk of functional UI. Diuretics, alcohol, and caffeine may produce urge incontinence, while anticholinergics, muscle relaxants, antiparkinsonism medications, and calcium channel blockers may increase the risk of urinary retention or overflow incontinence.

TABLE 9–1.   SYMPTOMS AND SUBTYPES OF URINARY INCONTINENCE

Type of UI	Definition	Pathophysiology	Symptoms and Signs
Urge	Involuntary loss of urine associated with a strong sensation of urinary urgency	Involuntary detrusor (bladder) contractions (detrusor instability [DI]) Detrusor hyperactivity with impaired bladder contractility (DHIC) Involuntary sphincter relaxation	Loss of urine with an abrupt and strong desire to void; usually loss of urine on way to bathroom Elevated postvoid residual (PVR) volume Involuntary loss of urine (without symptoms)
Stress	Urethral sphincter failure usually associated with increased intra-abdominal pressure	Urethral hypermobility due to anatomic changes or defects such as fascial detachments (hypermobility) Intrinsic urethral sphincter deficiency (ISD) failure of the sphincter at rest	Small amount of urine loss during coughing, sneezing, laughing, or other physical activities Continuous leak at rest or with minimal exertion (postural changes)
Mixed	Combination of urge and stress UI	Combination of urge and stress features as above Common in women, especially older women	Combinations of urge and stress UI symptoms as above; one symptom (urge or stress) often more bothersome to the patient than the other
Overflow	Bladder overdistention	Acontractile detrusor Hypotonic or underactive detrusor secondary to drugs, fecal impaction, diabetes, lower spinal cord injury, or disruption of the motor innervation of the detrusor muscle Obstruction due to fecal impaction, bladder stress, or bladder tumor	Variety of symptoms, including frequent or constant dribbling or urge or stress incontinence symptoms, as well as urgency and frequent urination

TABLE 9–1.   SYMPTOMS AND SUBTYPES OF URINARY INCONTINENCE (CONT.)

Type of UI	Definition	Pathophysiology	Symptoms and Signs
Overflow (cont.)		In men, secondary obstruction due to prostatic hyperplasia, prostatic carcinoma, or urethral stricture In women, obstruction due to severe genital prolapse or surgical overcorrection of urethral detachment	
Other			
Functional	Chronic impairments of physical and/or cognitive functioning	Chronic and functional mental disabilities	Urge incontinence or functional limitations
Unconscious or reflex	Neurologic dysfunction	Decreased bladder compliance with risk of vesicoureteral reflux and hydrone-phrosis Impaired voiding response in the pons—common in stroke and Parkinson's disease Secondary to radiation cystitis, inflammatory Parkinson's disease, bladder conditions, radical pelvic surgery, or myelomeningocele In many non-neuro-genic cases, no demonstrable DI	Postmicturitional or continual inconti-nence; severe urgency with bladder hypersensi-tivity (sensory urgency)

Source: Fantl, J. A., Newman, D. K., Collings, J., et al. (1996). Clinical Practice Guidelines: Managing Acute and Chronic Urinary Incontinence. Rockville, MD: U.S. Department of Health and Human Services, Agency for Health Care Policy and Research.

P Psychiatric issues. Depression ("Why bother?"); anger ("I'll show them. I'll wet the bed."); control ("I've lost control over my independence, but I will exert control by wetting the bed.")

E Endocrine. Fluid overload with resultant polyuria and changes in electrolyte balance may cause an overflow or functional incontinence.

TABLE 9–2.   CAUSES OF TRANSIENT URINARY CONTROL PROBLEMS

Problem	How Causes UI	How Tested

Infection and/or excessive excretion	Hyperglycemia can result in increased urine production. "Polyuria" and glucosuria can result in irritation of the bladder.
	
	Infections irritate the bladder lining, causing one to feel the need to urinate when there is only a small amount of urine present and can interfere with normal bladder control through urgency.
		Multiparameter dipstick for:
		  Leukocytes
		  Hematuria
		  Proteinuria
		  Glucosuria
		If positive, a clean-catch midstream specimen should be sent for culture and sensitivity with M.D. orders for treatment. Insure adequate fluid intake. Repeat dipstick after UTI treatment.

Excessive excretion	Cardiac problems can result in accumulating fluids. When one lies down, there is increased urine production and, thus, increased volume and frequency—often at night.	*History:* congestive heart failure, frequent voiding at night, shortness of breath at night, recent change to sleeping with head elevated. Use of diuretics: recent change, dosing schedule *PE:* monitor weight, dependent edema, pulmonary rales.
Mobility/dexterity	Time and energy required to transfer, walk to toilet/commode, pivot and balance to undress, and then safely lower oneself onto seat, exceeds time that individual can suppress the need to urinate.	Observe and roughly time how long it takes to complete full "dry (hopefully) run." Specifically watch transfer on and off toilet. Ask for demonstration of ability to button/unbutton.
Obstruction due to stool impaction/constipation	Fecal mass exerts pelvic pressure: • On the urethra. To move urine past that obstruction requires increased pressure inside the urinary system. This can lead to incomplete emptying and eventually to bladder dilatation, which further compromises emptying ability. Postvoid residuals are a setup for infections.	*History:* usual and current bowel pattern; complaints that bowel movements are hard, large, and/or relatively infrequent compared with usual pattern *PE:* rectal exam for impaction or hard stool

TABLE 9–2. CAUSES OF TRANSIENT URINARY CONTROL PROBLEMS (CONT.)

Problem	How Causes UI	How Tested
Obstruction due to stool impaction/constipation (cont.)	• On the bladder, this decreasing bladder capacity, creating the need to urinate frequently and sometimes urgently.	
Obstruction due to enlarged prostate	Overgrowth of prostate tissue causes a narrowing and compression of the urethra. To move urine past that obstruction requires increased pressure inside the urinary system. This can lead to incomplete emptying and eventually to bladder dilatation, which further compromises emptying ability. Postvoid residuals are a setup for infections, which further compromise normal function.	*History:* Prostate disease/surgery, difficulty starting urine stream, decreased stream force, dribbling *PE:* rectal exam for possible enlarged/tender/asymmetric/soft, boggy consistency on anterior rectal wall
Atrophic urethritis/vaginitis	Involution of perineal structures due to decreased estrogen can interfere with alignment of structure's compromising ability to control urination at will.	*History:* onset after menopause; noted dry vagina; frequent vaginal infections, symptoms of burning or itching *PE:* vaginal walls dry, pale, with few rugations
Pharmaceuticals	Altered sensorium, rapid increase in volume, weakened bladder contraction, increased outlet resistance, irritant to bladder mucosa, decreased sphincter control	Medication review: relationship of initiating drugs and onset of symptoms; see listing of drugs that commonly result in urinary symptoms.
Cognitive/mental issues	Inability to process and respond to neurological signals regarding need to urinate	History or family report, clinical observation, Folstein-Mini-Mental State Exam

R Restraints. Physical or environmental restraints such as bed bars, seat belts, or clothing that is difficult to remove quickly may result in functional incontinence.

S Stool impaction. Stool impaction can increase the risk of overflow incontinence by helping to create a situation in which the bladder does not empty completely.

Chronic or persistent UI can be related to one or several factors such as the following:

- Impaired cognitive functioning in which the individual is unable to recognize the signal to void or unable to sequence steps to toilet
- Physical impairments hindering self-toileting (inability to ambulate or decreased manual dexterity)
- Neurologic dysfunction resulting in an inability to control or initiate the voiding function
- Poor pelvic floor muscle tone that results in an involuntary loss of urine with any increase in intra-abdominal pressure (see Table 9–3)

Assessment

As UI is a symptom only, the management or correction of this problem requires the following:

- A focused assessment of the individual to determine the type of UI (see Fig. 9–1)
- Identification of risk factors (fluid volume taken, type of medication and time of day, bowel/bladder habits, previous bladder infections, surgery, instrumentation, diabetes) and reversible conditions
- Identification of the impact the condition has on the individual's life and his or her willingness to implement strategies to improve control
- Treatment of reversible conditions (acute infections, fecal impactions, atrophic vaginitis)
- Discussions of options for treatment (treatment of acute infections, improvement of bladder/bowel hygiene, dietary control, pelvic floor muscle education etc.)
- An effective, workable plan for management of the UI
- Education for management or prevention of UI for individuals, community members, or staff, depending on the setting in which you work

Figure 9–2 provides an algorithm for the evaluation and management of UI. Figure 9–3 reviews the overall process for assessing urinary control difficulties.

As in obtaining any health history, objective and subjective observations are not always consistent. The following are key assessment points that will help you:

- Most bothersome symptom reported by the individual
- Duration (length of time) problem has existed
- Frequency of voiding (continent and incontinent) and the time of day or night
- Presence of urinary tract symptoms (burning, urgency, volume/strength of urine stream, sensation of complete emptying of bladder)
- Daily fluid intake and bowel habits
- Protective devices used (incontinent briefs, shields, guards, etc.) and the frequency of changes per 24 hours
- The client's expectations (containment, cure or management)

The completion of a bladder record will help give detail to the UI problem (see Fig. 9–4). A week's record is desirable, but 2 to 3 days of recording can give you a baseline record of incontinence.

A physical exam, concentrated in the abdominal pelvic region, may be helpful in revealing problems associated with UI (weak rectal tone, abdominal distention,

TABLE 9–3.   FIVE TYPES OF PERSISTENT CAUSES FOR URINARY CONTROL DIFFICULTIES

Problem	Definition
Stress	Involuntary loss of urine (usually small amounts) with increases in intra-abdominal pressure (eg, coughing, sneezing, exercising, bending, or lifting)
Urge	Leaking because of inability to delay urinating after sensation of bladder fullness is perceived
Overflow (retention)	The bladder overfills until it finally overflows. This happens because of • Obstructions that prevent emptying • Muscle or nerve problems that let the bladder overfill without initiating the normal stimuli to empty
Functional	Leaking caused by inability to toilet because of a mobility, dexterity, environmental, or cognitive problem
Mixed	Some older individuals simultaneously have two or more types of problems leading to chronic UI

poor muscle tone in general). Obtaining a urinalysis and a postvoid residual (PVR) urine are also very helpful. Depending on one's setting, one may use a bladder scanner (eliminating need for catheterization) or do a simple cystometrogram to determine the muscle tone and strength in the perianal area as well as filling capacity of the bladder. (Insert catheter into empty bladder; fill bladder, noting amount when discomfort felt. Remove catheter. Have client stand, walk, and observe for leakage before emptying bladder.)

Points to pay attention to are as follows:

• *Hydration level.* Many community dwellers will limit the amount of fluid to prevent UI. This results in concentrated urine, which acts as an irritant to the bladder wall, causing contraction of the bladder (result is frequency or UI).

• *Bowel/fiber.* As previously mentioned, the bowel pattern of an individual may contribute to their UI. If stool is constipated, resulting in fecal impaction, the distention of the rectal vault can press against the urethra and may change the angle slightly, preventing complete emptying of the bladder. Always check the rectal vault even if the client reports frequent or daily soft stools.

• *Voiding intervals/habits.* Most people void upon rising, before bedtime, and at least once within that time frame. Often, people will void either before or after a meal. A greater number of voidings will guide you to look at possible physical causes or functional problems associated with voiding. Once the pattern is determined, a stated plan for frequency of toileting should be established by either the individual or the caregiver with a realistic goal in mind. This may mean that the individual is continent during the day hours only, or is kept dry at all times.

• *Pelvic muscle area fitness.* The tone of the pelvic floor muscle plays an important part in our ability to remain

Assessed by:_____   Date:_____
Client's name:_____   Date of birth:_____

Historical Data

Allergies:

Current medications	_____Sedative/hypnotic	_____Diuretic
	_____Tricyclic antidepressant	_____Antihistamine
	_____Anticholinergic	_____Decongestant
	_____Adrenergic agent	_____Calcium channel blocker
	_____Estrogen	
Surgical History	_____Neurologic	_____Colon
	_____Pelvic	_____Abdominal
	_____Rectal	
Mental Status	_____Depressed	_____Forgetful
	_____Anxious	_____None significant
	_____Confused	_____Mini-Mental State Exam Score
Neurologic history	_____Cerebrovascular accident	_____Parkinson's disease
	_____Spinal cord injury	_____Disk disease
	_____Multiple sclerosis	_____Dementia
Medical history	_____Diabetes	_____Glaucoma
	_____Hypertension	_____Cancer
	_____Congestive heart failure	_____Respiratory disease
	_____Arthritis	_____Depression
Gynecologic history	_____Number of pregnancies	_____Number of episiotomies
	_____Genital prolapse	_____Postmenopausal
	_____Vaginitis	_____Atrophic vaginitis
Urologic history	_____Urinary tract infection	_____Benign prostatic hypertrophy
	_____Calculi	_____Urinary procedures involving
	_____Tumor	bladder/urethra/prostate

Continence Description

Onset of urinary incontinence			
Daytime voiding pattern	Frequency		
Nighttime voiding pattern	Frequency		
Incontinence pattern	Frequency		
Previous treatment	_____No	_____Yes	_____Outcome
Absorbent product used	_____No	_____Yes	_____ Effective
Device used	_____External catheter	_____Pessary
	_____Intermittent catheter	_____Penile clamp
	_____Other	_____Effectiveness
Bowel pattern	_____Frequency	_____Consistency
	_____Use of laxatives	
Fluid intake pattern	_____Amount/24 hours	_____Alcohol
	_____Caffeine	_____Restricts fluids

Physical Examination

Mobility	_____Independent	_____Assistive device	
	_____Assistance required		
Transfer ability	_____Independent	_____Assistance required	
Manual dexterity	_____Independent	_____Assistance required	
Abdomen	_____Suprapubic distention	_____Tenderness/pain	

Female:
External genitalia/
  pelvic exam

	Labia/vaginal mucosa	_____ Dry	_____Moist
	Cyctocele	_____Yes	_____No
	Rectocele	_____Yes	_____No
	Urethral prolapse	_____Yes	_____No
	Uterine prolapse	_____Yes	_____No
	Perineal sensation	_____Normal	_____Decreased

Male:

Penis	Circumsized	_____Yes	_____No
	Freely movable foreskin	_____Yes	_____No
	Small retracted penis	_____Yes	_____No
	Penile discharge	_____Yes	_____No
Scrotum	Enlarged	_____Yes	_____No
	Tender	_____Yes	_____No
Prostate	Normal	_____Yes	_____No
Rectum	Hemorrhoids	_____Yes	_____No
	Anal wink each side	_____Yes	_____No
	Anal tone/strength	_____Firm	_____Weak
	Stool	_____None	_____Hard
		_____Soft	_____Impaction
	Guaiac	_____Not done	_____Positive
		_____Negative	

UA multiparameter dipstick results	_____Normal	_____ Abnormal	
	_____M.D. notified	_____Culture and sensitivity ordered	
Postvoid residual	_____Volume voided	_____PVR volume	_____$\geq$ 100 cc
Provoked stress maneuvers	_____Positive	_____Negative	
Simple uriflow	_____Normal stream	_____Abnormal stream	
Pelvic laxity assessment	_____Normal	_____Abnormal	

Environmental Assessment

Toileting distance from bed/favorite chair	_____Good	_____ Poor
Obstacle-free pathway	_____Yes	_____No
Accessible/adequate lighting	_____Yes	_____No
Adequate supports for balancing and pulling up	_____ Yes	_____No
Height of toilet/bed	_____Good	_____Poor

Figure 9–1. Continence Assessment Tool (cont.)

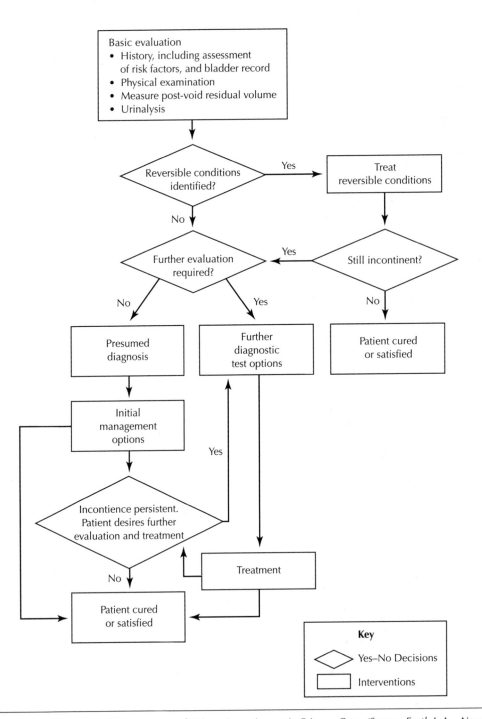

Figure 9–2. Evaluation and Management of Urinary Incontinence in Primary Care. *(Source: Fantl, J. A.,. Newman, D. K., Collings, J., et al. (1996). Clinical Practice Guidelines: Managing Acute and Chronic Urinary Incontinence. Rockville, MD: U.S. Department of Health and Human Services, Agency for Health Care Policy and Research.)*

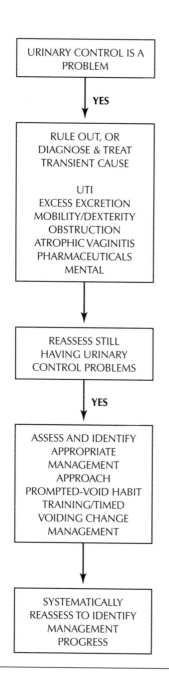

URINARY CONTROL IS A
PROBLEM

YES

RULE OUT, OR
DIAGNOSE & TREAT
TRANSIENT CAUSE

UTI
EXCESS EXCRETION
MOBILITY/DEXTERITY
OBSTRUCTION
ATROPHIC VAGINITIS
PHARMACEUTICALS
MENTAL

REASSESS STILL
HAVING URINARY
CONTROL PROBLEMS

YES

ASSESS AND IDENTIFY
APPROPRIATE
MANAGEMENT
APPROACH
PROMPTED-VOID HABIT
TRAINING/TIMED
VOIDING CHANGE
MANAGEMENT

SYSTEMATICALLY
REASSESS TO IDENTIFY
MANAGEMENT
PROGRESS

Figure 9–3. Assessment for Urinary Control Difficulties

continent. If muscle tone is weak due to obesity, previous surgery, or childbirth, exercise of these muscles will help to regain total or partial control of the UI. Most people need education/guidance in the proper technique of doing these exercises. Today, there are many aids/therapies available to help a person identify the proper muscles to exercise (vaginal cones, biofeedback techniques, or electrical stimulation) as well as monitor their progress in strengthening this area. Information as to professionals in one's area who may help you may be obtained by contacting the National Association for Continence, Spartanburg, SC, 29305. Pelvic floor muscle (Kegel) exercises can be one form of treatment of UI or a preventive technique for pre- and postmenopausal women (see Fig. 9–5).

- *Medications.* Prescription and over-the-counter (OTC) drugs must be looked at carefully for actions and side effects (see Table 9–4). An expected action of a diuretic is increased micturition, but an unexpected side effect, especially in an older man, of a common OTC cold medication may be urinary retention with incontinence. Types and frequency of medications must be considered when analyzing the urinary pattern, especially the incontinent episode.

Clinical Management

Behavioral interventions are usually the first management option for stress, urge, and mixed incontinence. Table 9–5 reviews the types of interventions, definitions, and target populations.

Name: _____

Date: _____

Fluid Intake			Bladder Function						Bowel Function	
Column 1		Column 2	Column 3	Column 4	Column 5 Amount of Leakage			Column 6	Column 7	Column 8
Time	Amount in Ounces	Type	Time	Amount of Urine Passed	Urge Only	Damp	Medium	Soaker	Cause or Location of Leakage	Absorbent Product Time Changed	Record Time of Bowel Movement

Figure 9-4. Fluid–Bladder/Bowel Activity Record

The pelvic floor musculature provides support to maintain the position and function of the internal pelvic organs. A weakened pelvic floor musculature loses its ability to adequately support the bladder and other internal pelvic organs. Consequently, the position of these organs may be altered, which in turn can interfere with adequate function. Additionally, sphincters (the sections of the pelvic floor musculature that surround the urethra and anus) also lose strength and tone and therefore cannot close tight nor stay tight enough to prevent leakage.

The purpose of pelvic floor muscle exercises is to help you improve and maintain the strength and tone of your pelvic floor musculature. Being consistent with regular exercise of the pelvic floor muscle can restore and maintain strength and tone and thus improve urinary control.

Getting Ready to Begin Pelvic Muscle Exercising

- First, empty your bladder.
- Adjust your clothing so that you are comfortable (loosen belts or garments that are tight around your abdomen).
- Find a quiet location (as exercise is mastered, it can be performed while doing other activities).
- Relax your entire body.
- When starting pelvic muscle exercising, find a position most comfortable for you. Later, as you master the pelvic floor muscle exercising, you will be encouraged to alternate positions.
- Positions: *Sit* upright in a straight-back chair, knees slightly apart, feet flat on the floor.
  Lie on your back, flat or with head slightly elevated, knees bent, and feet slightly apart.
  Stand by a chair, keep your back straight and knees slightly bent, feet slightly apart with toes slightly pointed outward.

Tune In: Locate and Isolate the Pelvic Floor Muscle

Pretend to be shutting off your urine flow or tightening your anus as to hold back gas. You should feel a sensation of closing and lifting. Concentrate, tighten (squeeze) only the pelvic floor muscle. *DO NOT* tighten leg muscles (thighs), buttocks, or abdomen. *DO NOT* hold your breath. Breathe normally.

- You can see that you need to concentrate to isolate the pelvic muscle from all your other muscles. It is important for you to isolate the pelvic muscle in order to experience the best exercising outcome. It takes a few practice sessions, but soon you will have it mastered.

Controlling the Pelvic Muscle

The proper exercise is a series of pelvic muscle tightening (squeezing and contracting are words also used) and relaxation.

- *One exercise* = tightening and relaxing.
- *Control* is achieved by timing oneself. oneself.
  Example: Tighten and hold for 3 seconds, relax for 3 seconds.
  It is equally important to control both muscle tightening and relaxing. Therefore, you should:
  (a) Relax for the same amount of time you tighten and hold.
  (b) *Relax completely* between each tightening.
- Slowly but steadily you'll build your ability to hold the tightening. It is important to build gradually, for example:
  First step   • 2 sessions per day
  • 3 seconds tightening and holding, 3 seconds relaxing
  • 10 repetitions (tightening/relaxing) at each session
(Follow this schedule for at least 1 week.)
  Second step   • 2 sessions per day
  • 5 seconds tightening and holding, 5 seconds relaxing
  • 10 repetitions (tightening/relaxing) at each session
(Follow this schedule for at least one week.)

Figure 9–5. Pelvic Floor Muscle Exercises *(Continues)*

Third step   • 2 sessions per day
             • 10 seconds tightening and holding, 10 seconds relaxing
             • 10 repetitions (tightening/relaxing) at each session
(Follow this schedule for at least one week.)
Fourth step   • 3 sessions per day
             • 10 seconds tightening and holding, 10 seconds relaxing
             • 15 repetitions (tightening/relaxing) at each session
(This is the targeted exercise schedule.)

Once this step is reached, it is followed until improved urinary control is achieved. The next step is to follow a maintenance schedule:

• 2 sessions per day
• 10 seconds tightening and holding, 10 seconds relaxing
• 15 repetitions (tightening/relaxing) at each session

Putting Pelvic Muscle Exercising Into Your Daily Life
The challenge is to consistently make pelvic muscle exercising a regular part of your life for the rest of your life. Although it is not easy, it is not impossible to:

Be determined.
Exercise regularly.
Develop a plan.
Record exercising—keep a diary.
"**Y**es, I can": *have confidence.*

Cautions:
• Do not stop and start urine flow as a form of exercising.
• Do not overexercise the pelvic muscle: start slow, build gradually.

Figure 9–5. Pelvic Floor Muscle Exercises (cont.)

• Prompted voiding is used in urge and functional incontinence. It employs a toileting schedule, verbal feedback and reinforcement, and is caregiver dependent.

• Habit training involves a schedule for toileting that is based on the client's 24-hour voiding pattern. It is used with cognitively impaired individuals with functional, urge, or mixed incontinence, who can cooperate with toileting.

• Bladder training, also known as bladder drill or bladder retraining, is used for urge incontinence. A fixed voiding schedule is determined (usually every 30 to 60 minutes), and if the urge occurs before the fixed time, suppression of the urge is controlled by relaxation or distraction techniques. A weekly increase (30 minutes) in fixed voiding time is established until the voiding pattern is every 3 or 4 hours.

• Pelvic muscle (Kegel) exercises are used for stress, urge, and mixed incontinence and for postprostatectomy patients. The client must learn to isolate and contract the muscles that control urination. These exercises must be performed on a regular schedule and done correctly. Frequent monitoring/guidance is needed initially to ensure that the proper muscle is being exercised. An audiotape of instructions is helpful to correctly perform exercises as are home training devices (such as

TABLE 9–4.   EFFECT OF MEDICATION ON THE URINARY SYSTEM

Type of Medication	Effect on Urinary System
Opiates Morphine, codeine, demerol, methadone	Weakens bladder contraction, causing incomplete bladder emptying, and alters ability to respond to need to urinate
Eyedrops containing atropine, cyclopentolate, or tropicamide (those used mainly for treating glaucoma)	Decreases bladder contractility, leading to urinary retention
Antiarrhythmics Norpace (disopyramide)	Weakens bladder contraction, leading to urinary hesitancy and potential retention
Calcium channel blockers Procardia, Calan, Cardizem	Inhibits bladder contractility potentially enhancing urinary retention
Decongestants (preparations containing phenylpropanolamine or pseudoephedrine, including nose drops/sprays) Allerest, Actifed, Sudafed, Sinutab, Dristan, Afrin	Relaxes smooth muscle, which causes relaxation of sphincter control (decreases sphincter resistance)
Antihypertensives Minipress, Catapres, Aldomet, Regitine (alpha-adrenergic blockers)	Relaxes smooth muscle, which causes relaxation of sphincter control (decreases sphincter resistance)
Alcohol Wine (especially white), beer, whiskey	Stimulates increase in urine volume load to bladder, leading to urgency and frequency; also decreases ability to sense urge to void
Caffeine-containing medications Aspirin, Darvon, Migral, Sinarest, Anacin, Cope, Bromo Seltzer, Excedrin, No-Doz, Vivarin, Dristan, Bromoquinine	Stimulates increase in urinary volume and is an irritant to the bladder mucosa, which can create urgency and frequency
Cerebral stimulant (amphetamine)	Increases urethral resistance, leading to urine retention

biofeedback therapy equipment). Electrical stimulation is another method in which the pelvic floor muscles are contracted artificially. Both biofeedback and electrical stimulation therapy need regular professional monitoring.

Pharmacologic Measures. Drugs are also used in the management of chronic UI.

Type of UI	Drug
Urge	Bentyl (dicyclamine) Urispas (flavoxate) Tofranil (imipramine) Ditropan (oxybutynin) Estrogen Tofranil (imipramine)

TABLE 9–5.   BEHAVIORAL INTERVENTIONS FOR STRESS, URGE, AND MIXED INCONTINENCE

Type of Intervention	Definition	Target Population
■ **TOILETING PROGRAMS**		
Scheduled toileting/habit training	Timed scheduled voiding Habit training scheduled to match client's voiding habits Caregiver dependent	Cognitively impaired Functionally disabled Incomplete bladder emptying Caregiver dependent
Prompted voiding	Scheduled voiding that requires prompting from caregiver Caregiver dependent	Functionally able to use toilet or toileting device Able to feel urge sensation Able to request toileting assistance Availability of caregiver
Bladder training	Systematic ability to delay voiding through the use of urge inhibition Active rehabilitation and education techniques	Cognitively intact Ability to discern urge sensation Cognitively able to understand or learn how to inhibit urge Able to toilet themselves or with assistance
■ **PELVIC MUSCLE REHABILITATION**		
Pelvic muscle exercises	Planned, active exercises of pelvic muscles to increase periurethral muscle strength Active rehabilitation and education techniques	Able to identify and contract pelvic muscles Compliance with instructions
Vaginal weight training	Active retention of increasing vaginal weights to induce increased pelvic muscle strength Active rehabilitation and education techniques Contraindication: pelvic organ prolapse	Cognitively intact Compliant with instructions Must be able to stand Must have sufficient pelvic floor strength to be able to contract muscle and retain lightest weight
Biofeedback	Electronic or mechanical instruments display information about neuromuscular and/or bladder activity, particularly with pelvic muscle exercises; can be used in association with other programs Active rehabilitation and education techniques	Ability to understand analog or digital signals using auditory or visual display Motivated persons who are able to learn voluntary control through observation of the biofeedback Health-care provider who can appropriately assess the UI problem and provide behavioral interventions

TABLE 9–5.   BEHAVIORAL INTERVENTIONS FOR STRESS, URGE, AND MIXED INCONTINENCE (CONT.)

Type of Intervention	Definition	Target Population
Electrical stimulation	Application of electrical current to sacral and pudendal afferent fibers via intra-anal and/or intravaginal electrodes to inhibit bladder instability and improve striated sphincter and levator ani contractility and efficiency Active rehabilitation and education techniques Contraindication: vaginal soreness, constipation, hematoma with needle stimulation	Useful as adjunct therapy in identification of pelvic muscles Ability to discern stimulation

Source: Fantl, J. A., Newman, D. K., Collings, J., et al. (1996). Clinical Practice Guidelines: Managing Acute and Chronic Urinary Incontinence. Rockville, MD: U.S. Department of Health and Human Services, Agency for Health Care Policy and Research.

Stress	Tofranil (imipramine) Nolamine (phenylpropanolamine) Sudafed (pseudoephedrine) Estrogen
Mixed	Same drugs as for urge or stress incontinence
Overflow	Urecholine (bethanechol)

Surgery may be used for those individuals unable to comply with other nonsurgical therapies (urge, stress). For those who have a sphincter deficiency, an artificial sphincter may be placed or periurethral bulking injections (Contigen Bard Collagen Implant, Bard Urological, Covington, Georgia) may be used for a man. Overflow incontinence from bladder neck or urethral obstruction can be relieved by a surgical procedure. A Credé maneuver or intermittent straight catheterization may be appropriate treatment for others.

Functional UI must be addressed at to its cause(s): mobility issues, decreased manual dexterity, sensory deficits, inadequate toilet facilities (eg, raised toilet seat) and elimination of physical restraints. Nursing staff (caregivers) play a key role in the optimal functioning and continence management of individuals with this problem.

Other measures that may be used are as follows:

- Intermittent catheterization for neurologic bladder problems or chronic urinary retention
- Indwelling catheters for those in whom other interventions are not possible
- Suprapubic catheters as an alternative to long-term catheter use
- External collection systems
- Pessaries for women with symptomatic pelvic organ prolapse

• Absorbent products as an adjunct to other therapies or for long-term care of chronic UI

A new option for the treatment of stress incontinence only is the Reliance Urinary Control Insert by UroMed Corp., Needham Mass. Smaller than a tampon, it is inserted into the urethra with an inflated balloon. It rests at the bladder neck and prevents the flow of urine. When the older adult needs to void, she pulls the attached string, the balloon deflates and the device is removed.

URINARY TRACT INFECTIONS

Urinary tract infections can be a common complication for older adults. They are more common in women; however, they can occur more frequently in men age 70 and older due to prostatic hypertrophy, leading to incomplete bladder emptying. Women are at a higher risk after menopause because of decreased vaginal glycogen and higher vaginal pH, which allow the colonization of gram-negative bacteria in the urinary tract. If an individual is institutionalized, the risk incidence rises to 50% for both men and women. Indwelling catheter use is the most common cause of UTIs in this population.

Clinical Presentation

The usual symptoms of a UTI are dysuria, urgency, frequency, lower abdominal pain, and fever. The often demonstrated presentations such as new-onset incontinence, loss of appetite, vomiting, falls, nocturia, difficulty urinating, or behavioral changes (eg, delirium, changes in mood/affect) are common symptoms of UTIs in the older adult. A urinalysis with white blood cells (WBCs) is an indicator of probable infection. A urine dipstick test can provide a quick screen. Usually, a positive leukocyte esterase and a positive nitrate can be correlated with a positive urine culture.

Diagnostic Studies

Urinalysis and urine culture are standard diagnostic tests for UTIs. Ten percent of older adults have a UTI annually. *Escherichia coli* (*E. coli*) pathogen is the most commonly isolated, with *Klebsiella pneumoniae* the second most common. *Proteus mirabilis, Proteus vulgaris,* and *Morganella morganii* are more common in men or in those who have been catheterized (Bruskewitz, 1995).

Asymptomatic UTIs have a greater than 10^5 colony count but have no other symptoms (dysuria, frequency, fever, etc.). There may be a small number of WBCs on urinalysis. Drug treatment should be instituted *only if symptomatic* or if the individual is at risk for developing more significant complications. New-onset or an exacerbation of urinary incontinence can be the only presenting symptom of a UTI in older adults and should be treated with appropriate antibiotics.

Clinical Management

Consider the pathogen, client's age, and other complicating factors (diabetes, renal insufficiency, immunosuppression, previous history of infection) when selecting the most appropriate antibiotic therapy. Antibiotics such as trimethoprim–sulfamethoxazole (Bactrim) (double strength), amoxicillin, cephalexin monohydrate, ceftriaxone sodium, ciprofloxacin hydrochloride and norfloxacin are usually appropriate choices for older adults. If the older adult is in the community with no previous history of UTI, consider using a short-course (3-day) treatment. If there is a history of previous UTIs, recent hospitalization, or diabetes, a 7 to 10-day course of therapy should be used.

Follow-up of a treated UTI is controversial. Some believe that follow-up (urine culture) should be done only if symptoms are unresolved or recur. Others believe that a repeat culture should be done 7 days after treatment regardless of symptoms.

The management of recurrent symptomatic UTIs in older adults depends on the frequency of recurrence. If the client has one to three UTIs per year, treat each occurrence appropriately. If more than three per year, consider long-term prophylactic therapy, such as Bactrim at night. Antibacterial agents (methenamine hippurate) can be effective in the prevention and suppression of chronic UTIs. For postmenopausal women whose vaginal microflora has been changed, estrogen cream can also decrease recurrence of infection.

An adequate amount of oral fluids is necessary to flush the bladder, especially when an infection is present. Cranberry juice and vitamin C have been found useful for prevention and treatment of UTIs, as it can acidify urine.

Client Education
Depending on the site of one's practice, education of the older adult or staff may be appropriate. Preventative behaviors include proper wiping from front to back after a bowel movement, urinating shortly after feeling the urge to void, changing wet clothing as quickly as possible, and avoiding scented vaginal sprays and sanitary pads (use incontinent pads/briefs, which wick urine away).

■ BENIGN PROSTATIC HYPERPLASIA

A palpable enlargement of the prostate is common in men over age 50. The enlargement does not necessarily correlate with the severity of symptoms or the degree of obstruction.

The symptoms of prostatism are frequent urination, nocturia, urgency, straining to urinate, hesitancy, weak or intermittent stream, and a sensation of incomplete emptying of the bladder.

Benign prostatic hyperplasia can result in urinary retention, renal insufficiency, UTI, gross hematuria, or bladder calculi over a long period of time.

ASSESSMENT

Obtain a detailed medical history, focusing on the urinary tract as well as general health issues to identify other causes of voiding dysfunction. Use of a voiding record (Fig. 9–4) can be helpful in determining the frequency and nature of the problem. Perform a physical exam, including a digital rectal exam, and urinalysis to rule out UTI and hematuria. Check the serum creatinine level to assess renal function. A prostate-specific antigen (PSA) test is optional. It may help detect early-stage cancer, but it does not discriminate very well among those with symptomatic BPH and those with prostate cancer.

CLINICAL MANAGEMENT

Asymptomatic BPH (lacking the usual symptoms of prostatism) does not require treatment.

Symptomatic BPH treatment includes the following:

- *"Watchful waiting."* At this time, there is no known progressive time line to this disease, so an annual follow-up is considered reasonable.
- *Surgery.* If the client is very bothered by the symptoms, surgery may be recommended.
    - TURP (transurethral resection of prostate) is the most common procedure.
    - TUIP (transurethral incision of the prostate) can be done in an ambulatory setting or during a 1-day hospitalization.
- *Balloon dilatation.* Dilatation of the urethra is less effective than surgery for relief of symptoms, but a temporary improvement of symptoms may last 2 years before recurring.
- *Medication.* Alpha blockers may cause a small increase in urinary flow rate and a small reduction in symptoms. Cardura (doxazosin), Proscar (Finasteride), Minipress (prazosin), and Hytrin (terazosin) are used, but the long-term effectiveness has not yet been determined. The side effects of these drugs (orthostatic hypotension, dizziness, tiredness, headache) must be considered in the treatment plan.
- *Transurethral hyperthermia,* in which heat is used to shrink the prostate and relieve obstruction, is being investigated at this time. This is a relatively new technique.

The care of older adults with GU problems can be complex. By combining medical and nursing skills, one can provide comfort, management, or cure.

CASE STUDY #1

Mr. Conner has come to your office for his annual physical exam. He is an 84-year-old retired executive of a large company who is concerned about the disruption his urinary problem has caused him over the years and his recent feelings of isolation. His physical exam is unremarkable for his age, with no significant medical history except for an inability to control his urine.

In focusing on his concern, you find a history of urinary frequency, urgency, and occasional incontinence that started many years ago when he was in the Navy. The problem is greatest during his waking hours, and, as he describes it, he could not drive for 45 minutes "without stopping at every gas station on the road." During his working years, he kept several pairs of trousers in his office in case of an "accident."

Mr. Conner denies burning on urination, weak stream, or difficulty starting urinary stream. He does have nocturia frequently. He has no previous history of UTI, although he has seen several urologists and taken medication with no relief of symp-

toms in the past. He now finds it difficult to play golf with friends due to
this problem.

A rectal exam shows fair sphincter
muscle tone. His PVR is 60 cc, and
urine dipstick is negative.

QUESTIONS

1. What other information will you need?

2. What recommendations would you make to him?

ANSWERS

1. A fluid–bladder bowel activity record for at least several days to a week would be helpful. Concentrate on fluid intake, amount, and time in relation to voiding pattern. Does there appear to be any bowel problem?

   It is apparent Mr. Conner takes an excessive amount of fluid at mealtimes (eg, two glasses of orange juice, two glasses of milk, three cups of coffee, and hot cereal for breakfast), drinks coffee throughout the day, and every evening has two cocktails.

2. Decrease bolus fluids at meals to a reasonable amount (be specific with type and quantity); change fluid between meals to noncaffeinated drinks and decrease amount; reduce to one drink at happy hour; point out the re-

lationship of fluid to voiding pattern. Monitor fluid–bladder–bowel activity record for several weeks until progress made. Consider recommending pelvic muscle exercises for better tone and using distraction techniques if he has urgency. Recommend a male disposable absorbent product until fluid volume and bladder tone are improved.

Impression: Urgency and occasional incontinence secondary to fluid overload and poor pelvic muscle tone.

Behavioral interventions are the first approach in management of a chronic urinary problem. Hydration can be a key issue. Usually, one finds the client to be dehydrated (limiting fluids in an attempt to control urgency or incontinence) rather than taking fluids in abundance. The value of a fluid–bladder–bowel activity record is highlighted in this situation. Working with an individual with this problem may take time, as frequent reinforcement of correct fluid–bladder pattern may be necessary. Also, instruction in pelvic muscle exercises and guidance with technique may require periodic follow-up visits.

CASE STUDY #2

Mrs. Ames is an 83-year-old woman in a nursing home with a history of dementia. She is independent in activities of daily living (ADL) and dependent in instrumental activities of daily living (IADLs). Nurses report weakness (new), two falls in 24 hours, and "feeling poorly."

Mrs. Ames is incontinent of urine (new onset), with a flushed face, afebrile, heart rate (100), and clear lungs. Her systolic blood pressure drops 24 points when she stands up. Her mental status is slightly impaired from her baseline (lethargic with some difficulty with details). A urinalysis is negative. Her WBC count is 8.0. She has no previous history of UTI or infection.

The next day, Mrs. Ames' WBC is 17.0. Her temperature is 99°F. Urinalysis is now grossly positive. Urine for culture and sensitivity is obtained. An antibiotic is started for a presumed UTI and PO fluids are encouraged.

In older adults, physical changes may precede any actual diagnostic data. The absence of a fever does not mean the absence of an infection, as this case of atypical UTI shows. Sudden onset or urinary incontinence may be the only sign of a UTI initially.

■ REFERENCES

Bruskewitz, R. C., & Wasson, J. (1995). Disorders of the lower genitourinary tract: Bladder, Prostate and testicles. In: Abrams, W. B., Beers, M. H., & Berkow, R. (Eds.). *The Merck manual of geriatrics* (2nd ed.) (pp. 785–795). Whitehouse Station, NJ: Merck Research Laboratories.

Fantl, J. A., Newman, D. K., Collings, J., et al. (1996). *Managing Acute and Chronic Urinary Incontinence.* Clinical Practice Guidelines No.2, 1996 update. AHCPR Publication No. 96-0686. Rockville, MD: U.S. Department of Health and Human Services, Public Health Service, Agency for Health Care Policy and Research.

Resnick, N. (1986). Urinary incontinence in the elderly. *Hosp Pract,* November 15, 1980.

10

TOPICS IN MUSCULOSKELETAL CARE

Geriann B. Gallagher • *Ann Marie Sommer*

■ INTRODUCTION

This chapter will discuss some of the most common musculoskeletal problems faced by older adults. These diseases can be insidious or abrupt in their presentation, but often lead to significant physical disability. In order to preserve maximum function, the advance practice nurse (APN) must have a thorough understanding of the assessment, diagnosis, and treatment of these conditions.

■ OSTEOARTHRITIS

Osteoarthritis (OA) is the most common joint disease and has an enormous economic impact. Arthritis is estimated to cost the United States approximately $54.6 billion including medical treatment, work loss, and disability (Ross, 1997). Osteoarthritis (OA) is defined as an inherently noninflammatory disorder of movable joints, characterized by dete-

rioration and abrasion of articular cartilage as well as by formation of new bone at the joint surfaces (McCarty, 1989).

AGE-RELATED CHANGES

Radiographic evidence of OA can be found at some site in the majority of people aged 65 years and older. More than 80% of people over 65 years of age are affected, and OA is the most common chronic disease affecting the elderly. Osteoarthritis is a major cause of disability, and the incidence of OA at all joints increases progressively with age.

CLINICAL PRESENTATION

Clinical features can include pain in the involved joint, stiffness after periods of immobility, enlargement of the joint, instability, limitation of motion, and functional impairment. Musculature surrounding the affected joint may become atrophied, and the associated weakness may contribute to disability. Pain in the early stages of OA occurs after joint use and is relieved by rest. As the disease progresses, pain occurs with minimal movement or even at rest.

Osteoarthritis is typically found in the hands, knees, hips, feet, and spine, and may be found in other joints as well.

Osteoarthritis of the hands may present with Heberden's nodes or spurs formed at the dorsolateral and medial aspects of the distal interphalangeal joints. The distal interphalangeal (DIP), proximal interphalangeal (PIP), and first carpometacarpal (CMC) joints are often affected.

Osteoarthritis of the knee may be characterized by local tenderness over various parts of the joint and pain with passive or active range of motion. Crepitus can often be detected, and muscle atrophy related to disuse may be present. Genu varus (bowleg) and genu valgus (knock-knee) deformities of the knee are often present.

In OA of the hip, there is an insidious onset of pain, which is often followed by a limp. Pain may be localized to the groin or along the inner aspect of the thigh. Pain may also be felt in the buttocks, sciatic region, or knee. Physical examination shows loss of hip motion, most notably on internal rotation or extension.

Osteoarthritis of the foot most often affects the first metatarsophalangeal (MTP) joint and is often aggravated by tight shoes. Irregularities in the shape of the joint and tenderness can often be palpated.

Osteoarthritis of the spine is most commonly seen in the L3–L4 area and results from involvement of the intervertebral disks, vertebral bodies, or posterior apophyseal articulations. Associated symptoms include radicular pain related to compression of contiguous nerve roots, and local pain and stiffness. The client may have spinal stenosis resulting from degenerative spurs, disk herniation, ligamentous hypertrophy, and spondylolisthesis.

ASSESSMENT

History

Assess for morning stiffness or stiffness after a long period of immobility, which usually subsides within 30 minutes. The client may complain of joint pain that occurs with motion, weight bearing, or activity. Assess family history, activity history, and any associated injury to the involved joints. Note precipitating and relieving factors, complaints of decreased motion, "crunching" or enlargement of the joint, or decrease in ambulation or of functional activity.

Physical Examination

Perform a thorough musculoskeletal exam. Assess for presence of Heberden's nodes at the DIP joints or the presence of Bouchard's nodes at the PIP joints. The affected joint may have the following changes: limited range of motion; bony enlargement; tenderness on palpation, with generally no increase in temperature and no associated erythema; crepitus; or mild swelling. Note any associated muscle weakness or spasm.

Diagnostic Studies

No specific diagnostic laboratory abnormalities exist in primary OA. The erythrocyte sedimentation rate, routine blood counts, urinalysis, and blood chemical determinations are normal and are important in excluding other forms of arthritis considered in the differential diagnosis. Radiologic studies are helpful to visualize the degenerative joint. In advancing disease, radiographs will reveal joint space narrowing and osteophyte formation.

CLINICAL MANAGEMENT

As with all treatments, the therapy must be individualized. Understand the goal of the individual for his or her treatment program. Is the program to increase function? To decrease pain? Therapy generally consists of a multidisciplinary approach addressing exercise; weight management, if indicated; drug therapy; and, finally, surgery.

Exercise may be facilitated through the guidance of a physical therapist. Protecting the joints from overuse is important. Use of assistive equipment such as a cane may assist in reducing pressure on the lower extremities when ambulating. It may be helpful to apply heat to the affected limb for 15 to 20 minutes prior to exercise. The goal of the exercise program is to preserve or improve range of motion and strengthen periarticular muscle.

Obesity has generally been accepted as a contributing factor in OA because of the excessive weight placed on the joint, although several studies indicate that it is not so simple. In general, maintaining ideal body weight and consuming a well-balanced diet are indicated.

Drug therapy is generally the most common treatment for OA. Treatment consists of analgesics, anti-inflammatory drugs, and narcotics. Analgesics such as acetaminophen administered on a regular basis are frequently effective. Acetaminophen can be given up to 1 gram four times a day. Methyl salicylate or capsaicin creams can also be used.

Narcotics should be used infrequently. Nonsteroidal anti-inflammatory drugs (NSAIDs) may also be helpful in the treatment of OA; however, side effects including rash, gastritis, gastroduodenal ulcers, renal insufficiency, and hepatic and neurologic toxicity may limit their usefulness. For high-risk clients, the administration of an H_2-receptor blocker may be helpful. Injection of corticosteroids into the joint may be beneficial but should be used infrequently. Pericapsular and ligamentous injections may provide relief for the joint.

Finally, if the disease is poorly controlled and the client is experiencing a decreased quality of life, function, or independence, referral to an orthopedic surgeon should be considered for consideration of joint replacement.

■ GOUT

Gout is defined as deposits of crystalline monosodium urate monohydrate (MSU) in the tissues. Several clinical manifestations may occur, including (1) recurrent attacks of severe acute or chronic articular and periarticular inflammation, also known as gouty arthritis; (2) accumulation of articular, osseous soft tissue and cartilaginous crystalline deposits, called tophi; (3) renal impairment also referred to as gouty nephropathy; and (4) uric acid calculi in the urinary tract (Schumacher et al., 1993). Gout is also a common cause of monarticular arthritis. It is noted by McCarty (1989) that while renal disease is common in gouty individuals, some evidence suggests that nephropathy in gout is usually secondary to associated conditions such as hypertension (HTN), vascular disease, or infection. The client may display hyperuricemia (generally above 7.0 mg/dL in males and 6.0 mg/dL in females), although this may often be insufficient for the expression of gout. Asymptomatic hyperuricemia in the absence of gout is not a disease state.

AGE-RELATED CHANGES

Elderly persons may experience gout related to the use of diuretics such as thiazides, which partially block the excretion of urates by the kidneys. The disease can cause significant short-term disability and occupational limitations, increasing the use of medical services.

CLINICAL PRESENTATION

The client may present with severe pain or tenderness over the involved joint, malaise, or chills. Objective findings include redness, pain, warmth, and swelling over the affected area. Presentation may also include a low-grade fever and the formation of tophi. The client may present in one of four stages of gout:

1. *Asymptomatic hyperuricemia.* Not all clients with hyperuricemia will develop gout.
2. *Acute gout arthritis.* The great toe is the most frequent spot for gout; however, it may occur in the knee, wrist, ankle, elbow bursa, heel, or fingers. The onset of the gouty attack is usually over a few hours, with the peak intensity in 24 to 36 hours, and will tend to spontaneously subside in 3 to 10 days without treatment.
3. *Intercritical gout.* This is defined as the interval between attacks. The client is generally without symptoms or abnormal physical findings.

4. *Chronic tophaceous gout.* Tophi are first noted an average of 10 years after the first episode of arthritis. Tophi occur in 95% of persons with chronic gout and may develop in the untreated client when the rate of urate production exceeds excretion. The rate of formation is related to the level and duration of hyperuricemia. The skin covering the tophus may ulcerate, causing drainage of crystals. Deforming arthritis can develop as a result of the erosion of cartilage and subchondral bone caused by the chronic inflammatory reaction and urate crystal deposition.

Acute attacks of gout may be triggered by a specific event such as trauma, alcohol, drugs, surgical stress, or acute medical illness. Some consider a diet high in purines to be a factor in gout attacks (Schumacher et al., 1993). However, McCarty (1989) notes that strict restriction of the intake of purine decreases the mean serum urate concentration by only 1.0 mg/dL.

ASSESSMENT

History
Assess symptom onset and character, location, radiation, quality, and timing of pain. Assess for any client or family history of gout, a diet that is high in purines, and use of diuretics, habitual alcohol intake, increased body weight, hypertriglyceridemia, and HTN—all risk factors for hyperuricemia and gout.

Physical Examination
Assess for malaise, fever, chills, and one or more red, warm, tender, and erythematous joints. The great toe is the most common site; however, a complete joint exam

is warranted. The client may also experience periarticular erythema, which should be differentiated from cellulitis, thrombophlebitis, septic arthritis, rheumatoid arthritis, OA, fracture, and dislocation.

Diagnostic Studies

Joint aspiration of fluid reveals rod- or needle-shaped crystals. The crystals can also be aspirated during the intercritical stage (or between attacks), and diagnosis can still be made.

X-rays are not usually helpful during the initial attack of gout except to exclude other causes and to note soft tissue swelling. With chronic gout, calcifications of the tophi and bony erosions may be noted.

Since the elevation of uric acid levels can be misleading, the demonstration of MSU crystals is generally helpful for establishing a diagnosis. Synovial fluid leukocytes are elevated in acute gouty arthritis, and effusions appear cloudy as a result of the high concentration of cells and crystals. Send the joint fluid for culture to rule out infection and check a complete blood count (CBC) triglyceride and uric acid level.

CLINICAL MANAGEMENT

It is noted by Yoshikawa et al. (1993) that while medication to reduce the uric acid level and prophylactic medication to prevent acute attacks are worthwhile, clients who are more than 70 years old when they develop their first attack of acute gout may be treated differently. Yoshikawa also suggests that since so few older men experience recurrent attacks of gout leading to chronic tophaceous gout, primary-care providers might elect to treat only acute attacks of gout. The average time for the

client to develop chronic gout is more than a decade from the first attack. Therefore the provider needs to consider the life expectancy of the client when developing a treatment plan.

After diagnosing gout, the goal of treatment should be to provide rapid and safe relief of the pain, prevent further attacks, and prevent destructive arthropathy and the formation of tophi or kidney stones.

Initial therapy should address diet and use of alcohol. Management of other medical problems such as obesity, hyperlipidemia, and HTN should be discussed.

Acute Gout

The common strategy for treating acute gout is the use of NSAIDs such as indomethacin 50 mg PO every 6 hours for 1 to 2 days, then 50 mg PO every 8 hours for 24 hours, and then 50 mg PO every 12 hours until the attack resolves (approximately 3 to 5 days). Other NSAIDs may be used as recommended by the manufacturer. Colchicine is often used; however, several sources (Schumacher et al., 1993; McCarty, 1989) note that this medication can be toxic in the elderly and cause gastrointestinal (GI) disturbances such as nausea, vomiting, and diarrhea. It should therefore be used with caution. NSAIDs also have a risk of GI problems such as gastritis, peptic ulceration, and GI bleeding.

According to Schumacher et al. (1993), corticosteroids and adrenocorticotropic hormone (ACTH) may be effective if the acute attack has failed treatment by colchicine or NSAIDs. Treat an episode of acute gout with a dose of 20 to 40 mg of prednisone by mouth daily for 3 to 4 days, and then gradually taper over 1 to 2 weeks.

Chronic Gout

According to McCarty (1989), before giving specific antihyperuricemic agents, the following criteria should be met:

1. All signs of acute inflammation should be absent.
2. The client should be educated regarding factors that may precipitate an acute attack and its prevention.
3. Treatment with prophylactic colchicine should be started.
4. The client should be educated that intermittent attacks of acute gout may occur.
5. The client should be given anti-inflammatory medication with instructions should an episode occur.

Probenecid, a uricosuric agent, can be started at 0.5 g/d and can be advanced slowly to not more than 1 g twice a day or until the targeted urate level of less than 6 mg/dL is reached. Common side effects include rash and GI upset.

Allopurinol, a xanthine oxidase inhibitor, is generally reserved for clients in whom there is urate overproduction, nephrolithiasis, or other contraindications to uricosuric therapy. Generally, a daily dose of 300 mg can be started initially; however, an initial dose of 100 mg may be appropriate for the elderly. It may be increased in 100-mg daily increments at weekly intervals, to a maximum of 800 mg/d and 300 mg/dose. It should be taken with food.

▪ RHEUMATOID ARTHRITIS

Rheumatoid arthritis (RA) is a systemic autoimmune disorder that can cause a chronic inflammatory disease. Other distinctive features include symmetric, erosive synovitis of peripheral joints. Although the cause of RA is unknown, it is possible that there is no single causative factor. Bacteria and viruses are still being studied as the focus of suspicion. The course of RA may include a series of exacerbations and remissions; however, the most common outcome of established disease is progressive development of various degrees of joint destruction, deformity, and disability.

AGE-RELATED CHANGES

The prevalence of RA increases with age for both males and females, with the prevalence being higher in females than in males. Diagnosis of RA in the older client may be difficult as several forms of arthritis may be present in the same person. In addition, OA and polymyalgia rheumatica are fairly common in the elderly and may make the differential diagnosis of RA difficult.

CLINICAL PRESENTATION

The clinical features of RA are heralded by polyarticular and symmetric joint inflammation, specifically pain; stiffness; limited motion; swelling; tenderness; and increased warmth. This usually starts in the PIP and metacarpophalangeal (MCP) joints and/or corresponding joints in the feet. Symptoms may spread in a varying pattern and degree to the hips, knees, wrists, shoulders, elbows, and spine. Clients usually experience morning stiffness lasting for an hour or more. Rheumatoid arthritis may not be confined to the joints and may involve the peripheral nerves, muscle, bone, pericardium, pleura, lung, eye, spleen, and blood. Clients may complain of constitutional symptoms such as fatigue, anorexia, weight loss, depression, generalized weakness, malaise, lymphadenopathy, and low-grade fever (Ross, 1997). An exacerbation of the disease may be preceded by emotional or physical stress.

Radiologic evidence of RA depends on the stage of the disease. Early changes are usually evident in the hands and feet. If the radiograph is examined closely, the line of demarcation of the engorged synovium can often be seen. The radiograph will also show localized subchondral osteoporosis and tiny erosions at the point of insertion of the synovium with the distal metaphysis.

The course of RA is characterized by periods of activity separated by intervals of disease inactivity. With each period of active disease, a certain amount of joint destruction will occur.

The practitioner should be aware of two complications in long-term RA. One is the sudden development of serious neurologic sequelae due to either atlantoaxial subluxation or subluxation of the cervical vertebrae themselves. The client may experience severe neck or occipital pain, inability to touch the chin to the sternum, numbness and tingling of hands or feet, a sense of limb tenderness, and urinary retention. Surgical reduction and fusion should be done as an emergency procedure.

The second complication is the development of sudden laryngeal obstruction due to rheumatoid synovitis of the cricoapophyseal joints. The client may experience voice change, dysphagia, and pain. This process may also be exacerbated by a superimposed infection or induction of anesthesia. The anesthesiologist should be made aware of the possibility of cervical cord involvement and laryngeal obstruction.

ASSESSMENT

History

The onset of RA may evolve insidiously over weeks to months, or it may be acute and develop virtually over night. The client may complain of morning stiffness that lasts longer than one hour. The morning stiffness tends to correlate with the level of inflammation and will decrease or disappear when the client is in remission.

Signs and symptoms of RA can vary from client to client. The client may experience pain, stiffness, or swelling, typically beginning in the peripheral joints, with the involvement usually being symmetric. The elderly may experience pain in the larger joints such as the shoulders and hips.

The client may also experience systemic symptoms as described above. Also, take the time to assess the client's perception of disease activity as well as social, emotional, financial, vocational, and family stressors. Depression is a common reaction to the losses imposed by RA.

Physical Examination

According to Schumacher et al. (1993), articular manifestations can be presented in two categories: (1) reversible signs and symptoms related to inflammatory synovitis and (2) irreversible structural damage brought on by synovitis. The resulting joint deformities are related to cartilage destruction and the client's attempt to avoid the pain of the process by posturing the joint in the least painful position. Joint deformities may develop as a result of joint immobilization (where the client may lose function), muscle spasm and shortening, bone and cartilage destruction, ligamentous laxity, and altered tendon function related to inflammation. As a result, the client may present with early morning stiffness.

Another physical finding is active synovitis. The joints (usually the superficial joints such as the PIP joints), have a warm and swollen appearance. Clients will also complain of general malaise and are easily fatigued. The practitioner should monitor the joints through physical examination and radiographs over time to evaluate progression of joint destruction. The structural damage to the joints is irreversible and cumulative, leading to progressive functional and anatomical deterioration.

Rheumatoid nodules, which are collections of inflammatory cells surrounding a center of cellular debris, may also be noted in 25% to 50% of clients. These nodules develop during active stages of RA along tendon sheaths and in bursae. The nodules may either disappear or involute over time.

Diagnostic Studies

Lab work includes a serum rheumatoid factor (RF), which is found in the serum of approximately 85% of clients with RA. Rheumatoid factor is positive in approximately 3% of healthy persons and increases with age. It may detect the presence of autoantibodies that are also elevated in sarcoidosis, endocarditis, chronic liver disease, and tuberculosis (Ross, 1997). Erythrocyte sedimentation rate (ESR) is almost always elevated. C-reactive protein (CRP) is one of the acute phase reactants but may also be used to monitor the level of inflammation over time. Antinuclear antibody (ANA) titer should be drawn especially if systemic lupus erythematosus (SLE) is part of the differential diagnosis.

It is also appropriate to obtain a baseline CBC and chemistry profile to assess renal and hepatic function should the client require any treatment. According to Schumacher et al. (1993), other laboratory abnormalities noted in RA include hypergammaglobulinemia, anemia, occasional hypocomplementemia, thrombocytosis, and eosinophilia. These abnormalities are often found in clients with more advanced disease.

Examination of synovial fluid aspirate will help in differentiating RA from OA, gout, calcium pyrophosphate deposition disease, and infection. Synovial fluid in RA is typically slightly cloudy and less viscous than normal with a white cell count in the range of 3000 to 25,000/mL.

Finally, radiographic evidence of the characteristic bony erosions, joint destruction, joint space narrowing and osteopenia assist with the diagnosis of RA. Because many of the extra-articular features of RA, such as the characteristic symmetry of inflammation and the typical serologic findings, may not be evident in the first month or two of the disease, the initial diagnosis of RA is usually presumptive early in its course.

CLINICAL MANAGEMENT

The goal of therapy is to minimize the damage caused by the disease process and avoid excess disability from the disease or the treatment. Management strategies may include bedrest early in the disease, progressive active exercises that are appropriate, NSAIDs, and remittive agents. However, in older adults, many of these treatments can be harmful. For example, bedrest for an extensive period may lead to a decrease in functional mobility related to deconditioning.

A team approach, including a physical and occupational therapist, orthopedist, podiatrist, nutritionist, and others can address the varied aspects of this complex disease process. The practitioner may want to initiate nonpharmacologic therapy, including exercise, orthopedic management, and psychosocial support. The goal of exercise includes the preservation of range of motion and lessening of deformities while maintaining muscle strength. The exercises should be done every day within the limits of pain. The pain should not last more than 3 to 5 minutes after the cessation of the exercise. As an acute exacerbation of RA subsides, more intense activity, such as anaerobic muscle-strengthening, stretching, and aerobic activity can be introduced. It is important for the client to commit to these exercises and may warrant a referral to the Arthritis Foundation and the Arthritis Self-Help Course. The Arthritis Self-Help Course is a 6-week educational program designed to teach people with arthritis how to take a more active role in their care.

Occupational therapy (OT) may assist with the management of acutely inflamed joints through the use of casts or splints worn during the night or part of the day to decrease the extent of inflammation and joint deformity. Splints are also used to preserve function in the joint and for comfort. Occupational therapy can also help to identify assistive devices for activities of daily living (ADL)

that will help the client to increase his or her independence and function.

The use of cold and heat modalities can assist with pain management. Cold can decrease swelling and provide analgesia. Heat treatments such as a warm bath or shower, heating pad, and hot packs can relax muscles and stimulate circulation. Client education should be done regarding safety when using these modalities (Ross, 1997).

Orthopedic surgery, such as joint replacement, reconstruction of extensor tendons, or incision of wrist tendons of a client with carpal tunnel syndrome may contribute to the maintenance of function and appearance.

Psychosocial and social support are critical in encouraging the client to cope more effectively with the disease. Clear explanation of the illness and prognosis, and a treatment plan that is mutually prepared may contribute to the client's self-confidence and adaptation to the disease.

Drug therapy may include NSAIDs as an initial treatment in clients with mild forms of the disease and with no radiographic changes. These drugs may act rapidly, provide a mild reduction in inflammation, and have an analgesic effect. However, the use of NSAIDs poses a risk to older individuals due to a propensity for gastropathy and decreased renal function. The NSAIDs may be started at a lower dosage to attempt to minimize the risk of GI bleeding and renal insufficiency. If the client has any additional risks for GI bleeding, the practitioner should consider concomitant administration of a prostaglandin antagonist.

Oral corticosteroids provide an anti-inflammatory and immunosuppressive effect but do not have disease modifica-

TABLE 10–1.   DOSING, EFFECTS, AND MONITORING STRATEGIES FOR DISEASE MODIFYING ANTIRHEUMATIC DRUGS

Drug	Action	Dose	Major Adverse Effects	Monitoring
Methotrexate (Rheumatrex)	Inhibits degradation of folic acid, resulting in inhibition of DNA synthesis of inflammatory cells	PO or IM 7.5 mg weekly up to 25 mg	Cirrhosis, pulmonary toxicity and infiltrates, stomatitis, leukopenia, renal insufficiency, thrombocytopenia, anemia, opportunistic infections	CXR (baseline), CBC every 1 to 2 months; creatinine, LFTs every 1 to 2 months
Hydroxychloroquine (Plaquenil)	Poorly understood, inhibits DNA synthesis	200 to 400 mg daily in 2 doses	Retinal toxicity (rare)	Eye exam every 12 months if age > 40 or history of eye disease
Sulfasalazine (Azulfidine)	Mechanism unknown	1 to 3 g daily in 2 doses	CNS and GI toxicity, leukopenia, anemia, neutropenia, Stevens-Johnson	CBC/LFT every 3 months
Gold (Ridaura, Solganal)	Suppresses immune response, unknown	25 to 50 mg IM weekly until 1 g, then 50 mg monthly	Dermatitis, stomatitis, proteinuria, enterocolitis, thrombocytopenia	CBC, UA before each dose
Azathioprine (Imuran)	Mechanism unknown	50 to 150 mg daily in 1 to 3 doses	Leukopenia, hepatitis, pancytopenia, pancreatitis	CBC every 1 to 2 months
D-penicillamine (Depen, Cuprimine)	Mechanism unknown	Start at 125 to 250 mg daily, maximum 1500 mg in 3 doses	Myasthenia gravis, Goodpasture syndrome, stomatitis, pemphigus	CBC, UA every 1 to 2 months

DNA, deoxyribonucleic acid; CXR, chest x-ray; CBC, complete blood count; LFTs, liver function tests; CNS, central nervous system; GI, gastrointestinal; U/A, urinalysis.

Source: Adapted and used with permission from Ross, C. (1997). A comparison of osteoarthritis and rheumatoid arthritis: Diagnosis and treatment. *Nurse Pract, 22* (9), 20–39. Copyright Springhouse Corporation.

tion potential. Due to the long-term complications of the steroids, they should be tapered as soon as possible.

Disease-modifying antirheumatic drugs (DMARDs) (such as gold, hydroxychloroquine, and sulfasalazine) are now generally recommended to be started early in the disease in clients with progressive polyarthritic involvement, persistent inflammation, elevated ESR or RF, or erosive changes in the joints on radiograph. The DMARDs should be started within 2 to 3 months if there is no relief with NSAIDs. Table 10–1 refers to the most commonly prescribed DMARDs.

According to Ross (1997), hydroxychloroquine and sulfasalazine are often recommended for mild cases, as they tend to be less toxic. Methotrexate has generally been indicated for more progressive disease. Sulfasalazine and methotrexate have an onset of action of approximately 3 to 6 weeks, while hydroxychloroquine, gold, azathioprine, and d-penicillamine may not have an onset for 3 to 6 months.

Combination drug therapy is becoming increasingly popular in the treatment of RA, as it allows lower doses of each drug than when used alone. The combination therapy may therefore decrease toxic side effects (Ross, 1997). Educating the client, setting mutual goals,

and discussing the plan of care is crucial. It should also be noted that many clients will try alternative therapies to relieve the pain of RA. A holistic and natural approach by the client and provider is encouraged; however, the provider should be knowledgeable of the treatment. Alert the client to be cautious of fad diets and remedies that "cure" arthritis.

■ POLYMYALGIA RHEUMATICA

Polymyalgia rheumatica (PMR) is a syndrome that is commonly found in the older population. It is a pain syndrome, often with a nondestructive synovitis, that may run a prolonged or recurring course. Clinical findings of PMR are characterized by pain, stiffness in the neck, shoulders, or hips that persists for at least one month Table 10–2. The onset of PMR may be abrupt. The client may go to bed feeling well and wake up stiff and sore the next day. The client may complain about how difficult it is to get out of bed in the morning, as gelling and morning stiffness are more pronounced. Generally, the symptoms are symmetric; however, the stiffness may start in one joint and slowly spread to another joint.

TABLE 10–2.   CLINICAL FINDINGS OF POLYMYALGIA RHEUMATICA

Onset	Insidious (may be abrupt)
Proximal girdle joints (shoulders and hips, neck)	Morning stiffness Pain, tenderness Symmetrical
Synovitis (15% of patients)	Limitation of joint movement

Source: Reproduced with permission from Dwolatzky, T., Sonnenblick, M., & Nesher, G. (1997). Giant cell arteritis and polymyalgia rheumatica: Clues to early diagnosis. *Geriatrics, 52*(6), 39–40. Copyright Advanstar Communications Inc.

The evidence of morning stiffness, gelling, and synovitis may make the diagnosis of PMR difficult to differentiate from RA, but RA is more likely to affect the small joints of the hands and feet, as opposed to the proximal distribution of PMR.

Polymyalgia rheumatica is often grouped with giant cell arteritis (GCA), also known as temporal arteritis. Giant cell arteritis is a chronic inflammatory process involving those arteries with elastic laminae, including the extracranial arteries. The classic and nonclassic features of GCA are presented in Table 10–3. These findings are a reflection of inflammation with resulting ischemia in the temporal artery. The client may show symptoms of visual compromise, with the most feared consequence being permanent visual loss.

The client may also present with constitutional symptoms such as fatigue, weakness, malaise, anorexia and weight loss, low-grade fever, night sweats, and depression (see Table 10–4). The clinician should be aware that both PMR and GCA may present atypically, suggesting an infectious, metabolic, or malignant syndrome.

The grouping of PMR and GCA occurs because 50% of clients with GCA have clinical features of PMR and 25% of clients with PMR have clinical or pathologic features of GCA. The etiology is unknown.

TABLE 10–3.   CLINICAL FINDINGS OF GIANT CELL ARTERITIS: CLASSIC AND NONCLASSIC

	Classic
Onset	Insidious (may be abrupt)
Headache	Common, severe
Vision	Visual loss (10% to 20% of patients)
	Ophthalmoplegia (diplopia, ptosis)
Vascular	Scalp tenderness
	Scalp arteries palpable, tender; absent or weak pulsations
	Bruits over large arteries
	Claudication (jaw, tongue, extremities)

	Nonclassic
Vascular	Myocardial infarction, angina pectoris
	Aortic dissection
Respiratory tract	Cough, sore throat, hoarseness
	Lung infiltrates
Renal	Portinuria, hematuria
Auditory system	Sensorineural hearing loss
Neurologic	Stroke/transient ischemic events
	Neuropathies
	Dementia

Source: Reproduced with permission from Dwolatzky, T., Sonnenblick, M., & Nesher, G. (1997). Giant cell arteritis and polymyalgia rheumatica: Clues to early diagnosis. *Geriatrics, 52*(6), 39–40. Copyright Advanstar Communications Inc.

TABLE 10–4.   CONSTITUTIONAL SYMPTOMS OF GIANT CELL ARTERITIS AND POLYMYALGIA RHEUMATICA

Low-grade fever

Night sweats

Anorexia

Weight loss

Malaise, fatigue

Depression

Source: Reproduced with permission from Dwolatzky, T., Sonnenblick, M., & Nesher, G. (1997). Giant cell arteritis and polymyalgia rheumatica: Clues to early diagnosis. *Geriatrics, 52*(6), 39–40. Copyright Advanstar Communications Inc.

AGE-RELATED CHANGES

Grouped together, GCA and PMR is twice as common in women as in men. The incidence increases with age and is 10 times more common in clients over 80 years of age. The incidence is also up to six times higher in Caucasians than in blacks. The client may have seen many other health-care providers and may have been told that his or her symptoms are a result of getting older.

ASSESSMENT

History

The client may complain of fever, malaise, depression, and weight loss. Commonly, pain is present in the neck, shoulders, upper arms, lower back, thighs, and hip girdles. The client may complain of weakness, although muscle testing generally shows good muscle strength. The features of GCA include temporal headache, which is usually unilateral, accompanied by temporal artery swelling and tenderness.

Physical Examination

The examination of the client may reveal tenderness and limited shoulder motions as a result of nonspecific inflammation in synovial tissues of the shoulders. The client may demonstrate difficulty with movement of the proximal joints such as rising out of a chair or moving the arms above the head. No joint damage is seen in PMR. The client may present with cachexia, fever, or anemia. In the client suspected of having GCA with transient loss of vision, a fundoscopic examination is normal. Transient loss of vision may precede permanent loss of vision for days or weeks, at which time the fundoscopic exam may reveal optic ischemia.

Diagnotic Studies

Common laboratory findings are presented in Table 10–5. The von Willebrand factor is synthesized in the vascular endothelium and may reflect endothelial inflammation and destruction. Other laboratory results such as RF and ANA are not present in significant amounts to be considered positive. Radiographs are typically normal; however, a bone scan may show increased uptake in the shoulder and hip joints.

Diagnosis of GCA is confirmed through biopsy of the temporal artery. According to Dwolatzky et al. (1997), an adequate biopsy of 2 to 3 cm with serial sections is essential. Bilateral biopsy will increase the rate of detection.

CLINICAL MANAGEMENT

The symptoms of PMR and GCA respond dramatically to small doses of prednisone. The response to the use of corticosteroids is often considered to be diagnostic of PMR. If there is no response

TABLE 10–5.   LABORATORY INVESTIGATIONS: FINDINGS IN GIANT CELL ARTERITIS AND POLYMYALGIA RHEUMATICA

Test	Finding
Acute phase reactants	↑↑ ESR
	↑ C-reactive protein
	↑ Fibrinogen
	↑ Alpha-2-globulins
	↑ Complement
Blood count	Anemia (normochromic)
	↑ Platelets
Liver function tests	↑ Alkaline phosphatase
	↑ Transaminases
	↑ Prothrombin time
	↓ Albumin
Synovial fluid (PMR)	1000 to 8000 WBCs
	(40% to 50% neutrophils)
Temporal artery biopsy (GCA)	Giant cell arteritis
Bone scan (PMR)	↑ Uptake shoulder and hips

Source: Reproduced with permission from Dwolatzky, T., Sonnenblick, M., & Nesher, G. (1997). Giant cell arteritis and polymyalgia rheumatica: Clues to early diagnosis. *Geriatrics, 52*(6) 39–40. Copyright Advanstar Communications Inc.

noted to prednisone within the first week, the diagnosis should be questioned. According to Schumacher et al. (1993), the usual starting dose of prednisone is 10 to 20 mg/d, which can be tapered by about 10% every week to a daily maintenance dose of 5 to 7.5 mg/d following clinical response. Dwolatzky et al. (1997) suggest an initial dose of 40 mg/d of prednisone in divided doses. It is suggested that the practitioner begin corticosteroid therapy early, even prior to temporal artery biopsy if there is a strong clinical suspicion of GCA, or if there are possible serious complications such as visual loss or other vascular events suspected. Some clients may be able to discontinue the prednisone after a year or two; however, approximately one third require long-term treatment to control inflammation. Keep in mind that there are potentially serious complications and side effects when treating an older client with steroids. This may include infections, osteoporotic fractures, difficulties in controlling diabetes, HTN, and mental changes (Dwolatzky et al., 1997).

■ OSTEOPOROSIS

Osteoporosis literally means porous bone and is commonly referred to as brittle bones. The skeletal system is ever changing through a process called bone remodeling. While it is not the intent of this book to provide detailed pathophysiology, a basic understanding of bone remodeling as well as calcium absorption is necessary to choose appropriate interventions and comprehend their mechanism of action.

At the cellular level, calcium uptake and release is conducted during bone remodeling. It is designed to prevent bones from becoming excessively thick or thin. Any interference in one of the four phases can lead to pathologic changes in bone mass. Bone remodeling starts when osteoclasts are activated upon the influence of a variety of stimuli. Bone resorption occurs and a cavity is formed secondary to the release of calcium. Immature osteoid is placed into the cavity during the bone formation phase. Finally, the osteoid is mineralized and the process is complete. It takes approximately 4 months to complete the cycle, and it is ongoing at different phases throughout the body. Osteoporosis occurs when there is an imbalance between bone formation and bone resorption, resulting in incompletely filled cavities within the bone matrix.

Fractures secondary to osteoporosis can occur at many sites within the musculoskeletal system, most commonly the hip, lumbar spine, and wrist. Other less common sites for fracture are the thoracic spine, pelvis, humerus, foot, and hand.

Osteoporosis has become a major health concern for the American public. It is one of the most prevalent chronic conditions among the elderly. Recent estimates suggest that more than half of the women in the United States will sustain an osteoporotic fracture in their lifetime. The risk of fracture for elderly men is 1 in 10. Such fractures cause a spiral of events to ensue, which may include (but is by no means limited to) prolonged acute-care stays, loss of independence, immobility, and possibly death. In addition, the economic costs associated with osteoporotic fractures is enormous. The annual cost for osteoporosis is estimated to exceed $10 billion.

Clinicians providing care for elders in virtually all settings have an opportunity to intervene and potentially interrupt the pathologic process of osteoporosis. It will be an investment in time, which can ultimately prevent or minimize the sequelae of this disease.

ASSESSMENT

History
Risk factor and possible symptom identification is the focus of the history component of the assessment. Two main factors have been identified in the development of osteoporosis: inadequate calcium intake over the life span and estrogen deficiency. Lifelong calcium intake should be assessed. While it is impossible to quantify lifelong calcium intake, inquiries regarding socioeconomic status, use of dietary supplements, and both the intake and tolerance of dairy products can assist in determining whether calcium intake has been markedly low or minimally sufficient. In addition, assess the client's overall nutritional state, especially vitamin D intake, which is essential for calcium absorption. In women, the next step is to identify the estrogen state. Questions regarding the onset of menopause (natural or induced) as well as the use of estrogen replacement are essential. The most rapid rate of bone loss occurs 5 to 7 years after menopause.

Identifying the client's race is necessary, as Caucasians and Asians have a higher incidence of osteoporosis. Body size (previous and current) is relevant, especially if there is a loss of height (> 2 in). A family history of osteoporosis is an important consideration. Clients may not be aware that osteoporosis existed in family members, but they can recall if a first-degree relative became shorter, fractured a hip, or had frequent episodes of acute back pain. Poor health habits, including alcohol abuse, tobacco smoking, and ingestion of large amounts of caffeinated and/or cola-colored beverages, are all relevant components of the assessment. Medications such as steroids, heparin, anticonvulsants (phenytoin, barbiturates), and overzealous thyroid supplementation adversely affect bone mass, whereas hormone replacement therapy (HRT) can have a protective effect on bones. Finally, periods of long-term inactivity contribute to bone loss and should be elucidated. Potential secondary causes of osteoporosis (hyperthyroidism, hyperparathyroidism, Cushing syndrome, multiple myeloma) may need to be ruled out.

Physical Examination

Osteoporotic changes in bone often progress without the typical symptomatology seen in other disease processes. In some instances, individuals may experience pain—most notably in the low back region—that prompts the clinician to investigate its source. Manual palpation of vertebral processes as well as paraspinal muscles can assist in confirming the presence of pain. However, bone mass may diminish and bone quality can deteriorate unnoticed until the client presents with a hip fracture, spinal crush fracture, or a Colles' fracture in the wrist. Hip fracture presents as acute pain occurring immediately prior to or after a fall. Joint disfigurement, edema, pain with range of motion, and shortening of the affected limb may be the result of an osteoporotic fracture.

Diagnostic Studies

Laboratory data is of limited value in diagnosing this disease. Osteoporosis progresses as calcium is removed from bone to maintain adequate serum calcium levels, thus making serum calcium a useless test. Biochemical markers of bone resorption and formation exist, but these only indirectly measure bone mass. They are not commonly used but may become increasingly useful as more specific assays are developed.

In men, a hypogonadal state contributes to low bone mass. Serum testosterone levels should be obtained in men with low bone mass, as testosterone replacement can aid in reversing the bone loss.

The best available noninvasive technique to quantify bone mass is dual x-ray absorptiometry (DEXA). Women with identified risk factors entering menopause should be encouraged to undergo bone densiometry in order to establish a baseline bone mineral density (BMD). The test quantifies bone mass at the wrist, spine, and hip. It is noninvasive, requires short scan times, and has low radiation exposure. The cost is approximately $200. It is covered by most insurers, including Medicare, when ordered with the proper diagnosis—estrogen deficiency.

Results of BMD are interpreted in standard deviations (SD) from the young adult reference mean and are used as a guide for interventions. Individuals within 1 SD of the mean are considered to have normal BMD. Osteopenia (low bone mass) is the diagnosis if the results are 1 to 2.5 SD below the young adult mean. Bone mineral density greater than 2.5 SD below the mean is diagnostic of osteoporosis.

Clinical indicators for recommending a DEXA scan include the following:

- Presence of strong risk factors (premature menopause, family history of osteoporosis, loss of height, low calcium intake, corticosteroid therapy, long-term inactivity)
- Evidence of vertebral deformity or osteopenia on x-ray
- Previous fracture suspicious for osteoporosis
- Consideration of HRT at onset of menopause
- Monitoring osteoporosis therapy

CLINICAL MANAGEMENT

Pharmacologic Measures

Numerous medications are now available for the management of osteoporosis. Consideration of other risk factors and disease processes will assist in guiding the clinician's decision-making process as to which medication(s) are most appropriate.

Hormone replacement therapy with estrogen for postmenopausal women and testosterone for hypogonadal men has shown to be effective in slowing bone loss. The optimal dose of estrogen is 0.625 mg/d and can be given unopposed for those whose uterus has been removed. Due to the risk of endometrial cancer, progestin should be added for women with an intact uterus. Hormone replacement therapy is contraindicated with a history of breast cancer. Estrogen supplementation is available in both oral and topical form. In addition, a product known as Prempro combines estrogen and progesterone in one oral tablet. The most bothersome side effect with HRT is unpredictable monthly vaginal bleeding.

Cycling progestin for 10 to 14 days at the beginning of the month will result in predictable vaginal bleeding.

Testosterone is available via a dermal patch, and the recommended dose is 2.5 mg/d. The benefits of this medication on bone mass may be offset by exacerbation of prostatic hypertrophy and an adverse effect on lipid profiles.

The availability of intranasal calcitonin has increased its popularity, as side effects are minimized. Clients use two puffs per day and alternate nares with each administration. Rhinorrhea is the most common side effect of this preparation. Short-term pain relief, especially in the lumbar spine, is an added benefit of this drug. Its approximate cost is $50 per month.

Alendronate (Fosamax) is the first in the bisphosphonate class of drugs, which has received U.S. Food and Drug Administration (FDA) approval for treating as well as preventing osteoporosis. It has been shown to increase BMD and decrease the risk of fracture. The dosage for prevention is 5 mg/d and for treatment is 10 mg/d. Erosive esophagitis, a serious side effect, can be avoided by following the manufacturer's instructions to drink a full 8 oz of water and remain upright for 1 hour after ingesting the tablet. Less serious but nonetheless distressing is the common complaint of stomach upset and bloating. The drug's absorption is inhibited by food; therefore, it should be taken upon arising in the morning, at least 30 minutes and ideally 1 hour before eating. It is priced similar to calcitonin at $50 monthly.

Calcitonin/estrogen and alendronate/estrogen combination therapy are being used in clinical practice as well as being investigated in research studies.

They are not currently FDA approved for use in combination.

The most dramatic increase in BMD is seen in the first year of HRT. Bone mineral density can increase by 5% to 12% with leveling off thereafter (Miller, 1996). Use of calcitonin and alendronate confer additional benefits over a longer period as they both increase BMD at both the femoral neck and spine (6.9% to 8.8%). However, the rate of increase is greater with alendronate (Bellantoni, 1996). All prescription medications for osteoporosis must be used in combination with adequate daily calcium and vitamin D intake.

In November 1997, the FDA recommended approval of raloxifene. It is the first in a new class of drugs known as selective estrogen receptor modulators (SERMs). These drugs mimic the effects of estrogen in some parts of the body (for example, the bones), while not necessarily increasing the risk of cancer. Initial 2-year research data shows that raloxifene increases bone density by 2% to 3% and that women taking the medication have a 60% lower probability of getting breast cancer than expected. Longer studies examining outcomes, risks, and possible cardioprotective effects are continuing.

Nonpharmacologic Measures

The most promising approach to treating osteoporosis is to prevent its occurrence. Osteoporosis affects mostly women, and preventive efforts should be aimed at this population. Prevention must begin premenopausally when bone mass is accruing and approaching its peak. Peak bone mass is achieved around the age of thirty. Efforts initiated during this time will enhance peak bone mass

and provide an increased margin for bone loss without resulting in osteoporosis. Many of the mechanisms used to prevent osteoporosis are the same as those used to treat it.

It is important to acknowledge that bone loss accelerates with age. Clients may believe that after age 65 it is too late for treatment, which is untrue. Elderly persons at any age can benefit from treatment. There are now more options than ever before for clinicians to choose from.

Adequate calcium intake is the foundation for treating osteoporosis. Postmenopausal women 50 to 65 years of age on estrogen should consume 1000 mg of calcium per day. This is also recommended for men in this age group. According to the government recommended daily allowance (RDA), all individuals older than 65 years of age should consume 1000 to 1500 mg of calcium daily unless there is a history of renal dysfunction and/or calculi. The most common side effect is constipation, which can be alleviated with a magnesium supplement. Calcium supplementation costs approximately $3 to $15 monthly, depending on the type purchased.

Adequate serum levels of vitamin D (25-hydroxy) are necessary for absorption of calcium, yet many individuals are deficient due to poor intake and/or minimal sun exposure. Ingestion of 400 to 800 IU of vitamin D is required to reverse the deficiency. It costs approximately $3 to $6 monthly.

Dietary Interventions

Good dietary sources of both calcium and vitamin D are listed below. If adequate supplementation is not achieved through diet, over-the-counter (OTC) supplements should be recommended.

Calcium (mg)
- Yogurt, 8 oz (415)
- Milk, 8 oz (300)
- Kale, $^1/_2$ cup (179)
- Broccoli, 1 spear (82)

Vitamin D (IU)
- Cod liver oil, 1 tsp (835)
- Herring, pickled, 1 oz (190)
- Milk, 8 oz (100)
- Cold cereal, fortified, 1 oz (39)
- Egg yolk (25)

Exercise

Moderate weight-bearing exercise increases the stress on bones and assists in bone formation. In addition, exercise promotes strength, flexibility, and balance, which are valuable in fall prevention. There is an ongoing debate surrounding the required intensity, duration, and frequency of exercise to aid in bone mass improvements. An acceptable recommendation for most individuals is that weight-bearing exercise should be conducted for at least 20 minutes three to four times a week. Tailoring programs according to a person's other conditions (cardiac, arthritic, etc.) is advisable. Frequent encouragement and support is necessary to promote compliance with this life-style change.

Life Style

Other life-style changes that are recommended, if applicable, include eliminating or decreasing the use of substances believed to interfere with bone remodeling. Caffeine, alcohol, and cola-type soft drinks all deplete calcium stores in the skeleton, and their consumption should be minimized. Cigarettes accelerate bone resorption; thus, their use should be decreased and hopefully discontinued.

▪ FRACTURES

COLLES' FRACTURE

Fractures of the distal radius occur most often from falls on an outstretched hand. Colles' fracture, or fracture of the distal radius, is the most common fracture, primarily affecting older females. Colles' fracture involves the distal metaphysis of the radius, which presents with dorsal angulation and displacement, radial angulation, and shortening. Figure 10–1 depicts the typical "overturned dinner fork deformity." Because of the dorsal displacement, the median nerve is at significant risk for injury. A thorough neurovascular examination is crucial. Approximately 60% of the time, there is an accompanying fracture of the ulnar styloid.

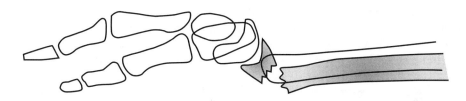

Figure 10–1. Colles' fracture. This fracture of the distal radius is the most common fracture primarily affecting older females. Radiographs typically reveal the "overturned dinner fork deformity," as illustrated here.

Fractures of the wrist can be broadly classified as extra-articular or intra-articular. A Colles' fracture is extra-articular. According to Rockwood et al. (1991), treatment is based on the extent of potential instability. Stable fractures are usually extra-articular, with mild to moderated displacement. When these fractures are reduced, they do not redisplace to the original deformity. The more unstable fractures are commonly comminuted, shortened, and have articular fractures that involve the radiocarpal joint and the distal radioulnar joint.

Age-Related Changes

As the client ages, there is an increased risk of falls, osteoporosis, gait changes, and mental status changes, which may increase the client's risk for a fracture.

Assessment

Physical Examination. Examination reveals an obvious deformity of the wrist, with dorsal displacement of the hand. The dorsum of the hand and wrist are generally swollen and ecchymotic. The wrist should be examined for tenderness at the radial fracture site, the distal ulna, elbow, and shoulder. The examiner may also note crepitus on examination of the wrist and pain when the client moves the fingers. A thorough neurovascular exam is important and should include testing for circulatory and sensory functions such as pain, paresthesia, paralysis, pallor, or pulselessness. The function of the median nerve and the flexor and extensor tendons should be tested. The practitioner should consider local or regional anesthesia prior to assessment of instability. The most common injury associated with a Colles' fracture is damage to the median nerve. This can be as a result of stretching of the nerve, displaced fracture fragments, delayed or inadequate reduction, or hematoma formation and increased compartment pressure. Prompt reduction of the fracture can help reduce median nerve involvement.

Diagnostic Studies. Radiographic studies are warranted. The two most important views are the anteroposterior and the lateral views in neutral position. Additional views include posteroanterior views in maximal radial deviation, maximal flexion, and maximal extension. Computed tomography (CT) scans and magnetic resonance imaging (MRI) are two other methods of diagnosing a fracture.

Clinical Management

Initially, the wrist should be iced, elevated, and immobilized. Ice packs can be applied for 20 minutes on and 20 minutes off for the first 24 hours.

Nondisplaced Colles' Fractures. The elderly have a large percentage of nondisplaced fractures. The goal of treatment in this situation is to protect the fracture site from further injury and to mobilize the hand and wrist as soon as symptoms allow. Generally, the client is either casted or splinted. The length of the client's immobilization may vary from 3 to 6 weeks. After the arm is casted, the client may wear a sling to elevate the arm above the level of the heart. Instruct the client on cast care and to monitor for neurovascular changes.

Displaced Colles' Fracture. The goal of management of a displaced fracture is to obtain anatomic reduction and to maintain that reduction with appropriate methods of immobilization. Cast immobilization is generally preferred. However, more complicated fractures may warrant external fixation, percutaneous pin fixation, or open reduction.

VERTEBRAL COMPRESSION FRACTURE

Vertebral compression fractures can result in a significant loss of general health, mobility, and quality of life. According to Rockwood et al. (1991), compression fractures are a result of anterior or lateral flexion causing fracture of the anterior column. Vertebral compression fractures can occur from movements such as putting a load on outstretched arms, such as raising a window or lifting a small child. Clients with severe osteoporosis may sustain a fracture with coughing or sneezing. Radiographically, the anterior, or central height of the vertebral body is diminished, while the posterior height remains normal. These fractures are normally stable and rarely involve neurologic compromise. According to Lukert (1994), solitary wedge fractures seldom occur above the seventh thoracic vertebra, and causes other than osteoporosis, such as metastatic or infectious disease, must be suspected in these circumstances.

Assessment

History. The client will complain of acute back pain. The pain can be incapacitating for a few weeks. The pain will usually diminish in severity but can remain intense for 2 to 3 months. Chronic pain may persist, related to deformity of the vertebra, alterations of joint articula-

tion, and the development of degenerative joint disease (DJD).

The history should include any transient paralysis and numbness or tingling of an extremity that would suggest spinal involvement. Inversely, if the client has no feeling or suddenly develops a period of altered sensation, this may suggest an incomplete spinal cord injury. Also note the client's history of osteoporosis, falls, pain, and medications.

Physical Examination. Compression fractures are easiest to diagnose in clients who present with acute pain and an identifiable deformity of a vertebra corresponding to the area of pain. Carefully observe the motion of the client's extremities. Inspect and palpate the entire spine to locate the area of pain. The physical should include a complete neurologic exam, including motor function by nerve root level involving proprioception and pain/temperature pathways. Cord compression is rare; however, examine for signs and symptoms, including bilateral leg pain, paresthesias, urinary or stool incontinence, ileus and motor weakness. Include a digital rectal exam for voluntary or reflex anal sphincter contraction. Assess and grade the strength of each muscle, and record deficits.

The client may experience a loss of height and changes in postural alignment. As a result, the client will have a reduction in the size of the abdominal and thoracic cavities and may develop a protuberant abdomen and a feeling of abdominal distention. Early satiety is a common complaint and may lead to weight loss. Over the course of time, the ribs may overlap the iliac crests and cause discomfort. Spinal muscles that are involved in extension become weak and promote worsening of kyphosis. This results in the client's becoming easily fatigued and limited in his or her activities. As the volume of the thoracic cage decreases, the client has diminished lung volume and restrictive pulmonary disease (Lukert, 1994). Additionally, the client may develop sleep disturbances, fibromyalgia, depression, and spinal stenosis.

Diagnostic Studies. Plain x-rays of the anteroposterior and lateral view of the thoracic lumbar spine form the basis of examination in most clients. Computed tomography scans allow better visualization of the vertebral body. Magnetic resonance imaging permits visualization of the spinal cord. Bone scan will reveal increased uptake at the site of a recent fracture.

Labwork may include a CBC and a chemistry profile. The results are expected to be normal except for an elevation in alkaline phosphatase for 2 to 3 months following the fracture.

Clinical Management

Educating the client regarding the course of the pain may help to reassure him or her that the pain is not permanent and will diminish over time. Clients can be managed as outpatients unless they experience an ileus, urinary retention, or neurologic complications.

Compression fractures are generally stable and rarely involve neurologic compromise. The client is generally treated symptomatically. In the acute phase of a compression fracture, the treatment may include bedrest, local analgesia, systemic analgesia, and narcotics for 1 to 2 weeks. The client may find it difficult to sleep lying flat and may need to be positioned in a hospital bed or a lounge chair/recliner for comfort (Lukert, 1994).

Local analgesia may include ice massage to the point of numbness, which may give pain relief for a few hours. In a few weeks, moist heat can be applied for 20 minutes every few hours to relieve muscle spasm.

Systemic analgesics include NSAIDs. Bear in mind the previously mentioned side effects of NSAIDs in the elderly population. Muscle relaxants are poorly tolerated in the elderly. Narcotics may be indicated in the acute phase of a compression fracture. Unfortunately, narcotics also have serious side effects and need to be monitored closely. Lukert (1994) utilizes hydrocodone bitartrate 7.5 mg with acetaminophen 750 mg (Vicodin ES) and codeine phosphate 30 mg with acetaminophen (Tylenol #3). However, methods of pain control vary.

Providing a brace for the client may allow for early ambulation by stabilizing the spine and preventing movements that aggravate the pain. Bracing may also help alleviate back fatigue. According to Lukert (1994), a wide lumbar support with Velcro closures is frequently adequate for lower lumbar fractures. For fractures of the lower thoracic vertebrae, a cruciform brace that has pressure points on the symphysis pubis and the sternum may be helpful. Finally, for a higher thoracic fracture, a modified Taylor brace (a lightweight brace with paraspinous plastic or metal supports extending to the upper thoracic region and straps going up over the shoulder) maintains extension of the thoracic spine.

Management of a vertebral compression fracture also includes treating the underlying osteoporosis, if appropriate, to prevent further fractures. Some clients may benefit from calcitonin–salmon injections. Calcitonin has been shown to have an analgesic effect and has been useful in clients with acute vertebral compression fractures. Calcitonin can be given 25 units subcutaneously for a few days, with a gradual increase to 50 to 100 units daily for 2 months tapered then to every other day. Treatment usually lasts up to 1 year.

As soon as the fracture heals, the client should begin exercise. A physical therapist should be able to assist the client to develop an exercise program which includes strategies to promote back safety.

If there is a loss of more than 50% vertebral body height, angulation of more than 20%, or multiple adjacent compression fractures, the injury is considered to be potentially unstable. The client is usually treated in a hyperextension cast or, if necessary, with an open reduction and internal fixation (ORIF) using posterior instrumentation and fusion.

HIP FRACTURE

Hip fractures generally involve the femoral neck or the trochanteric processes. In the elderly, a fractured hip is a common complication of falls and gait instability and is a leading cause of disability among the elderly. Hip fractures are one of the many acute health events that may lead to permanent changes in the level of functioning of an older person (Bradley & Kozak, 1995). Risk factors for a hip fracture are listed in Table 10–6.

Age-related Changes

Approximately 5% of falls in elderly persons result in a fracture. Many of the fractures are thought to be due to osteo-

TABLE 10–6. HIP FRACTURE: WHAT INCREASES THE RISK

- Osteoporosis
- Low body weight
- Old age
- Minimal weight-bearing activity, such as walking
- Diet low in calcium and vitamin D
- Diet high in protein, caffeine, and alcohol
- Smoking
- Cancer of the bone or metastases to the bone
- Confusion or altered orientation
- Parkinson's disease
- Prolonged bedrest
- Stroke
- Urinary retention
- Decreased sensation in legs and feet

Source: Used with permission from Pellino, T. (1994). How to manage hip fractures. *AJN, 94*(4), 49.

porosis. According to Menkes et al. (1989), the client may fall, but the fall does not necessarily cause the fracture. In many cases, the fracture causes the fall. Older persons have the highest rate of hospitalization for acute injuries.

Hip fractures are a serious complication of a fall. More than 250,000 hip fractures occur each year in clients over 65 years of age. The risk for a hip fracture increases dramatically with age and is highest in white women. Persons of Caucasian heritage have approximately twice the rate of hip fractures of persons of other races.

Approximately 5% of elderly persons who suffer a hip fracture will die during hospitalization. Of the elders who are hospitalized for a fall, only 50% will live for 1 year after. An additional 12% to 67%, depending on the population studied, will die within 24 months following a hip fracture. Of those who survive the fracture, many will suffer a decreased quality of life. About half will not be able to walk after a fracture, and many will be unable to live independently. There is a high rate of long-term institutional placement following this surgery.

Assessment

History. The client may report a history of trauma or a fall and will complain of persistent groin pain, especially with weight bearing. Some fractures, such as a femoral neck fracture, may be more occult and the client may not have a deformity on examination.

Physical Examination. Generally, the elderly client will present with groin pain on the affected side; however, occasionally, the pain can be referred to the knee. Due to pain, the client will be unable or unwilling to walk or sit upright. The affected leg may be shortened, bruised, externally rotated, and slightly flexed. The client may also present with soft tissue injuries such as edema about the hip and thigh from hemorrhage and multiple bone fragments. Some injuries may be extensive. If a hip fracture is suspected, minimize movement of the hip to prevent further damage.

Assess the client's neurovascular status of the entire leg below the injury and compare to the opposite side. Check pulses, temperature, capillary refill time, skin color, and sensory and motor nerve functions. Assess for chest pain, shortness of breath, and possible internal bleeding at the fracture site as well as signs of shock. Medicating the client for pain is crucial.

Next, an assessment of the cause of the fracture must be completed. Assess for medical problems such as syncope, osteoporosis, and visual changes that may have led to a fall. In addition, the environment should be surveyed to help to determine its contribution to the etiology of the fall.

Diagnostic Studies. Radiographs of the hip are warranted. Anteroposterior and lateral views of the hip, CT scans, bone scans, or MRIs may also reveal a fracture. According to Menkes et al. (1989), a subcapital fracture may be more difficult to see radiographically, and the only clinical sign may be pain with range of motion. If complications, such as hemorrhage, occur or are suspected, hematologic studies are appropriate.

Clinical Management

Hip fractures are generally treated surgically. Depending on the type of fracture and the client's activity level and general health, he or she will undergo operative stabilization through an ORIF or a prosthetic replacement. Traction can produce healing, but the process can take from 4 to 8 weeks and the client may suffer complications from bedrest and immobilization.

Standard postoperative care is recommended. Generally, the client must follow precautions outlined by the orthopedist to avoid dislocation. These may include avoiding adduction, rotation of the hip internally or externally, and flexing the hip more than 90 degrees. Referring the client to acute/subacute rehabilitation may maximize his or her functional level and may facilitate the return to independence and into the community.

CASE STUDY

Mrs. Kowalski is a 95-year-old Polish immigrant who lives in her own three-family home with a live-in companion. She has early to midstage Alzheimer's dementia, affecting short-term memory and time/place orientation. She is otherwise very healthy and is independent in activities of daily living (ADL). Her live-in companion assists with instrumental activities of daily living (IADL) and monitors Mrs. Kowalski's whereabouts, since she has a tendency to descend three flights of stairs and wander outdoors occasionally at night.

Mrs. Kowalski got up in the middle of the night for her usual snack and use of the bathroom. She fell to the floor, landing on her left hip and hitting her head on the door frame. Her companion was unable to lift her off the floor, so she called 911. Mrs. Kowalski was assessed at the local emergency room, where she was found to have no serious injuries. X-rays of her left hip were negative and she was discharged home that morning.

Over the next few days, Mrs. Kowalski became less active in her personal care, although she could ambulate at baseline with a walker. She denied pain but was restless at night, sleeping very little. Her appetite declined, and she ate few of her favorite foods. She became more confused, mistaking her caregiver for her sister, who has been dead for many years. Her caregiver became very concerned and called the advanced practice nurse (APN) who sees her in the geriatric clinic for her input.

QUESTIONS

1. How would you proceed in your workup of Mrs. Kowalski?
2. What are your differential diagnoses?

ANSWERS

1. Mrs. Kowalski's decline in cognitive and functional status following a fall are of utmost concern. Conducting formal mental status and functional exams to compare with baseline results is extremely helpful to objectively measure changes from her prefall status. A thorough medication history is necessary to identify potential pharmacologic contributors. A detailed physical exam to rule out any disease pathology is indicated, with focus on the neuromuscular system. Based on your physical findings, appropriate diagnostic studies should follow. At minimum, CBC with differential, chemistry panel, and urinalysis would be indicated.

2. A fall that involves a blow to the head and cognitive changes raises the possibility of a subdural hematoma. Delirium from a subdural hematoma may not appear until up to several weeks following the fall due to the increased space between the atrophied brain and skull of older adults. A fracture of the hip must still be considered in spite of the initial negative x-ray. Some hip fractures are obscured and may be present only on bone scan. If a person continues to show a significant change from functional baseline following a blow to the hip, serial x-rays may be required to detect the fracture. Other fractures (spine, pelvis) should also be considered. A urinary tract infection may be responsible for cognitive and functional changes, even in the absence of fever, dysuria, and leukocytosis. Other infections may also present atypically (bronchitis, pneumonia). Acute cardiac disease (myocardial infarction, congestive heart failure) can have altered presentations and should be pursued if suspicion arises.

Mrs. Kowalski was found to have an intertrochanteric fracture of her left hip on repeat x-ray. It was thought that the weight bearing she performed postfall, ambulating about her apartment with the walker, aggravated the initial fracture, making it visible only on the second x-ray. Even though she did not complain of a great deal of pain from the hip fracture, her delirium was thought to be an expression of this injury. Persons with dementia are at risk of developing delirium with even minor changes in health status. She underwent a surgical repair and remained delirious initially following the procedure, but after one week regained her cognitive baseline. She returned home with her live-in companion following a brief stay at a rehabilitative facility at her previous level of function.

■ REFERENCES

Bellantoni, M. F. (1996). Osteoporosis prevention and treatment. *Am Fam Phys, 54,* 986–992, 995–996.

Bradley, C. F., & Kozak, C. (1995). Nursing care and management of the elderly: The elderly hip fractured patient. *J Gerontol Nurs, 21*(8), 15–22.

Dwolatzky, T., Sonnenblick, M., & Nesher, G. (1997). Giant cell arteritis and polymyalgia rheumatica: Clues to early diagnosis. *Geriatrics, 52*(6), 38–44.

Lukert, B. P. (1994). Vertebral compression fractures: How to manage pain, avoid disability. *Geriatrics, 49*(2), 22–26.

McCarty, D. J. (1989). *Arthritis and allied conditions* (11th ed.). Philadelphia: Lea & Febiger.

Menkes, J. S., Nygaard, A., & Rogers, L. F. (1989). Easy-to-miss fractures. *Patient Care, 23,* 151–174.

Miller, K. L. Hormone replacement therapy in the elderly. *Clin Obstet Gynecol, 39,* 912–932.

Rockwood, C. A., Green, D. P., & Bucholz, R. W. (1991). *Rockwood and Green's fractures in adults* (3rd ed.). New York: J. B. Lippincott.

Ross, C. (1997). A comparison of osteoarthritis and rheumatoid arthritis: Diagnosis and treatment. *Nurse Pract, 22*(9), 20–39.

Schumacher, H. R., Klippel, J. H., & Koopman, W. J. (Eds.). (1993). *Primer of the rheumatic diseases.* Atlanta: Arthritis Foundation.

Yoshikawa, T. T., Cobbs, E. L., & Brummel-Smith, K. (1993). *Ambulatory geriatric care.* St. Louis: Mosby.

11

TOPICS IN NEUROLOGIC CARE

Claudia Kling • Christine Marek Waszynski

■ INTRODUCTION

Pathologic changes in the structure and function of the nervous system may result in subtle to severe changes in a person's mobility, balance, coordination, sensory interpretations, level of consciousness, intellectual performance, personality, communication, comprehension of stimuli and concepts, emotional responses, behaviors, and thought processes.

Some neurologic signs and symptoms are associated with normal aging. These are usually bilateral and symmetric; therefore, abnormal findings that are unilateral or asymmetric should increase suspicion of an underlying pathology. Changes in neurologic function or behaviors should never be assumed to be a part of normal aging until a full neurologic evaluation of the complaint has been completed.

The neurologic system is affected by several normal aging changes. These changes can be summarized as a general slowing of neurologic responses. As one ages, fewer neurons are available to provide sensory and motor messages in and out of the central nervous system (CNS). The remaining neurons function at a less-than-optimal capacity due to myelin sheath degeneration and decreased amounts of available neural transmitters. This results in slower reaction times.

On examination of the older client, some or all of the following findings may be exhibited:

- Reduced sense of smell and taste
- Reduced sense of pain, light touch, and temperature
- Reduced visual acuity
- Pupils may be small, slow to react to light and accommodate
- Slowed movement, motor reaction time, and deep tendon reflex
- Decreased muscle strength, muscle mass, and fine motor coordination
- Decreased balance and coordination

• Reduced reflexes and vibratory sense, particularly at the ankle

Coupled with normal aging changes in other systems, it is clear that synergistic factors can threaten the balance of functional abilities and deficits necessary for independent activities of daily living (ADL). Attempts to minimize the impact of these age-related presentations is a focus of the advanced practice nurse (APN) and is a theme throughout the text of this book.

When subtle deficits caused by acute or chronic pathology are superimposed on normal aging changes, neurologic assessment and diagnosis becomes extremely challenging. This chapter on common neurologic problems found in the elderly population will demonstrate this. It will focus on the nuances of disease presentation and the management of neurologic conditions commonly encountered in the geriatric patient. The reader is referred to texts of primary care and neurology for complete information regarding pathophysiology, differential diagnosis, and treatment and for information regarding neurologic changes that are not covered in this chapter. A "quickie" neurologic evaluation guide is found in Appendix F at the back of this book.

It is important to note that improved imaging techniques which are now available allow the demonstration of a specific source of the neurologic deficit, which can lead to a definitive diagnosis and more specific treatment. However, because CNS tissue does not regenerate, even with the knowledge of the specific source of the neurologic deficit, full recovery is often not the outcome of treatment.

■ CEREBROVASCULAR ACCIDENT (STROKE)

Strokes are one of the most common neurologic problems in the elderly. A stroke is defined as a rapidly developing vascular deficit in the brain, which causes a focal disturbance of brain function for more than 24 hours. A focal deficit of vascular origin that resolves in less than 24 hours is defined as a transient ischemic attack (TIA). TIAs are often due to platelet emboli from the heart; 25% to 40% of patients who have had TIAs go on to have a major cerebrovascular accident (CVA). A focal deficit of vascular origin which lasts longer than 24 hours, but resolves completely is defined as a reversable ischemic neurologic deficit (RIND).

Strokes are the third most common cause of death in industrialized countries. Approximately 20% of stroke patients die within a month of the CVA; approximately 50% of stroke survivors have significant, permanent disabilities that require them to have assistance and supervision; approximately 30% of stroke survivors have obvious neurologic deficits but are able to live an independent life.

Seventy percent of CVAs occur in persons over 65 years old. Hypertension is a contributing factor in 70% of CVAs; diabetes mellitus doubles the risk of CVAs. Other risk factors for stroke are cardiac disease, including atrial fibrillation, valvular heart disease, cardiac failure, ischemic heart disease, and atherosclerotic vascular disease; oral contraceptives; severe anemias; and (particularly in the elderly) hypotension.

ASSESSMENT

Physical Examination

Past medical history is important, as certain predisposing factors contribute to each type of stroke. A history of angina or claudication indicates the presence of atherosclerosis, which may contribute to thrombosis. Cardiac valve disease or atrial fibrillation may contribute to embolic disease, and hypertension (HTN) may be a precursor of hemorrhagic disease.

The two major causes of CVAs are: (1) hemorrhages due to hematomas and aneurysms that bleed into the brain, causing displacement of and pressure on brain structures, which leads to destruction of the tissue of the brain; and (2) ischemia due to thrombosis and embolism in which a lack of blood to an area of the brain causes lack of oxygenation and destruction of the brain tissue.

When the cerebral blood supply is interrupted by hemorrhage or ischemia, tissue destruction results. The symptoms that occur are directly related to the vessels where the circulation has been interrupted and the function of the anatomic area of the brain affected. The history and progression of the stroke is important, as certain patterns of onset and progression may suggest different causes of the CVA (Table 11–1).

The brain is perfused by two major vascular systems: the carotid artery system and the vertebrobasilar artery system. The carotid artery system, which perfuses the anterior two thirds of the cerebral hemispheres, is comprised of two branches of the internal carotid artery, specifically, the midcerebral artery and the anterior cerebral artery. The vertebrobasilar artery system, which supplies the posterior cerebral circulation, is comprised of the vertebrobasilar artery and the posterior cerebral artery. The location of the CVA will correspond to an identifiable vessel, with certain uniformity of symptoms (Table 11–2).

Lacunar infarcts are small infarcts in

TABLE 11–1. PRESENTATION OF STROKE

History/Progression	Probable Cause
Abrupt onset followed by rapid improvement	Embolus
Abrupt onset with stepwise progression; onset may be during sleep; improvement over a day to a few weeks	Thrombosis
Onset associated with headache or altered consciousness, with rapid deterioration over several hours	Hemorrhage
Focal neurologic symptoms lasting only minutes to 24 hours	Transient ischemic attack
Visual disturbances (ie, amaurosis fugax: a monocular blindness of short duration)	Carotid artery disease (ie, embolism to the ophthalmic artery, which is the first branch of the internal carotid artery)
Disturbance of equilibrium	Posterior cerebral circulation damage
Spastic hemiparesis and lower facial weakness	Cerebral hemisphere damage due to carotid artery disease

TABLE 11–2. ANATOMIC AREAS SUPPLIED BY CEREBRAL ARTERIES AND ASSOCIATED SYMPTOMS RELATED TO THE LOCATION OF CEREBROVASCULAR ACCIDENTS

Vessel	Anatomic Area	Associated Symptoms
Internal carotid artery	Anterior two thirds of the cerebral hemispheres	Contralateral hemiplegia and hemianesthesia Aphasia (global) Hemianopsia Contralateral neglect[a] Visual–spatial agnosia[a] Constructional apraxia[a]
Midcerebral artery	Lateral aspect of the cerebral hemispheres	Contralateral hemiplegia and hemianesthesia Hemianopsia Aphasia (expressive more than receptive) Contralateral neglect[b] Constructional apraxia[b] Sensory inattention[b] Loss of geographic orientation[b]
Anterior cerebral artery	Medial aspect of the cerebral hemispheres	Contralateral hemiparesis with greater involvement of lower extremities than upper extermities or face Behavioral changes/emotional liability Grasp reflex on the affected side Expressive (Broca's) aphasia Dementia with apathy and paranoia[c] Incontinence[c] Gait disturbances[c] Bilateral grasp reflexes[c] Akinetic mutism[c]
Posterior cerebral artery[d]	Upper brain stem Midbrain Thalamus Inferior and medial aspect of the temporal lobe Medial aspect of the occipital lobe	Contralateral sensory loss and/or painful dysesthesias Contralateral neglect Homonymous hemianopsia Visual agnosia Vertical gaze palsy Ocular and constructional apraxia Sensory inattention

TABLE 11–2.   ANATOMICAL AREAS SUPPLIED BY CEREBRAL ARTERIES AND ASSOCIATED SYMPTOMS RELATED TO THE LOCATION OF CEREBROVASCULAR ACCIDENTS (CONT.)

Vessel	Anatomic Area	Associated Symptoms

Vertebrobasilar artery	Medulla
	Most rostral portion of the
	   spinal cord
		Fatal coma
		Quadriplegia
		Loss of brain stem reflexes
		   (survival with "locked-in"
		   syndrome)

[a] A dominant hemisphere infarct will cause aphasia; a nondominant hemisphere infarct will cause spatial and perceptual disorders.
[b] A dominant hemisphere infarct will cause aphasia; a nondominant hemisphere infarct will additionally cause parietal symptoms.
[c] Anterior cerebral artery infarcts may be bilateral, causing these additional symptoms.
[d] If the posterior cerebral artery receives its main vascular supply from the internal cerebral artery rather than the basilar artery, there will be occlusion or hemorrhage of the internal areas supplied by the posterior cerebral artery, with the additional neurologic symptoms. This is not common, but it is possible.

deeper, noncortical areas of the cerebral hemispheres and brain stem. Their symptoms result from occlusion or hemorrhage of the small, distal, penetrating branches of the larger arteries. Common lacunar infarct syndromes include:

- Posterior thalamic infarction, causing only sensory deficits
- Infarction of the posterior limb of the internal capsule, lower basal pontine, or a peduncular infarction, causing only motor deficits
- Basal pontine infarction, causing hemiparesis with ataxia of individual extremities
- Pontine infarction, causing facial weakness, dysarthria, dysphagia, and mild ataxia and hemiparesis of one hand

Lacunar infarcts are often multiple and may cumulatively lead to severe neurologic deficits, specifically multi-infarct dementia.

Diagnostic Studies

A computed tomography (CT) scan should be done on every stroke client as soon as possible. The CT scan will differentiate between hemorrhage and infarct. If the stroke is due to hemorrhage, anticoagulation should not be prescribed; if the CT scan shows an infarct or is within normal limits, evaluation of the cerebral vasculature should ensue and anticoagulation may be prescribed. The findings on the CT scan must correlate with the client's neurologic exam. There might be old or clinically silent infarctions that are not relevant to the current diagnosis but show up on the scan.

Magnetic resonance imaging (MRI) may identify abnormalities not visible on CT scan (ie, lacunar infarcts, posterior fossa abnormalities, plaques of multiple sclerosis), which may be important for final/differential diagnosis.

There is a high correlation between cerebral infarction and cardiac abnormalities. More than one third of persons with CVAs will show electrocardiographic (ECG) abnormalities at some time within the first 24 hours. Continuous monitoring during the first days poststroke should be considered.

CLINICAL MANAGEMENT

A stroke client may continue to show improvement for 6 to 12 months, sometimes longer with appropriate rehabilitation. Function may return as cerebral ischemia subsides and collateral circulation provides blood supply to areas of ischemia. Prevention of secondary disabilities and proper initial medical management are necessary to allow the client to take advantage of the skills to be learned in rehabilitation and to promote any spontaneous improvement that may occur.

Pharmacologic Measures

Approximately 48 hours after infarction, cerebral edema may occur, causing the client's condition to deteriorate. Steroid administration is a part of the early treatment of a CVA. Dexamethesone 4 to 20 mg every 4 hours may be prescribed. The dose should be rapidly tapered and continued for no more than 7 to 10 days.

If no hemorrhage is evident on CT scan or MRI, anticoagulation (initially with heparin, and later with warfarin) should be prescribed to prevent further emboli. Long term anticoagulation may be achieved with enteric-coated aspirin 325 mg one tablet PO per day or with warfarin.

Nonpharmacologic Measures

Aneurysms, subdural hematomas, tumors, and abcesses found on CT scan or MRI should be referred to a neurosurgeon. With 80% stenosis of the carotid artery and symptoms, a carotid endarterectomy is generally recommended. If there is carotid stenosis without symptoms, carotid endarterectomy may not be recommended, and treatment with an enteric-coated aspirin 325 mg PO per day should begin.

Rehabilitation should be started as soon as a diagnosis is made to prevent contractures; to improve range of motion, strength, coordination, and balance; to decrease spasticity; to prevent subluxation of the affected shoulder; to provide evaluation for speech and language training; and to provide evaluation for training to reduce perceptual dysfunction. Emphasis is placed on prevention of secondary disabilities, retraining toward maximum independence in ADL, and providing adaptive equipment, which will allow the patient to reach full functional potential.

Nursing management should focus on monitoring for changes in physical and neurologic status; providing care and assistance for dysfunctional body systems (eg, skin, bladder, bowels, respiratory system, and gastrointestinal system); prevention of secondary disabilities (eg, pressure sores, urinary tract infection [UTI], constipation, pneumonia, contractures, and malnutrition). Assisting with rehabilitation by providing teaching and training which will allow clients to reach their maximum functional potential and understand their disability and functional capabilities.

Physical therapists and occupational therapists should work with the client and family on skills of mobility, independence in ADL, and safety within the home. Adaptive equipment can assist with goal achievement. A psychologist can assist with identification and treatment of poststroke depression, as well as providing psychologic testing to determine the severity of a client's mental status deficits and improvement. This is of particular importance because of problems in speech and communication, which can be mistaken for a dementia. A speech therapist can assist with issues of speech, comprehension, communication, and swallowing. A modified barium swallow may be ordered if there is a question of aspiration, to determine what types of foods and liquids the client can safely swallow.

Home care may be necessary in order for a client to remain in the home. This may include a home health aide to assist with ADL, rehabilitative specialists to assess for needs and provide ongoing therapy and a social worker to assist with social and familial issues. If a client's care becomes too great for home care, a long-term care facility that provides access to an active multidisciplinary team should be carefully selected to allow the client to continue to function at the highest possible level.

REHABILITATION

Due to the functional impairments caused by diseases of the nervous system, treatment must be carried out by a multidisciplinary team whose goal is to restore the client's function and to maintain the highest and most independent level of functioning in a safe, unrestricted, and (if possible) noninstitutional setting. If the client is to go home, the family must be taught how to assist the client and to understand the abilities and limitations that result from the neurologic deficit.

The multidisciplinary team may include some or all of the following members:

- Physician (neurologist, physiatrist, and other specialists) as necessary
- Registered Nurse specializing in neurologic or rehabilitation nursing
- Physical Therapist
- Occupational Therapist
- Speech Therapist
- Recreational Therapist
- Dietitian
- Social Worker
- Vocational Counselor
- Psychologist

Initially, the team's focus will be to restore as much function as possible. This will include gaining strength, improving communication, regaining mobility, relearning ADL, resuming social roles and activities, and controlling the effects of incontinence.

Assistive devices may be necessary for a client to attain the highest level of function, and the family must understand how to properly set the client up to use these devices. The family should also be able to recognize when to help and when to allow the client to struggle a bit to achieve further independence. Maintaining the client's maximum level of function requires continuous vigilance to prevent deterioration of an unaffected part and protect against further deterioration or injury to an affected part. Prevention is a continuous aspect of care throughout the life of any person with a chronic neurologic disease, and the family must understand the possible complications and how to prevent further injury or loss of function.

All members of the multidisciplinary team should be teachers and should help the client and his or her family to become experts and able to function again independently with the limitations and new competencies necessitated by the impairments created by a neurologic disease.

■ PARKINSON'S DISEASE

Parkinson's disease is an idiopathic degenerative process of the pigmented dopaminergic neurons of the substantia nigra, which may be caused by various pathologic disease processes that interrupt or reduce the neurotransmission of dopamines.

Parkinson's disease is the most frequent extrapyramidal movement disorder seen in patients over 50 years old and is thought to affect about 1% of all persons over 50 years old.

CLINICAL PRESENTATION

Parkinson's disease is a movement disorder that is characterized by the slow development of the following neurologic changes:

- Decreased voluntary movement
- Increased involuntary movements
- Impaired muscle tone
- Impaired postural reflexes

Initially, the symptoms are unilateral, but within 1 to 2 years, as they progress, they become bilateral (Table 11–3). Reactive depression is common as the disabilities caused by Parkinson's disease become increasingly severe.

The history may include reports of the following:

- Decreased strength
- Increased fatigue and lethargy, with slowing of all movements
- Difficulty walking; with increased rigidity and tremors, uneven shuffling gait, and difficulty stopping
- Increased falls
- Difficulty maintaining balance (particularly in a crowd)
- Difficulty rising from a low position or a soft surface
- Difficulty turning over in bed
- Inability to maintain an upright position

- Dressing and undressing takes an extended amount of time
- Difficulty getting into/out of an automobile
- Difficulty buttoning clothes, fastening hooks and snaps
- Changes in handwriting
- Changes in voice quality
- Difficulty swallowing
- Drooling
- Difficulty cutting food
- Blank facial expression
- Mental status changes
- Weight loss
- Tremor at rest

CLINICAL MANAGEMENT

The stages and progression of this disease are outlined in Table 11–4. Replenishing the dopamine stores in the brain is the goal of treatment. Since dopamine cannot cross the blood–brain barrier, therapy consists of administering levodopa (its metabolic precursor), which can cross the blood–brain barrier, or attempting to stimulate the release of dopamine from the substantia nigra.

PHARMACOLOGIC MEASURES

Amantadine (Symmetrel) resembles anticholinergic drugs and is often the first medication used for treatment. It releases dopamine from the cells of the substantia nigra and decreases rigidity, tremors, and bradykinesia. It is effective in 50% of patients treated with it. The usual dose is 100 mg PO twice a day. Side effects include discoloration of the skin, swelling of the feet, confusion, delusions, and hallucinations. All are temporary and will resolve when medication is discontinued.

TABLE 11–3.   PARKINSON'S DISEASE: CHANGES ON PHYSICAL EXAMINATION

Findings	Description
Rigidity with cogwheeling	Increased tone with a rachetlike sensation, palpated during flexion and extension. This silent finding can be brought out by asking the client to draw circles in the air with one arm while examining the other for cogwheeling
Festinant gait	An uneven, shuffling gait that changes from walking to a running pace, or may freeze and stop
	Upper limbs may be carried in a slightly flexed position, resulting in little or absent arm swing
Retropulsion	Steps or falls backwards if gently pushed; unable to resist the push and stay in place
Involuntary tremulous motions with decreased muscle power	
Intention tremor	Tremors that may increase with anxiety and when attempting to complete a task
Resting tremor	Tremors that may increase with anxiety or increase with purposeful movement which do not when attempting to complete a task
	Resting tremors may also involve the muscles of the face or the tongue but are most common in the hands
Pill rolling	The most characteristic movement of Parkinson's disease is the movement of the fingers and thumb, described as "pill rolling"
	The wrist is in a flexed position, with the fingers extended and the thumb abducted. There is an oscillating movement of the fingers and thumb
Bradykinesia	Slowed voluntary muscle movement that deteriorates with repetition and may cause the client to freeze (ie, drooling/difficulty swallowing, changes in handwriting, blank facial expression, changes in voice quality)
	Contributes to the fixed facial expression, rigidity during tasks and movements, slowed speech and decreased voice volume, and problems with swallowing and drooling
Poor postural reflexes	A posture which bends forward, with poor balance and slow postural adjustment, contributing to falls

(Continues)

TABLE 11–3.   PARKINSON'S DISEASE: CHANGES ON PHYSICAL EXAMINATION (CONT.)

Findings	Description
Poor postural reflexes (cont.)	Decreased ability to right oneself and not lose one's balance after a slight postural disturbance Difficulty turning around/changing direction while walking
Mental status changes	
Weight loss	
Contractures	
Seborrheic dermatitis of eyebrows, ears or scalp line	

Levodopa–carbidopa (Sinemet) and Levodopa–benserazide (Madopar) are peripheral, noncompetitive dopa decarboxylase inhibitors that block the peripheral decarboxylation of levodopa, therefore slowing its conversion to dopamine in the extracerebral tissues (ie, stomach, intestines, walls of the blood vessels). Because it cannot cross the blood–brain barrier, it does not prevent the conver-

TABLE 11–4.   STAGES OF PARKINSON'S DISEASE

Stage I	Unilateral involvement Tremors of upper extremities Mild rigidity Uneven gait, with affected arm in a flexed position and posture leaning toward the unaffected side Blank facial expression
Stage II	Bilateral involvement Slow, shuffling gait, with stooped position Slowing of all movements (bradykinesia)
Stage III	Postural instability with tendency to fall Retropulsion and propulsion Assistance with ADL becomes necessary
Stage IV	Rigidity and bradykinesia become disabling, requiring substantial assistance with ADL Standing is unstable, falls are frequent Retropulsion and propulsion become severe Use of a wheelchair becomes necessary
Stage V	Bradykinesia and rigidity become severe, leaving the person unable to move Facial expression becomes fixed and staring Speech becomes difficult to understand Difficulty swallowing Total assistance is required with all ADL and movement Walking is no longer possible

sion of levodopa to dopamine in the brain. This allows increased availability of dopamine in the brain, where it is necessary, but prevents the conversion of levodopa to dopamine outside the brain, where increased levels are not necessary and will cause only unwanted side effects. Levodopa is the precursor of dopamine and is considered the cornerstone of symptomatic treatment. Side effects include increased involuntary movements, mental status changes, and dizziness. Over time the response to levadopa may decrease, requiring a higher dose to achieve effect. For this reason, use of this medication is delayed until symptoms have a significant impact on mobility and quality of life.

Cogentin (benztropine mesylate), Artane (trihexyphenidyl), and Akineton (bigeriden) are anticholinergics that block the action of the transmitter acetylcholine, which (particularly in the early stages of the disease) may decrease rigidity and tremors. They may prolong dopamine effects by blocking dopamine reuptake and storage at central receptor sites. They help to balance the cholinergic activity in the basal ganglia by blocking the central cholinergic receptors. In addition, these medications lessen rigidity, tremors, and drooling. The usual dose is as follows: Cogentin, 0.5 to 6 mg/d PO; Artane, 6 to 10 mg/d PO in 3 to 4 divided doses; and Akineton, 2 to 4 mg PO twice a day or four times a day. Side effects include dry mouth, blurred vision, constipation, difficulty voiding, and mental status changes.

Bromocriptine (Parlodel) and Pergolide (Permar) are dopamine receptor antagonists given as an adjunct to Sinemet (when used in combination, less Sinemet may be used to get acceptable symptom control). These drugs mimic the effects of dopamine by bypassing the degenerating cells in the substantia nigra and stimulating the dopamine receptors directly. (They do not need to be changed to dopamine before being able to be effective.) The usual dose is as follows: Parlodel, 1.25 mg PO twice a day with meals, which may be increased every 14 to 28 days up to 100 mg/d or when the maximum therapeutic effect has been reached. For Pergolide, begin dosing at 0.5 mg/d PO, which may be increased by 0.1 to 1.5 mg every third day to a up to 3 mg/d or when the maximum therapeutic effect has been reached. Side effects include nausea, dizziness, and mental status changes.

Eldepryl (selegiline hydrochloride) is a monoamine oxidase inhibitor (MAOI) that is given as an adjunct to or prior to beginning Sinemet. It may directly increase dopaminergic activity by decreasing the uptake of dopamine into the nerve cells. The usual dose is 5 mg PO twice a day, with breakfast and lunch.

NONPHARMACOLOGIC MEASURES

There is no cure for Parkinson's disease, so the treatment is symptomatic. The goal is to decrease the progression of the disease and keep the patient active and mobile for as long as possible.

Physical therapy and occupational therapy are necessary to keep the client mobile, independent, and safe. A speech therapist will be able to assist with issues of swallowing and drooling, and concerns regarding which types of foods and liquids the client can safely swallow. A dietitian can assist to assure sufficient caloric intake to prevent severe weight loss and related complications.

Home care may be necessary in order for a client to remain in the home, including a home health aide to assist with ADL and a social worker to assist with social and familial issues as the client's mental status and physical capabilities diminish. If a client's care becomes too great for home care, a long-term care facility that provides access to an active multidisciplinary team should be carefully selected to allow the client to continue to function at the highest possible level.

There are local chapters of national organizations to provide ongoing support and education to persons with Parkinson's disease and their families. The APN should have this information readily available.

■ TEMPORAL ARTERITIS

Temporal arteritis (also known as giant cell arteritis) is a vasculitic disorder of the cranial arteries. It is called temporal arteritis because it produces temporal headaches and temporal artery biopsy shows distinctive inflammatory changes. When an elderly person develops a headache, it is important to test him or her for temporal arteritis, a condition that is rare in persons under 60 years old.

CLINICAL PRESENTATION

Clients will present with a headache, local tenderness to palpation of the forehead, and temporal arteries and possibly visual loss. The tenderness to palpation of the forehead is caused by a granulomatous inflammation of lymphocytes and giant cells in the cranial arteries. Systemic complaints such as weight loss, anorexia, weakness, and a low-grade fever may precede complaints of headaches and local tenderness.

ASSESSMENT
Diagnostic Studies
The erythrocyte sedimentation rate (ESR) is elevated, and there is a polyclonal increase in serum globulins. The diagnosis is confirmed by a temporal artery biopsy.

CLINICAL MANAGEMENT
Pharmacologic Measures
Treatment includes *immediate* initiation of high-dose steroid treatment. This will produce relief of the headache and systemic symptoms normalizing the ESR in about 4 weeks. The initiation of treatment should not await final confirmation of the temporal artery biopsy.

Temporal arteritis should be considered a medical emergency, as there may be ischemic symptoms which can cause blindness due to retinal infarct, myocardial infarction (MI) or CVA.

Temporal arteritis is generally considered self-limiting, and many clients are free of recurrent episodes after 1 to 2 years of treatment. However, some will repeatedly relapse, requiring maintenance with low doses of steroids. These clients must be closely monitored for complications of long-term steroid use, but this risk is considered acceptable because of the greater risks of untreated temporal arteritis.

■ DIZZINESS

Dizziness is the most common complaint among persons age 75 and older (Koch & Smith, 1985). Although 80% of patients suffering from dizziness reported the symptom to the primary-care provider, only 56% received treatment (Jonsson & Lipsitz, 1994). Of those treated, 90% received a prescription for meclizine (Sloane, 1989). Disorders of balance are often multifactorial in the older adult. The history can be complex or vague, and causes can be related to normal aging changes or disease states in various systems simultaneously. The implications, however, can be devastating, leading to falls with injuries and/or decreased functional ability. Of patients aged 60 and older, 20% have experienced dizziness severe enough to affect ADL (Sloane, 1989; Boult et al., 1991).

AGE-RELATED CHANGES

The normal aging changes within the ear that may affect balance include presbycusis with or without tinnitus and a loss of sensory epithial cells, vascular nerve fibers, and otoconia. Cupular deposits in the semicircular canal can produce short, sudden gravity-like responses that cause a sensation of imbalance. Other expected sensory losses, including presbyopia and decreased proprioception, may also accompany normal aging. Abrupt positional changes can create sensations of disequilibrium due to diminished carotid body response or saccular atrophy. A decreased ability to maintain homeostasis in the pulmonary and cardiovascular systems under stress, as well as previously described neurologic slowing, can all contribute to a loss of equilibrium in the older adult.

CLINICAL PRESENTATION

There are several categories of control and balance disturbance. Disequilibrium can be defined as spatial disorientation, disturbed balance, feelings of unsteadiness, fainting, clumsiness, near falling, or disturbed walking. It is not caused by an inner ear problem but by diseases or disturbances in other systems. Please refer to Table 11–5, which categorizes a variety of disorders that may present with disequilibrium.

The term *disequilibrium* can be further delineated into dizziness/lightheadedness, ataxia, and near syncope. Dizziness/lightheadedness is often described as sensations of numbness, wooziness, swimming, or floating. Ataxia is an inability to perform smooth, coordinated motions for walking, resulting in clumsiness or instability. Near syncope is a feeling of sinking, blacking out, or fainting, often related to cardiovascular and peripheral vascular disorders.

Vertigo and nystagmus are symptoms specifically related to the vestibular system: (1) right and left peripheral vestibular labyrinths, each with three semicircular canals and utriculosaccular organs; (2) the lower CNS vestibular pathways; and (3) the higher, integrative CNS vestibular pathways, involving cerebellar or cerebral functions (Goodhill, 1979). When these systems work harmoniously, equilibrium is maintained. A disorder of the peripheral vestibular system would involve the inner ear (labyrinth) or the vestibular nerve. A disorder of the central vestibular system would involve vascular or nonvascular pathways to the brain stem, cerebellum, and spinal cord (see Fig. 11–1 and Table 11–5).

Vertigo is defined as a spatial disorientation, characterized as a sensation of rotational movement involving the individual and/or the surroundings. It is often described as a feeling of being pulled to one side. Nystagmus is an involuntary movement of the eye that accompanies

TABLE 11–5. CHARACTERIZATIONS OF CONTROL/BALANCE DISORDERS

Disease/Syndrome	Dizziness	Ataxia	Near Syncope	Vertigo	Nystagmus	Hearing Loss	Tinnitus	Nausea/Vomitting	Positional/Provoked	Comments
■ PERIPHERAL VESTIBULAR DISORDERS										
Benign positional vertigo				X	X				X	Symptoms last less than 1 minute, extinguish; resolves within weeks
Ménière's disease				X	X	X	X	X		Symptoms last hours, resolve within weeks; hearing loss unilateral
Herpes zoster				X	X	X				Vesicles present in ear canal
Vestibular neuronitis				X	X		X	X		Symptoms last days; often follows upper respiratory infection
Acute labyrinthitis (due to infection, influenza, or meningitis)				X	X					
Labyrinthine damage (due to drug toxicity)				X	X	X	X			
Labyrinthine trauma				X	X					Includes temporal bone fracture
Acoustic neuroma (8th nerve tumors)				X	X	X				Do not extinguish
■ CENTRAL VESTIBULAR DISORDERS										
Vertebrobasilar insufficiency	X	X		X	X	±			x	Symptoms last minutes to days; also experience diplopia, dysarthria, dysphasia
Brain tumors				X	X	X		X		
Brain stem infarction		X		X	X					Other neurologic findings
Cerebellar ischemia		X		X	X			X		
Meningitis encephalitis				X	X					
Multiple sclerosis				X	X					

TABLE 11–5. CHARACTERIZATIONS OF CONTROL/BALANCE DISORDERS (CONT.)

Disease/Syndrome	Dizziness	Ataxia	Near Syncope	Vertigo	Nystagmus	Hearing Loss	Tinnitus	Nausea/Vomitting	Positional/Provoked	Comments
■ CARDIOVASCULAR DISORDERS										
Valvular disorders			X							
Arrhythmias			X							
Orthostatic hypotension			X						X	
Vasovagal attacks			X						X	
Carotid sinus hypersensitivity			X							
CVA/TIA (nonposterior circulation)	X	X	X							
■ BRAIN/THOUGHT DISORDERS										
Depression	X									
Anxiety/panic attacks	X									
Somatization disorder	X									
Substance abuse	X	X								
Parkinson's disease		X								
Alzheimer's disease		X								
■ SENSORY DEFICITS										
Visual impairment	X									
Auditory impairment	X									
Position sense disorder	X	X								
Neuropathy	X	X								
Spinocerebellar disorders	X	X								
■ OTHER										
Drugs	X	X	X	X	X	X	X	X	X	
Motion sickness			X	X	X			X		
Cough syncope			X						X	
Micturation syncope			X						X	
Anemia			X							
Hypoglycemia	X		X							
Thyroid disorder	X		X							
Systemic infecton	X									
Dehydraton	X		X							
Trauma (nonlabyrinthine)	X	X	X							
Syphilis			X				X			
Nicotine withdrawal	X		X							Headache

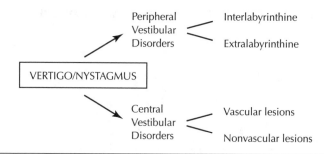

Figure 11–1. Effects of Vestibular System Disorders

vertigo. Nystagmus can be horizontal, vertical, diagonal, or rotary. Vertigo may also be accompanied by nausea and vomiting, hearing loss, and tinnitus, depending on the disease entity (Table 11–5).

ASSESSMENT

History

A comprehensive history is necessary to determine the elements surrounding the complaint of dizziness. History alone is the key component for accurate diagnosis in the majority of cases (Prestwood, 1991). Barker et al. (1986) list more than 30 terms used by patients to describe their complaint of spatial disorientation. This is why a thorough characterization of the problem is required. Figure 11–2 is an example of a questionnaire that may be used to gather data from a client (Ross & Robinson, 1984). Assessing the effect of symptoms on day-to-day function is essential for its appropriate management. The Dizziness Handicap Inventory (Jacobson & Newman, 1990) is an example of a tool that can help the examiner to assess the physical, emotional, and functional components of the complaint. An objective tool to establish a baseline cognitive and mood profile will also supplement the examiner's database.

Physical Examination

- Eyes: Visual acuity (central and peripheral), extraocular movements (observe for nystagmus; disregard if only a few beats present at extreme lateral gaze)
- Fundoscopic exam (cataracts, glaucoma, macular degeneration)
- Ears: Hearing acuity (preferably with audiometer), cerumen impaction, Weber and Rinne tests
- Cardiovascular: Lying, sitting, and standing blood pressure and apical pulse; carotid and abdominal bruits; extra heart sounds or murmurs
- Full neurologic exam: Cranial nerves, reflexes, motor and sensory testing, cerebellar and balance testing
- Special maneuvers: Hallpike–Dix maneuver (Fig. 11–3)

In a study of 120 male patients with dizziness, the Hallpike–Dix maneuver was positive in 44% of the cases, making it the most common abnormal finding (Davis, 1994). The Hallpike–Dix maneuver is used to detect vertigo and nystagmus, which accompany benign positional vertigo (BPV) and other syndromes with positional symptomatology. Benign positional vertigo is a commonly missed treatable

Please complete statements, circle letter, and check blank spaces that apply to your dizziness.

A. DESCRIPTION OF DIZZINESS
   1. Describe briefly, in your own words, your last dizzy spell.

   _____

   _____

   2. Words that describe my dizziness:
      a. lightheaded, woozy, swimming in head
      b. blacking out or loss of consciousness
      c. sinking feeling
      d. tendency to fall
         _____to right   _____to left
         _____forward   _____backward
      e. unsteadiness on feet or loss of balance
         _____to right   _____to left
         _____forward   _____backward
      f. hurled into space, to ground or floor
      g. room or objects spin around me
      h. feel I'm turning or rocking
      i. headache
      j. nausea or vomiting
      k. numb feeling
      l. pressure in head
      m. other

B. CHARACTERISTICS OF DIZZINESS
   1. My present dizziness began _____
                                    (approximate date, time—AM/PM)
   2. Very first occurrence of dizzy spells

   _____

   3. Warning sign that dizziness will start _____
   4. Have you ever had this illness before?
      _____No _____Yes If yes, the date _____
   5. Dizziness comes on suddenly _____ gradually _____
   6. Dizziness is continuous _____ in spells or episodes _____
   7. My dizziness each time usually lasts:
      flash_____   seconds_____   minutes_____   hours_____   other_____
   8. Dizzy spells now are:
      worse_____   better_____   more often_____   less often _____
   9. What seems to bring on or aggravate your dizziness?
      a. turning in bed, moving side to side (state side_____), moving backward
      b. lying down (state side_____) or on my back _____
      c. changes from lying or sitting to standing position
      d. other _____
   10. What seems to help?
      a. keeping head in one position
      b. resting
      c. moving more slowly
      d. taking less medication
      e. lying down
      f. better in morning after moving around
      g. closing my eyes

Figure 11–2. Dizziness Questionnaire *(Continues)*

     h. different glasses
     i. other
11. I recently had one more of the following:
     a. infection: other sickness (specify) _____ when _____
     b. new drug or medications (specify) _____
     c. fall or head injury (specify) _____
     d. other _____
12. In addition to dizziness, I notice:
     a. hearing loss: left_____, right _____, both sides _____
     b. blockage or fullness in my ear: one side _____, both sides _____
     c. spots before my eyes
     d. blurred vision _____, double vision_____, blindness _____
     e. numbness or tingling in my arms and legs (specify) _____
     f. difficulty talking
     g. difficulty swallowing
     h. tendency to fall or drop
     i. jerking, rotating, or quivering of my eyes
     j. confusion
     k. clumsiness in arms or legs
     l. weakness in arms/legs
     m. pain in neck or shoulder
     n. trouble walking in dark
13. All medications I am now taking (prescribed and otherwise):

_____
_____

(use back if needed)
14. Use of:
     alcohol_____ when_____
     tobacco_____ when_____
15. Allergies:
     a. drugs _____
     b. foods _____
     c. other _____
16. What I think causes or changes my dizziness:
     a. allergies (specify) _____
     b. activity or lack of activity (specify) _____
     c. irritating fumes, paints, etc. _____
     d. stress _____, fatigue _____, hunger _____, menstrual period _____
     e. medications (specify) _____
     f. head injury _____when_____, unconscious _____
     g. other _____

Figure 11–2. Dizziness Questionnaire. (cont.) *(Reprinted with permission from Ross, V., & Robinson, B. (1984). "Dizziness: causes, prevention and management."* Geriatr Nurs, *September/October, pp. 73–74.*

condition, with an incidence of 64 per 100,000 population per year (Froehling et al., 1990). In BPV, the nystagmus is rotary and directed toward the undermost ear, has a latency of 3 to 30 seconds after the stimulus and lasts less than 60 seconds, fatigues (decreased intensity and duration of vertigo and nystagmus), and eventually is eliminated with repetition of the maneuver. In other syndromes that may pro-

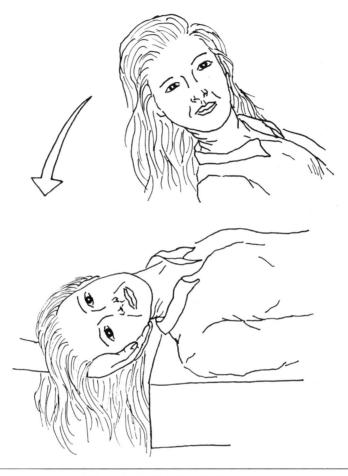

Figure 11–3. Hallpike–Dix Maneuver

duce nystagmus and vertigo with positioning (see Table 11–5), the nystagmus may be persistent (nonextinguishable) and up-beating or horizontal in direction, without latency. Any case of positional vertigo and nystagmus that does not meet the criteria for BPV should be referred for further neurologic investigation.

To perform the Hallpike–Dix maneuver, follow these nine steps:

1. Explain the maneuver to the client before beginning.

2. Seat the client on a bed or table so that when the client lies back, his or her head will extend over the side.

3. Instruct the client to look upward with eyes open and head tilted backward.

4. Grasp the client's head firmly with your two hands and guide him or her into a lying position.

5. Quickly turn the client's head to the right and observe for nystag-

mus (note time of onset, duration, and direction of nystagmus) and report of vertigo.

6. After 1 minute, return the client to the sitting position.
7. Repeat steps 4 through 6 with head turned to the left.
8. Repeat steps 4 through 6 with head hyperextended over the edge of the bed or table.
9. Continue to repeat any maneuver that causes vertigo or nystagmus. Observe for either fatigue and eventual disappearance of symptoms or persistence of symptoms.

Diagnostic Studies

The laboratory tests ordered for the workup of dizziness are often specific to the symptoms or suspected etiology. They are as follows: complete blood count (CBC) with differential, ESR, Mono spot test, chemistry profile, thyroid function studies, rapid plasma reagin/Venereal Disease Research Laboratory (RPR/VDRL), fluorescent treponemal antibody-absorption test for syphilis (FTA-ABS), lipid studies, and antinuclear antibody (ANA) rheumatoid factor. Davis (1994) found that routine blood tests yielded little assistance in the differential diagnosis of dizziness, even though they were frequently abnormal.

An audiogram should be performed. If abnormal, a brain stem evoked response audiometry (BERA), which examines the conduction capacity of the cochlear nerve, should follow.

Electronystagmography records a response to caloric stimuli, testing the function of the labyrinth. Crude caloric testing can be done in the office setting by the instillation of ice water into the external canal and the observation of nystagmus beating away from the tested ear, which would be the expected normal response. Absent or asymmetric responses would indicate impaired labyrinthine function.

Computed tomography may be considered if tumor is suspected. Magnetic resonance imaging can additionally reveal trauma or malformations, as well as lesions.

Harmonic acceleration testing examines one's ability to maintain equilibrium during rotational movement, and posturography assesses movements and muscle activities to maintain and restore balance.

If warranted, electroencephalogram (EEG), ECG, Holter monitoring, event monitoring, cervical spine x-rays, or peripheral nerve conduction velocities may be considered.

CLINICAL MANAGEMENT

The treatment and management of the disequilibrium is determined by assessing the cause and the degree of disability resulting in the condition. Due to the often multifactorial or complex etiology of disequilibrium, a variety of interventions may be considered.

In general, pharmacologic measures to treat symptoms are reserved for the most severe presentations. These drugs may be helpful in suppressing the nausea, vomiting, and feelings of imbalance that may occur intermittently but are not effective during acute episodes. When using these medications, begin with a low dose and assess positive and negative effects of the drug before making any adjustments. The suggested drugs are meclizine hydrochloride 25 mg every 6 to 8 hours as needed or promethazine hydrochloride 25 mg every 6 hours as needed. If no benefit is derived from these medications, discontinuation is recommended due to their potential side effect profile.

Environmental considerations can supplement a treatment plan to minimize the risk of falling.

CLINICAL PEARL

Avoiding sudden head or entire body movements, and standing for a short time before beginning to walk are body mechanics the client can learn to implement in day-to-day life.

Assistive devices for support, balance, or ease of movement can facilitate safety and optimize functional abilities. Improving sensory input through visual enhancement (glasses, visual aids, color contrast, lighting, cataract extraction), auditory enhancement (cerumen impaction removal, hearing aids, amplification devices), and tactile enhancement (grips on slippery surfaces, avoiding uneven surfaces, wearing well-fitting shoes) are important considerations.

Interventions specific to contributing diagnoses are as follows: For BPV, the treatment is based on theories of its cause. The Cupulolithiasis Theory suggests that basophilic deposits develop and attach to the cupula in the semicircular canal, causing it to become weighted down and pulled. This action is thought to be the etiology of nystagmus and vertigo, especially with position change. The Canalithiasis Theory proposes that basophilic deposits form and free float within the endolymph. With movement, the symptoms appear (Herdman, 1990; Parnes & McClure, 1992).

Traditional treatment involves head positioning exercises performed multiple times each day for several weeks. Fujino et al. (1994) showed that these exercises improved the signs and symptoms of vertigo and nystagmus more effectively than use of medication. These exercises are thought to rid the ear canals of debris, by directing it out of the canal and into the utricle, and have been found to accelerate remissions in most cases of BPV (Brandt & Daroff, 1980). These exercises are usually carried out by a physical therapist. Client compliance with the regimen can be problematic, as the exercises initially invoke the symptoms it is treating. The practitioner may consider the judicious use of antivertiginous medications during the initial exercise sessions to assist the client in tolerating the symptoms until the treatment takes hold. Once the client is well into the course of therapy, a home exercise program may be designed.

Cawthorne–Cooksey exercises (Baloh, 1984) are an example of a structured program that an individual could perform at home, once the initial maneuvers are performed by a physical therapist. In addition, posturography is a tool that can assist in the treatment of BPV by giving feedback to the individual as he or she is tilted in different positions.

Researchers have looked at the duration of exercise therapy needed to benefit persons suffering from BPV (Herdman et al., 1993). They examined two single-treatment approaches and compared them with the effectiveness of the traditional series of repeated maneuvers.

The single-treatment maneuvers were found to be equally as effective as the repeated maneuvers in 90% of the cases in improving or extinguishing the symptoms of vertigo and nystagmus.

Surgical treatment is reserved for the most recalcitrant cases, which severely affect function. It involves a fusion of structures within the ear to prevent the traveling of the deposits. It remains controversial.

Ménière's disease is thought to be related to an accumulation of fluid in the endolymphatic space, leading to a distention of this contained area. This results in the symptoms of vertigo, nystagmus, unilateral hearing loss, tinnitus, nausea, and vomiting. Therefore, many of the proposed treatments are aimed at the prevention or reduction of this accumulation of fluid. Diets restricted in sodium (2 g), caffeine, tobacco, alcohol, and fluid, as well as a course of diuretic therapy, have proven to be useful in decreasing the frequency and severity of attacks. Referral to an otolaryngologist is often necessary. Surgical treatment (labyrinthectomy) is controversial in its efficacy.

Orthostatic hypotension can occur as a part of normal aging but can be exacerbated by other contributing factors such as dehydration and medications (antihypertensives, diuretics, tricyclic antidepressants, phenothiazines, and others with anticholenergic properties). Orthostatic hypotension is defined as a drop in blood pressure of at least 20 mm Hg systolic and/or 10 mm Hg diastolic. Changes in pulse rates of less than 5 or greater than 10 beats per minute with position change from lying to standing may also contribute to this syndrome. Interventions include rehydration; alteration in medication regimen if an of-

fending agent is suspected; application of elastic hose and/or abdominal binders to prevent pooling of blood; avoidance of rapid, abrupt position changes; and the administration of caffeine, salt, and/or Florinef (fludrocortisone) 0.1 mg daily.

CLINICAL PEARL

Suggest sitting on the side of the bed and saying a little prayer before getting up. Some older adults may find this suggestion easy to relate to.

Once appropriately diagnosed, management of cardiac arrhythmias depends on the etiology of the underlying disorder. Pacemaker insertion can be helpful in conduction disorders. Medications to control other rate and rhythm disorders may be indicated.

Psychiatric disorders often present with chronic, unexplained dizziness. Appropriate treatment of the underlying psychiatric disorder with behavioral and/or pharmacologic intervention can improve symptoms.

Control of risk factors such as hyperlipidemia, hypertension, and hyperglycemia may prevent or minimize the development of disequilibrium. This can be accomplished by encouraging maximum exercise, healthy diets, smoking cessation, and life-style choices to achieve emotional satisfaction.

SETTING-SPECIFIC ISSUES

Disequilibrium can be especially challenging for the functionally independent community-dwelling elder. This symptom generally mandates cessation of driving (at least temporarily) and taxes one's abilities to remain self-sufficient in the arena of instrumental activities of daily living (IADL). Creative strategies must be implemented to ensure safe and appropriate assistance. Formal help may be required, such as a driving service, companion, or personal attendant to replace or supplement informal assistance from family and friends. These interventions may be short term, as most of these disorders resolve in time with proper diagnosis and intervention.

The presenting signs of disequilibrium may be unsteadiness and falls. In all settings, a thorough workup should be launched for reversible or treatable causes. The APN must always strive to understand the etiology and minimize its effect on function, and avoid treating only the consequences (increasing supervision or limiting the mobility of an unsteady client).

■ SEIZURE DISORDERS

The incidence of seizures significantly increases in the population over the age of 60. This is primarily due to the incidence of conditions associated with seizures which increase with age. These conditions include the following:

- Cerebrovascular disease (hemorrhagic and ischemic CVA)
- Brain tumor
- Head injury (subdural hematoma)
- Metabolic disorders (diabetes, renal failure, hepatic failure)
- Dementia (Alzheimer's type and others)

- Ingestion or exposure to convulsive or toxic substances (alcohol, carbon monoxide, strychnine)
- Withdrawal from addictive substances
- Heatstroke

Cerebrovascular accidents remain the most common cause of seizures in the elderly. It is unclear whether epilepsy is in turn a risk factor for stroke. An isolated seizure occurring early in the poststroke period is often related to acute injury and may not recur, as opposed to seizures occurring later in the recovery phase, which are more likely to proceed to epilepsy. Luhdorf et al. (1986) found that 75% of persons with new-onset seizures had at least one recurrence and were then treated with anticonvulsant medications. The majority of persons with onset of seizure after age 60 either remained seizure free or experienced fewer than 10 seizures per year once anticonvulsant therapy was instituted (Luhdorf et al., 1986; Scheuer & Cohen, 1993). Two factors that increase the risk of seizure recurrence are an underlying neurologic abnormality and having experienced a partial rather than a generalized seizure. Persons over age 60 with a seizure disorder with a known cause have a higher mortality rate than those with unknown cause or those without a seizure history. This is thought to be due to the underlying illness, rather than epilepsy. Luhdorf et al. (1986) found that the time interval between seizures decreases in untreated epileptics.

CLINICAL PRESENTATION

Usual Presentation of Disease
The terminology used to characterize the type of seizure disorder demon-

strated by the patient has been revised in recent years. Figure 11–4 displays the categories of seizures and their presentation.

Partial seizures are more common than generalized seizures. It is important to recognize that simple partial seizures can evolve into complex partial seizures, which may further evolve into generalized seizures. Although one can sometimes presume to characterize the type of seizure based on its presentation, this is confirmed by the results of an EEG. The abnormal neuronal discharge in a partial seizure originates in a localized area of the brain, while in a generalized seizure it arises bilaterally and synchronously from both hemispheres. Some seizures are unclassified due to incomplete data or not meeting diagnostic criteria for either category.

CLINICAL PEARL

Up to one third of persons experiencing a seizure may have a normal EEG. Use of anticonvulsant therapy may affect the EEG result.

Atypical Presentation of Disease

Acute illness in older adults often presents with a lack of expected symptoms or with unusual symptoms. Many conditions such as UTI or other infections can

Partial (focal)		Generalized	
Originates in a localized area of the brain		Originates BILATERALLY, symetrically in the brain	
Simple Partial	Complex Partial	Convulsive	Nonconvulsive
• No change in level of consciousness	• Altered level of consciousness	• Altered level of consciousness	• Altered level of consciousness
• Conclusive, marching, jerky movements may be present	• Unusual or inappropriate behaviors Automatisms	• Tonic/clonic (grand mal): sustained contraction followed by rhythmic contractions of all four extremities	• Absence seizure (petite mal): brief lapse of consciousness and/or posture
• Abnormal sensations may be present Tingling Strange smell or taste Colors or flashing lights	• Often accompanied by movements or sensations of simple partial seizures		• Minor motor seizure: repetitive muscle contractions (myoclonus)

Figure 11–4. Types of Classified Seizures

present with syncope, which can be misdiagnosed as seizure or may truly trigger a seizure in a patient with well-controlled epilepsy or a predisposition for seizure.

Absence seizures or simple partial seizures can be misdiagnosed as dementia. When a history suggests fluctuations in function and cognition, consider a seizure workup.

ASSESSMENT

History
This should include reports from the patient and witnesses regarding aura, level of consciousness, presence of abnormal movements, duration, frequency, patterns, and triggers for seizure activity. Drug (therapeutic and recreational) and alcohol intake must be scrutinized. Some medications may cause seizures, and others may increase a preexisting risk. Perform a thorough review of past and/or chronic medical conditions such as stroke, TIA, cardiac arrhythmias, hypertension, malignancy, dementia, diabetes mellitus, renal disease, headache, or head trauma. It is important to note that a family history of seizure is significant in lifelong epilepsy but rarely contributes to new-onset seizure disorders among the geriatric population.

Physical Examination
- General: Vital signs with temperature and weight
- Head: Inspect for head trauma
- Eyes: Fundoscopic exam to look for papilledema (increased intracranial pressure [ICP]) or hemorrhages (increased blood pressure [BP])
- Neck: Check range of motion (ROM) for pain/stiffness (meningitis) and carotid vessels for bruits

- Cardiac: Heart assessment for arrhythmias or valvular abnormalities
- Abdomen: Assess for hepatomegaly (alcohol), ascites and vascular bruits (increased BP)
- Neuro: Complete exam for evidence of focal findings or gait abnormalities
- Mental status: Folstein Mini-Mental State Exam (Folstein et al., 1975, Appendix A) or another standardized tool for a baseline measurement

CLINICAL PEARL

Serial mental status exams can be helpful in the diagnosis of dementia related seizures, the identification of adverse side effects of anticonvulsants in the realm of cognition, and a person's functional ability to be compliant with a plan of care.

Diagnostic Studies
There is some disagreement in the literature regarding the essential elements of a seizure workup. Most agree, however, that minimum studies include serum glucose, electrolytes, and an EEG. The EEG should be done within 36 hours of the seizure. A CT scan of the head and a panel of bloodwork including serum blood urea nitrogen (BUN), creatinine, ionized calcium, liver function tests, magnesium, ammonia, and phosphorus should be obtained. Additionally, drug levels, toxicology screens, CBC, bacterial/viral cultures, VDRL, urinalysis, lumbar puncture, MRI, sleep study, and chest

x-ray (specifically to rule out malignancy) may be included in the panel of essential diagnostic tools. According to a study done by Henneman et al. (1994), one half of all persons with new-onset seizure require hospital admission.

The differential diagnosis of seizure includes TIA; syncope; cardiac arrhythmias; brain stem ischemia; pseudoseizure; transient global amnesia; panic attacks; rage attacks; and sleep disorders, specifically rapid eye movement (REM) behavior disorder.

CLINICAL MANAGEMENT

Pharmacologic Measures

There are basic premises concerning the use of anticonvulsants in the geriatric client. In new-onset seizure disorders, a decision must be made regarding when and if to begin pharmacologic therapy. The literature suggests the following:

- In a healthy client free of a history of cerebral insult, with a normal or abnormal EEG depicting generalized seizure activity, forego therapy unless a second seizure occurs.
- Consider anticonvulsant medications after the first seizure if the EEG shows partial (focal) rather than generalized seizure and if neurologic abnormalities are found on examination.
- If the seizure is due to an illness or chemical imbalance, treat the underlying cause rather than the seizure. Discontinue anticonvulsants as soon as the temporary catalyst is removed (seizures secondary to alcohol withdrawal).

Table 11–6 lists the most commonly prescribed anticonvulsants, their indications, benefits, concerns, recommended dosages for older adults, and special considerations. Almost all of these agents can cause dose-related neurotoxic side effects such as ataxia, delirium, and visual and behavioral manifestations. Older adults generally require lower doses than younger adults to achieve seizure control (Treiman, 1993).

- Strive for single-dose therapy; increasing the dose of the drug before adding another if seizures are occurring. If a drug is proven ineffective, start a second drug and begin withdrawing the first.
- Control seizures at the lowest dose of medication possible; start low, titrate up slowly, monitoring the effect and side effects.
- Titrate the drug to control seizures, not to achieve blood levels within the therapeutic range.
- Check blood levels of drug only when a seizure occurs, adverse effects are present, or compliance is in question. Many of the anticonvulsants are highly protein bound and require a free drug level rather than total serum drug level.
- Weigh the side effects and potential interactions of drug therapy against the consequences of further seizures.
- Consider a gradual withdrawal (2 to 6 months) of the anticonvulsant in the client who is seizure free for at least 2 years; this is extended to 5 years in a client with known neurologic abnormalities.
- Minimize routine monitoring of liver function and blood counts; check if problem suspected.

TABLE 11–6. PHARMACOLOGIC TREATMENT OF SEIZURES IN THE ELDERLY

Drug	Indications	Benefits	Concerns	Dosage	Considerations
Phenytoin	Tonic/clonic Partial	Most commonly used anticonvulsant Well-known efficacy and side effect profile	90% protein bound Many drug interactions; decreased insulin release, decreased quinidine effect Accelerates osteoporosis Gingival hyperplasia; megaloblastic anemia	Single daily dose Begin with 100 mg/d; may increase to 200 mg/d after 1 week with 50-mg increases as needed	Check free levels if toxicity is suspected (1–2 normal free level) Many dosage-related side effects Drug of chice for indicated seizure type Check CBC occasionally
	Status epilepticus		Watch for hypotension, bradycardia, arrhythmias, respiratory depression with IV use	IV 5–25 mg/min	
Diazepam	Status epilepticus		Watch for hypotension and respiratory depression with IV use	IV 5–10 mg, may repeat at 15-minute intervals to max of 30 mg total	
Lorazepam	Status epilepticus		Watch for hypotension and respiratory depression with IV use	IV 1–2 mg	
Valproic acid	All except status epilepticus	Good efficacy Limited side effect profile	Highly protein bound Few studies in elderly, especially regarding adverse effects —weight gain, hair loss, hepatotoxicity	250 mg bid; increase by 250 mg q5d prn up to 500 mg tid	Check free levels if toxicity suspected May become drug of choice for most seizure types when more experience gained Occasional LFTs

(Continues)

TABLE 11–6. PHARMACOLOGIC TREATMENT OF SEIZURES IN THE ELDERLY (CONT.)

Drug	Indications	Benefits	Concerns	Dosage	Considerations
Carbamazepine	Tonic/clonic Partial	Wide use	Many drug interactions—increases metabolism of other anticonvulsants Short half-life—tid dosing Accelerates osteoporosis May cause heart block, bradycardia; SIADH Increased risk of aplastic anemia; agranulocytosis	Begin with 100 mg/d in 2 or 3 divided doses; increase by 100 mg/d q4–7d	Use cautiously in person with underlying conduction system disease Obtain baseline ECG to rule out conduction disorder before first dose Check CBC and LFTs occasionally
Ethosuximide	Absence seizures		Affects serum levels of other anticonvulsants if used simultaneously	100 mg/d in 2 divided doses; increase prn by 50-mg doses	Drug of choice in absence seizures
Clonazepam	Absence seizures Myoclonic			1.5 mg/d in 3 divided doses	Contraindicated in narrow-angle glaucoma Occasional LFTs
Phenobarbital	Tonic/clonic Partial		Many drug interactions Accelerates osteoporosis	1/3–1/2 recommended adult dosage	Try to avoid in elderly Identified as a risk factor for falls
Primadone	Tonic/clonic Partial		Accelerates osteoporosis	750–1500 mg/d	

CBC, complete blood count; LFTs, liver function tests; ECG, electrocardiogram; SIADH, syndrome of inappropriate diuretic hormone.

CLIENT EDUCATION

Older adults must be educated on a variety of aspects of their condition for successful management. The goal is to preserve quality of life by balancing seizure control with functional independence. The seizure disorder itself or its cause can pose challenges to meet this goal.

- Help clients to identify triggers for seizure activity: alcohol, caffeine, tobacco, stress, heat (environment or fever), sleep deprivation, medication noncompliance, poor blood sugar control, hyponatremia.
- Identify safety issues: driving (know your state law regarding epileptic drivers), avoid swimming alone, encourage showering instead of tub bathing, avoid heights and dangerous equipment.
- Discuss side effects of medications or any change in health status promptly with a health-care provider; do not self-adjust or stop anticonvulsants; carry list of medications, dosages, and interactions in wallet; wear an identification bracelet with name, address, and indication of seizure disorder.
- Educate family members regarding positioning and care during and following a seizure; teach recognition of subtle changes in the client's physical, cognitive, functional, or emotional health, which can be an indication of poor seizure management; toxic effect of medication, impending illness, or difficulty coping with the implications of the seizure disorder.

vignette

Mr. Taylor is accompanied by his son and daughter to the memory loss clinic. His family reports that Mr. Taylor has been acting strangely for several months. He displays periods of time when he does not recognize his surroundings or family. During these episodes, which can last a few hours, Mr. Taylor can become quite agitated and aggressive. He usually falls asleep after a while, waking up to his normal baseline cognitive status with no recollection of the event. He tests 29/30 on the Folstein Mini-Mental State Exam today, displaying an excellent attention span. His family asks if he has Alzheimer's disease. Due to the history of recent onset and extremes in performance and behavior, you consult with your collaborating physician and perform an EEG, which shows complex partial seizures in the parietal lobe. You begin phenytoin 100 mg/d, gradually titrating to 100 mg tid, with good effect of seizure activity and a stable, oriented demeanor for Mr. Taylor.

■ BELL'S PALSY

Bell's palsy is an idiopathic paralysis of the seventh cranial nerve. It is the most common cause of facial paralysis and has an increased incidence in persons ages 30 to 40 and over 70. Persons with diabetes mellitus, arterial HTN, and serum lipid disturbances are at increased risk of developing this condition (Paolino et al., 1985). The APN working with geriatric clients will see many individuals who fit this risk and symptom profile. Therefore, a brief discussion of this condition is warranted to assist with prevention, early recognition, differential diagnosis, and prompt treatment. Education and measures to prevent, detect, and optimally manage diabetes mellitus, HTN, and hyperlipidemia are the focus of preventative efforts for Bell's palsy.

CLINICAL PRESENTATION

The onset is acute and evolves to its peak within hours. Common symptoms may include an inability to close the eye, eye pain and tearing, drooling, hyperacusis (sound distortion), tinnitus, ear pain, fever, and loss of taste. The presence of these symptoms, which are usually unilateral, will vary among individuals, based on the level of the lesion that is preventing transmission of nerve impulses down the facial nerve, but should always involve the innervation of the forehead, eye, and mouth. The etiology of the lesion is unclear, but it is known to cause anoxia and swelling of the facial nerve.

ASSESSMENT

History

- Thorough discussion of the onset, evolution, and presentation of symptoms and their effect upon day-to-day function
- Presence and control of diabetes mellitus, HTN, and hyperlipidemia
- Recent herpes zoster infection (may be ear involvement).

Physical Exam

- Neurologic exam: Cranial nerves; look for unilateral decreased/absent forehead wrinkling, inability to close the eye, tearing, lack of corneal reflex, flattening of the nasolabial fold, drooling, food collecting between the cheek and gum, loss of deep facial sensation, inability to puff out cheek, distorted smile.
- Cardiovascular exam: Check blood pressure.
- Ear exam: Examine ear canal, tympanic membrane, and behind the ear for herpetic lesions. Perform gross hearing, Weber, Rinne, and audiometric testing to assess for hearing loss and tinnitus.

Diagnostic Studies

- CBC with differential
- ESR
- Serum cholesterol and triglycerides
- Fasting blood sugar (hemoglobin aminoimidazole carboxamide [AIC] in known diabetics)
- Tonogram (rule out space-occupying lesions or bony destruction of middle and inner ear)
- Lyme titer (if risk factors or other suspicious symptoms are present)
- Electromyography (EMG) between days 14 and 18; evidence of nerve degeneration suggests a prolonged and incomplete recovery

Look for infectious etiologies (otitis media, herpes zoster, Lyme disease), neoplastic lesions (acoustic neuromas, parotid tumors, and others), additional neurologic causes (CVA, supranuclear palsy, Guillain–Barre syndrome, and others), and trauma.

CLINICAL MANAGEMENT

Most clients with Bell's palsy will recover either totally or to an acceptable degree cosmetically and functionally. Increasing age is a risk factor for a less-than-complete recovery.

Pharmacologic Measures

Instill methylcellulose drops at morning, midday, and bedtime until the eye can close to prevent corneal injury. Administer corticosteroids, 60 mg days 1 through 3, then taper by 10 mg/d for 6 days to increase the chance of a successful recovery, as well as decrease pain if started within 3 days of onset of symptoms. Since the majority of persons with Bell's palsy will recover adequately without corticosteroid treatment, this therapy is most appropriate in clients who present with severe paralysis and pain. Use cautiously in diabetics, with close monitoring of blood sugars.

Nonpharmacologic Measures

Patch or tape down the affected eye at night to prevent injury until lid function returns. Controversy exists surrounding the use of surgical procedures, which include facial nerve decompression, facial nerve graft, and nerve anastomosis. Refer to an otolaryngologist or neurosurgeon if these procedures are to be considered. Electromyography stimulation will prevent muscle atrophy (physical therapy referral).

CLIENT EDUCATION

- Application of eye patch or tape
- Diet counseling for underlying conditions (hyperlipidemia, HTN, diabetes)
- Review medication regimen used to treat Bell's palsy and underlying conditions
- Avoid factors which may cause decreased circulation to the face (cold, pressure)

- Gentle facial massage 2 to 3 times per day for 10 minutes to maintain muscle tone
- Support of facial tissues with tape, pulling the skin and musculature near mouth and cheek up toward the ear

■ FALLS

Falls are due to a complex interaction between age-related changes, diseases, and the environment. Most are multifactorial and pose a serious threat to the health of older adults. Falls are the leading cause of injury-related death due the fall itself or the complications resulting from it. Potential consequences of falls include death, fracture, soft tissue injury, fallophobia, and subdural hematoma. Persons rendered incapacitated and stranded without help for long periods of time before being found following a fall often suffer from dehydration, hypothermia, pressure sores, pneumonia, UTI, and rhabdomyolysis. Alexander et al. (1992) found fall-related trauma to account for 5.3% of hospitalizations. Smallegan (1983) reported that falls contribute to 40% of all nursing home admissions.

Falls are common among the older population—35% to 40% of community-dwelling individuals over the age of 65 fall at least once per year. This statistic increases to 45% in the nursing home population, with 50% of all falls occurring during attempts to meet physical needs.

CLINICAL PRESENTATION

Recently, studies have recognized falls as an indicator of acute illness or an exacerbation of chronic illness (Lawrence

& Maher, 1992). It is often the only symptom in an atypical presentation of disease.

vignette

Mr. Taraschke is a 92-year-old, fiercely independent, community-dwelling gentleman with insulin-dependent diabetes mellitus (IDDM), chronic obstructive pulmonary disease (COPD), glaucoma, coronary artery disease (CAD), atrial fibrillation, and benign prostatic hypertrophy (BPH). He reports falling eight times within a 3-day span. This gentleman rarely falls and is demonstrating a change in baseline physical function. On examination, his lungs are clear, with normal vesicular breath sounds (breath sounds are usually decreased bilaterally), and his vital signs are within his baseline. He is afebrile, with blood sugars 120 to 150 qid. He denies visual change, cough, dizziness, vertigo, or urinary symptoms. Due to his history of COPD, a chest x-ray is ordered, which reveals bilateral infiltrates. He is treated with cefuroxime axetil (Ceftin) 250 mg bid for 10 days with a return to baseline status within 24 hours of treatment initiation.

ASSESSMENT

All elders should be assessed at least yearly for fall risk. The APN should focus on age-related changes, disease status and environmental precipitants. The assessment should include a review of risk factors, a detailed exploration of the cause and consequences of any fall, an observation of gait and balance, and an assessment of the living environment whenever possible. (See Table 11–7.)

History

Many older adults are hesitant to admit to a fall due to its potential implications for independent living. Family and health-care professionals often become concerned when a fall occurs. The older adult may see this concern as unwarranted, possibly leading to intrusions in life style (increased supervision, pressure to use an assistive device, limitations upon activities).

CLINICAL PEARL

Phrase your fall history to assume that the older person has fallen, thereby eliminating a value judgment and presenting falls as the common occurrence that they are. "Tell me about the last time you've fallen."

Inquire about the following facts surrounding the fall: perceived cause, witnesses, health status at time of fall, time of day, activity engaged in at time of fall, location, environmental contributors, clothing contributors, use of assistive device at time of fall, direction of fall, position landed in, and injury or other consequences of the fall. A thorough medication review is warranted. A review of all chronic illnesses that may contribute to falls is indicated for prevention.

Physical Examination

A complete physical examination is necessary to assess for potential risk factors for falls. Emphasis is placed on sensory impairments, cardiopulmonary function, neuromuscular function, cognitive status, and endocrine abnormalities. Direct observation of gait and mobility is extremely useful to characterize abilities and deficits, to establish a baseline, and to assess improvement or decline overtime. Tinetti et al. (1995) found abnormalities in gait and balance to be more sensitive than neurologic or muscle testing in predicting falls. Examples of formalized testing include the "get up and go" test (Mathais et al., 1986) and the Tinetti Balance and Gait Evaluation (Tinetti et al., 1995). Both involve observing the individual rise from a chair, ambulate a short distance, turn, and sit back down. The Tinetti tool also involves a sternal nudge to observe the person's ability to "right" himself. The observation of these components of mobility can assist the APN to identify specific realms of impairment, raising questions of the etiology, treatment and management of the problem, striving to meet the goals of correcting reversible deficits, and supporting chronic impairments to maximize function.

Diagnostic Studies

These studies should be individualized, based on the specific history and physical examination findings encountered.

········ *vignette* ········

Mr. Powers reports a history of difficulty standing from a sitting position, resulting in several falls from his bed, kitchen chair, and toilet. This weakness has been gradually increasing over the past several months, limiting Mr. Powers' ability to drive due to difficulty getting out of the car. He denies pain, dizziness, vertigo, or paresthesias. He is an insulin-dependent diabetic of 5 years' duration, with

excellent control of his blood sugar and physical health. He has gained 7 pounds over the past 6 months, which he attributes to occasional overindulgence and decreased activity related to his chief complaint. On physical examination, you detect proximal muscle weakness in the upper and lower extremities. This is also demonstrated when he makes repeated attempts to rise from the chair. When questioned directly, Mr. Powers does admit to difficulty putting his arms in his sleeves and combing his hair. You discover a hung-up tendon reflex in the patellar testing. There is no evidence of orthostatic hypotension or any other significant abnormalities. You order a thyroid-stimulating hormone (TSH) and discover that Mr. Powers is severely hypothyroid (TSH = 12). After consulting with your collaborating physician, you start him on a small dose (0.25 μg) of levothyroxine sodium (Synthroid) and observe cardiac status carefully for tolerance to this medication. You refer Mr. Powers to the physical therapist for muscle strengthening exercises and prescribe the rental of a lift chair and elevated toilet seat with bars to assist with function and safety. In 6 weeks, the TSH has fallen to 6. The client has shown improvement in proximal muscle strength. You continue to follow his lab values with minor adjustments in his thyroid medication until his TSH returns to normal and his physical function follows suit.

CLINICAL MANAGEMENT

Management is specific to the issues detected from assessment. The primary goal for the APN is to maximize independence and mobility opportunities while attempting to identify and treat potentially reversible or modifiable conditions. This

TABLE 11–7. FALL RISK INDICATORS

Normal Aging Changes by System	Pathology	Assessment	Interventions
■ **CARDIOVASCULAR**			
Orthostatic hypotension due to decreased baroreceptor response	Postprandial hypotension (1 hr after meals); orthostatic hypotension worsened by: Volume depletion Drugs Shy–Drager syndrome Parkinson's disease Diabetes mellitus Prolonged immobility Anemia Varicosities Arrhythmias SSS Heart blocks Tachycardia Bradycardia CHF MI	Cardiac rate and rhythm: Check for S$_3$ or S$_4$ Positional BP and HR (lying, sitting, standing); watch for ↑ or ↓ HR and BP measurements ECG, Holter monitor if arrythmia or syncope is involved	Positional vitals changes: Elevate head of bed at least 30° at all times, change position slowly, support hose, monitor and correct salt and fluid status, review meds for contributing effects, ankle pumping and hand clenching exercise prior to ambulation or with prolonged standing, lie down for 1 hour after meals, avoid antihypertensives within one hour of meals, avoid hot showers and baths, avoid prolonged bedrest. Consider caffeine, fludrocortisone to assist with correction if indicated
■ **CEREBROVASCULAR**			
None	Vertebrobasilar insufficiency; CVA, TIA leads to decreased seizure threshold Carotid artery insufficiency	Vertebrobasilar insufficiency: dizziness, ataxia, visual hallucinations, diplopia, visual field cuts.	Effect on function: remind client of functional limitations from CVA; use visual reminders for clients with

neglect or impaired judgment; modify environment; consult PT, OT

Dizziness: balance exercises, assistive ambulation devices; review meds for effects

Vertigo: remind client to change position slowly, avoid tilting head backward or turning sharply side to side; soft collar; prism lenses; vestibular exercises

Carotid artery insufficiency, syncope, dizziness, vertigo

Touch: assess for inability to perceive uneven floor/terrain; inspect feet for lesion that might contribute to fall

Position sense: assess dependence on visual cues

Communication: expressive and receptive

Vestibular function: assess for:
Nystagmus
Tremors
Decreased grasp
History of ear infections
Head trauma
Ear surgery
Furosemide
Aminoglycosides
Quinidine
Gait changes
Decreased position sense

Vestibular dysfunction

Normal pressure hydrocephalus, peripheral neuropathy, Parkinson's disease, seizure disorder, paresis, paralysis

---

Highlight uneven floor surfaces with colored tape (stairs, thresholds)

Trim toenails; refer to podiatrist if foot pathology is impairing gait

Balance exercises (consult PT), assistive walking device

Ensure good lighting

Use alternative methods to spoken word, consult ST

Parkinson's: adapt environment to compensate for deficits in mobility and perception, exercise therapy, monitor side effects of anticholinergics

Seizure disorder: seizure precautions, observe for precursors to seizure to

---

■ NEUROLOGIC

Changes in touch, position sense, communication—receptive or expressive

Decreased righting time, increased reaction time

(Continues)

345

TABLE 11–7. FALL RISK INDICATORS (CONT.)

Normal Aging Changes by System	Pathology	Assessment	Interventions
■ NEUROLOGIC (CONT.)			
		Decreased sensory awareness of feet	secure safe environment prior to episode Paralysis: modify environment for physical support in mobility
■ MUSCULOSKELETAL			
Gait changes: increased body sway, female waddle, male broad gait, ↓ steppage, ↓ arm swing, ↓ height	Degenerative joint disease Osteoporosis Cervical spondylosis Foot deformities Proximal muscle weakness Pain/joint immobility Osteomalacia Hypo/hyperthyroid PMR	Inspect feet Clothing too long as height decreases Check blood work for metabolic or endocrine imbalance Perform gait and balance screens	Transfer/gait problems: refer to PT; hip and quadriceps exercises; transfer training; adaptive equipment; motorized recliner chair; remove environmental obstacles and moveable objects with wheels, which may be grabbed for support Arthritis: modify environment, exercises and assistive devices, balance rest with activity Weakness: environmental stabilizers, balance rest with activity, physical therapy for strengthening exercises Pain/joint immobility: modify environment, balance rest with activity to promote healing while minimizing disability, monitor side effects of analgesics

■ VISION

Decreased visual acuity
Decreased peripheral vision
Decreased adaptation (↓ pupil size)
Decreased depth perception
Decreased color discrimination
Increased lens opacity—decreased glare tolerance

Macular degeneration
Cataracts
Glaucoma

Visual acuity (with and without correction)
Peripheral vision
EOMs
Accomodation
Fundoscopic exam

Podiatric factors: inspect footwear, pad painful areas, refer to podiatrist, refer to PT for gait training if foot deformity

Note: when visual deficits are suddenly treated, new sensory input may disorient person leading to falls (takes 1 month to 1 year to adapt); corrective lenses, proper lighting, arrange furniture to maximize function, fluorescent tape marking on floors (caution areas), interdisciplinary evaluation

■ HEARING

Decreased auditory acuity, presbycusis

8th cranial nerve impairment
Cerumen impaction
Otitis externa
Otitis media

Whisper test
Weber and Rinne tests
Otoscopic exam
Audiometry

Note: when hearing deficits are suddenly treated, new sensory input may disorient person leading to falls (takes 1 month to 1 year to adapt); wear hearing aids, inspect ears for cerumen impaction, remove impaction; use good communication techniques—speak slowly, in low tones, enunciate, speaker in good

(Continues)

347

TABLE 11–7. FALL RISK INDICATORS (CONT.)

Normal Aging Changes by System	Pathology	Assessment	Interventions
■ **HEARING (CONT.)**			light in client's view, use amplifier, gesture, written words
■ **UROLOGIC** Decreased bladder capacity, decreased ability to postpone voiding	Urge incontinence Micturition hypotension	Observe client's behavior when urgency occurs Decreased BP after voiding large amount	Remove environmental impediments in route to bathroom, promote easy access to toileting facility/appliances, night light, fluorescent tape leading path to bathroom, assistive devices within reach, easily removable clothing, continence management program
■ **GASTROINTESTINAL** Slowing of gastromotility	Bleeding Diarrhea Fecal incontinence	Abdominal assessment Rectal exam for tone and impaction/lesions Lab work: electrolytes, CBC, stool for blood	Bowel management program (see urologic incontinence above) Anemia workup: referral to GI specialist for further studies if bleeding/anemia is found
■ **PSYCHOLOGIC** Longer time to process and learn new things	Dementia Delirium Depression Anxiety Impulsiveness Psychosis	Assess for decreased awareness of limits, safety neglect, risk taking, obsessive–compulsive behavior Perform cognitive and psychosocial screening exams	Anxiety: explore previous coping mechanisms, use problem-solving approach to uncover fears, identify misperceptions, use reassurance and empathic responses,

| Character disorder (eg, obsessve–compulsive behavior) | (Folstein Mini-Mental State Exam; attentional testing; Geriatric Depression Scale) | relaxation techniques, psych liaison, refer to PT if anxiety is related to falls
Impulsivity: discuss client's desire to remain safe, visual and verbal reminders of restrictions and precautions, give positive feedback for attempts at compliance
Depression: explore desire to remain safe, assess mobility level for agitation or psychomotor retardation, contract with patient regarding goals for safe ambulation, consult regarding side effects of psych meds
Psychosis: explore hallucinations/delusions, which may lead to falls
Character disorder—dependent: reinforce attempts at independent mobility, break down tasks into simple components to promote accomplishment, provide requested assistance without positive reinforcement, withdraw attention when client exhibits dependent/attention seeking behaviors
Character disorder—obsessive–compulsive: identify ritualistic behavior that puts client at risk for falls, interfere only if extreme risk |

(Continues)

TABLE 11–7. FALL RISK INDICATORS (CONT.)

Normal Aging Changes by System	Pathology	Assessment	Interventions
■ **METABOLIC/ENDOCRINE** ↓ Glucose tolerance	Thyroid disorder Diabetes	Assess for tremor, fatigue, aching, weak muscles, lethargy, nervousness, apathy, peripheral neuropathy, visual impairment Assess heart rate at rest and during activity Perform neurologic, visual, peripheral vascular, and musculoskeletal exam Assess over/under treatment of thyroid disorder via TSH Assess glucose levels for signs of hyper/hypoglycemia via FBS, fingerstick blood sugars, urine for microalbuminemia, hemoglobin AIC	Thyroid: remind client of limitations from disorder, plan to balance rest with activity, monitor for adverse effects of sedatives and narcotics Diabetes: remind of functional limitations, monitor effects of other meds on glucose control (hypoglycemics, steroids, beta blockers), refer to podiatrist for foot lesions; refer to ophthalmologist for visual deficits

BP, blood pressure; HR, heart rate; ECG, electrocardiogram; SSS, sick sinus syndrome; CHF, congestive heart failure; MI, myocardial infarction; CVA, cerebrovascular accident; TIA, transient ischemic attack; PT, physical therapist; OT, occupational therapist; PMR, polymyalgia rheumatica; EOMs, extrocular movements; TSH, thyroid-stimulating hormone; FBS, fasting blood sugar.

EQUIPMENT AND DEVICES
All product information is based on company literature as of 11/4/96. Prices may vary.

ALERT-CARE PRODUCTS

ITEM	DESCRIPTION	COST
Ambularm	Alerting device; attaches to thigh and emits an intermittent sound when wearer swings leg over edge of bed. Lifelong battery.	$185.00
Walk Alerts	Nonskid, bright blue slippers; alert any health-care giver that wearer should be assisted if seen ambulating alone.	$82.20/pack (4 dozen, one size fits all)
Door Exit Sensor	Attach to closed door and door frame. Works with alarm portion of Ambularm to alert caregiver when door is opened.	$27.00 plus $185 for Ambularm
Tether Alarm	Similar to door exit sensor but allows door to be partially open. Attach to door and door frame; tether will disconnect, sounding alarm when door is opened beyond tether length.	$160.00 introductory price (will be $185)

Available from: Alert-Care, Inc.
Shelterpoint Business Center
591 Redwood Highway
Mill Valley, CA 94941
Maria Barrios, Customer Service Manager, 1-800-826-7444

BED-CHECK CORP. PRODUCTS

ITEM	DESCRIPTION	COST
Bed Check	Bed sensor mat. Connects to nurse call bell system to alert staff when individual moves off mat. Also available in chair size.	$315.00 alarm unit $20.00 each sensor

Available from: Bed Check Corp.
Distributor: Future Med 1–800–510–6024

CLOCK MEDICAL SUPPLY PRODUCTS

ITEM	DESCRIPTION	COST
STOPPER Kit	8″ high × 54′ long mesh strip to Velcro across doorway to visually cue person not to enter. Comes with STOP sign to apply on mesh strip, and Velcro to attach all components.	$24.95
STOP Sign	12″ STOP sign made of thick poster-board attaches to surface with adhesive strips.	$5.00
Johnson Displacement Cushion	Antislider beanbag cushion. For person to sit on—prevents sliding.	$37.95
Cheese Leaner	Bolster cushion to fit in between side of wheelchair and person to prevent leaning to side.	$31.95
Deluxe Wedge Cushion	Foam wedge to sit on in chair—prevents sliding.	$29.50
The Foot Lift	Cushions for foot pedals of wheelchair when legs are too short for chair and feet dangle—allows user to rest feet on cushion.	$29.95 pair

Available from: Clock Medical Supply, Inc. 1–800–362–1314

POSEY PRODUCTS

ITEM	DESCRIPTION	COST
Personal Alarm	Alarm mounts with Velcro to chair or bed and cord attaches to person's clothing. When wearer	$149.95

Figure 11–5. Resources to Prevent Falls/Enhance Safety *(Continues)*

POSEY PRODUCTS (CONT.)

ITEM	DESCRIPTION	COST
	moves beyond cord length (you adjust length), alarm will sound.	
Posey Sitter Bed/Chair Exit Monitor	Pressure sensor with portable alarm/battery device. Versions for chair or bed.	$470–600+ according to model
Posey Grip Slip Resistant Matting	Thin matting cut from roll to size needed. To be placed under seating cushion to prevent sliding, under tray on bedside table to prevent sliding while eating, directly under person (clothing between body and matting) to prevent sliding. Washable, reusable, nontoxic.	$12.24 each 12″ × 120″ roll

Available from Posey: 1-800-447-6739 M–F (5 A.M.–5 P.M. Pacific)

SNYDER ELECTRONICS PRODUCTS

ITEM	DESCRIPTION	COST
Bed Alert	Sensor mat placed under mattress, will sound when user gets out of bed. Alarm receiver unit can be plugged in up to 100 feet away. Another receiver option is battery powered and has a belt clip to be worn by attendant.	$109.11
Wireless Annunciator	Infrared battery-operated detector mounted on wall over a door to detect body heat of person entering the monitored area. Chime sounds at remote receiver, which plugs in up to 100 feet away.	$124.95
Ray-O-Matic PIR Annunciator	Infrared detector as above that is wired to AC current rather than battery operated.	$98.95
Medalert Mats	Battery-powered wireless pressure-sensitive mat. Vinyl surface or carpeted surface, or thin under-carpet style.	$63.69 plus annunciator Wireless, $80 A/C, $30

Available from: SNYDER Electronics
2082 Lincoln Ave.
Altadena, CA 91001
Phone: (818) 794-7139   Fax: (818) 794-8844

ALIMED PRODUCTS

ITEM	DESCRIPTION	COST
Easy Release Soft Wheelchair Belt	Soft wide belt over waist with Velcro closure and large hand loop for wearer to self-release. Marketed as "meeting OBRA requirements for patient accessible release." Item # 8780	$14.95
Anterior Posture Cushion	Vinyl covered foam cushion placed over wheelchair user's lap, fits under armrests. Helps prevent forward leaning, may remind not to get up without help. Item # 8769	$32.29 (27″ × 10″ × 4″)
Lap Top Cushion	Similar to above. Available in 2 1/2″ thick or 4″ thick. (These cushions are considered to be a restraint if patient is unable to remove it without assistance.) Item # 8788, 8789	$19.95 $22.95
Roll Control Bed Bolster	Wedge-shaped soft bolsters to prevent person from rolling too far to either side in bed when side rail not in use. Item # 8790	$76.95 set

Figure 11–5. Resources to Prevent Falls/Enhance Safety *(Continues)*

ALIMED PRODUCTS (CONT.)

ITEM	DESCRIPTION	COST
Walker Skis	Nylon ski glides to place on back legs of any wheeled walker to increase mobility without drag or friction. 1 1/2 " diameter. Item # 73092 (also available 1")	$24.95 pair
Anti-Tipper Device	Attaches to wheelchair frame and extends slightly behind chair on floor to prevent tipping backward. Item # 8432	$79.95 pair
Easy Grasp Reacher	Hand grasp trigger activates grabber jaw on end of 26" handle. Different styles and sizes available. Item # 8326	$15.95 and up

Available from: AliMed Inc.
Phone: (800) 225-2610
8:00 A.M.–8:00 P.M. ET M–F
24-hour Fax: (617) 329–8392

SECURE CARE PRODUCTS

ITEM	DESCRIPTION	COST
SmartLoc	Security Exit System; wrist/ankle band, automatic door lock when band wearer attempts to exit.	Call for system pricing
Bed Tender and Chair Tender	Small pressure sensitive pads and portable alarm units.	Bed control unit, $299.00 Mat $34.00 Each (single patient use) or mats, $299.00 (Box of 10) Chair control unit, $134.65 Mat, $36.00 Each (single patient use) or $319.00 (box of 10)

Available from: Sani-Med Distributors
Phone: (800) 899-7264

RADIO SHACK PRODUCTS

ITEM	DESCRIPTION	COST
Personal Alarm	Attach alarm to person's clothing and string to chair/bed. When attempting to get up, string is pulled and loud alarm sounds.	$9.99
Door Alarm/Entry Chime	Alerts with alarm or chime when door is opened. Battery operated.	$25.99
Motion Detector	Will sense motion in the room—entrance, exit, or moving about in room.	$35.00

Available at Radio Shack stores

COMPUMED, INC. PRODUCTS

ITEM	DESCRIPTION	COST
CompuMed Automated Medication Dispenser	Automated medication dispenser to address compliance issues. Contains med tray that holds meds for one week. Programmable to dispense at selected times—buzzer sounds continuously until med drawer is opened and replaced. Also available with flashing light. Tamper proof. Can	$40.00 per month rental With monitoring, $55.00 per month NOT covered by Medicare

Figure 11–5. Resources to Prevent Falls/Enhance Safety *(Continues)*

COMPUMED, INC. PRODUCTS

ITEM	DESCRIPTION	COST
	arrange med monitoring which will notify caregiver in case of noncompliance.	

Available from: Distributors: Colonial Medical Alert Systems
Phone: (800) 323–6794

RAINTECH PRODUCTS

ITEM	DESCRIPTION	COST
Roam Alert	Wrist or ankle band transmitter that is waterproof, has long-life battery lasting 4 years. Signal can alert a remote alarm, pocket pager, voice paging, door lock.	Call for pricing

Available from: Raintech Sound & Communications, Inc.
Manchester, CT
(203) 649–8122

MAGELLAN PRODUCTS

ITEM	DESCRIPTION	COST
Limelite	Night light—2 1/4 " square, 1/4 " deep. Gives off soft green glow like a computer screen. Stays cool to the touch. Low profile. Inexpensive to operate, lifetime guarantee. Many varieties to choose from.	$19.95 for 2 If ordering additional lights, no shipping fee

Available from: Magellan
(800) 644–8100

SERVICE MERCHANDISE PRODUCTS

ITEM	DESCRIPTION	COST
Portable Door Lock	Turns any door into a locked door. Portable design provides protection when away from home. Fits all standard doors. Item # SPDL1PEF	$7.99 each
Vibration Door Alarm	Hangs on door knob and emits alarm when attempt to open door is made. Uses 9-V battery. Item # 85TKL	$14.99

Available from: Service Merchandise
(800)435–5826

Figure 11–5.   Resources to Prevent Falls/Enhance Safety (cont.) *(Chris Waszynski 1996.)*

can be a challenge, particularly in acute-care settings where OBRA (Omnibus Budget and Reconciliation Act of 1987) regulations on restraint reduction do not currently apply. The historical nursing paradigm of utilizing restraints to maintain client safety still influences the nurs-ing community. The APN is in an ideal position to educate, support, and encourage creative nursing interventions in the care of older adults with the potential for falls. See Fig. 11–5 for products that enhance client autonomy and promote function rather than immobilization.

CASE STUDY #1

Mrs. Blake lived in a congregate living center with mild Alzheimer's disease. She fell in her apartment when she tripped on her long bathrobe and fractured her left hip. She had a surgical repair, following which she became and remained delirious. She was discharged from the hospital to an extended care facility, where she was labeled as "confused" and put in an upper torso restraint. The nurses justified this as a safety measure since she often would try to stand from her bed and chair, forgetting that she had recently broken her hip.

QUESTIONS

1. What strategies could you use to assist the nursing staff to be more creative in their interventions for Mrs. Blake's gait instability?

2. What are alternatives to restraints that might be recommended in this situation?

ANSWERS

1. Nurses often become defensive to suggestions made by other care providers to release or decrease restraints. This may be due to the false beliefs that restraints maintain safety and decrease supervision time. Studies show that restraints actually increase nursing care time if the release and reapplication is performed every 2 hours. Restraints put the client at risk for incontinence, skin breakdown, depression, agitation, further immobility, deconditioning, and falls with injury. Nurses will often respond if they are encouraged to participate in the designing of a creative care plan to minimize restraints and maximize function. Empowering the nurse with increased knowledge and support can be very successful. Close and frequent observation for positive responses in the client to a care plan that minimizes restraints can increase the nurse's confidence level in attempting further reductions.

2. Assess the client's mental status with a Folstein Mini-Mental State Exam to determine her ability to register and retain spoken and written information. If she is able to read, a large note in her lap or taped to an object in her direct view that says "REMAIN SEATED" may be sufficient to discourage her from standing alone. For persons who are unable to read and comprehend written instructions due to delirium, dementia, or some other cause of mental status impairment, a tape recording with intermittent spoken reminders with or without a re-

movable seatbelt or ribbon/yarn tied across the front of the chair as a visual reminder can be useful. A bed or chair monitor will alert the caregiver

that the person is attempting to stand without prohibiting it from occurring. The focus is increased function rather than stifled movement.

 ## CASE STUDY #2

Mrs. Collier is a 100-year-old, community-dwelling woman, who is referred to you by her case manager. Mrs. Collier has fallen three times in her apartment within the past week. She has been brought to the emergency room after each incident, given a clean bill of health, and returned to

her apartment only to fall again. You make a home visit to Mrs. Collier, who comes to the door approximately 4 minutes after you ring the bell. She is using a walker but displays an unusual gait. She is bearing weight on the ball of her left foot and the lateral aspect of her right foot.

QUESTIONS

1. How would you proceed in your assessment?

2. What are the most likely differential diagnoses for the abnormal gait pattern described in the case study?

ANSWERS

1. A close look for the etiology of Mrs. Collier's gait disturbance is the focus of your assessment. The reason her problem was not found in the emergency room is that she was examined only for injury and not for source of fall. She was examined only on a stretcher, never asked to walk, and never asked to take off her shoes.

2. Podiatric problems were the source of her gait disturbance. A large plantar wart on the bottom of her left heel made weight bearing painful, as did an infected bunion of her right medial metatarsal. Treatment of these conditions led to a restabilized gait.

■ REFERENCES

Alexander, B., Rivara, F., & Wolf, M. (1992). The cost and frequency of hospitalization for fall-related injuries in older adults. *Am J Pub Health, 82*(7), 1020–1023.

Baloh, R. W. (1984). *Dizziness, hearing and tinnitus: The essentials of neurology.* Philadelphia: F. A. Davis.

Barker, R. L., Gordon, B., & Moses, H. (1986). In Barker, R. L., Burton, & Zieve (Eds.). *Principles on ambulatory care.* (pp. 841–859). Baltimore: Williams & Wilkins.

Boult, C., Murphy, J., Sloane, P., et al. (1991). The relationship of dizziness to functional decline. *J Am Geriatr Soc, 39,* 858–861.

Brandt, T., & Daroff, R. B. (1980). Physical therapy for benign paroxysmal positional vertigo. *Arch Otolaryngol, 106,* 484.

Davis, L. E. (1994). Dizziness in elderly men. *J Am Geriatr Soc, 42,* 1184–1188.

Folstein, M., Folstein, S., McHugh, P. (1975). Mini-Mental State: A practical method for grading the cognitive state of patients for the clinician. *J Psych Res, 12,* 189–198.

Froehling, D. A., Silverstein, M. D., Mohr, D. N., Beatty, C. W., Offord, K. P., & Ballard D. J. (1991). Benign positional vertigo: incidence and prognosis in a population-based study in Olmsted County, Minnesoa. *Mayo Clin Proc, 66,* 596–601.

Fujino, A., Tokumasu, K., Yosio, S., et al. (1994). Vestibular training for benign paroxysmal positional vertigo. *Arch Otolaryngol Head Neck Surg, 120,* 497–504.

Goodhill, V. (1979). *Ear diseases, deafness and dizziness.* (p. 187). New York: Harper & Row.

Henneman, P., Deroos, F., & Lewis, R. (1994). Determining the need for admission in patients with new-onset seizures. *Ann Emerg Med, 24,* 1108–1114.

Herdman, S. J., Tusa, R. J., Zee, D. S., Proctor, L. R. & Mattor, D. E. (1993). Single treatment approaches to benign paroxysmal positional vertigo. *Arch Otolaryngol Head Neck Surg, 119,* April, p. 450–454.

Herdman, S. J. (1990). Treatment of benign paroxysmal positional vertigo. *Phys Ther, 70*(6) 381–388.

Jacobson, G., & Newman, C. (1990). The development of the Dizziness Handicap Inventory. *Arch Otolaryngol Head Neck Surg, 116,* 424–427.

Jonsson, P., & Lipsitz, L. (1994). Dizziness and syncope: In Hazzard, W., Bierman, J., Blass, J., & Halter, W. (Eds.). *Principles of geriatric medicine and gerontology* (3rd ed.). New York: McGraw-Hill.

Koch, H., & Smith, M. C. (1985). Office-based ambulatory care for patients 75 years old and over. *National ambulatory medical care survey 1980 & 1981,* NCHC Advance Data No. 110. National Center for Health Statistics, Public Health Service. Hyattsville, MD: U.S. Government Printing Office.

Lawrence, J., & Maher, P. (1992). An interdisciplinary falls consult team: A collaborative approach to patient falls. *J Nurs Care Qual, 6*(3), 21–29.

Luhdorf, K., Jensen, L. D., & Plesner, A. M. (1986). Epilepsy in the elderly. *Epilepsia, 74,* 409.

Mathias, S., Nayak, U. S., Isaacs, B. (1986). Balance in elderly patients: The "get up and go" test. *Arch Phys Med Rehab, 67,* 387–389.

Paolino, E., Granieri, E., Tola, M. R., et al. (1985). Predisposin factors in Bell's palsy: A case-controlled study. *J Neurol, 232*(6), 363–365.

Parnes, L. S., & McClure, J. A. (1992). Free-floating endolymph particles: A new operative finding during posterior semicircular canal occlusion. *Laryngoscope, 102,* 988–992.

Prestwood, K. (1991). Dizziness in older adults. *Geri Ed Cen News, V,*(2) 1–3.

Ross, V., & Robinson, B. (1984). Dizziness: Causes, prevention and management. *Geriatr Nurs,* Sept/Oct, 70–85.

Scheuer, M. I., & Cohen, J. (1993). Seizure and epilepsy in the elderly. *Neurol Clin, 11,* 787–804.

Sloane, P. D. (1989). Dizziness in primary care: Results from the national ambulatory medical care survey. *J Fam Pract, 29,* 33–38.

Smallegan, M. (1983). How families decide on nursing home admission. *Geriatr Consult, 1,* 21–24.

Tinetti, M., Inouye, S., Gill, T., & Doucette, J. (1995). Shared risk factors for falls, incontinence and functional dependence. *JAMA, 273*(17), 1348–1353.

Treiman, D. M. (1993). Current treatment strategies in selected situations in epilepsy. *Epilepsia, 34*(Suppl), S17–S23.

12

TOPICS IN ENDOCRINE AND HEMATOLOGIC CARE

Mary Armetta • Sheila L. Molony

■ INTRODUCTION

Endocrine and hematologic disorders in the older adult represent potentially hidden sources of morbidity and mortality. Diabetes mellitus, thyroid disease, and anemia often progress silently until the disease process is severe or significant secondary pathology has resulted. These syndromes may be discovered incidentally during a routine examination or during the workup of another condition. This chapter reviews the diagnosis and management of these common conditions.

■ DIABETES

According to the American Diabetes Association (ADA) (1997a), there are four classifications associated with glucose intolerance: diabetes mellitus (DM), impaired fasting glucose, impaired glucose

tolerance, and gestational diabetes. There are three types of diabetes mellitus:

1. Type 1 (approximately 10% of currently diagnosed diabetes) is characterized by insulin deficiency as a result of pancreatic islet cell loss. Ketosis is common with uncontrolled type 1 diabetes mellitus. There is a strong genetic component, with environmental factors playing a lesser role.

2. Type 2 is characterized by insulin resistance, with an increase in the production of insulin early in the process of the illness in an attempt to overcome the insulin resistance. This is usually followed by dysfunction of the pancreatic beta cell. There is a genetic component, but environmental factors play a large role (ie, obesity, sedentary life style). Ketosis is not present with type 2.

3. The third type of diabetes occurs in relation to other diseases, pancreatic diseases, drug or chemical use

endocrinopathies, insulin receptor disorders, and certain genetic syndromes (ADA, 1997a).

The second classification is impaired fasting glucose. The fasting glucose levels are 110 mg/dL or above but less than 126 mg/dL and confirmed by repeat testing.

The third classification is impaired glucose tolerance. The glucose levels are 140 mg/dL or above but less than 200 mg/dL at the 2-hour point of the oral glucose tolerance test.

The fourth classification is gestational diabetes. Individuals with gestational diabetes are at risk for developing type 2 diabetes within 10 years.

CLINICAL PRESENTATION

Usual Presentation of Disease

The classic signs and symptoms of diabetes are related to a blood glucose level above 140 mg/dL. These include polyuria, polydipsia, polyphagia, lethargy, blurred vision, weight loss, and dry skin. The onset of signs and symptoms in individuals with type I diabetes is usually over a shorter time span and more dramatic. The presentation may include ketoacidosis.

The presentation of type 2 diabetes is usually more subtle. Individuals may have diabetes for more than a year before it is actually diagnosed. It maybe diagnosed at the time of a routine physical exam or suspected as a result of an optometrist visit secondary to blurred vision or at the time of gynecologic exam secondary to dysuria or yeast infection.

Atypical Presentation of Disease

The presenting signs and symptoms of diabetes in the older adult may not be the obvious polyuria, polyphagia, and polydipsia. Some individuals with undiagnosed diabetes are asymptomatic; others present with evidence of long-term complications. In the older adult, the presenting symptoms may be nonspecific and attributed to normal aging, such as mild weight loss; fatigue; blurred vision; anorexia; depression; incontinence; decreasing memory; mild, recurrent infections; falls; nocturia; sleep pattern changes; and peripheral neuropathies.

AGE-RELATED CHANGES

The increased incidence of hyperglycemia and glucose intolerance in individuals over age 60 was identified as early as 1921 (Spence, 1921). Diabetes is a common condition among older adults. Recent statistics for the prevalence of diabetes in the age group 65 through 74 are 17.9% to 26.4%, depending on the race of the individual (Finucane, 1995). The prevalence is higher in the Hispanic and black communities. Research has identified several possible mechanisms for glucose intolerance, which occur with age (Stout, 1995). These include decreased insulin secretion, peripheral insulin insensitivity, and hormonal changes (glucagon and catecholamines). The practitioner needs to be aware that obesity, sedentary life style, decreased kidney function, and polypharmacy may worsen glucose intolerance.

PRIMARY PREVENTION

The main area to be addressed in primary prevention is nutrition. There is a strong association between obesity and type 2 diabetes. As little as a 10- to 15-lb weight loss can normalize blood sugar levels in some obese individuals. Obesity is defined as greater than 20% above desirable weight.

Calorie restriction should be individualized to prevent malnutrition. The ideal dietary composition has not been determined, but some general guidelines that appear to make sense include taking in approximately 55% to 60% of calories from carbohydrates, less than 30% from fat (10% saturated fat), 15% from protein, low cholesterol, and less than 2 g sodium. The role of zinc, chromium, magnesium, vitamin E, and other micronutrients is currently being studied, related to management and prevention. Activity and exercise may also play a role in diabetes prevention. It has been demonstrated that increased physical activity improves insulin sensitivity and decreases glucose intolerance. As societies have become more sedentary, the incidence of type 2 diabetes has increased (Villareal & Morley, 1995). The exercise prescription should be individualized, but most people would benefit from walking 20 to 30 minutes five to seven times a week.

ASSESSMENT

History
Assess presence/absence of symptoms; if present, note duration and character. Obtain family history, psychosocial history, exercise history, nutritional history (24-hour or 3-day recall), weight history, medications, economic situation, and tobacco/alcohol history, as well as a standard review of systems.

Physical Examination
Check height and weight, and blood pressure (orthostatic); perform an ophthalmoscopic exam, thyroid palpation, oral exam, cardiac exam (including pulses), skin/foot exam, and neurologic exam (sensory/vibratory) (ADA, 1998).

Diagnostic Studies
Check fasting glucose, glycated hemoglobin, fasting lipids, and urine for microalbumin; perform an electrocardiogram (ECG) and urine culture and sensitivities; and test thyroid function if indicated (ADA, 1998).

The oral glucose tolerance test is of little value in the older adult. The individual may have impaired glucose tolerance but not diabetes. When obtaining the nutritional history, do not assume the person eats three meals a day or that he or she avoids eating during the night. Initially, triglyceride levels may be elevated due to the insulin resistance, and once glucose levels are within normal range, the triglyceride level will also decrease.

CLINICAL MANAGEMENT

Diabetes is a chronic illness, and the individual/significant other must learn to manage it on a daily basis. For this reason, education is key. The older adult needs to learn survival skills: information related to basic nutrition, acute complications (eg, hypo/hyperglycemia), medication administration and side effects, and monitoring. With any teaching that is done, written information should also be provided. For nutritional education, a referral should be made to a registered dietitian. Nutrition is the cornerstone of diabetes management. An individualized meal plan needs to be established with

CLINICAL PEARL

Ask the client to bring in a grocery receipt if he or she is unable to remember what was eaten.

CLINICAL PEARL

Dietary intervention should be discussed at every visit with the health-care provider. It is not to be viewed as a one-time instruction.

the client. It must take into consideration the client's likes/dislikes, economic situation, cooking facilities, and overall life style.

The principles for motivating change need to be incorporated. A 50-lb weight loss may be overwhelming to an individual, but a pound a week loss could be managed. Also, the client may be willing to change one thing in his or her diet (ie, switch from potato chips to hot-air-popped popcorn or increase daily amount of vegetables). Once the client succeeds with that change, he or she is more receptive to other changes. Physical activity/exercise is recommended in the management of diabetes. Regular exercise will decrease insulin resistance, improve blood glucose levels, assist with weight loss, decrease stress levels, and improve overall feeling of health. The client's exercise prescription needs to be individualized. Factors to be considered include current exercise program, physical limitations, presence of long-term diabetes complications (retinopathy, peripheral and autonomic neuropathy), cardiovascular disease, other medical condition, motivation, and exercise preferences. For example, a person with proliferative retinopathy should not be doing exercises that would increase intraocular pressure such as heavy lifting or bouncing (Maynard, 1991). With the increased risk of peripheral neuropathy,

properly fitting footwear, cotton socks, and foot inspections are important.

Individuals taking medication (sulfonylureas/insulin) to lower glucose levels need to be instructed about the risk of hypoglycemia and steps to take to avoid it. This is especially true when starting an exercise program. The steps may include but are not limited to checking glucose levels pre- and postexercise, carrying a carbohydrate source, eating a snack before exercise, exercising at least 30 minutes after eating, and not exercising alone. Walking is easy, inexpensive, and beneficial. Regular walking at least three times a week for 15 to 20 minutes is a starting point. It is recommended that the client have a stress test prior to beginning an exercise program. A recent study reported that individuals with type II diabetes may not see the importance of exercise because health-care providers do not provide guidance and reinforcement (Kayima et al., 1995). Therefore, exercise should be discussed at each visit and the individual assisted with establishing goals and rewards.

Pharmacologic Measures

Nutrition and exercise play a continued role in diabetes management. An approach in the management of the newly diagnosed individual may be focused solely on nutrition and exercise. The initial recommended therapies are nutrition and exercise for 2 to 3 months for newly diagnosed type 2 individuals who are asymptomatic, obese, and have a fasting glucose level under 200 mg/dL and a random glucose level under 240 mg/dL.

Pharmacologic therapy is recommended after failure with nutrition and exercise change. It is also recommended for newly diagnosed individuals with type 2 diabetes who are symptomatic and/or nonobese with a fasting glucose level above 200 mg/dL and/or random glucose levels above 240 mg/dL. At the present time, available drug classes include sulfonylureas, alpha-glucosidase inhibitors, biguanide, thiazolidinedione, insulin and insulin analogues (see Table 12–1). Refer to a basic pharmacology book for the mechanism of action of each of the drugs. Pharmacologic therapy is initiated in approximately 85% of type 2 patients who are unable to achieve glucose control with nutrition medical therapy and exercise (Lebovitz, 1995).

There are factors to consider before initiating pharmacologic therapy for type 2 diabetes. These factors include age, duration of diabetes, history of previous insulin therapy, coexisting medical conditions, weight, current glucose level, and polypharmacy.

General guidelines for the use of sulfonylureas in the older adult require that the health-care practitioner be aware

that sulfonylureas, oral hypoglycemic agents (OHAs), can cause hypoglycemia. Oral hypoglycemic agents work primarily by increasing the release of insulin by the beta cells. These drugs also have a glucose-lowering effect by decreasing peripheral insulin resistance. There must be functioning beta cells for OHAs to be effective. Oral hypoglycemic agents are primarily metabolized by the liver and excreted by the kidney. Since the process of aging decreases hepatic blood flow and renal filtration function, a shorter-acting OHA such as tolbutamide or low-dose glipizide should be prescribed. Oral hypoglycemic agents should be prescribed with caution in individuals with hepatic and renal disease. The unpredictability of action and high risk of hypoglycemia due to extended duration of action with chlorpropamide outweigh the benefits. There is a severe interaction with chlorpropamide and alcohol that is similiar to that seen with disulfiram (Antabuse). Oral hypoglycemic agents have been reported to be responsible for

TABLE 12–1.   ANTIHYPERGLYCEMIC AGENTS

Drug Name	Class	Duration of Action (hr)	Dosage Range (mg/24 hr)
Tolazamide	First-generation sulfonylurea	16–24	100–1000
Tolbutamide	First-generation sulfonylurea	6–10	500–3000
Chlorpropamide[a]	First-generation sulfonylurea	48–60	100–500
Glipizide	Second-generation sulfonylurea	10–24	2.5–40
Glyburide	Second-generation sulfonylurea	16–24	1.25–20
Glimepiride	Third-generation sulfonylurea	24	1–8
Acarbose	Alpha-glucosidase inhibitor	14–24	75–300[b]
Metformin	Biguanide	3–6	500–2500
Troglitazone	Thiazolidinedione	16–24	200–600

[a] Chlorpropamide is not recommended for the older adult due to duration of action.
[b] Maximum acarbose dose for individuals < 60 kg is 50 mg tid.

a 5- to 7-lb weight gain in a year. In addition to hypoglycemia, gastrointestinal upset and skin rash have been reported side effects with OHAs. The presence of skin rash may necessitate the discontinuation of the OHA secondary to sulfa allergy. This drug class would be appropriate for the newly diagnosed nonobese individual with glucose levels under 200 mg/dL, with no known hepatic or renal disease.

Acarbose, an alpha-glucosidase inhibitor, acts in the small intestine, slowing down the digestion of complex carbohydrates. The slowed-down digestion delays the absorption of glucose, blunting the postprandial rise in blood glucose levels of individuals with diabetes. "Postprandial hyperglycemia persists in more than 60% of type 2 individuals, and evidence exists that the cumulative effects of episodic postprandial hyperglycemia account for sustained increases in glycoslated hemoglobin" (Taylor, 1993).

Acarbose should be administered with the first bite of each meal. Common side effects of acarbose are gastrointestinal (GI) discomfort, bloating, abdominal cramps, and increased flatulence. For this reason, the dosage should be gradually increased. The use of over-the-counter (OTC) antiflatulence products may be helpful.

Acarbose is indicated as monotherapy for individuals with type II diabetes, as well as in combination with OHAs, metformin, or insulin (Chaisson et al., 1994). Liver function tests (LFTs) should be obtained prior to initiation of acarbose therapy. The LFTs should be obtained every 6 months if the client is taking 100 mg three times a day, as a

dose-related elevation in LFTs has occurred in some patients during clinical trials (Bayer Pharmaceuticals, 1996). Acarbose is contraindicated in individuals with inflammatory bowel disease, obstructive bowel disease, and chronic intestinal disorders that may worsen with intestinal gas formation (Bayer Pharmaceuticals, 1996). Acarbose as monotherapy is contraindicated in clients with type 1 diabetes. It is also advised not to prescribe acarbose in clients with serum creatinine levels above 2.0 mg/dL, due to a reported increase in acarbose plasma concentration, although data from long-term studies is not currently available (Bayer Pharmaceuticals, 1996).

Individuals taking acarbose and OHAs should treat hypoglycemia with commercial glucose preparations (dextrose) or milk. This is necessary because the acarbose would slow down the digestion/absorption of sucrose in juices, soda, honey, and so forth.

Metformin is a biguanide antihyperglycemic agent that is effective in the treatment of some individuals with type 2 diabetes. Metformin works by inhibiting hepatic glucose production and promoting muscle tissue uptake of glucose (DeFronzo et al., 1995). Hypoglycemia is not a risk in a person taking metformin as monotherapy. The reported weight gain with OHAs has not occurred with metformin. For this reason, metformin is recommended for obese individuals with type 2 diabetes (if not contraindicated; see below). Reductions in total serum cholesterol, low-density lipoprotein (LDL), and triglycerides have occurred in metformin-treated patients (DeFronzo et al., 1995). Common side effects involve the gastrointestinal (GI) system, such as nausea, abdominal cramps, and diarrhea. In most cases, these are dose related and manageable by slow titration of the dosage (adding 500 mg/d every 10 to 14 days as needed). Metformin is contraindicated in clients with a history of lactic acidosis, alcohol abuse, hepatic or renal disease (serum creatinine levels above 1.4 in females and above 1.5 in males) (DeFronzo et al., 1995). When iodine containing contrast is used, the client's renal status requires monitoring postprocedure as well as observation for signs/symptoms of lactic acidosis.

Treatment options include metformin as monotherapy, metformin/sulfonylurea, metformin/acarbose, and metformin/insulin. When metformin is added to sulfonylurea or insulin regimens, the client needs to be reminded of the risk of hypoglycemia secondary to sulfonylurea or insulin action.

Troglitazone is an antihyperglycemic agent that acts by decreasing insulin resistance. This agent was approved by the U.S. Food and Drug Administration (FDA) in early 1997. In clinical trials, "troglitazone improves sensitivity to insulin in muscle and adipose tissue and inhibits hepatic gluconeogenesis" (Warner-Lambert, 1997). Troglitazone action is dependent on the presence of endogenous insulin. Indications for troglitazone are for the management of clients with type 2 diabetes currently on insulin therapy of more than 30 units of insulin per day with hemoglobin A_{1c} greater than 8.5%, combination therapy with sulfonylureas, biguanide or monotherapy (Warner-Lambert, 1997). Troglitazone should be used with caution in clients with New York Heart Association (NYHA) class 3 or 4 cardiac status (Warner-

Lambert, 1997). Heart enlargement without microscopic changes was observed in rodents. Individuals with NYHA class 3 or 4 were not included in clinical trials (Warner-Lambert, 1997). Troglitazone should not be initiated in clients who exhibit clinical or laboratory evidence of active hepatic disease. Prior to initiation of troglitazone therapy a serum transaminase level should be obtained and rechecked frequently. Adjustments in the insulin dosage must be made to reduce the risk of hypoglycemia. A suggested schedule for dosage reduction is 20%, and the client needs to perform home glucose monitoring. In clinical trial data provided by the drug company, there was no significant difference in efficacy in geriatric patients (Warner-Lambert, 1997). There are no special considerations when prescribing troglitazone in the older adult.

Exogenous insulin has been a treatment plan for diabetes since 1922. Insulin lowers fasting blood glucose levels as well as postprandial blood glucose levels. Insulin type, dose, level of insulin resistance, and individual activity level all affect the amount of lowering of glucose levels. Lispro (Humalog) is a recently approved rapid-acting insulin analogue. Lispro effectively lowers postprandial glucose levels (Table 12–2).

Insulin therapy may be required initially with clients whose fasting blood glucose is above 300 mg/dL or random glucose is above 350 mg/dL. Insulin would also be initiated in cases of oral agent failure. Guidelines to be used in this case are preprandial blood glucose above 140 mg/dL consistently, random blood glucose above 160 mg/dL consistently, and a hemoglobin A_{1c} of more than 8%

TABLE 12–2.   INSULIN ACTIONS

Type	Onset (hr)	Peak (hr)	Therapeutic Duration (hr)
Lispro (insulin analogue)	< 1/2	1	4
Regular	1/2	1–2	6–8
Neutral protamine Hagedorn (NPH), Lente	1–2	6–12	16–24
Ultralente	4–6	16–18	24–36
Premixed 70/30, 50/50	1/2	1–2, 6–8	16–24

(ADA, 1998). Weight gain does occur with insulin therapy. The risk of hypoglycemia is of concern with the older adult. The older adult may not consistently eat an evening meal, and this presents a problem with neutral protamine Hagedorn (NPH) administered in the morning.

A recommended starting dose for insulin is 0.2 U/kg/d, with titration of 2 to 5 units every 3 to 5 days until fasting glucose is under 130 mg/dL. (Cefalu, 1996). Hypoglycemia is a risk with tightening of glycemic control, but this should not prevent the clinician from initiating insulin if needed. In the past, the goals of diabetes management in the older adult were to provide relief from symptoms and prevent hypoglycemia. This usually meant keeping blood glucose levels above 140 mg/dL and below 250 mg/dL. This philosophy has changed with increased life expectancy. Older adults are at risk for developing long-term complications that possibly could be prevented with improved glucose control (above 100 mg/dL and under 180 mg/dL with hemoglobin A_{1c} less than 8%).

The following drugs are associated with hypoglycemia: alcohol, beta-adren-ergic antagonists, pentamidine, phenylbutazone, salicylates, sulfonamides (White et al., 1993). The following drugs are associated with hyperglycemia: amiodarone, beta-adrenergic antagonists, corticosteroids, diuretics (thiazide/loop), lithium, phenytoin, theophylline (White et al., 1993).

Continuing Care

As stated earlier, the target glycemic level is the same for the older adult, as outlined by the ADA (Table 12–3).

The results of the Diabetes Control and Complications Trial (DCCT) proved that individuals who maintained a glycated hemoglobin under 7.1% significantly decreased their risk of development or progression of nephropathy, retinopathy, and neuropathy (Diabetes Control and Complications Trial Research Group, 1993). This study was conducted with type I individuals. Research with Type 2 individuals is currently underway. After diagnosis, the individual needs to be assessed for the presence of complications/coexisting disease (retinopathy, neuropathy, nephropathy, cardiovascular disease, foot ulceration). Results of the assessment need to be included in the treatment plan. Evidence

TABLE 12–3.   **RECOMMENDED GLYCEMIC CONTROL FOR INDIVIDUALS WITH DIABETES**

Biochemical Index	Goal	Action Suggested	
Fasting glucose (mg/dL)	80–120	< 80	> 140
Bedtime glucose (mg/dL)	100–140	< 100	> 160
Glycated hemoglobin (%)*	< 7	> 8	

*Glycated hemoglobin level for nondiabetic 4–6%.

Adapted with permission from American Diabetes Association, Clinical Practice Recommendations 1997. Standards for Medical Care for Patients with Diabetes Mellitus.

exists that the use of angiotensin-converting enzyme (ACE) inhibitors will delay and/or slow the progression of nephropathy. Therefore, if not contraindicated, these should be included in the treatment regimen. Hypertension and hyperlipidemia management require inclusion in the diabetes treatment plan.

Education is a key component in diabetes management. The older adult may require shorter sessions, adaptive aids, follow-up telephone contact, and visiting nurse referral. Blood glucose monitoring performed by the client, family, or caregiver should be initiated soon after diagnosis. Urine glucose testing maybe considered as an alternative only if the client is unable or unwilling to perform blood glucose monitoring or if the only goal is avoidance of symptomatic hyperglycemia. The results of urine glucose testing are affected by the renal threshold for glucose. This level varies in individuals between 150 and 300 mg/dL serum glucose. An individual with a serum glucose level of 299 mg/dL may have a urine glucose test result of negative.

The schedule for home glucose monitoring is dependent on the pharmacologic therapy, other medical conditions, glucose levels, and stability. During times of illness, the individual must perform blood glucose monitoring more frequently. Testing is recommended to be four times a day, including a 3 A.M. test. A recommended testing schedule for an individual started on insulin is fasting, bedtime, and before lunch or dinner every day while the dose is titrated. Once glucose levels are stabilized, daily testing before breakfast/dinner can be alternated with before breakfast/bedtime a week at a time.

If the client is on oral agents initially, a recommended testing schedule is fasting, before dinner, and at bedtime three times a week until glucose levels are stabilized. Once stabilized, testing before breakfast/dinner can be alternated with before breakfast/bedtime at least twice a week.

For the client with nonpharmacologic therapy, testing frequency can be decreased to at least weekly. Remember that obtaining only fasting glucose levels does not provide the necessary information to adjust therapies. What is the client's glucose level the other 23 hours and 59 minutes? If the client is unwilling to test 2 to 3 times every day, suggest 2 to 3 times every other day. The cost of home glucose monitoring is a factor for some individuals on a fixed income. There should be investigation of insurance coverage for supplies and promotional offers by suppliers. Consultations with certified diabetes educators, pharmacists, and/or medical suppliers can yield the information. The individual should bring his or her home glucose monitor to the medical appointment so that the results can be correlated with lab results and the technique can be observed.

The provider and client/significant other need to establish short- and long-term goals. The goals need to take into consideration the client's age, physical limitations, social situations, eating patterns, and other medical conditions. The older adult client's preferences and expectations have a significant impact on the outcome of an educational session (Ahroni, 1996). The quality of information is more important than the quantity. As a rule, rituals and habits are important to the older adult; therefore, if possible, the practitioner must incorporate the diabetes regimen into the client's routine. Directions should be specific and concrete.

The client should have at least a yearly review of nutrition education. Whenever there is a change in the client's glucose levels, questions regarding eating patterns must be asked. This includes asking about portion size of "diet," "sugar-free," and "low-fat" foods. Some sugar-free foods have a higher fat content, and eating more than a serving size can cause increased glucose levels. Referral for counseling related to stress management, adaptation to living with chronic illness, support, and so on is beneficial.

Continuing care is critical for an individual with diabetes. The frequency of follow-up visits depends on the type of diabetes, level of glycemic control, presence of complications, and presence of other illnesses (hypertension [HTN], hyperlipidemia) (ADA, 1998). Clients receiving insulin should have follow-up at least quarterly, and other clients at least semiannually. At follow-up visits, perform a history review, highlighting any changes since the last visit; medication review; physical exam, including blood pressure; fundoscopic exam; sensory/vibratory exam; foot exam; and laboratory testing for glycated hemoglobin, annual fasting lipid profile, and annual microalbumin measurement/urinalysis for protein (ADA, 1998). The follow-up visit is more effective if the labwork is obtained about 2 weeks before the visit. This allows for discussion of the results and adjustment in the treatment regimen at the time of the visit. The individual should be asked about any difficulties with diabetes management. The ADA recommends that individuals over the age of 30 receive a comprehensive dilated-eye exam annually (ADA, 1998).

SETTING-SPECIFIC ISSUES

When an individual with diabetes is hospitalized, glucose levels generally rise. Explanations include infection, required medications, stress, and medical condition. A hospitalized individual with diabetes requires blood glucose monitoring every 4 hours or before meals and at bedtime depending on acuity. Insulin administration may be required to maintain glucose levels under 200 mg/dL. Acute complications of hyperglycemia are diabetic ketoacidosis (DKA) (type 1) and hyperglycemic hyperosmolar nonketotic (HHNK) coma (type 2). In most of these cases, hospitalization is required, as well as referral to an internist/endocrinologist. The signs and symptoms may occur over hours or days. These include increased urinary output, dehydration, weakness, hyperglycemia, dry skin, lethargy, and mental status changes. Treatment includes intensive monitoring of electrolytes and blood gases, administration of intravenous fluids and insulin, and management of the underlying cause. The recognition and prevention of DKA and HHNK is critical. The individual should be educated about the signs and symptoms and possible treatment plans to prevent recurrence or worsening.

The nutritional status of long-term care facility residents with diabetes should be evaluated. "Malnutrition, not obesity, is the more prevalent nutrition-related problem of the older adult" (Franz, 1994). The diet of the resident needs to be palatable, simple, and not necessarily calorie restricted. Age-related changes predispose the older adult to dehydration. This fluid imbalance is a risk factor for hyperglycemia in individuals with diabetes. Dehydration, malnutrition, and diabetes have a negative impact on wound healing and infection-fighting ability. All residents with diabetes should have blood glucose monitoring according to guidelines discussed earlier. One must also remember that the resident probably will not be able to verbalize sign/symptoms of hypo/hyperglycemia; therefore, monitoring is key.

■ THYROID DISORDERS

The hormones that are synthesized by the thyroid gland have a general effect on metabolism and growth. These hormones are thyroxine (T_4) and triiodothy-ronine (T_3). Disorders of the thyroid gland include hypothyroidism, hyperthyroidism, and thyroid nodules. Thyroid disorders are the second most common endocrine disorder, surpassed only by diabetes (Kaiser, 1995).

Thyroid hormone production is controlled by a negative feedback mechanism involving the hypothalamus, anterior pituitary, and thyroid. The follicular cells of the thyroid produce thyroglobulin (a glycoprotein). The thyroglobulin then undergoes iodination. Dietary intake at least 50 µg/d of iodine is necessary. Once the iodination occurs, T_4 and T_3 are produced. The ratio of T_4 to T_3 is 13:1 (Kaiser, 1995). There is peripheral conversion of T_4 to T_3, primarily in the kidney and liver. The thyroid hormones are released into the bloodstream, and almost immediately a majority of the hormones are bound to proteins. Only 0.05% of total T_4 and 0.5% of total T_3 are free.

The level of free thyroid hormones stimulate or suppress the thyrotropin-releasing hormone (TRH) from the hypothalamus in a negative feedback mechanism. The presence of TRH stimulates the anterior pituitary to release thyroid-stimulating hormone (TSH), which in turn activates the thyroid gland to produce thyroglobulin.

The adult thyroid gland weighs approximately 20 g, with asymmetric lobes (right larger than left). It is usually larger in women. The lobes are connected by an isthmus. The upper edge of the isthmus is just below the cricoid cartilage. "The thyroid gland has a bloodflow which is estimated to range from 4 to 6 mL/min/g of tissue, which is nearly twice that of the kidneys" (Brook & Marshall, 1996).

The thyroid gland can store as much as a 2-month supply of hormone in the gland. As a result, a disorder involving decreased production of hormone or decreased iodine intake will not be apparent immediately.

The amount of total thyroid hormones can be increased or decreased by factors that affect thyroid-binding proteins. Cordarone interferes with T_4 metabolism, either lowering or raising free T_4 levels. Lithium can block secretion of T_4 and T_3, as well as elevate TSH in euthyroid individuals (Brody & Reichard, 1995).

AGE-RELATED CHANGES

The production of T_4 and T_3 by the thyroid gland is reduced by about 25% in the older adult. This decreased production appears to be a result of thyroid hormone degradation and excretion (Mooradian, 1995). It is not known whether these changes are inherent to aging or a response to thyroid tissue damage (Mooradian, 1995). The overall homeostasis is maintained in the healthy older adult.

There is an increase in "macroscopic and microscopic nodules and in interfollicular fibrous tissue and a decrease in the uptake of iodine" in the aging thyroid gland (Finucane, 1995).

HYPOTHYROIDISM

Clinical Presentation

Usual Presentation of Disease. Hypothyroidism is an endocrine disorder with a decrease in circulating thyroid hormones (T_3 and T_4), resulting in overall decreased metabolism. Hypothyroidism can be classified as primary or

secondary, depending on the cause of decreased thyroid hormone. Mechanisms of primary hypothyroidism are blockade of TSH receptors, impaired thyroxine production, and inhibition of thyroxine release.

Secondary hypothyroidism is a result of pituitary or hypothalamic pathology. The individual will present with additional signs/symptoms related to pituitary/hypothalamic dysfunction.

The typical presentation is related to decreased metabolism. The onset of hypothyroidism is insidious, initially related to the fact that there is a supply of thyroid hormone in the gland as the body tries to maintain homeostasis. Initial presentation may include complaints of lethargy, fatigue, constipation, cold intolerance, dry skin, coarse hair, weight gain, and depression. Second-level onset sign/symptoms include muscle weakness, decreased left ventricular function, arthralgias, carpal tunnel syndrome, slowing of intellectual activity, decreasing memory, goiter or atrophic gland, and delayed relaxation of deep tendon reflexes. Late-onset signs/symptoms include congestive heart failure (CHF), pericardial effusions, bowel obstruction, sleep apnea, respiratory muscle weakness, hyponatremia, hypothermia, and stupor.

Atypical Presentation of Disease. The prevalence of hypothyroidism is reported to be 5% to 7% of individuals over the age of 60. The older adult rarely presents with the initial signs/symptoms of hypothyroidism. If the individual does have these initial complaints, health-care providers have been known to attribute the complaints to aging (eg, cold intolerance, dry skin, and constipation). The older adult may initially present with the second-level signs/symptoms and may progress to myxedema coma before the diagnosis of hypothyroidism is made.

Anemia, hypercholesterolemia, and elevated creatine phosphokinase (CPK) levels without other signs/symptoms have been reported to reveal hypothyroidism on thyroid function testing (Barzel, 1995).

Older adults with an underlying autoimmune thyroiditis are susceptible to hypothyroidism when exposed to iodine-containing drugs/solutions. These include but are not limited to amiodarone, cough preparations, povidone–iodine (Betadine), and long-term lithium therapy (Barzel, 1995).

Since the presentation of hypothyroidism in the older adult may be atypical, it should be considered in an individual with a past history of hyperthyroidism, subacute thyroiditis, treated head/neck cancer (radiation), Addison's disease, and pernicious anemia (Sawin, 1991).

Subclinical hypothyroidism may present without overt symptoms and is diagnosed by laboratory studies. On questioning, the individual may admit to constipation, memory loss, and fatigue. Subclinical hypothyroidism is more prevalent in women than in men. There is approximately a 20% risk of clinical hypothyroidism in the 5 years after diagnosis with subclinical hypothyroidism. The TSH level is elevated slightly less than 10 μ/mL, and the T_4 level is at the low end of normal.

Assessment

The practitioner should question the older adult about the presence of signs/symptoms of hypothyroidism at each visit. The individual's history relative to hyperthyroidism, subacute thyroiditis, previous head/neck radiation, and family history of thyroid disease must be obtained. The physical exam should focus on general appearance, weight, skin/hair, hearing exam, neck exam (thyroid enlargement/nodules), cardiovascular (bradycardia, CHF), GI (constipation), muscle strength, deep tendon reflexes, and Mini-Mental State Exam (MMSE). Hypothyroidism can adversely affect performance on mental status exams (Osterweil et al., 1992).

Because the onset of hypothyroidism is insidious, it is recommended that TSH levels be obtained on a yearly basis for individuals over the age of 60.

If hypothyroidism is suspected based on physical exam, a TSH and free T_4 should be obtained. Primary hypothyroidism is diagnosed when the TSH level is high and the free T_4 level is low. In cases of subclinical hypothyroidism, the TSH is elevated and the free T_4 is low normal.

Hypothyroidism is treated by the oral administration of levothyroxine. The starting dose is 25 to 50 μg/d for the older adult. For individuals who have preexisting coronary disease, the dose should be started at 12.5 μg/d. The lower starting dose is recommended due to the reduced metabolic clearance of thyroid hormone by the older adult. Dosage adjustments are made at 4- to 6-week intervals, with a goal of achievement and maintainence of a normal TSH level. Dosages are increased by 12.5 or 25 μg. It may take 3 to 4 months before the proper dosage is reached. Clinical signs and symptoms and repeat TSH levels are used to determine dose adjustment.

Individuals with a coronary disease history require careful monitoring for reports of increased angina attacks. Levothyroxine increases the individual's basal metabolism, leading to an increased oxygen demand and increased workload on the heart. The older adult needs to be educated about this possibility and the importance of notifying the practitioner of increased angina frequency. The practitioner in turn needs to ask the individual about angina attack frequency at each contact, and appropriate antianginal therapy must be undertaken. Previously undiagnosed angina may become evident during therapy.

An individual with adrenal insufficiency is at risk for adrenal crisis when levothyroxine therapy is initiated. Therefore, Addison's disease should be ruled out before starting levothyroxine. If Addison's disease is present, it should be treated first.

It has been reported that excessive thyroid hormone administration has been associated with decreased bone density (Barzel, 1995) and increased risk for osteoporosis. Therefore, proper dosing of levothyroxine is critical. Levothyroxine absorption may be decreased when it is taken at the same time as ferrous sulfate (Barzel, 1995). The brand name preparation of levothyroxine is preferable because each dose strength is a different color, which facilitates the older adult's easily knowing what dosage is being taken.

The older adult will usually demonstrate improvement in signs/symptoms within the first month of treatment. This includes improvement in cognitive abilities previously affected by low thyroxine levels. Referral to an endocrinologist is recommended if there is no trend toward a decreasing TSH level with levothyroxine therapy.

Setting-specific Issues

Acute Care. An extreme presentation of hypothyroidism is myxedema coma. There is an increased incidence in the older adult. It may present related to infection, exposure to cold, or drugs.

Classic signs and symptoms are depressed mental status, hypothermia, periorbital edema, hypotension, bradycardia, pleural or pericardial effusions, bowel obstruction, respiratory failure, hyponatremia, hypoglycemia, and hypercalcemia (Isley, 1993).

Treatment of myxedema coma focuses on maintaining the airway, hypotension treatment with isotonic IV fluids with glucose, client warming, IV corticosteroids, IV levothyroxine, and identification and treatment of underlying cause.

Long-term Care. Individuals in long-term care settings receiving treatment for hypothyroidism require monitoring for possible myxedema onset. These individuals should have mental status changes investigated. Thyroid-stimulating hormone levels should be checked every 6 months. Some practitioners will also obtain a T_4 level. These levels may change as a result of other medications and decreased renal function.

Community Setting. Medication compliance is always a question with older adults. On routine monitoring, a normal or raised T_4 level and a raised TSH level in a person on levothyroxine therapy may indicate erratic medication administration. A malabsorption problem should be considered if the person is reliable with medication administration.

In terms of cost, levothyroxine is relatively inexpensive, but the cost of TSH monitoring twice a year can exceed $200.

HYPERTHYROIDISM (THYROXICOSIS)

Clinical Presentation

Usual Presentation of Disease. Hyperthyroidism is an endocrine disorder with an increase in circulating thyroid hormones (T_4 and T_3), resulting in overall increased metabolism. Major causes of hyperthyroidism are Graves' disease (thyroid-stimulating immunoglobulin G [IgG] antibody), toxic multinodular goiter (increased endogenous production and release of T_4), single toxic nodule ("hot" nodule evident on scan), thyroiditis (transient hyperthyroidism, then hypothyroidism), overproduction of TSH (pituitary adenoma), and increased intake of exogenous hormone (overtreatment of hypothyroidism or treatment for obesity, fatigue).

The typical presentation is related to increased metabolism. Initial presentation may include heat intolerance; weight loss; sweating; nervousness; deficits in memory, attention, and problem solving; tremor, increased appetite; lid lag; goiter, tachycardia; muscle weakness; and diarrhea. In addition, individuals with Graves' disease may exhibit upper eyelid retraction, periorbital edema, exophthalmos, thickening of skin over the lower tibia, and patchy depigmentation of the skin (Brook & Marshall, 1996).

Atypical Presentation of Disease. The older adult presents in a nonspecific manner that is not as dramatic as the presentation in younger individuals. It is reported that as high as 20% of hyperthyroid older adults do not have an enlarged or palpable thyroid gland (Gambert & Escher, 1988). The prevalence of

hyperthyroidism in the older adult is 1%. Toxic multinodular goiter is the most common cause in the older adult. Infiltrative ophthalmopathy is not common in the older adult.

The older adult may present with coarse skin; coarse tremors; correction of a preexisting constipation; weight loss; decreased appetite; reduced muscle mass, leading to a functional decline in proximal muscles (inability to stand from sitting position); CHF; atrial fibrillation; new or worsening angina; and changes in mental status.

Apathetic thyrotoxicosis is a form of hyperthyroidism in which the older adult does not present with the classic signs and symptoms. The individual may be withdrawn, depressed, and lethargic, though weight loss and muscle weakness is evident (Gambert & Escher, 1988). There is usually cardiac dysfunction.

Assessment

A basic history should be obtained, with a focus on family history of hyperthyroidism or other autoimmune diseases, recent increased dietary iodine intake, and medications such as amiodarone. Individuals receiving treatment for hypothyroidism need to be questioned regarding dosage and change from brand name to generic and vice versa. A complete physical exam with focus on mentation, cardiovascular (CHF, atrial fibrillation), GI, muscular, and neck–thyroid palpation is indicated.

The initial diagnostic studies are TSH and T_4. A low TSH with elevated T_4 is diagnostic of hyperthyroidism. If the TSH level is low and T_4 normal and hyperthyroidism is still suspected, a T_3 level should be obtained (elevated level indicative of T_3 thyrotoxicosis).

Thyroid scans can be performed in the case of suspicious nodules and to rule out thyroiditis. There is a low or absent uptake of radioisotopes in thyroiditis and a high uptake in Graves' disease or toxic nodules (Gambert, 1995).

Thyroid Function Tests. The sensitive TSH assay is an effective measure of thyroid function. Medications that can lower TSH levels include dopamine hydrochloride and glucocorticoids. Lithium can increase TSH levels (Brody & Reichard, 1995).

Total T_4 levels reflect free and bound thyroxine. Total T_4 levels can be affected by certain medications. It can be raised by estrogens, tamoxifen, and opiates. The levels can be lowered with carbamazepine, iodinated cough preparations, lithium, phenytoin, and salicylates (Brody & Reichard, 1995). Therefore, it is recommended to obtain free thyroxine levels when one is evaluating thyroid function by labwork.

Total T_3 levels are useful in determining the type of hyperthyroidism. This is the case when the TSH level is low and free T_4 is normal but the individual is presenting clinically with hyperthyroidism. Total T_3 level is lowered by glucocorticoids, lithium, and propranolol (Brody & Reichard, 1995).

A thyroid autoantibody panel consists of serum antithyroglobulin and antimicrosomal antibody titers (Brody & Reichard, 1995). These titers are elevated with Hashimoto's thyroiditis. Thyroid-stimulating IgG antibody is elevated in Graves' disease.

Clinical Management

Hyperthyroidism can be managed with antithyroid drugs, radioiodine or surgery. Available antithyroid drugs are propylthiouracil (PTU) or methimazole (Tapazole). These drugs act by inhibiting hormone formation and conversion of T_4 to T_3. The antithyroid drugs have no effect on the stored thyroid hormone. Therefore, it may be 2 to 3 weeks before an improvement in signs/symptoms is seen.

The starting dose of antithyroid drugs is 75 to 100 mg every 8 hours of PTU, or 10 mg every 8 hours of Tapazole. Tapazole has a longer half-life, and 20 mg once a day may be prescribed. The individual should have every 3 to 4 week monitoring of TSH and T_4 levels. Once the individual is euthyroid, the medication dosage should be decreased 30% to 50%, with thyroid function monitoring every 3 months. A maintenance dose may be as low as 50 mg/d of PTU or 10 mg/d of Tapazole (Gambert, 1995).

A baseline leukocyte count should be obtained as granulocytosis can be a severe side effect, which occurs in less than 0.5% of cases (Gambert, 1995). It is recommended to be rechecked with any sign of infection, as it is a sudden change that routine monitoring may not reveal. Some practitioners choose to monitor the leukocyte count every month for 4 months.

Antithyroid drug therapy is continued for 12 months once the individual is euthyroid. The drug is then discontinued, and monitoring of thyroid function is done every 3 months for 1 year, then yearly for 2 to 3 years, and then at increasing intervals. If hyperthyroidism recurs, radioactive iodine or surgery is the treatment.

Hypothyroidism is a possible side effect of antithyroid drug therapy. Therefore, the individual should be educated about and monitored for hypothyroidism.

Radioactive iodine (I^{131}) is a treatment option for hyperthyroidism. It is the recommended treatment for toxic thyroid nodule. Since most hyperthyroidism in the older adult is caused by toxic nodule, I^{131} is a common treatment. The long-term effects of the radiation are not a major concern with the older adult.

When treating an older adult with radioisotopes, there is a small risk of causing severe thyrotoxicosis if the client is not euthyroid. This occurs as a result of a transient release of stored thyroid hormone (Gambert, 1995). For this reason, antithyroid drugs are usually administered prior to and after radioisotope therapy. The advantages of radioisotope therapy are proven results, less expense, low side effect profile, and ease of administration.

Hypothyroidism is a common side effect, and the older adult will require lifetime monitoring of thyroid function and thyroid hormone replacement as needed. Approximately 20% of individuals with ophthalmopathy will have a worsening of the condition with radioisotope therapy.

An adjunct to therapy is the use of beta blockers for the associated hyperadrenergic symptoms. Beta blockers do not have an effect on thyroid hormone levels. Cardioselective beta blockers (short-acting beta blockers such as Brevibloc [esmolol hydrochloride]) should be used with caution in individuals with asthma, diabetes, and chronic CHF. Digoxin and anticoagulation therapy may be required if the individual presents with atrial fibrillation.

With the increased rate of metabolism associated with thyrotoxicosis, there is an increased rate of bone turnover and serum calcium level. This results in the older adult's being at risk for osteoporosis. Once the individual is euthyroid, it is recommended that calcium and vitamin D supplementation for females be prescribed.

Subtotal or total thyroidectomy is a treatment option for hyperthyroidism. It is not recommended for the older adult. The risk of injury to the parathyroids or vocal cords outweighs the benefits, especially since more conservative treatments are available.

Setting-specific Issues

Thyroid storm is an acute presentation of hyperthyroidism. The signs and symptoms are exaggerated, along with fever and altered mental status. There is usually a concurrent illness, but it may occur following cessation of antithyroid drugs or after I^{131} treatment (Singer et al., 1995). Treatment is provided in the intensive care setting. An endocrinologist must be involved in the care of the individual. Treatment for thyroid storm as recommended by the Standards of Care Committee of the American Thyroid Association is directed toward "drugs that inhibit thyroid hormone biosynthesis (PTU/Tapazole), drugs that inhibit release of thyroid hormone from the gland (potassium iodide, lithium carbonate), and agents that decrease the peripheral effects of thyroid hormone (corticosteroids, ipodate)." (Singer et al., 1995) Treatment also includes supportive measures and symptom and precipitating cause management. Aspirin should be avoided, as it may replace thyroid hormone at binding protein sites, causing an increased free thyroid hormone level (Isley, 1993).

THYROID NODULES

Age-related Changes

Thyroid nodules may be localized (solitary thyroid nodule) or multiple and uneven (multinodular goiter). Thyroid nodules are more common in the older adult, especially females (Rolla, 1995). There is a greater chance of malignancy than in the younger individual.

Clinical Presentation

The older adult may present with signs/symptoms of hyperthyroidism, neck pain, shortness of breath, hoarseness, or goiter, or the individual may be asymptomatic. For asymptomatic presentation, thyroid palpation and TSH monitoring annually is necessary. Thyroid nodules may be single or multiple (Goroll, 1995).

Single-nodular

Type	Features
Colloid	Approximately 60% of thyroid nodules, poorly demarcated from rest of gland, tend to be hypofunctioning
Benign adenomas	Approximately 30% of thyroid nodules, well demarcated by fibrous capsule, may be "hot" or "cold" on scan, usually macrofollicular by aspiration biopsy
Carcinomas (papillary, follicular, anaplastic medullary, lymphoma)	Approximately 10% of thyroid nodules, very firm on palpation, "cold" on scan
Thyroid cysts	Usually "cold" on scan; epithelial-lined, hemorrhagic or necrotic; clear, amber, or hemorrhagic aspirate

A multinodular gland may be caused by Hashimoto's thyroiditis, multinodular goiter, or cancer (uncommon cause).

Assessment

The individual's history should be obtained, with a focus on family history of thyroid cancer, history of head/neck irradiation, symptoms of local invasion (hoarseness, dysphagia), and symptoms of hypo/hyperthyroidism.

The physical exam should focus on presence of signs of hypo/hyperthyroidism, palpation of the thyroid gland (noting the size, number, and consistency of nodules), and presence/absence of lymph node enlargement in the surrounding area. Thyroid-stimulating hormone and T_4 levels should be obtained. Pharmacologic therapy is initiated if indicated by results, followed by fine-needle aspiration biopsy. In most cases, referral is made to an endocrinologist for this procedure. Fine-needle aspiration biopsy has a sensitivity of greater than 95% and a specificity of 70% to 90% (Goroll, 1995). Benign nodules should be monitored yearly with thyroid function testing, palpation/examination, and repeat fine-needle biopsy as indicated. Malignant nodules should be removed surgically with follow-up by an endocrinologist. Approximately 10% of all biopsies are classified as "suspicious" or indeterminate (Rolla, 1995). These individuals should have a radionuclide scan of the thyroid. This will demonstrate the uptake by the nodule compared to the rest of the gland. The nodule would be classified as cold, warm, or hot. Most thyroid cancers present as a "cold" nodule (Rolla, 1995). An individual with a nodule that is suspicious on biopsy, or cold or warm on scan, should be referred for surgery.

A thyroid ultrasound is performed to differentiate solid versus cystic nodule and to assist with localization for biopsy.

Clinical Management

Malignant nodules are removed surgically. Toxic nodules and multinodular goiters are treated with radioisotopes in the older adult. These individuals are at risk for hyperthyroidism and the associated osteoporosis and cardiac manifestations. Monitoring for hypothyroidism as previously discussed is needed.

Controversy currently exists regarding the treatment of an older adult with a benign solitary nodule who is euthyroid. Treatment with levothyroxine for suppression is indicated in the younger adult. Two key issues are (1) that the older the individual/nodule, the more resistant to shrinkage from suppression therapy; and (2) that suppression therapy may precipitate thyrotoxicosis (Rolla, 1995).

Diagnosis of thyroid disease in the older adult requires awareness on the part of the practitioner of atypical presentation. A TSH level is invaluable. It may save the individual unnecessary testing. Thyroid disease is easily managed.

■ ANEMIAS

Anemia is defined as a hemoglobin of less than 13 in males or less than 12 in females, and a hematocrit of less than 42 in males and less than 36 in females (Goroll, May, & Mulley, 1995). Anemia is a common disorder in the elderly, particularly in the institutionalized population. Over two thirds of all anemias in the elderly are attributable to iron deficiency or the anemia of chronic disease (Small & Damon, 1996). Vitamin B_{12} deficiency, folate deficiency, and hemolytic anemias are also prevalent in older adults.

AGE-RELATED CHANGES

A slight decrease in hemoglobin may occur with aging, but all anemias must be investigated rather than attributed to normal aging. Silent blood loss, organ failure or disease, and nutritional deficiencies occur with increased frequency in advanced age and represent potential sources of clinically significant anemia.

PREVENTION

Efforts at primary prevention of anemias should focus on judicious use of aspirin and nonsteroidal anti-inflammatory drugs (NSAIDs) in clinical practice, particularly in older adults with a past history of gastritis, ulcer, or GI bleeding. Secondary prevention involves screening for signs and symptoms of anemia outlined below, screening for occult fecal blood loss yearly, and reviewing dietary intake and substance use for vitamin deficiency risks.

CLINICAL PEARL

Clients with neurologic changes such as confusion, depression, change in personality, or paresthesias should be screened for vitamin B_{12} and folate deficiencies, even in the absence of demonstrable anemia.

PRESENTATION OF DISEASE

Usual Presentation of Disease

Symptoms of anemia are listed in Table 12–4. The presence and severity of these symptoms is dependent on the severity of the anemia, the acuity of onset, the client's underlying cardiorespiratory reserve, and the overall oxygen demand.

Atypical Presentation of Disease

Weakness, fatigue, and dyspnea on exertion are common presenting signs of anemia, but may be masked in older adults with sedentary life styles. Exacerbations of CHF may be treated without a search for underlying anemia. Neurologic and GI symptoms may be misinter-

TABLE 12–4.   SIGNS AND SYMPTOMS OF ANEMIA*

Symptoms	Signs
■ **GENERAL**	
Weakness, fatigue	Orthostasis, tachycardia
Headache, tinnitus	Pallor (hemoglobin < 7–8)
Anorexia, nausea, vague abdominal discomfort	Pale conjunctivae and mucous membranes
Palpitations, chest pain	Early systolic murmur
Dyspnea, orthostasis	Signs of congestive heart failure
■ **IRON DEFICIENCY**	
Dysphagia (only in severe cases)	Angular cheilitis
Tarry stools	Guaiac-positive stools
■ **VITAMIN B$_{12}$ Deficiency**	
Burning tongue	Glossitis
Digestive disturbances	Decreased position and vibration sense
Paresthesias, poor concentration	Dysesthesia
Irritability, depression	Ataxia, poor coordination
	Cognitive impairment
■ **HEMOLYTIC ANEMIA**	
Fever, chills (acute)	Fever
Abdominal or back pain (acute)	Scleral icterus
Dark urine, jaundice	Hepatosplenomegaly
■ **OTHER**	
Abdominal pain, neuropsychiatric symptoms (lead toxicity)	
Lymphadenopathy (infection or malignancy, chronic disease)	
Weight loss, night sweats (infection, chronic disease)	
Splenomegaly (malignancy, infection, sideroblastic anemia)	

*Symptoms are categorized to simplify diagnostic reasoning, but the presence of any given symptom is *not* diagnostic of the *type* of anemia. Significant overlap does occur, and most anemias are found in the asymptomatic client. Laboratory findings provide the primary mechanism of differential diagnosis and should be correlated with the clinical findings.

preted as age-related sequelae or attributed to other illnesses.

ASSESSMENT

History
Features of the clinical history that may assist in diagnosis are listed in Fig. 12–1.

Review of Symptoms
Assess for symptoms listed in Table 12–4.

Physical Examination
Assess for pallor of skin, conjunctivae, mucous membranes (especially important for darkly pigmented skin), and nailbeds. Examine sclera for icterus or cyanosis and tongue for glossitis. Look for tachycardia and early systolic murmur. Check for hepatosplenomegaly. Assess Romberg, position sense, vibration sense, and Babinski reflex. Check for orthostatic hypotension. Assess stool for occult blood.

Diagnostic Studies
The initial workup is based on the complete blood count (CBC) and red blood cell (RBC) indices, particularly mean corpuscular volume (MCV), which reflects RBC size, and mean corpuscular hemoglobin concentration (MCHC), which reflects cell color. Anemia may be masked by dehydration, which falsely elevates hemoglobin and hematocrit. Table 12–5 reviews anemia classification based on cell size. Additional labwork such as iron studies, B_{12}, folate, and reticulocyte counts are used to confirm the diagnosis and differentiate between anemias with similar findings on peripheral smear. A reticulocyte count should be assessed for all normocytic or macrocytic anemias. Diagnosis of microcytic anemia warrants iron studies. Table 12–6 differentiates microcytic anemias.

MICROCYTIC ANEMIA

Iron Deficiency
Iron deficiency anemia in the elderly is almost always due to blood loss and warrants testing stools for occult blood with referral for possible endoscopic examination of the GI tract. Causes of GI bleeding include ulcer disease, gastritis, polyps, diverticulosis, and neoplasms. Other possible contributing causes of iron deficiency include dietary insufficiency and decreased absorption due to gastric surgery or heavy antacid use. Iatrogenic causes include frequent blood draws and surgical blood loss.

Family history:	Blood disorders, anemias (thalassemias, sickle cell, hemoglobinopathy, hereditary spherocytosis), autoimmune disorders (aplastic anemia, pernicious anemia, autoimmune hemolytic anemia), hypothyroidism
Past medical history:	Partial or total gastrectomy (pernicious anemia, malabsorption), chronic infection, malignancy (anemia of chronic disease), hypothyroidism, renal disease, adrenal or pituitary disease
Medication history:	NSAIDs (GI bleeding), prescription drugs (hemolysis)
Nutritional history:	Pica (iron deficiency anemia), vegan diet (B_{12} deficiency, iron deficiency), no fruits or vegetables (folate deficiency)
Psychosocial history:	Occupation (lead poisoning), alcohol use (folate and B_{12} deficiency, anemia due to liver disease, bone marrow depression), age of home (before 1950, lead paint)

Figure 12–1. Clinical History for Workup of Anemia

TABLE 12–5.   ANEMIA CLASSIFICATION[a]

Microcytic (MCV < 87)	Normocytic (MCV 87–103)	Macrocytic (MCV > 103)
Iron deficiency (late)	Iron deficiency (early)	B_{12} deficiency
Anemia of chronic disease (late)	Anemia of chronic disease (early)	Folate deficiency
Sideroblastic anemia	Hemolytic anemia	Chemotherapy and other meds[c]
Lead toxicity (rare)	Iron deficiency + B_{12} deficiency	Liver disease
	Renal disease[b]	Myelodysplasia
	Thyroid disease	Thyroid disease

[a] The higher the red cell width, the greater the variability of cell size and the less accurate the classification based on MCV.
[b] Renal failure often coexists with folate and iron deficiency, especially in the dialysis client.
[c] Macrocytic anemias may be caused by alcohol, colchicine, trimethoprim–sulfamethoxazole (Bactrim); phenytoin (Dilantin), zidovudine, and many other agents.

Assessment. The differential diagnosis of iron deficiency anemia warrants additional lab studies. Iron losses are reflected in diagnostic studies in sequential order, with serum iron and ferritin levels dropping first, followed by an increase in total iron-binding capacity (TIBC) and decline in transferrin saturation. Finally, the losses are reflected in the hemoglobin count and RBC indices, demonstrating a microcytic, hypochromic anemia. Some authors cite ferritin as the single best indicator of iron deficiency (Guyatt et al., 1992; Richer, 1997; Massey, 1992; Shine, 1997), but it should be noted that ferritin will rise in the presence of coexistent inflammatory disease (Payne, & Wheby, 1995). Serum iron, TIBC, and transferrin saturation are used to further clarify the diagnosis. Iron deficiency anemia begins as a normocytic anemia and becomes microcytic and hypochromic as the hemoglobin decreases.

Clinical Management. Ferrous sulfate 325 mg PO three times a day is usually prescribed and continued until the he-

TABLE 12–6.   DIFFERENTIATION OF MICROCYTIC ANEMIAS

	Iron Deficiency	Anemia of Chronic Disease	Sideroblastic (rare)
Serum iron	↓	↓	↑
Ferritin[a]	↓	N or ↑	N
Total iron-binding capacity (TIBC)	↑	↓	N
Transferrin saturation	↓	↓	↑

N, normal.
[a] Ferritin increases in the presence of inflammation, malignancy, fever, and other chronic diseases; a cutoff of < 10–15 ng/mL is used as diagnostic of iron deficiency, but in persons with known inflammatory disease, a higher cutoff of 50–60 ng/mL has been suggested; serum iron, TIBC, and transferrin saturation are needed to assist the clinician in diagnosing iron deficiency in these clients.

moglobin level returns to normal, followed by 3 to 6 months of twice-a-day dosing to replenish ferritin stores. Initiating therapy with once-a-day dosing (325 mg) and gradually titrating upward may help minimize GI intolerance. Lower doses may be used to decrease constipation. The addition of vitamin C to the regimen potentiates iron absorption. A reticulocyte count should be drawn 1 to 2 weeks after therapy if the anemia is severe or bone marrow activity is in question (an increase in reticulocytes is expected). The hemoglobin should be reassessed after 3 to 4 weeks to document improvement. The hemoglobin should return to normal in 6 to 8 weeks, but therapy should continue (with twice-a-day dosing) until ferritin stores are replenished (3 to 6 months). Failure of the hemoglobin to respond to treatment suggests misdiagnosis, malabsorption, noncompliance, or unrelenting blood loss. Nonresponders should be referred to a physician. Assessment of the reticulocyte count and erythrocyte sedimentation rate (ESR) may assist in clarifying the diagnosis.

Client Education. Instruct the client to avoid taking iron with milk products or antacids. Taking with orange juice may improve absorption. Advise that stools will look darker in color. Recommend an increase in fluid and fiber intake to prevent constipation (see Chapter 7 for further measures). Encourage foods high in iron, including lean meats; egg yolks; shellfish; apricots; peaches; prunes; grapes; raisins; green, leafy vegetables; and iron-fortified breads and cereals. Counsel regarding the cause of the anemia and any measures to prevent recurrence.

NORMOCYTIC ANEMIAS

Anemia of Chronic Disease

Anemia often accompanies chronic inflammation or malignancy due to decreased RBC longevity and decreased erythropoiesis. Potential causes include autoimmune disease, chronic infection (tuberculosis, endocarditis, human immunodeficiency virus [HIV]) and malignancy. Liver disease and chronic renal failure may produce a similar anemia. The anemia of chronic disease (ACD) is normocytic but may become hypochromic or microcytic over time. It rarely causes the hemoglobin and hematocrit to drop below 9 and 25, respectively, unless accompanied by coexisting pathology. Iron deficiency frequently coexists with ACD. Like iron deficiency, the serum iron and transferrin saturation will be low in ACD, but unlike iron deficiency, ferritin is normal or increased and TIBC is low. The reticulocyte count should also be assessed.

Clinical Management. Treatment is aimed at the underlying disease process, and physician consultation should be sought. If the hemoglobin is less than 9 or the hematocrit is less than 25, look for coexisting pathology (B_{12}, iron deficiency, multiple myeloma, etc.). Symptomatic clients with renal failure may be treated with erythropoietin and will also require adequate vitamin C, vitamin E, and iron intake to assist with RBC synthesis. Hypothyroidism may also result in a normocytic anemia, and the clinician should consider assessing thyroid function. An empiric trial of iron is often beneficial to treat any coexistent iron deficiency.

Sideroblastic Anemia

Sideroblastic anemia is characterized by the accumulation of iron deposits in red blood cell mitochondria, producing "ringed sideroblasts" in the bone marrow. The condition may be due to chronic alcoholism, lead poisoning, preleukemic myelodysplasia, pyridoxine deficiency, and other causes. The anemia may be normocytic, macrocytic, or occasionally microcytic, and is characterized by elevated serum iron and transferrin saturation. The lactic dehydrogenase (LDH) level will be elevated, and hepatic or splenic enlargement may be found on exam. Bone marrow examination is required, and such clients should be referred to the physician.

Aplastic Anemia

Aplasia (absence of cell production) may affect RBCs exclusively or may impact all cell lines, resulting in pancytopenia. Aplasia may stem from medications, malignancies, infections, severe alcohol abuse, autoimmune disease, or idiopathic causes. Aplasia presents as a severe normocytic anemia, with negligible or absent reticulocyte count. Physician referral and bone marrow biopsy is warranted.

Hemolytic Anemia

Hemolytic anemia presents with a progressive normocytic anemia despite adequate or brisk reticulocytosis as the bone marrow attempts to replace cells that are rapidly being destroyed. Total and indirect bilirubin are elevated, and jaundice may be present as the liver attempts to process the byproducts of the hemolyzed red cells. Causes include glucose-6-phosphate dehydrogenase (G6PD) deficiency, sickle cell or hereditary spherocytosis, medication-induced hemolysis, and autoimmune disease. Drugs that may prompt a hemolytic response include methyldopa, penicillin, quinidine, and sulfa drugs. Acute hemolysis presents with fever, chills, back pain, abdominal pain, and hemoglobinuria. A Coombs' test is needed to differentiate autoimmune phenomena from other nonautoimmune hemolytic diseases. Physician referral is warranted in all cases of suspected hemolytic anemia. Definitive therapy depends on the cause of the hemolysis.

MACROCYTIC ANEMIAS

The most common cause of macrocytosis is alcohol abuse. B_{12} and folate deficiency account for one third of all macrocytic anemias. Thyroid disease, liver disease, and many medications (including trimethoprim–sulfamethoxasole, phenytoin, and zidovudine) can also cause macrocytosis. Macrocytic anemia not found to be caused by one of these conditions represents possible myelodysplasia. Physician consultation is warranted in all cases.

Vitamin B_{12} Deficiency

The most common cause of B_{12} deficiency is pernicious anemia, a chronic, progressive, macrocytic anemia caused by a deficiency in intrinsic factor, a substance necessary for B_{12} absorption in the GI tract. (Davenport, 1996) Pernicious anemia is believed to be an autoimmune disease, most common in women aged 35 to 60 of Northern or Eastern European ancestry. Less common causes of B_{12} deficiency include gastric surgery (gastrectomy or ileal resection), Crohn's disease, pancreatic insufficiency, or dietary insufficiency. Dietary deficiency is uncommon and is found primarily in persons who consume no animal or dairy products.

Clinical Presentation. Initial symptoms of B_{12} deficiency include change in taste, anorexia, mouth soreness, nausea, and bowel changes. The individual may experience irritability, memory changes, mood swings, and paresthesias. Objective findings include neurologic abnormalities and glossitis (see Table 12–4). Lab studies reveal normal or elevated MCV, slightly elevated bilirubin, and decreased reticulocyte count. Lactic dehydrogenase may be elevated, and if the B_{12} deficiency is severe, white blood cells (WBCs) and platelets may also be depressed. The Schilling test is used to differentiate pernicious anemia from other causes of B_{12} deficiency. Folic acid levels should be assessed in all cases.

Clinical Management. Treatment is initiated with 100 μg of B_{12} given intramuscularly on a daily basis for 1 week, followed by a weekly dose for 1 month, and subsequently a monthly dose for life. The first few days of treatment produce a brisk reticulocytosis and cellular production, which places the older adult at risk for CHF and hypokalemia, as potassium is used in the formation of new cells. Folate and iron stores may also require supplementation.

Collboration and Referral. Physician consultation is recommended during the initial diagnosis and treatment phase. Collaboration regarding appropriate follow-up is also warranted, since persons with pernicious anemia are at increased risk for gastric atrophy and gastric carcinoma and may require regular endoscopic exams. Community resources should be sought for individuals and families who are unable to self-administer B_{12} injections.

Folic Acid Deficiency

Folic acid is found in most fruits, vegetables, meats, and dairy products and may be deficient due to inadequate intake (common in elderly alcoholics), chronic ingestion of overcooked foods or increased body requirements (malignancy, hemolytic anemia, severe exfoliative psoriasis). Medications such as phenytoin, methotrexate, triamterene, and trimethoprim may also promote deficiency. The disease presents with macrocytic anemia and low serum folate levels. B_{12} should always be assessed in the presence of folate deficiency, since folate replacement will mask the hematologic findings but not prevent the neurological sequelae caused by coexistent B_{12} deficiency. Clinical management includes treating the underlying cause and supplementing folic acid (usually 1 mg PO qd) until the deficiency resolves.

Anemia represents a clinically significant herald of underlying pathology in the older adult and poses a threat to organ systems with minimal functional reserve. Appropriate diagnosis and treatment will minimize morbidity and mortality in this population.

CASE STUDY #1

Mr. Zimmerman is a 63-year-old retired machine operator, whose past medical history includes type 2 DM for 7 years, myocardial infarction (MI) 9 years ago, HTN, prostate cancer s/p prostatectomy and radiation treatment (6 months prior). Current medications are glyburide 10 mg bid, lisinopril 10 mg qd, and acetylsalicylic acid (ASA) qd. His height is 5'11" and his weight is 186 lb. He reports following a 1600 calorie ADA diet. Mr. Zimmerman is being seen for his quarterly visit. He reports increased fatigue and blurry vision. Self blood glucose monitoring results are fasting 175 to 190 mg/dL, and predinner 235 to 280 mg/dL. Results of laboratory tests obtained 1 week prior to visit are sodium 136, potassium 4.1, chloride 105, CO_2 26, blood urea nitrogen (BUN) 28, creatinine 1.8, and glycated hemoglobin 9.6% (7.2% previously). Mr. Zimmerman denies any change in his routine. He continues to walk 1 mile a day.

QUESTIONS

1. What should the practitioner do to address this apparently sudden increase in Mr. Zimmerman's glucose level without any reported change on his part?

2. Since it appears that the cause of increased glucose levels is due to change in insulin resistance, what medication changes should be considered?

ANSWERS

1. The practitioner should realize that possible explanations include (1) oral agent failure (as he has been on oral agents for 7 years), (2) increased insulin resistance, (3) medication non-compliance or additional OTC medications (ie, vitamins; patient recently diagnosed with cancer), and (4) increased food intake/change in activity.

   Initially, the client should be asked to test his blood sugar before each meal and at bedtime for 1 week. The practitioner should review with the client all medications he is taking and schedule checking for increased sugar content in any vitamins. A referral should be made to a registered dietitian for medical nutrition review.

   Mr. Zimmerman returns to the office in 2 weeks, with similar blood sugar readings as noted previously. He has a correct understanding of his medications and is not taking any OTC products that contain sugar. Mr. Zimmerman consults with the dietitian and reports that he has been "pretty much following the recommended diet."

2. Mr. Zimmerman is not a candidate for metformin due to his elevated creatinine level. Since acarbose has the greatest effect on postprandial glucose levels, it would not be beneficial in Mr. Zimmerman's case of elevated fasting and premeal glucose levels. Troglitazone and insulin are appropriate options for Mr. Zimmerman. The plan was to start him on bedtime NPH insulin (5 to 8 units) while he remained on glyburide. While discussing NPH insulin action, peak, and duration, it was learned that checking a blood sugar level at 3 A.M. would not be a problem for the client. He apparently gets up about this time every night to let his dog out for a walk. While he was up waiting for the dog to return, he would eat half of a breakfast coffee cake because he was hungry. He only mentioned this when specifically asked about activity during the night. He was willing to change his snacking habits and was able to continue on his glyburide, and a repeat glycated hemoglobin result was 7.4%. The importance of inquiring about an individual's 24-hour schedule should not be overlooked.

 ## CASE STUDY #2

Mrs. Welch is an 85-year-old white female who lives alone in a senior center housing complex. Her nearest family member lives 75 miles away. She is in the mild–moderate stage of multi-infarct dementia. She displays deficits in short-term memory and time orientation. She has had type 2 DM for 16 years and been taking insulin for 5 years. Her insulin prescription is 28 units of 70/30 insulin in the arm. On random blood sugar testing, her glucoses are 200 to 350 mg/dL, with a glycated hemoglobin of 11.4%. The elevated glucose levels are related to the fact that Mrs. Welch sometimes forgets to take her insulin. Since having cataract surgery, Mrs. Welch is more involved with the activities at the senior center and taking walks to visit her friends. During the practitioner's weekly visit, Mrs. Welch is found to be hallucinating and is unable to recognize the clinician or her apartment. A random fingerstick blood glucose is 135 mg/dL. She is given a 15-g carbohydrate snack, and a repeat fingerstick is 189 mg/dL. At this point, her mental status returns to her baseline.

QUESTION

1. What changes should the practitioner make in Mrs. Welch's diabetes management?

ANSWER

1. Mrs. Welch had an episode of hypoglycemia, even though her glucose was in the normal range at 135 mg/dL. The reason is that individuals can experience hypoglycemic signs and symptoms when there is a rapid decrease in blood glucose from the individual's usual level. Changes in mental status may be the only sign/symptom of hypoglycemia that an older adult experiences.

Mrs. Welch's insulin requirements need to be reassessed, as she is now more active and at risk for hypoglycemia. The adjustments would be decreases of 2 units every 3 days until glucose levels are stabilized. Principles for medication reminders should be instituted.

■ REFERENCES

Ahroni, J. (1996). Strategies for teaching elders from a human development perspective. *Diabetes Educator, 22,* 47–52.

American Diabetes Association. (1997a). Guide to diagnosis and classification of diabetes mellitus and other categories of glucose intolerance. *Diabetes Care, 20*(Suppl 1), 21.

American Diabetes Association. (1998). Standards of medical care for patients with diabetes mellitus. *Diabetes Care, 21*(Suppl 1), 23–31.

Barzel, U. (1995). Hypothyroidism diagnosis and management. *Clin Geriatr Med, 11* 239–249.

Bayer Pharmaceuticals. (1996). Precose package insert.

Brody, M., & Reichard, R. (1995). Thyroid screening—how to interpret and apply the results. *Postgrad Med, 98,* 54–68.

Brook, C., & Marshall, N. (1996). *Essential endocrinology.* London: Blackwell Science.

Cefalu, W. (1996). Non insulin dependent diabetes: Clinical considerations. *Clin Rev,* March, 69–87.

Chiasson, J. L., Josse, R., Hunt, J., et al. (1994). The efficacy of acarbose in the treatment of patients with non-insulin dependent diabetes mellitus—a multicenter controlled clinical trial. *Ann Intern Med, 121,* 928–935.

Davenport, J. (1996). Macrocytic anemia. *Am Fam Phys, 53*(1), 155–162.

DeFronzo, R., Goodman, A., & Multicenter Metformin Study Group. (1995). Efficacy of metformin in patients with non-insulin dependent diabetes mellitus. *N Engl J Med, 333,* 541–549.

Diabetes Control and Complications Trial Research Group. (1993). The effects of intensive treatment of diabetes on the development and progression of long-term complications in insulin-dependent diabetes mellitus. *N Engl J Med, 329,* 977–986.

Finucane, P. (1995). Abnormal glucose tolerance in old age: The scale of the problem. In Finucane, P., & Sinclair, A. (Eds.). *Diabetes in old age.* (pp. 12–19). West Sussex, England: John Wiley & Sons.

Franz, M. (1994). Summary and commentary. *Diabetes Spectrum, 7,* 375–376.

Gambert, S., & Escher, J. (1988). Atypical presentation of endocrine disorders in the elderly. *Geriatrics, 43,* 69–78.

Gambert, S. (1995). Hyperthyroidism in the elderly. *Clin Geriatr Med, 11,* 181–188.

Goroll, A. H., May, L. A. & Mulley Jr., A. G. (1995). *Primary care medicine* (3rd ed.). Philadelphia: J. B. Lippincott. 529–534, 447–455.

Guyatt, G. H., Oxman, A. D., Ali, M., et al. (1992). Laboratory diagnosis of iron-deficiency anemia: An overview. *J Gen Intern Med, 7,* 145–153.

Isley, W. (1993). Thyroid dysfunction in the severly ill and elderly—forget the classic signs and symptoms. *Postgrad Med, 94*(3) 111–128.

Kaiser, F. (1995). Thyroid function tests. *Clin Geriatr Med, 11,* 171–179.

Kamiya, A., Ohsewa, I., Fujii, T., et al. (1995). A clinical survey on the compliance of exercise therapy for diabetic outpatients. *Diabetes Res Clin Pract, 27,* 141–145.

Lebovitz, H. (1995). Rationale in the management of non-insulin dependent diabetes. In Leslie, R., & Robbins, D. (Eds.). *Diabetes: Clinical science in practice.* (pp. 450–461). Cambridge, England: Cambridge University Press.

Massey, A. C. (1992). Microcytic anemia: Differential diagnosis and management of iron deficiency anemia. *Med Clin North Am, 76,* 549–566.

Maynard, T. (1991). Part II. Translating the exercise prescription. *Diabetes Educator, 5,* 384–393.

Mooradian, A. (1995). Normal age related changes in thyroid hormone economy. *Clin Geriatr Med, 11,* 159–169.

Osterweil, D., Syndulko, K., Cohen, S., (1992). Cognitive function in non-demented older adults with hypothyroidism. *J Am Geriatr Soc, 40,* 325–335.

Payne, S. K., & Wheby, M. S. (1995). Anemia: How to streamline the diagnosis: Identify reversible causes. *Consultant,* November, 1685–1692.

Richer, S. (1997). A practical guide for differentiating between iron deficiency anemia and anemia of chronic disease in children and adults. *Nurse Pract, 22*(4), 82–103.

Rolla, A. (1995). Thyroid nodules in the elderly. *Clin Geriatr Med, 11,* 259–269.

Sawin, C. (1991). Thyroid dysfunction in older persons. *Adv Intern Med, 37,* 223–248.

Shine, J. (1997). Microcytic anemia. *Am Fam Phys, 55*(7), 2455–2462.

Singer, P., Cooper, D., Levy, E., (1995). Treatment guidelines for patients with hyperthyroidism and hypothyroidism. *JAMA, 273,* 808–812.

Small, E. J., & Damon, L. E. (1996). Blood (Ch 18). In Lonergan, E. T. (Ed.). *Geriatrics: A Lange clinical manual.* Stamford, CT: Appleton & Lange.

Spence, J. C. (1921). Some observations on sugar tolerance with special reference to variations found at different ages. *Q J Med, 14,* 314–326.

Stout, R. (1995). Ageing and glucose tolerance. In Finucane, P. & Sinclair, A. (Eds.). *Diabetes in old age.* (pp. 21–44). New York: John Wiley & Sons.

Taylor, R. (1993). Post-prandial hyperglycemia and diabetic complications. *Pract Diabetes Suppl, 10,* 10–14.

Villareal, D., & Morley, J. (1995). Prevention of diabetes in elderly people. In Finucane, P., & Sinclair, A. (Eds.). *Diabetes in old age.* (pp. 45–67). New York: John Wiley & Sons.

Warner-Lambert Co. (1997). Rezulin package insert.

White, J., Hartman, J., & Campbell, R. K. (1993). Drug interactions in diabetic patients. *Postgrad Med, 93,* 130–142.

13

TOPICS IN ONCOLOGY CARE

Gail A. Rogers • Joan Flaherty

■ INTRODUCTION

Advancing age is the greatest risk factor for developing cancer. Sixty percent of all malignancies will occur in persons 65 years of age and older (Kennedy & Cohen, 1996). Many of these cancers will be diagnosed at a later stage, as the elderly often delay seeking care for their symptoms.

Myths continue to exist that cancer in the elderly is a less serious disease than that in a younger individual. Many believe it should not be treated aggressively, if at all. Cancer in the elderly is similar to other age groups, with the exception that the elderly may also be faced with comorbid diseases.

Treatment decisions should be made, with careful attention paid to comorbid disease states. Age alone should never disqualify the elderly individual from receiving appropriate cancer treatment. Many clinical trials, however, continue to exclude the elderly. Clearly, this treat-

ment bias needs to be addressed. Maintaining quality of life during and after cancer treatment is essential in the elderly patient. Diagnostic tests and/or procedures associated with little probability of a positive outcome may be justified if they are associated with little to no harmful effect and/or cost (McKenna, 1994). In contrast, testing associated with a high mortality/morbidity rate is justified only if patient survival is improved (McKenna, 1994).

■ PROSTATE CANCER

According to the American Cancer Society (ACS), 334,000 new cases of prostate cancer will be detected in 1997; with the incidence higher for African-American men than for white men. The incidence of prostate cancer increases with age, with 80% of all prostate cancer diagnosed in men over age 65. Incidence rates are expected to increase with further widespread use of prostate serum screening tests.

Prostatic tumors are usually slow growing and indolent. Autopsy results reveal that more men will die with this disease than from it (Littrup, 1994), indicating that sometimes these tumors may not manifest obvious clinical symptoms.

Criticism and debate have surrounded the widespread use of prostate-specific antigen (PSA) as a screening tool. While the specificity of PSA is considered good compared with other tumor markers, improvement is needed. Elevation of PSA is common with diseases of the prostate other than cancer: benign prostatic hyperplasia, acute or chronic prostatitis, and prostatic infarction. Such conditions cannot be identified based on clinical findings, and prostate biopsy is the only present means to detect prostate cancer (Montie & Meyers, 1997).

The use of PSA as a screening modality has increased diagnosis at an earlier stage and probably prolonged survival but has not demonstrated a sustained decrease in mortality (Stenman, 1997; Benson, 1997). The mortality rate after the first increase in PSA is relatively low during the first 10 years after the tumor becomes detectable. Mortality rates rise 15 to 20 years after diagnosis. Therefore, according to Stenman (1997), patients with an expected lifetime of 15 to 20 years would benefit from successful treatment at an early stage. Screening men over 70 years of age may not reduce prostate cancer mortality but may still reduce morbidity.

Quality-of-life issues need to be considered when screening for prostate cancer. False-positive results in a screening program cause considerable cost and worry to the client (Herr, 1997). An important goal in screening is to avoid overtreatment; treat only the tumors that need to be and can be treated successfully, minimizing harm to the client.

AGE-RELATED CHANGES

Beginning about the fifth decade, enlargement of the prostate is common as the gland becomes hyperplastic.

ASSESSMENT

History

Review genitourinary (GU) system: Assess for weak or interrupted urine flow; inability to urinate, feelings of incomplete emptying, or difficulty starting or stopping the urine flow; the need to urinate frequently, especially at night; pain or burning on urination; and blood in the urine. Most of these symptoms are nonspecific and may be similar to those caused by benign conditions such as infection or prostatic enlargement. Unfortunately, some men may experience their first symptoms from metastases. These signs may include lumbosacral pain (radiating to hips and upper thighs), weight loss, and anemia. Assess for family history of prostate cancer. Review dietary fat intake and possible occupational exposure, especially cadmium. Cadmium is a nonessential trace element and a zinc antagonist. Zinc is an essential trace element, needed for cell growth and found in high concentration in the prostate. An exposure to cadmium can result in accumulation in the prostate and an interruption of normal cell growth. Only a small number of cases of prostate cancer can be linked to cadmium exposure (Groenwald et al., 1993).

Physical Examination

Perform a digital rectal exam.

Diagnostic Studies

As discussed earlier, there is much controversy surrounding the use of PSA for screening. Elevations of PSA have been linked to other prostatic conditions; therefore, diagnosis of prostate cancer cannot be made solely on the results of PSA. For a definitive diagnosis, a referral to a urologist and other diagnostic studies are needed. Transrectal ultrasound (TRUS) imaging and biopsy technology provide accurate guidance for directed biopsies of prostate abnormalities, while minimizing the discomfort and risk of biopsy.

CLINICAL MANAGEMENT

Currently, treatment options for localized prostate cancer include observation, radical prostatectomy, external beam radiation, and brachytherapy. Hormones and chemotherapy, or combinations of these options, might be considered for more widespread or metastatic disease. Careful observation without immediate active treatment may be appropriate, particularly for older individuals with low-grade and/or early-stage tumors.

Radical prostatectomy refers to the surgical removal of the entire prostate, including the seminal vesicles and part of the bladder neck. Considerations of the client's age, stage of cancer, and other medical conditions of the client should be made in conjunction with the physician.

The toxicity of radiation treatment does not appear to be increased with age (Olmi, 1997). In the elderly, limiting the volume to the prostate and total dose obtains good local control.

Some prostate cancers depend on androgens for growth. Luteinizing hormone from the pituitary gland stimulates the testes to synthesize testosterone. Estrogen blocks the release of luteinizing hormone. With estrogen therapy, clients are at increased risk for cardiogenic complications and thrombophlebitis. Flutamide is an antiandrogen used to interfere with androgen activity in the cell.

Chemotherapy is primarily used in clients with hormone-resistant cancers. Estramustine phosphate is an agent that combines a hormonal agent with an antineoplastic drug.

Prostate-specific antigen at this point is useful in monitoring the course of the disease or response to therapy.

CLIENT EDUCATION

As might be expected because of the organs involved, a high degree of sexual dysfunction is reported among prostate cancer survivors, especially following radical prostatectomy and radiation therapy (Herr, 1997). Sexual dysfunction includes the loss of erectile potency and absence of emission and ejaculation, which result from damage to the nerves and muscle tissue surrounding the prostate following surgery. Obtaining a brief sexual assessment regarding the client's and his partner's physical and emotional states, what they want to know, and what they need to know can lead to successful nursing intervention (Groenwald et al., 1993). The client and his partner must be reminded that only they can determine what is sexually fulfilling. Sexual alternatives, experimentation with their partner, and communication of what is enjoyable to each partner are successful strategies. Referral to a qualified therapist can be made for those who choose it.

■ BREAST CANCER

An estimated 180,000 new cases of breast cancer among women will be diagnosed in the United States during 1997 (ACS, 1997), and approximately 44% of these new cases will be in women 65 years or older (Newschaffer et al., 1996). It should be noted that about 1% of new cases will be diagnosed in men. A recent rise in incidence rates among women has been observed, but is believed to be due to increases in mammography utilization, allowing for early detection of breast cancers before they become clinically apparent (ACS, 1997). Early detection and improved treatment account for recent declines in mortality rates.

AGE-RELATED CHANGES

Breasts tend to diminish in size as glandular tissue is replaced by fat. The ducts around the nipple are more palpable as firm, stringy strands.

ASSESSMENT

The etiology of breast cancer is unknown, but many risk factors have been identified. The incidence of disease has been linked to genetic, hormonal, and biochemical factors.

Age, coupled with hormonal factors, has been implicated in the etiology of breast cancer. Prolonged exposure to estrogens (early menarche/late menopause) is considered high risk. In women, three estrogens are found: estradiol, estrone, and estriol. Estradiol and estrone are potent estrogens with some carcinogenic actions. Estriol behaves antagonistically to the carcinogenic actions of the other two estrogens. Levels of estriol increase dramatically during pregnancy.

Studies indicate that a woman has at least a twofold risk of developing breast cancer (as compared with the general population) if a first-degree relative (mother, sister, aunt) had breast cancer (ACS, 1997). The case for a genetic connection with breast cancer recently became stronger with the discovery of the "breast cancer gene," BRCA 1 (Myriad Genetic Laboratories, Salt Lake City, UT). BRCA 1, the first major gene to be isolated, is a large gene found on chromosome 17. The BRCA 1 gene codes for a protein that has a tumor suppressor function. Loss of this function may result in tumor development. Inherited loss of BRCA 1 function confers an increased susceptibility to both breast and ovarian cancer (Claus et al., 1996).

Fibrocystic disease is a common breast lesion found in women. The relationship of fibrocystic disease to breast cancer is disputed. However, compared with the general population, the incidence of breast cancer among these women is higher (Groenwald et al., 1993).

Dietary factors may contribute to their risk of breast cancer. Although inconsistencies exist in studies between individual dietary fat intake and breast cancer, obesity is related to breast cancer. It has been suggested that a hormonal component of excessive body weight might affect breast cancer growth and metastasis (Byers, 1994).

In studies, alcohol has more consistently shown an increased risk for breast cancer. This may be due to the effect on the endocrine system, including affecting estrogen metabolism in the liver.

History

Review breast health (ie, any forms of benign breast disease, self-breast examination). Assess for personal or family history of breast cancer, early menarche, late menopause, lengthy exposure to postmenopausal estrogens, and never having children or having the first live birth at a late age. Assess for history of chest wall radiation and ovarian, endometrial, or colon cancer. Review alcohol, tobacco, and dietary fat intake.

Physical

Perform breast examination, assessing for breast lump or thickening; dimpling of skin, nipple retraction or deviation, and asymmetry of breast; scaling skin on nipple or areola; peau d'orange skin; and bloody nipple discharge or breast ulceration. Palpate for enlarged nodes in supraclavicular and axillary regions.

Diagnostic Studies

Screening mammography can identify breast abnormalities before physical symptoms develop. The ACS recommends that screening mammography begin at age 40, with mammograms every 1 to 2 years until age 50, then every year at age 50 or over. However, in 1990, the National Cancer Institute and the National Institute on Aging supported the recommendations of a forum on breast cancer screening in older women: For women aged 65 to 74, mammography should be performed at regular intervals of approximately every 2 years. For women aged 75 and older whose general health and life expectancy are good, mammography should be performed at regular intervals of approximately every 2 years.

Studies have reported that screening for breast cancer is less widespread in women older than 65 than in those younger than 65 (Costanza, 1994). A number of barriers related to mammography have been identified: lack of knowledge that screening mammography is needed, particularly in the absence of symptoms; lack of belief in the benefit of mammography; lack of physician recommendation; cost; access (lack of transportation or remoteness of mammography facility); lower levels of education and low income; and not having a regular physician.

When a suspicious lump is detected or a suspicious area is identified on mammogram, diagnostic mammography can help determine whether additional tests are needed if there are other lesions too small to be felt in the same or opposite breast. *All* suspicious lumps should be biopsied for definitive diagnosis; therefore, a surgical referral is necessary.

CLINICAL MANAGEMENT

Treatment of breast cancer should take into account the medical situation and the client's preferences. Denying proper diagnostic and prognostic evaluations and appropriate surgical or other modalities of treatment on the basis of age in inappropriate. Treatment may involve breast-conserving surgery (lumpectomy), modified radical mastectomy with or without reconstruction, radiation therapy, chemotherapy, or hormone therapy (tamoxifen). Often, two or more methods are used in combination.

Mastectomy has a low operative mortality rate in women over age 65 and provides excellent control. There is no survival benefit for mastectomy over lumpectomy and radiotherapy (Berger & Roslyn, 1997). Axillary dissection is regarded as a staging procedure and a method of local control, but its use is decreasing among older women with clinically negative axillae. When it comes to surgical management of breast cancer, many older women are anxious to preserve their breasts and should be given this option.

Radiation therapy, after surgery, increases local control and is well tolerated. Disease relapse in patients with radiation after conservative surgery ranges 0.3% to 13% versus 8% to 34% with patients treated with surgery alone (Olmi et al., 1997).

Chemotherapy for patients with breast cancer was introduced in the 1960s and rapidly developed from treatment with single agents to combination regimens. Paclitaxel, a new agent, has demonstrated antitumor activity when used as a single agent or in combination with doxorubicin. Over the years, combination chemotherapy regimens have become the standard of care for the treatment of breast cancer (Hortobagyi, 1995). The most commonly used front-line combination regimens include cyclophosphamide–methotrexate–fluorouracil (CMF), fluorouracil–doxorubicin–cyclophosphamide (FAC), and cyclophosphamide–doxorubicin–fluorouracil (CAF).

Manipulation of the endocrine system is the oldest form of systemic breast cancer therapy. The discovery of estrogen receptors on breast cancer tumors cells has enhanced the understanding of the endocrine system in the disease. Approximately 50% of all malignant breast diseases are estrogen receptor positive and 50% to 60% of patients with estrogen receptor–positive tumors respond to hormonal therapy (Chlebowski et al., 1993). Tamoxifen, an estrogen-blocking drug, is now commonly used in used in women with hormonal-responsive tumors. Tamoxifen's side effects are usually mild but may include hot flashes, nausea, and vaginal dryness. Occassionally, it can cause visual disturbances, including corneal changes, cataracts, and retinopathy.

CLIENT EDUCATION

Mammography is only one strategy employed in the early detection of breast cancer. Clinical breast examination and breast self-examination are other important screening techniques. Ninety percent of breast cancers are found by either the client on breast self-examination or by the physician during routine evaluation (Schonwetter, 1992). Women older than 65 are reluctant to examine their own breasts for a variety of reasons: fear and anxiety of cancer, lack of knowledge of how to perform breast self-exam and interpret results, and ignorance of the importance of monthly breast self-exam as a supplement to physical examination.

Further education on breast self-examination can be accomplished through a variety of approaches. Rimer (1994) has identified types of interventions that aid in this task: individual-directed interventions (mailed reminders, telephone counseling); system-directed or physician-directed interventions (prompts, manual or computer-generated reminders); access-enhancing interventions (mobile vans or provision of transportation); social network interventions (peer-group leaders); and multistrategy interventions (combination of interventions). Not only should the general population be educated on breast cancer screening, but efforts need to be focused on health-care providers as well.

DELIRIUM IN THE OLDER PERSON WITH CANCER

It is well known that elderly individuals may exhibit signs and symptoms of illness atypically, meaning that underlying problems may not be recognizable in a traditional manner. Delirium is a presenting feature of acute physical illness, or it may be drug related. Delirium is a difficult diagnostic problem and is most often mistaken for schizophrenia or dementia. It is reported that physicians often fail to detect delirium; they document its signs and symptoms in only 30% to 50% of affected clients (Francis, 1992). The fluctuating nature of delirium makes it difficult to detect, particularly when physicians spend only a brief time with the client. Even when physicians notice behavioral disturbances, they may fail to realize their significance.

Delirium is a serious consequence affecting many older adults with cancer. Cancer can cause delirium through space-occupying lesions, metastasis, cerebral edema, encephalitis, hemorrhage, and metabolic abnormalities. Cognitive impairment and depression may be presenting signs of malignancy. Three of the most common cancers in older adults— lung, breast, and prostate cancer—have an increased propensity to metastasize to the brain (Weinrich & Sarna, 1994).

Cancer treatments, chemotherapy, radiation therapy, and surgery can contribute to the etiology of delirium. Side effects of treatment that can cause delirium include infection, fever, fluid and electrolyte imbalance, organ failure, medication toxicity, and compromised nutritional status. For diagnosis and management of delirium, see Chapter 3.

■ LUNG CANCER

Lung cancer continues to be a major health problem in the United States. The ACS is estimating 178,000 new cases of lung cancer in 1998, accounting for 13% of cancer diagnoses, and an estimated 160,400 deaths in 1998, accounting for 29% of all cancer deaths. Early detection of lung cancer is difficult because symptoms often do not appear until the disease is advanced. Because of inadequate early detection techniques, efforts should be focused on decreasing or eliminating risk factors.

AGE-RELATED CHANGES

With age, tissues in the lung lose their elasticity, resulting in a decreased number of collapsible small airways. There is also a decrease in the functioning of the mucous/ciliary clearance in the trachea and small airways. These airways are lined with columnar epithelial cells, which are either mucus-secreting goblet cells, ciliated cells, or brush cells. With years of irritation or environmental assault, these cells are shed from the surface.

CLINICAL PRESENTATION

Clinical presentation of lung cancer depends on the location and extent of the tumor. Presenting pulmonary symptoms such as dyspnea, cough, and hemoptysis are similar to those of other lung conditions (pneumonia, chronic obstructive lung disease) and are not appreciated as symptoms of an oncologic process. Symptoms of local spread include hoarseness (tumor against or involving the larynx), chest or shoulder pain, dysphagia (tumor against or involving the esophagus), or head and neck swelling (tumor against the superior vena cava).

ASSESSMENT

History
Review respiratory, cardiac, and upper gastrointestinal (GI) symptoms. Assess history of tobacco use and history of tuberculosis or pulmonary inflammatory process. Assess exposure to certain industrial substances such as arsenic, radon, and asbestos, as well as radiation exposure from occupational, medical, and environmental sources. Assess for family history of lung cancer.

Physical Examination
Perform a respiratory, cardiac, and upper GI examination.

Diagnostic Studies
Obtain a chest x-ray and sputum cytology; refer the client to physician. Suspicious results of x-ray and sputum may need to be further investigated through bronchoscopy (centrally located tumors) and percutaneous needle biopsy (peripherally located tumors).

CLINICAL MANAGEMENT

Management of lung cancer is dependent on the type and stage of cancer. For many localized cancers, surgery is usually the treatment of choice. According to Schonwetter (1992), there is an inverse relationship with age to the stage of lung cancer at the time of diagnosis; that is, older people have a higher incidence of localized lung cancer at the time of diagnosis and tolerate resections of lung carcinomas as a result. Radiation therapy and chemotherapy are used in combination when disease is advanced. Radiation therapy is effective in symptomatic control of dyspnea and edema from superior vena cava syndrome and in pain management. Locally advanced lung cancer may be treated with a combination of radiotherapy and cisplatin-containing chemotherapy.

■ CERVICAL CANCER

Cervical cancer continues to be the leading cause of avoidable deaths among older women. Women over age 65 constitute 13% of the total U.S. female population but account for 25% of new cases and 41% of deaths from this disease (Mandelblatt & Phillips, 1996). Cervical cancer can be detected early through Papanicolaou (Pap) tests, which can be performed as part of a routine exam. Historically, older women are underrepresented in screening programs for cervical cancer.

Most professional organizations, the ACS and the National Cancer Institute included, recommend Pap smears for all women, with no upper age limit, and most agree that after several annual negative smears, screening frequency can be changed to every 3 years. However, there are cases in which screening can cease at age 65, but only if there is a documented history of regular screening with technically adequate and negative smears (Mandelblatt & Phillips, 1996). Women who have never been screened, who have infrequent Pap smears, or who have a history of human papillomavirus should receive priority for screening. Because most older women visit their physicians once a year, there is an opportunity to increase screening rates by incorporating pelvic exams and Pap smears into the annual exam.

AGE-RELATED CHANGES

The vagina narrows and shortens, and its mucosa becomes thin, pale, and dry. The cervix undergoes atrophic changes.

ASSESSMENT

History

Assess for age of menopause, postmenopausal bleeding, abnormal vaginal discharge, and history of sexually transmitted disease and their treatments. Inquire about the client's last Pap test and how often screened, as well as sexual practices (multiple sexual partners or partners who have had multiple sexual partners).

Physical Examination

Perform a speculum exam, visualizing the vagina and cervix. Note the color of the cervix, characteristics of the surface, and any ulcerations, nodules, masses, bleeding, or discharge. Swab a sample of cells from the endocervix and exocervix (Pap test).

At this time, a pelvic exam may be incorporated to detect ovarian and/or retroperitoneal masses. Ovarian cancer is often "silent," showing no obvious signs or symptoms until late in its development. The most common sign is enlargement of the abdomen, caused by fluid accumulation, or vague digestive disturbances (stomach discomfort, gas distention). Any palpable mass should be referred to a physician for follow-up.

CLINICAL MANAGEMENT

An understanding of the cytologic results of the Pap smear is needed in order to manage treatment and follow-up. A class I report is normal. A class II report shows atypia, usually due to inflammation. The results of this report should be followed up in 2 weeks and any infection treated. Class III (dysplasia) and class IV (carcinoma in situ) reports need an inspection via colposcopy. The colposcope is able to visualize the epithelium of the cervix, magnified 8 to 18 times, and abnormal areas are biopsied.

Invasive cervical cancers generally are treated by surgery (hysterectomy) or radiation, or by a combination of the two. Chemotherapy is used generally when there is systemic involvement. Changes in the cervix during in situ cancer stages may be treated by cryotherapy (destruction of cells by extreme cold), by electrocoagulation (destruction of cells by electric current), laser ablation, or local surgery (cold knife cone biopsy).

According to White et al. (1993), age-related changes may make it difficult to adequately perform a Pap test. The following suggestions have been offered to facilitate:

- Using a metal speculum lubricated with warm water
- Using a pediatric-sized, narrow speculum
- Using an upside-down fracture pan to lift the buttocks when performing the exam on a client who is in bed

■ COLORECTAL CANCER

It is estimated that cancer of the colon and rectum will be diagnosed in 131,200 Americans in 1997 (Parker et al., 1997). Colorectal cancer is the third most common cancer in men and women and the second leading cause of cancer-related mortality.

The incidence of colorectal cancer rises dramatically after age 50 and doubles with each successive decade of life (Cohen, 1996). Peak incidence occurs in the seventh decade. Early detection and treatment can achieve cure rates of 80% to 90% (Cohen, 1996).

AGE-RELATED CHANGES

Anatomic changes associated with the aging of the large intestine include: (1) atrophy of the mucosa, (2) proliferation of connective tissue, and (3) vascular changes, primarily atherosclerosis (Timiris, 1994).

CLINICAL PRESENTATION

Signs and symptoms of colorectal cancer in its early stages are typically vague. Clinical presentations depend on the portion and function of colon that is affected by the tumor (Table 13–1).

ASSESSMENT

History

Review GI system. Assess for personal and family history of colorectal cancer, adenomatous polyps, familial adenomatous polyposis, and Gardner's syndrome. Assess for personal history of breast or uterine cancer, Crohn's disease, ulcera-

TABLE 13–1.   COLORECTAL CANCER DISEASE PRESENTATION

Anatomic Location	Early Symptoms	Late Symptoms
Right side (ascending colon)	Usually no signs/symptoms of obstruction Black, tarry stools Anemia Abdominal aching, pressure, cramping	Weakness Fatigue Dyspnea Vertigo Diarrhea Obstipation Anorexia, weight loss, vomiting Signs/symptoms of intestinal obstruction Tumor may be palpable on right side
Left side (descending colon)	Signs/symptoms of intestinal obstruction Rectal bleeding Intermittent abdominal fullness Cramping Rectal pressure	Obstipation Change in appearance of stool (ribbon- or pencil-like) Bleeding with bowel movements
Rectum	Urgency Obstipation alternating with diarrhea Blood or mucus in stool Feeling of incomplete evacuation	Rectal fullness Aching, pain in area of rectum and/or scrotum

tive colitis, and hereditary nonpolyposis cancer syndrome. Indviduals with a positive history of any of the preceding have a higher risk of developing colorectal cancer. Review dietary habits, including alcohol and fat intake. Discuss tobacco use, bowel patterns, and history of laxative use.

Physical Examination
Check vital signs, height, and weight. Assess abdomen; tumors involving the ascending colon may have a palpable mass in the right upper or lower quadrants. Perform a digital rectal exam, and check stool for occult blood.

Diagnostic Studies
Check CBC. Perform serial stool sampling for fecal occult blood. Instruct clients to avoid rare red meat, raw vegetable, vitamin C, aspirin, and iron supplements 2 days before testing and until sample collection is completed to avoid false-positive results. Individuals testing positive for fecal occult blood should be referred for a colonoscopy or the combination of a sigmoidoscopy plus air contrast barium enema (Goroll et al., 1995). Perform liver function tests (LFTs) if metastatic disease is suspected.

Carcinoembryonic antigen (CEA) is not sensitive enough to aid in early diagnosis. This blood test is used primarily for monitoring clients before and after treatment to detect metastasis or disease recurrence.

CLINICAL MANAGEMENT

Surgery
Colorectal surgery is currently safe in the elderly, with the mortality rate being less than 10% in most studies (Berger &

Roslyn, 1997). The type of surgery performed, along with the need for an ostomy, depends on the location and extent of the tumor. Curative surgery includes the removal of the malignancy, allowing for adequate surgical margins plus the draining lymphatic nodal basins. Palliative surgery should be used to alleviate distressing symptoms such as obstruction and/or hemorrhage. Approximately 25% to 33% of colorectal cancer patients will develop liver metastasis (Berger & Roslyn, 1997). Twenty-five to thirty-three percent of these patients will have metastases that can be surgically removed (Berger & Roslyn, 1997). Of the elderly patients who undergo liver resection, postoperative mortality remains the same as in younger patients (Fong et al., 1995).

Radiation Therapy
External beam radiation therapy, either pre- or postoperatively, is used as an adjuvant treatment in rectal cancer. Radiation therapy has not been generally used for cancers of the colon. Thirty to fifty percent of rectal cancers that have penetrated the bowel wall will recur locally (Goroll et al., 1995). The application of postoperative radiation has significantly reduced the rate of recurrence.

Chemotherapy
Chemotherapy will be used as an adjuvant to surgery when positive lymph nodes are detected and/or the tumor has penetrated deeply into the bowel wall. Chemotherapy is also indicated for clients with metastases. Common chemotherapeutic agents include fluorouracil with levamisole, leucovorin, methotrexate, or streptozocin.

■ SKIN CANCER

The incidence of basal and squamous cell cancers of the skin rise with age. Sun exposure is the primary risk factor for developing skin cancer. Melanoma of the skin also increases in incidence with advancing age. Nodular melanomas and acral lentiginous melanomas occur more frequently in the aged population.

AGE-RELATED CHANGES

As one ages, there is a 50% decrease in the epidermal turnover rate between the third and seventh decades of life (Timiris, 1994). Basal cells therefore take longer to reach the stratum corneum to be exfoliated. This slowed movement and decreased turnover prolongs the exposure of epidermal cells to carcinogens. This in turn increases an individual's chances of developing skin cancer.

There is a decreased production of melanocytes and Langerhans' cells with age. This contributes to an overall decline in the skin's cell-mediated immunity. The distribution of melanocytes is altered, reducing the protective mechanisms of melanin on the skin. This, combined with the reduced inflammatory warning signs and decreased cell-mediated immunity, increases the risk for skin cancer.

CLINICAL PRESENTATION

Basal Cell Carcinoma

The following three types of basal cell carcinomas may occur:

- Noduloulcerative lesions
    Location: face, forehead, eyelid margins, and nasolabial folds
    Appearance: smooth, translucent papule with telangiectasias over the surface
    Occasionally pigmented. As lesions grow the center will become depressed and ulcerate. The borders become firm and elevated and are pearly in color. May be pigmented in darker-skinned individuals.
- Superficial basal cell carcinoma
    Location: chest and back, several lesions usually present
    Appearance: typically have the appearance of an erythematous plaque. May be oval in shape or irregular. Borders tend to be sharply defined, and slightly elevated. Plaques are lightly pigmented.
- Sclerosing basal cell carcinoma
    Location: head and neck
    Appearance: have the appearance of small patches of scleroderma. Sclerotic, waxy, yellow to white lesions. Borders are indistinct.

Squamous Cell Carcinoma

Often preceded by actinic keratosis (see Chapter 14), squamous cell carcinoma is an invasive skin cancer with metastatic potential.

- Squamous cell cancer in situ or Bowen's disease
    Location: face, ears, dorsa of the hands, forearms, any sun-damaged skin
    Appearance: a chronic, nonhealing, slowly enlarging erythematous patch, usually with a sharp/irregular outline. Lesions may also be flesh-colored nodules

that grow slowly on a firm, indurated base (Foley et al., 1996).

- Advanced squamous cell carcinoma
  Location: as above
  Appearance: a flesh-colored, asymptomatic nodule that may ulcerate and form a cutaneous horn. The lesion may look warty in appearance, dull, or red, and may bleed. Lesion may invade underlying structures. Regional lymph nodes can become involved.

Melanoma

Four types of melanoma exist. Superficial spreading melanoma has an irregular border, with pigmentation pattern and coloration. Colors may include brown, tan, red, white, blue, black, pink, purple, or gray. The nodular type arise independently or within existing nevi and will appear as a blue-black or gray nodule. Lentigo maligna has a marked irregular border and pigmentation pattern and

arise from a freckle-like lesion. Acral lentiginous melanoma will occur on the palms, soles, subungual areas, and mucous membranes. These lesions have the hallmark characteristics of an irregular border and pigment pattern (see Table 13–2).

ASSESSMENT

History

Review the integumentary system and history of sun exposure, as well as the client's profession (does he or she work out of doors?). Assess for history of arsenic exposure, radiodermatitis secondary to x-ray exposure, thermal burns, polycyclic hydrocarbon exposure, mucosal disease, pyogenic ulcers, and human papillomavirus. Assess for personal and family history of basal cell nevus syndrome, dysplastic nevus syndrome, congenital melanocytic nevus, and actinic keratosis. Assess for skin lesions and/or moles that have changed in size or are sore, oozing, cracked, itchy, or bleeding and not healing.

TABLE 13–2. DEFINING CHARACTERISTICS OF MALIGNANT MELANOMA

Type	Characteristics
Superficial spreading	Irregular border, pigmentation pattern, and coloration. Colors may include brown, tan, red, white, blue, black, pink, purple, or gray Irregular surface with elevated nodule Lesion may bleed, ulcerate
Nodular	Arise independently or within existing nevi Polypoidal nodule that is blue-black or gray
Lentigo maligna	Arise from a "freckle-like" lesion Marked irregular border and pigmentation pattern Slow growth, may eventually ulcerate Typically found on the dorsa of the hands, face, and under the fingernails
Acral lentiginous	Hallmark characteristics of irregular border and pigmentation pattern Occur in the subungual areas, mucous membranes, and on the palms or soles of feet

Physical Examination

Perform a skin exam, including hair-covered regions, palms, soles, subungual areas, and mucous membranes. Basal and squamous cell carcinomas can occur in scars left from radiation dermatitis or thermal burns.

Diagnostic Studies

Refer to a physician, dermatologist, or surgeon for biopsy if skin cancer is suspected.

CLINICAL MANAGEMENT

Basal cell carcinoma can be treated with local excision, cryosurgery, electrodesiccation, Mohs' micrographic surgery, and radiation therapy. Individuals who have been diagnosed with one basal cell cancer are at greater risk for developing another one. Annual skin exams should be done to detect new lesions at their earliest stage. Squamous cell carcinoma treatment consists of local excision, cryosurgery, electrodesiccation, and Mohs' micrography surgery. Melanoma treatment includes wide local excision with or without regional lymph node dissection. Surgery may be followed up with radiation therapy, chemotherapy, and/or hormonal therapy. Skin exams should be done every 6 months to yearly to detect new lesions. Family members should be educated regarding their need for skin exams.

■ PAIN IN THE ELDERLY

In the institutionalized elderly, over 70% complain of moderate to severe pain (Ferrell et al., 1990). The prevalence of pain in the elderly population is twice that of the population under age 60 (250/1000 vs. 125/1000) (Crook et al., 1984). Although advances have been made in the area of pain control, the special needs of the elderly continues to be a neglected area.

Several special issues arise when treating the elderly individual with pain. The elderly frequently have multiple sources of pain. The elderly have an increased susceptibility to painful conditions due to normal aging changes and chronic illness. Compression fractures and back pain result from decreased bone mass. Joint pain results from the greater incidence of degenerative joint disease (DJD). A decreased immune system can predispose the individual to herpes zoster, temporal arteritis, and polymyalgia rheumatica. Ischemic limb pain can occur secondary to peripheral vascular disease.

Older individuals tend to have numerous areas and types of pain, all of which need individualized attention. Drug–drug interactions along with drug–disease interactions can also make pain control difficult. Research on pain management in the elderly continues to be rare. Pain management techniques are based primarily on those of a younger population. Misconceptions regarding pain in the elderly are numerous, as can be seen in Table 13–3. These misconceptions place elderly individuals at risk for the undertreatment of their pain.

AGE-RELATED CHANGES

A number of factors alter the pharmacokinetics in the elderly individual. Absorption is altered due to changes in blood flow, decreased gastric motility, and changes in gastric pH. Drug distribution

TABLE 13–3.   MISCONCEPTIONS REGARDING PAIN IN THE ELDERLY

Misconception	Correction
Pain is part of the aging process.	Pain is not a natural part of aging. Complaints of pain should be followed up with careful assessment, diagnosis, and treatment.
Elderly people do not feel pain.	Although elders may have atypical presentations of pain in some conditions, this cannot be generalized to all types of pain.
Narcotic side effects are too dangerous in the elderly.	With careful monitoring and evaluation, narcotics can be safely used in the elderly.
An elder who is easily distracted from pain does not have much pain.	The elderly will learn to divert their attention to activities such as reading, needlepoint, watching TV, or listening to the radio.
Depression causes pain in the elderly.	It is normal to be depressed if you are experiencing chronic, unrelieved pain.
Narcotics should be used only for cancer pain.	Narcotics can be used safely for nonmalignant pain.

Source: Adapted from McCaffery, M. & Beebe, A. (1989). *Pain: Clinical manual for nursing practice.* Philadelphia: C. V. Mosby.

is altered by a decrease in lean body weight, water content, and body mass. Decreased hepatic mass and decreased enzymatic activity causes a decrease in the metabolism of drugs. Elimination is slowed secondary to a decrease in the glomerular filtration rate. Dehydration and cardiac disease may also add to a reduction in renal function (McCaffery & Beebe, 1989).

ASSESSMENT

Cognitive and Sensory Impairments

Numerous issues make pain assessment difficult in the elderly population. Cognitive and sensory impairments may interfere with assessment. The visual analog scale (Acute Pain Management Guideline Panel, 1992) (see Fig. 13–1) has not been validated in the elderly. Reports from family and caregivers regarding

their loved one's physical and emotional changes, which indicate pain or pain relief, may be the only guide the professional has in treating the elder's pain. Observations of a client's change in level of function or behavior become the cornerstone of assessment, such as a change in gait, guarding of a body part, decreased level of activity, diminished ability to perform activities of daily living (ADL), decreased appetite, and increased anxiety or agitation.

········ *vignette* ·····················

Mrs. Riley leans drastically to the right side in her wheelchair. No complaints of pain are offered. She is found to have a 9 × 12-cm mass in the left upper and lower quadrants of the abdomen. The family wished no workup of the tumor, and the client was made "Comfort Mea-

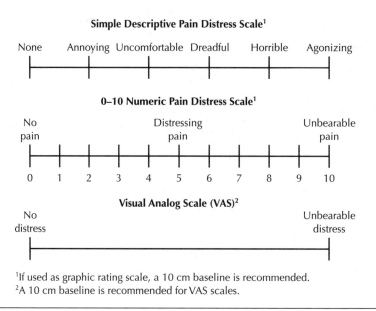

[1]If used as graphic rating scale, a 10 cm baseline is recommended.
[2]A 10 cm baseline is recommended for VAS scales.

Figure 13–1. Pain Distress Scales. *(Source: Acute Pain Management Guideline Panel, 1992.)*

sures Only" status. A pain medication regimen consisting of acetaminophen with codeine (Tylenol #3) one tablet every 4 hours was instituted. Improvement in the woman's posture was seen shortly after starting the pain medication. In addition, her appetite increased slightly and she became more cooperative with transfers.

The vignette points out that in some instances, a pain medication trial should be implemented even though there are no verbal complaints of pain. Her overall improved status after the initiation of the Tylenol #3 leads one to believe that pain was a significant problem.

The elderly client with confusion and pain presents a challenging situation. Some may be able to accurately report their pain, while others will use different words that are unique to the individual. Research on the elderly nursing home population shows that many people with

mild to moderate cognitive impairment are able to reliably report their pain at the moment it is occurring, but once it has passed they are unable to recall the experience (McCaffery & Beebe, 1989). Assessments therefore need to be done frequently, approximately every 1 to 2 hours, to capture data about the pain, as shown in the following example: An elderly client has Alzheimer's disease. After a fall, she described severe pain in her right leg this way, "The head broke off . . . WOW!" When pressed for more information about her pain, she became increasingly unclear in her reports due to significant word-finding difficulty.

Asking detailed questions can lead to frustration and anxiety. Try to keep questions simple. Use of body language can be helpful. For example, while asking, "Does it hurt here?," point to the client's body part; or ask the client to "point to where it hurts."

Underreporting of Pain

Elders may deny that they have pain when asked. Many older people do not use the word "pain" to describe how they are feeling. Words such as achiness, pressure, discomfort, hurt, throbbing, and soreness may better describe the pain, and the individual may be more comfortable and familiar with the terminology.

Some elders may believe that pain is just a natural part of becoming old and that reporting pain or expecting treatment of the pain is inappropriate. Cultural factors may also add to an individual's underreporting of pain. Pain may be underreported and deliberately covered up due to fear of invasive, painful testing, hospitalizations, and increased medical expenses (McCaffery & Beebe, 1989). Individuals may fear the addition of new medications and the need to alter daily routines or living circumstances.

Pain Assessment Tools

Figure 13–2 contains an excellent pain assessment tool developed by McCaffery and Beebe (1989). Aspects that are of particular importance for the elderly client include the following:

1. Location: Document all areas of pain, as the client may be suffering with a number of different types of pain, such as arthritic pain, cancer pain, and pain secondary to peripheral vascular disease.
2. Intensity: Use a numerical scale or the "faces" scale often used with children (Figure 13–3).
3. Quality: Use the client's words—"My hip feels like a creaky old horse."
4. Onset, duration, variation, rhythms: How are daily activities altered?
5. Manner of expressing pain: Can the client readily communicate or

do you need to rely on body language?
6. What relieves the pain: Question old "remedies" used in the past, (menthol creams or ointments, plasters, an alcoholic beverage).
7. What other symptoms accompany the pain: Nausea, diarrhea, increased anxiety, and so on.
8. What activity or activities causes the pain.
9. What would the elder be doing if he or she had no pain or if the pain were reduced? What does the pain prevent the client from doing?

PAIN CONTROL INTERVENTIONS

Three concepts are essential in achieving adequate pain control: (1) use a preventative approach, (2) titrate to effect, and (3) use client-controlled analgesia (McCaffery & Beebe, 1989). For individuals experiencing consistent pain, around-the-clock dosing should be implemented. This preventative approach to pain management will avoid the peaks and troughs that can occur with prn dosing. An oral drug should be used if possible, as it is the most convenient and economical. When oral drugs cannot be taken, use rectal and/or transdermal routes. Intramuscular and subcutaneous drug absorption is highly variable and likely to be diminished due to deconditioning, poor nutrition, or dehydration and diminished peripheral circulation. Doses can then be titrated to effect, respecting the individual's report of pain. Differences can and will occur between clients in their requirements for medications. There is no contraindication for the use of narcotics in the elderly popu-

Date_____

Patient's Name_____ Age_____ Room_____

Diagnosis_____ Physician_____

Nurse_____

I. LOCATION: Patient or nurse mark drawing.

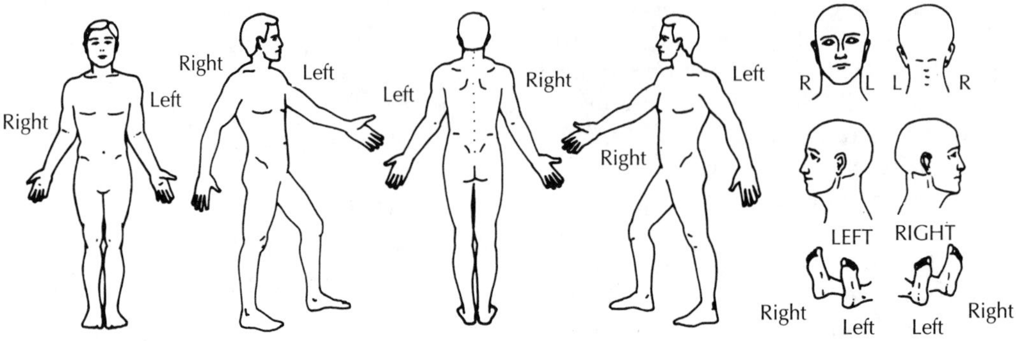

II. INTENSITY: Patient rates the pain. Scale used _____
     Present: _____
     Worst pain gets:_____
     Best pain gets: _____
     Acceptable level of pain: _____

III. QUALTIY: (Use patient's own words, eg, prick, ache, burn, throb, pull, sharp)_____
     _____

IV. ONSET, DURATION VARIATIONS, RHYTHMS: _____
     _____

V. MANNER OF EXPRESSING PAIN: _____
     _____
     _____

VI. WHAT RELIEVES THE PAIN?_____
     _____
     _____

VII. WHAT CAUSES OR INCREASES THE PAIN?_____
     _____
     _____

VIII. EFFECTS OF PAIN: (Note decreased function, decreased quality of life.)
     Accompanying symptoms (e.g. nausea) _____
     Sleep_____
     Appetite _____
     Physical activity_____
     Relationship with others (eg, irritability)_____
     Emotions (eg, anger, suicidal, crying) _____
     Concentration _____
     Other_____

IX. OTHER COMMENTS: _____
     _____

X. PLAN: _____
     _____
     _____

Figure 13–2. Initial pain assessment tool. *(Source: McCaffery, M., & Beebe, A. (1989).* Pain: Clinical manual for nursing practice. *St. Louis: C. V. Mosby. Used with permission.)*

1) Explain to the child that each face is for a person who feels happy because he has no pain (hurt, or whatever word the child uses) or feels sad because he has some or a lot of pain.

2) Point to the appropriate face and state, "This face is...":
0—"very happy because he doesn't hurt at all."
1—"hurts just a little bit."
2—"hurts a little more."
3—"hurts even more."
4—"hurts a whole lot."
5—"hurts as much as you can imagine, although you don't have to be crying to feel this bad."

3) Ask the child to choose the face that best describes how he feels. Be specific about which pain (eg, "shot" or incision) and what time (e.g. now? earlier before lunch?)

Figure 13–3. Wong/Baker Faces Rating Scale. *(Source: Wong, D., & Whaley, L. [1986]. Clinical handbook of pediatric nursing [2nd ed.]. St. Louis: C. V. Mosby. Used with permission.)*

lation. In addition, there is no data supporting the myth that elderly people need lower doses of narcotics (McCaffery & Beebe, 1989). Age should not be used to determine the initial dose, as it has been found that frequency of dosing rather than dosage is affected by age (Kaiko et al., 1982). Dose cannot be accurately calculated by using height, weight, or body surface area either (Bellville et al., 1971). The only safe way to administer analgesics is to monitor the effect a certain dose has on the individual. Ineffective pain control should lead to a rapid titrating upward of a drug, while untoward side effects warrant a decrease in dose. A flow sheet (Fig. 13–4) and daily diary (Fig. 13–5) should be used for all individuals monitoring such parameters as respiratory rate, the individual's pain rating, and dosage of pain medication. Of note, there is *no* ceiling to analgesic dosage with opioids except

to limit adverse effects. Opioid milligrams per client can be increased indefinitely until the desired effect is achieved.

Whenever possible, clients should be encouraged to self-medicate. Pain is subjective, and the client is the authority on his or her pain. When mental status changes make self-administration impossible, caregivers must be keen observers of behavior or functional indicators of pain control.

Non-narcotic Analgesics

Non-narcotic analgesics are often underused and undervalued. Of note is the fact that two aspirin or acetaminophen tablets are equivalent to the pain relief obtained from codeine 30 mg orally, meperidine hydrochloride (Demerol) 50 mg orally, or propoxyphene napsylate (Darvon-N) one tablet.

Combining a non-narcotic with a nar-

Patient_____   Date_____

*Pain rating scale used_____

Purpose: To evaluate the safety and effectiveness of the analgesic(s)

Analgesic(s) prescribed:_____

Time	Pain rating	Analgesic	R	P	BP	Level of arousal	Other†	Plan & comments

*Pain rating: A number of different scales may be used. Indicate which scale is used and use the same one each time. For example, 0–10 (0 = no pain, 10= worst pain).

†Possibilities for other columns: bowel function, activities, nausea and vomitting, other pain relief measures. Identify the side effects of greatest concern to patient, family, physician, nurses.

Figure 13–4. Flow Sheet—Pain. *(Source: McCaffery, M., & Beebe, A. (1989).* Pain: Clinical manual for nursing practice. *St. Louis: C. V. Mosby. Used with permission.)*

Name_____   Date_____

Time	Pain rating scale	Medication type & amount taken	Other pain relief measures tried or anything that influences your pain	Major activity being done: lying sitting standing/walking
12 MIDNIGHT				
1 am				
2				
3				
4				
5				
6				
7				
8				
9				
10				
11				
12 NOON				
1				
2				
3				
4				
5				
6				
7				
8				
9				
10				
11				

Comments: _____

_____

_____

Figure 13–5. Daily diary. *(Source: McCaffery, M., & Beebe, A. (1989). Pain: Clinical manual for nursing practice. St. Louis: C. V. Mosby. Used with permission.)*

cotic can provide safe and effective pain management. In the elderly person, the addition of a non-narcotic analgesic to the narcotic may result in increased analgesia without increasing side effects. This is of particular importance in the elderly population.

Around-the-clock dosing with acetaminophen is a first-line pain control regimen. If not adequate to relieve pain, the addition of salicylates and/or nonsteroidal anti-inflammatory drugs (NSAIDs) may be necessary. Due to the potential GI, central nervous system (CNS), and renal side effects, NSAIDs, acetaminophen, or a combination of acetaminophen with salicylates or NSAIDs is desirable. NSAIDs are an excellent choice for bone pain. When pain persists or increases, an opioid should be added, not substituted, to the NSAID regime.

Older adults using NSAIDs need to be monitored closely for changes in renal function, electrolytes, mental status, hematocrit and hemoglobin, and stool for occult blood.

Narcotic Analgesics

The clearance of morphine plasma levels decreases with age. Elderly clients may be more sensitive to the analgesic effects of opioids, experiencing higher peak effect and longer duration of action. "Start low and go slow" is a good rule of thumb in the dosing and administration of narcotics. See Table 13–4 for equianalgesic charts when switching clients from one narcotic to another.

Oxycodone is used for moderate pain. It is effective when used in combination with acetaminophen (Percocet) or aspirin (Percodan). It is also available alone in an immediate-release tablet and a sustained-release tablet. The usual start-

ing dose is 5 mg orally every 6 hours. When pain has been successfully managed with the immediate-release tablet, the client can then be converted over to the sustained-release preparation for ease of administration. Oxycodone has no ceiling to the maximum 24-hour dose when used alone. When combined with acetaminophen or aspirin, one would need to adhere to the maximum daily doses for those drugs.

Codeine is used for moderate pain. It is potentiated by acetaminophen or aspirin. The usual starting dose is 15 mg orally every 4 hours. As with oxycodone, codeine has no maximum 24-hour dose when used alone.

Morphine is an excellent drug for moderate to severe pain. It has a half-life of 2 to 3 hours and a duration of action of 4 to 6 hours. It can accumulate in clients with renal and/or hepatic impairment. It is available in a wide variety of dosing forms, including immediate-release tablet, sustained-release tablet, oral elixir, parenteral form, and rectal suppositories. There is no ceiling to the maximum 24-hour dose. Patients should be started on immediate-release tablets 10 mg orally every 4 to 6 hours and then converted over to the sustained-release form (duration of action 8 to 12 hours) when pain has been managed. This allows for ease of administration. Sustained-release tablets should always be ordered in combination with immediate-release tablets for breakthrough pain.

Hydromorphone (Dilaudid) is an excellent second choice for moderate to severe pain. It has a half-life of 1 to 3 hours and a duration of action of 4 to 6 hours. There is no ceiling to the maximum 24-hour dose. It is available in tablet, rectal suppository, and parenteral forms. Clients

TABLE 13–4.   EQUIANALGESIC CHART: APPROXIMATE EQUIVALENT DOSES OF IM AND PO ANALGESICS FOR MODERATE AND SEVERE PAIN[a]

Analgesic	IM Route (mg)[b]	PO Route (mg)[c]	Comments
Morphine	10	60 (30)[d]	Both IM and PO doses of morphine have a duration of action of about 4 to 6 hr. Sustained-release tablets, rectal suppositories, and preservative-free spinal analgesia are also available. The PO dose is 3 to 6 times the IM dose. The lower PO dose is suggested by several clinicians and is based on anecdotal evidence, not experimental research; it may be appropriate for some clients, especially elderly clients with chronic cancer pain. *All IM and PO doses in this chart are considered equivalent to 10 mg of IM morphine in analgesic effect.*
Buprenorphine (Buprenex)	0.4 (0.3)	—	A narcotic agonist–antagonist that may precipitate withdrawal in clients *very* physically dependent on narcotics. Dose for the sublingual form (not available in the United States) is 0.8 mg. Compared with morphine, this drug is longer acting and more likely to produce nausea and vomiting. Respiratory depression is rare but serious because it is not readily reversed by naloxone. Not available in Canada.
Butorphanol (Stadol)	2	—	A narcotic agonist–antagonist that may produce withdrawal in clients physically dependent on narcotics. May also produce psychotomimetic effects such as hallucinations. Not available in Canada.
Codeine	130	200	Relatively more toxic in high doses than morphine, causing more nausea and vomiting and considerable constipation. The PO dose is about 1.5 times the IM dose.
Fentanyl (Sublimaze)	0.05	—	Most common use is for anesthesia, given IV. Onset of action when given IM is about 15 min; duration of action, about 90 min. Analgesic effect is not significantly increased by droperidol. Has been used as a substitute for high-dose IV morphine in terminally ill patients when morphine caused excitation. Used IV in neonates and for brief procedures.
Hydromorphone (Dilaudid)	1.5	7.5	Somewhat shorter acting than morphine. Also available as rectal suppository and in high-potency injectable form (10 mg/mL). The PO dose is 5 times the IM dose.

(Continues)

TABLE 13–4.   EQUIANALGESIC CHART: APPROXIMATE EQUIVALENT DOSES OF IM AND PO ANALGESICS FOR MODERATE AND SEVERE PAIN[a] (CONT.)

Analgesic	IM Route (mg)[b]	PO Route (mg)[c]	Comments
Levorphanol (Levo-Dromoran)	2	4	Longer acting than morphine when given in repeated, regular doses. Useful alternative to PO methadone. Careful titration required because drug accumulates; both dose and interval must be adjusted. Onset of action with PO dose occurs within 1 1/2 hr. Because drug accumulates, analgesic effect may increase with repeated doses. *Initial* PO dose is twice the injectable dose. (The SC route is recommended over the IM route.)
Meperidine (Demerol)	75	300	Shorter acting (2 to 4 hr) than morphine. Watch for toxic effects on the central nervous system (CNS) caused by accumulation of the active metabolite normeperidine, which produces neuroexcitability. Use with caution in clients with renal disease. *Because of the risk to the CNS, 300 mg PO is not recommended.* Since normeperidine has a long half-life (15 hr or longer), decreasing the dose in clients exhibiting a toxic reaction may increase CNS excitability, causing seizures. Effects of normeperidine are increased (not reversed) by naloxone. The PO dose is 4 times the IM dose.
Methadone (Dolophine)	10	20	Longer acting than morphine when given in repeated, regular doses. Careful titration required because drug accumulates; both dose and interval must be adjusted. Onset with PO dose occurs within 1 hr. Because drug accumulates, analgesic effect may increase with repeated doses. *Initial* PO dose is twice the IM dose.
Methotrimeprazine (Levoprome)	20	—	A phenothiazine (non-narcotic) drug. Duration of action is 4 to 5 hr. Common adverse effect is hypotension; not recommended for ambulatory clients.
Nalbuphine (Nubain)	10 (20)	—	A narcotic agonist–antagonist that may produce withdrawal in clients physically dependent on narcotics. Longer acting and less likely to cause hypotension than morphine. In doses above 10 mg/70 kg, it causes no additional respiratory depression, so client may be started on a high dose.
Opium (Pantopon, opium tincture)	20 (13.3)	(6 ml)	Infrequently used. Pantopon is the injectable form; opium tincture, the oral form. Pantopon 20 mg equals 10 mg of IM morphine or 15 mg of IM morphine. Opium tincture contains 1% morphine, that is, 0.6 mL equals 6 mg of PO morphine. Therefore 6 mL equals 60 mg of PO morphine.

TABLE 13–4.   EQUIANALGESIC CHART: APPROXIMATE EQUIVALENT DOSES OF IM AND PO ANALGESICS FOR MODERATE AND SEVERE PAIN[a] (CONT.)

Analgesic	IM Route (mg)[b]	PO Route (mg)[c]	Comments
Oxycodone	—	30 (15)	Has faster onset and higher peak effect than most PO narcotics; duration of action is up to 6 hr. In one study of postoperative pain, a preparation similar to the old formulation of Percodan (containing oxycodone, aspirin, phenacetin, and caffeine) was more effective and caused fewer adverse reactions than 90 mg of PO codeine or 75 mg of PO pentazocine, and was almost equivalent to 12.5 mg of IM morphine.
Oxymorphone (Numorphan)	1 (1.5)	—	Also available as rectal suppository; 10 mg given rectally equals 10 mg of IM morphine. Up to 1.5 mg IM is now recommended as equal to 10 mg of IM morphine.
Pentazocine (Talwin)	60	180	Narcotic agonist–antagonist that may produce withdrawal in clients physically dependent on narcotics. Could produce psychotomimetic effects. The PO dose is 3 times the IM dose.
Propoxyphene HCl (Darvon)	—	500	The one recognized use is for mild to moderate pain unrelieved by non-narcotics. *Never give as much as 500 mg PO;* only low PO doses (65 to 130 mg) are recommended. The IM form is not available in the United States.

[a] The equianalgesic doses in this chart are based primarily on recommendations of the Analgesic Study Section, Sloan-Kettering Institute for Cancer Research, New York, based on double-blind analgesic research. This format is adapted from McCaffery, M. (1987). A practical, portable chart of equianalgesic doses. *Nursing, 17* 56–57.
[b] Based on clinical experience, many consider the IM and IV dose equianalgesic. However, some recommend using one-half the IM dose for the IV dose.
[c] Initial PO doses are usually lower than those listed here, especially for mild to moderate pain.
[d] Values in parentheses refer to differences of opinion among clinicians.
A guide to using the equianalgesic chart:
- Equianalgesic means *approximately* the same pain relief. Onset, peak effect, and duration of analgesia for each drug often differ and may also vary with individual people.
- Variability among individuals may be due to differences in absorption, organ dysfunction, or tolerance to one narcotic and not to another.
- An equianalgesic chart is a *guideline.* The individual client's response must be observed. Doses and intervals between doses are then titrated according to the individual's response.
- An equianalgesic chart is helpful when (1) switching from one drug to another or (2) switching from one route of administration to another.
- Dosages in this chart are *not* necessarily starting doses. They suggest the *ratio* for comparing the analgesia of one drug with another.
- Based on clinical experience, the IV dose is approximately the same as the IM dose. Dose adjustments are then made according to the individual's response. Some clinicians suggest approximately one-half the IM dose equals the IV dose.

Source: Adapted from McCaffery, M., & Beebe, A. (1989). *Pain: Clinical manual for nursing practice.* St. Louis: C. V. Mosby. Used with permission.

should be started on 1 mg intravenously or 4 mg orally every 4 to 6 hours.

Methadone and levorphanol tartrate (Levo-Dromoran) are narcotics with long half-lives and delayed toxicity. Effective titration of these drugs is difficult. Methadone's half-life is 24 hours, and Levo-Dromoran's half-life is from 12 to 16 hours. Both are poor drug choices for the elderly, as the plasma levels of these drugs rise over many days. As a result, delayed toxicity may be encountered.

Transdermal fentanyl is currently the only opioid available for transdermal use. It is 100 times more potent than morphine. Each patch contains a 72-hour supply of drug, which is passively absorbed by the skin over 12 to 18 hours. The elimination half-life is 21 hours, making transdermal fentanyl unsuitable for rapid dose titration. The fentanyl patch should be considered when clients already on opioid therapy have relatively constant pain with infrequent episodes of breakthrough pain, such that rapid increases or decreases in pain intensity are not anticipated. Patients should *not* be started on this drug as a first-line defense against pain. Titration should be made three days after the initial dose. The use of breakthrough medication should be encouraged during times of increased pain (see Table 13–5).

Narcotic Side Effects

Respiratory Depression. Respiratory depression can occur in individuals who are just beginning opioid therapy or in individuals with pulmonary disease. Respiratory depression is not a common side effect in those who have been on long-term opioid therapy. In these instances, individuals usually develop a tolerance to the respiratory-depressant effects of the opioid (Jacox et al., 1994). Occasionally, respiratory depression can occur once a client's pain has been relieved, as the sedative effects of the opioid are no longer opposed by the constant pain (Hanks et al., 1981).

Many clinicians are concerned that high doses of narcotics will cause harm or even death to their clients. It is important to remember that when death is imminent due to the progression of disease, the benefit of pain relief and painless death outweighs increased risk of earlier death. It is at this time that the clinician has the ethical duty to relieve pain by increasing the doses to provide pain relief.

Constipation. Constipation is a commonly occurring side effect associated with the use of opioids. Tolerance to this side effect generally does not occur; therefore, bowel regimens are mandatory. Mild constipation can be relieved by addition of fiber and a mild laxative such as magnesium hydroxide (Milk of Magnesia). When constipation is severe, stimulating cathartic drugs such as senna (Senokot) (1 to 2 tablets bid) are added to the above regimen as necessary. Individuals should also be assessed for common conditions that cause constipation (eg, ileus, dehydration, anorexia). The above processes may add to the constipating effects of the opioids.

Confusion (Delirium). Occasionally, confusion occurs with opioid therapy. Try not to immediately blame the narcotic, as polypharmacy, multiple medical problems, and age-related changes may also contribute to the confusion the client is displaying. Therefore, all drugs and their interactions and physical causes such as

TABLE 13–5. TRANSDERMAL FENTANYL: ADVANTAGES AND DISADVANTAGES

Advantages	Disadvantages
Convenient	Fever or external heat (waterbed, heating pad) can increase absorption from patch
Continuous delivery system	Lag period of 12–18 hr
Single application can maintain plasma levels for up to 72 hr	Persistent effect 12–18 hr after patch is removed
Useful for clients with impaired alimentary function or access	Opioid side effects possible
Lack of bowel contact makes it less constipating than other opiates	Not for pediatric clients, postoperative pain, or clients with unstable pain

electrolyte imbalance, disease progression, and metastasis should be explored as explanations for the delirium.

Nausea and Vomiting. When individuals complain of nausea and vomiting after opioid administration, it is often helpful to begin antiemetics on a fixed schedule for several days. After this, as-needed dosage is usually adequate. This should not be viewed as an adverse reaction, but rather as a side effect that can be effectively managed.

Tolerance. Over time, a given dose of narcotic loses its effectiveness necessitating larger doses to manage pain. The first indication of tolerance is decreased duration of action followed by decreased analgesic effect (Jaffe, 1985). Tolerance does not indicate addiction.

Adjuvant Analgesics

Adjuvant analgesics are drugs that are not specifically classified as analgesics but are used alone or in combination with other analgesics to effectively relieve pain.

Tricyclic Antidepressants

Tricyclic antidepressants (TCAs) are presumed to increase efficacy of endogenous antinociceptive pathways. The mechanisms of pain relief include mood elevation, potentiation or enhancement of opioid analgesia, and direct analgesic effect. Tricyclic antidepressants are especially useful when treating neuropathic pain, as well as pain caused by surgery, chemotherapy, and nerve infiltration.

Amitriptyline is used most frequently as an adjuvant pain medication. Amitriptyline should be started at 10 to 25 mg at bedtime and increased by 10 to 25 mg every 2 to 4 days until a maximum of 150 mg/d has been reached. Side effects include sedation, dry mouth, urinary retention, visual changes, and orthostatic hypotension. Agitation can occur in some clients.

Anticonvulsants

Anticonvulsants are useful for neuropathic pain, especially the type that produces a burning, lancinating, or shooting pain. Drugs used are phenytoin (Dilantin), carbamazepine (Tegretol), valproic acid, and gabapentin (Neurotin). They suppress spontaneous neuronal firing and are used to control lancinating pain. Doses of the above medications are the same as with anticonvulsant therapy, and serum levels should be checked monthly in the stable client.

Steroids

Steroids can be added to opioids for the management of pain in brachial or lumbosacral plexopathy. Dexamethasone (16 to 24 mg/d) or prednisone (40 to 100 mg/d) can be added to the existing pain management regimen (Jacox et al., 1994). Steroids are also beneficial in the management of cancer cachexia/anorexia in terminal illness and can re-

duce cerebral/spinal cord edema in the emergency treatment of increased intracranial pressure. Side effects include myopathy, hyperglycemia, weight gain, and dysphoria.

Adjuvant Medications

Adjuvant medications are drugs which treat symptoms that commonly accompany pain.

Anxiolytic Sedatives

Anxiolytic sedatives are used to ease the anxiety associated with pain. Lorazepam (Ativan) and alprazolam (Xanax) are given in the same doses recommended for antianxiety and or sedation.

 CASE STUDY

Mrs. Allison was an 89-year-old white female with a history of paranoid schizophrenia, which was well controlled on haloperidol (Haldol). She detected a lump in her breast while bathing. She was erroneously encouraged by the fact that it did not hurt when she pressed on it. On inspection, a 3-cm lump (hard, nonmobile, nontender) was found, with the overlying skin having a peau d'orange appearance. She had not been offered a mammogram by her primary-

care practitioner. On biopsy, the mass was found to be cancerous. She underwent a lumpectomy followed by radiation therapy.

Approximately a year and a half later, Mrs. Allison became increasingly paranoid and disoriented. Her primary-care physician referred her to her psychiatrist, who increased her Haldol without effect. Four months later, Mrs. Allison was diagnosed with metastatic cancer to the brain and died shortly thereafter.

QUESTIONS

1. What health maintenance/promoting issues are involved in Mrs. Allison's case?

2. Could Mrs. A's disorientation and paranoia be handled differently? If so, how?

ANSWERS

1. Mrs. Allison discovered her lump through self-exam while bathing. It is not clear whether she engaged in this practice regularly, but the practice needs to be encouraged in all older women. Mrs. Allison was falsely reassured that her lump was benign because it was nontender. It should be emphasized that *all* lumps need to be evaluated. Education of health-care providers regarding screening mammograms is needed. Mrs. Allison's age should not be a factor for screening.

2. Acute changes in mental status, especially in older individuals, need to be evaluated. Given that her Haldol was increased without effect, investigation into possible reversible causes (other meds, metabolic/endocrine disorders, metastasis/other space-occupying lesions) is warranted. There is nothing normal about cognitive and functional impairment in older adults.

■ REFERENCES

Acute Pain Management Guideline Panel. (1992). *Acute pain management: Operative or medical procedures and trauma.* Clinical Practice Guideline. AHCPR Pub. No. 920032. Rockville, MD: Agency for Health Care Policy and Research, U.S. Department of Health and Human Services, Public Health Service.

American Cancer Society. (1997). *Cancer facts and figures—1997*, Atlanta, GA.

Bellville, J. W., Forrest, W. H., Miller, E., & Brown, B. W. (1971). Influence of age on pain relief from analgesics. *JAMA, 217,* 1835–1841.

Benson, M. C. (1997). Prostate specific antigen. *J Urol, 157,* 2197–2198.

Berger, D. H. and Roslyn, J. J. (1997). Cancer surgery in the elderly. *Clin Geriatr Med, 13*(1), 119–139.

Byers, T. (1994). Nutritional risk factors for breast cancer. *Cancer, 74*(1), 288–293.

Chlebowski, R. T., Butler, J., Nelson, A., et al. (1993). Breast cancer chemoprevention. Tamoxifen: Current issues and future prospective. *Cancer, 72,* 1032–1037.

Claus, E. B., Schildkraut, J. M., Thompson, W. D., et al. (1996). The genetic attributable risk of breast and ovarian cancer. *Cancer, 77,* 2318–2324.

Cohen, L. B. (1996). Colorectal cancer: A primary care approach to screening. *Geriatrics, 51,*(12), 45–49.

Costanza, M. E. (1994). The extent of breast cancer screening in older women. *Cancer, 74,* 2046–2049.

Crook, J., Rideout, E., & Browne, G. (1984). The prevalence of pain complaints in a general population. *Pain, 18*(3), 299–314.

Ferrell, B. A., Ferrell, B. R., & Osterweil, D. (1990). Pain in the nursing home. *J Am Geriatr Soc, 38*(4), 409–414.

Foley, M., Schilling, J., & Tscheschlog, B. (1996). *Handbook of diseases.* Springhouse, PA: Springhouse Corporation.

Fong, Y., Blumgart, L. H., Fortner, J. G., & Brennan, M. F. (1995). Pancreatic or liver resection is safe and effective for the elderly. *Ann Surg, 222,* 426.

Francis, J. (1992). Delirium in older patients. *J Am Geriatr Soc, 40,* 829–838.

Goroll, A. H., May, L. A., & Mulley, A. G. (1995). *Primary care medicine.* Philadelphia, PA: J. B. Lippincott.

Groenwald, S., Frogge, M., Goodman, M., & Yarbro, C. (Eds.). *Cancer nursing: Principles and practice.* Boston: Jones and Bartlett.

Hanks, G. W., Twycross, R. G., & Lloyd, J. W. (1981). Unexpected complication of successful nerve block. Morphine induced respiratory depression precipitated by removal of severe pain. *Anaesthesia, 36*(1), 37–39.

Herr, H. W. (1997). Quality of life in prostate cancer patients. *CA: A Cancer Journal for Clinicians, 47*(4), 207–217.

Hortobagyi, G. N. (1995). Management of breast cancer: Status and future trends. *Sem Oncol, 22*(12), 108–116.

Jacox, A., Carr, D. B., Payne, R., et al. (1994). *Management of cancer pain.* Clinical Practice Guidelines No. 9. AHCPR Publication No 94-0592. Rockville MD: Agency for Health Care Policy and Research, U.S. Department of Health and Human Services, Public Health Service, March.

Jaffe, J. H. (1985). Drug addiction and drug abuse. In Gilman, A. G., Goodman, L. S., Rall, T. W., & Murad, F. (Eds.). *The pharmacological basis of therapeutics.* (7th ed.). New York: Macmillan.

Kaiko, R. F., Wallenstein, S. L., Rogers, A., et al. (1982). Narcotics in the elderly. *Med Clin North Am, 66,* 1079–1089.

Kennedy, B. J., & Cohen, H. J. (1996). Geriatric oncology. *Cancer, 77*(6), 1017–1019.

Littrup, P. J. (1994). Prostate cancer screening: Appropriate choices? *Cancer, 74*(7), 2016–2022.

Mandelblatt, J. S., & Phillips, R. N. (1996).

Cervical cancer: How often—and why—to screen older women. *Geriatrics, 51*(6), 45–48.

McCaffery, M., & Beebe, A. (1989). *Pain: Clinical manual for nursing practice.* Philadelphia: C. V. Mosby.

McKenna, R. J. (1994). Clinical aspects of cancer in the elderly. *Cancer, 74*(7), 2107–2115.

Montie, J. E., & Meyers, S. E. (1997). Defining the ideal tumor marker for prostate cancer. *Urol Clin North Am, 24*(2), 247–252.

Newschaffer, C. J., Penberthy, L., Desch, C. C., et al. (1996). The effect of age and comorbidity in the treatment of elderly with nonmetastatic breast cancer. *Arch Intern Med, 156,* 85–90.

Olmi, P., et al. (1997). Radiotherapy in the aged. *Clin Geriatr Med, 13*(1), 143–163.

Parker, S. L., Tong, T., Bolden, S., & Wingo, P. A. (1997). Cancer statistics. *CA: A Cancer Journal for Clinicians, 47*(1), 5–27.

Rimer, B. K. (1994). Interventions to increase breast screening. *Cancer, 74*(1), 323–327.

Schonwetter, R. S. (1992). Geriatric oncology. *Primary Care, 19*(3), 451–463.

Stenman, U. H. (1997). Prostate specific antigen, clinical use and staging: An overview. *Br J Urol, 79*(1), 53–60.

Timiris, P. (Ed.). (1994). *Physiological basis of aging and geriatrics.* Ann Arbor, MI: CRC Press.

Weinrich, S., & Sarna, L. (1994). Delirium in the older person with cancer. *Cancer, 74*(7), 2079–2088.

White, J. E., Begg, L., Fishman, N.W., et al. (1993). Increasing cervical cancer screening among minority elderly. *J Gerontol Nurs, 19*(5), 28–34.

14

INTEGUMENTARY ISSUES

Lori J. O'Connor

■ INTRODUCTION

The skin is the largest organ in the body, covering 300 square inches of body surface area, weighing approximately 6 pounds, and receiving one third of the body's circulating blood supply. The skin provides the human body with a number of key functions. It defines who we are, helps to maintain thermoregulation, synthesizes vitamin D, supports underlying body surfaces, and provides us protection from the environment and infectious organisms. This chapter will focus on the most common skin disorders that a practicing clinician may encounter when caring for an older adult in a variety of settings.

■ INTEGUMENTARY CHANGES IN AGING SKIN

It is common knowledge that our skin changes with age. Age-related changes and clinical implications are outlined in Table

14–1. Although research in this area has greatly increased in the last 10 years, the distinction between age-associated skin changes and environmental damage from chemical or mechanical wear and tear is unclear. From a clinical perspective, research has concluded that a distinct difference exists between skin that has aged because of exposure to the environment, known as "photoaging," and that of the aging process itself (Kligman, 1986). These findings provide clinicians with a framework of care based on two broad concepts:

1. Changes in skin do not necessarily represent normal aging.
2. Prevention and early detection of various skin conditions can enhance quality of life and prevent increased morbidity and mortality.

ASSESSMENT

The assessment process of the integumentary system in an older adult is similar in format to that of other age groups.

TABLE 14–1.   PHYSIOLOGIC CHANGES AND CLINICAL IMPLICATIONS OF AGING SKIN

Physiologic Change	Clinical Implication
The dermis undergoes structural changes in elastic fibers. This is especially pronounced on sun-exposed areas. Atrophy of the subcutaneous tissue occurs.	These changes cause sagging of the skin and contribute to underlying tissue injury following trauma. This condition is most visible on the hands and forearms. There may be an increased prevalence of foot ulcerations due to loss of subcutaneous tissue.
The dermis becomes relatively avascular.	The patient appears pale. There is a decrease in surface temperature. A decrease in perception of temperature changes occur.
The dermis is slower in clearing foreign material. This leads to a blunted inflammatory response. There is a delay in the immune response.	These changes result in an increased incidence of contact dermatitis. Older adults develop blisters and wheals more readily. There is a potential delay in patch test reactions. Immune changes may result in an increase risk of infections and malignancy.
There is a decrease in nail plate thickness.	The nails are pink in color, and vasculature is easily visible in the nail bed. Nails may break and frequently become soft and fragile.
There is a decline in melanocytes.	Graying hair develops. Tanning becomes more uneven. There is a possible increased risk of skin cancers.
There is a decline in pacinian and Meissner cutaneous organ receptors which are responsible for touch and pressure.	There is an increased risk of serious injury. The patient may lack the ability to report sensation of burning associated with pressure ulcers.
There are changes in both eccrine and apocrine glands.	The sweating response is diminished. Changes in gland secretion may contribute to xerosis and thermoregulatory alteration.
There is a decrease in androgen–testosterone levels.	This causes coarseness in the texture of the hair. Additional hairs develop on eyebrows, nose, and ears.
There is a decreased epidermal turnover, decrease in tensile strength, delay in cell proliferation, decline in collagen remodeling and wound reepithelization.	Wound healing is prolonged. There is a possible increase in the risk of secondary infections.
There is a decreased ability to produce vitamin D.	This change may contribute to osteomalacia.

Source: Fenske & Lober; Kurban & Kurban, 1993; Grove, 1989.

A suggested format for evaluation is outlined in Table 14–2. A general review of the persons overall health is essential in identifying previous medical and family history associated with integumentary changes. Skin cancer, as well as diseases affecting the endocrine, renal, and hepatic systems, may all present with various skin conditions. Adequate lighting is essential during the skin examination. The use of a microscope called an Episcope is helpful in illuminating the skin surface. This provides a close-up look at skin lesions.

Environmental and Photoaging Changes

Both the physical environment and the individual's genetic makeup are responsible for the variety of skin changes reflecting the aging process. Among the most common features of aging skin are wrinkling, yellowing, and changes in texture. Frequently observed benign sun-induced lesions are discussed later in this chapter. In general, it is well documented that environmental exposure takes many years to accumulate and cause visible skin damage. Research into photoaging has demonstrated that the use of sunscreens and avoidance of sun will limit further damage. Therefore, older adults should be provided with preventive health information such as avoiding the sun during the more intense times of the season and day and using a sunscreen of at least sun protection factor (SPF)-15 in strength.

Cosmetic Effects

Dermatologic cosmetic research has become an explosive industry. This is partially based on our culture's preoccupation with a youthful appearance and driven by aging statistics. Population de-

TABLE 14–2.   GUIDE FOR ASSESSING THE INTEGUMENTARY SYSTEM

Present complaint	Reason for visit: Onset, course, local symptoms
	Treatment of current and past:
	    Systemic symptoms
	    Symptoms of remission or exacerbations

Skin-care practices	Frequency of bathing, lack of bathing facilities Past and present exposure to sun Soaps, lotions, emollients
Patient profile	Occupational history and chemical exposure Hobbies, life-style, travel history Family history, ethnic background, genetic history
Appearance of skin	Skin changes, itching, warmth, color, turgor Lesion's appearance past and present
Past medical history	Chronic disease History of allergic reactions Previous type of lesions Contact with individuals with similar skin conditions Nutritional deficits
Drug history	Medication, including prescription and over-the-counter

mographics predict that 22% of the U.S. population will be over 65 by the year 2025. Many of the products advertised to reverse the signs of aging skin are simply expensive moisturizers. Topical 8% glycolic acid and 8% L-lactic acid creams have been shown to reduce the signs of chronic cutaneous photo damage and are available without a prescription. Tretinoin 1%, and recently estrogen, have shown promise in the treatment of photoaging (Weiss et al., 1988; Dunn et al., 1997). Older adults should receive education regarding the effectiveness of cosmetic products and the need for routine daily skin inspection. There remains a therapeutic role for routine cosmetic makeovers, which may positively impact self-image (Kligman & Graham, 1989).

NONCANCEROUS SKIN LESIONS/CONDITIONS

There are a variety of skin lesions that frequently occur in older adults that are noncancerous. Many of the lesions are due to a lifetime of sun exposure. Table 14–3 outlines assessment and management of these various lesions.

■ PRURITUS

Pruritus is a fairly common symptom in the elderly and can result from a host of local conditions that are rather irritating but nevertheless benign. In approximately 10% to 50% of patients who report generalized pruritus, a serious underlying medical condition was found to coexist (Gilchrest, 1986). Itching, regardless of its cause, can have an adverse effect on daily function. Frequently, the

sleep pattern is interrupted and this may lead to irritability and mental status changes. Older adults commonly seek advice from family and friends. Therefore, the pruritus may be exacerbated by a variety of home remedies. Certain health conditions or social circumstances such as psychiatric disorders, cognitive impairment, limited income, embarrassment, or lack of education may further delay medical care. When itching is prolonged, a chronic itch–scratch cycle occurs, which may contribute to secondary skin infection and makes diagnosis more difficult. Table 14–4 lists conditions which cause itching without subsequent rash.

vignette

Mrs. Smith is an 86-year-old woman who resides in a nursing facility. She has dementia and is unable to communicate. The main complaint of the nursing staff is that Mrs. Smith continues to scratch at multiple seborrheic lesions on her back, rendering most of her clothes and sheets bloody. Mrs. Smith is bathed daily because of both urine and stool incontinence. The nursing staff have placed mitts on Mrs. Smith's hands because she continues to scratch. Mrs. Smith has become quite agitated, especially at night, and psychiatry has prescribed an anxiolytic prn for agitation and a hypnotic at night for sleep.

This case illustrates how irritated seborrheic lesions, compounded by low humidity and drying soaps, may lead to the potential iatrogenic effects, including restraints, agitation, insomnia, polypharmacy, and potential skin infections. The clinician should consider the use of a

TABLE 14–3. NONCANCEROUS SKIN LESIONS

Condition & Description	Assessment	Clinical Management	Other Considerations
■ SENILE LENTIGOS Termed liver spots, solar lentigos, or senile freckles. *Description:* Well-defined hyperpigmented tan to dark brown macular benign lesions presenting on exposed areas such as the back of the hands and forearms of older adults. *Size:* The lesions can range in size from 1 mm to 2 mm.	Differentiate from lentigo maligna, which have irregular borders and variation in pigmentation. These lesions are generally found on the face. Lentigo maligna are melanoma in situ and require aggressive treatment and close dermatologic follow-up.	If the lesions are felt to be cosmetically unpleasant, the client should be referred to a dermatologist for removal. *Pharmacologic:* Treatment with topical tretinoin has also been found to fade the color of the lesion. *Nonpharmacologic:* The current treatment is removal by liquid nitrogen.	
■ SKIN TAGS Also known as fibro-epithelial polyp or acrochordons. They are benign, fleshy, penduculated papules frequently found on the neck, upper eyelid, and intertriginous areas of the body.	Skin tags increase in number up to age 50 and are readily identified by direct observation.	Skin tags are benign lesions and do not require treatment. *Nonpharmacologic:* Cosmetic treatment includes scissor excision or electro-desiccation by a dermatologist.	*Client education:* The literature identifies an association between skin tags and an increase in colon cancer. Although this association is not necessarily agreed upon by all clinicians, enough evidence to support the following preventative health monitoring exists. Current treatment recommendations include: 1. Obtain a stool for occult blood. 2. Referral for flexible sigmoidoscopy if a family history of the colon cancer is reported (Habif, 1990).

(Continues)

TABLE 14–3. NONCANCEROUS SKIN LESIONS (CONT.)

Condition & Description	Assessment	Clinical Management	Other Considerations

■ **ACTINIC KERATOSIS** (see Figure 1 of Color Plate within this chapter)

Condition & Description	Assessment	Clinical Management	Other Considerations
Acitinic keratoses, also termed solar keratoses, are precancerous lesions. *Location:* Sun-exposed areas of the body. The face, forehead, ears, hands, and the heads of bald men are common sites. *Size:* The lesions can range from a few millimeters to 1 cm in size. *Description:* Color range—tan to red; well-demarcated; scaly, gritty, rough surface. A yellow crust will eventually form, and the lesion will bleed when the crust is removed. (see color plate) *Variations:* The lesions are more common in light-skinned individuals and are rarely found in the black population.	Differentiate from rough, dry, or unevenly tanned skin. A history of sun exposure is usually elicited and a previous history of skin cancers is common. Approximately 12%–25% of actinic keratosis lesions will progress to squamous cell cancer (Lin et al., 1989). (See Chapter 13 for a discussion of skin cancer in older adults.)	Determined by the extent of the lesion and the client's overall physical health and functional ability. *Pharmacologic:* Treatments include the use of retinoid creams, high concentration of alpha-hydroxy acids, and 5-fluorouracil. *Nonpharmacologic:* Dermatologic interventions include cryotherapy, curettage, and electrodesiccation.	*Client education:* The lesions are closely associated with sun exposure, and the client should be educated on avoiding the sun, regular use of a sunscreen, and the precancerous nature of the lesion. Topical treatments are expensive and may be discontinued before a beneficial effect is delivered.

■ **SEBORRHEIC KERATOSIS**

Condition & Description	Assessment	Clinical Management	Other Considerations
Description: Seborrheic keratoses are benign lesions. Frequent areas are reported to be on the back, chest, and face. *Color:* Lesions vary in color from light brown to dark brown/black. The surface of the lesion can take on a greasy, crusty, bumpy ap-	Consider size, shape, color, number, adherence to the skin, and effect on daily function (eg, rubbing on clothing) and personal apearance. Lesions that are repeatedly irritated by clothing or suspicious should be considered for dermatologic removal.	Seborrheic keratoses are benign lesions that are relatively common in the elderly, developing in middle age, and generally do not require treatment. *Nonpharmacologic:* Seborrheic keratosis can be a great source of annoyance for older adults. Coup-	A large number of lesions upward of one to several hundred tend to run in families (Shelley & Shelley, 1982). A sudden proliferation of lesions could be indicative of an underlying neoplastic condition known as Leser–Trelat sign.

TABLE 14–3.   NONCANCEROUS SKIN LESIONS (CONT.)

Condition & Description	Assessment	Clinical Management	Other Considerations
■ SEBORRHEIC KERATOSIS (CONT.)			
pearance (see Fig. 14–1). *Size:* The lesions may range from 2 mm to 4 cm. *Atypical presentation:* Several variant forms of seborrheic keratosis exist. Stucco keratoses are white plaques which can be frequently found on the extremities of older adults. Dermatosis papulosa nigra is a smaller, dark lesion, primarily found in large numbers on the face of dark-skinned individuals.	The variations of the presentation of the lesion frequently make them difficult to distinguish between melanomas and basal cell carcinomas.	led with drying skin, the lesions itch, crack, and bleed. This may be particularly problematic in individuals who reside in nursing homes, where their skin may be exposed to harsh, irritating soaps and low environmental humidity (see clinical management of pruritis). Liquid nitrogen, curettage, or light electrodesiccation. *Pharmacology:* Early dermatologic treatment includes the use of alpha-hydroxy acid cream.	This proliferation of lesions is frequently accompanied by pruritis (Holdiness, 1988).
■ CHERRY ANGIOMAS			
Cherry angiomas are also called DeMorgan's spots, senile angiomas, or senile hemangiomas. *Description:* Cherry-red benign lesions *Size:* From 0.5 to 5 mm and are caused by vascular malformation.	The lesions are most frequent on the trunk, but may be present on the extremities, and are common in individuals over the age of 40.	*Nonpharmacologic:* The lesions are benign and do not require treatment unless requested by the client. Successful treatment by a dermatologist includes shave excision, electrodesiccation, and cryosurgery.	
■ VENOUS LAKES			
Venous lakes are dark blue, raised lesions caused by a dilated, blood-filled venous channel (see Figure 14–2). They are seen primarily on the lips, ears, and face of older adults.	Venous lake lesions are easily identifiable by direct observation. If trauma occurs to the direct area, they may bleed.	*Nonpharmacologic:* Treatment if desired by the client includes the use of electrodesiccation, and shave excision by a dermatologist.	

(Continues)

TABLE 14–3. NONCANCEROUS SKIN LESIONS (CONT.)

Condition & Description	Assessment	Clinical Management	Other Considerations
■ SENILE PURPURA Also called Bateman's purpura. *Description:* Dark red areas that occur over the forearms or hands of older adults. The lesions result from a thinning of the dermis and underlying shearing and subsequent trauma to the blood vessels. These lesions may occur with little or no trauma.	A history should include evidence of bleeding disorders or recent trauma. The use of steroids thins the subcutaneous tissue and predisposes individuals to this condition. *Laboratory values:* Evaluation of a completed blood count and liver profile is necessary to rule out any bleeding abnormalities.	There is no required clinical treatment for this condition. Protection of the hands may include the use of gloves.	*Setting-specific issues:* Protection to the hands and arms of clients in long-term care facilities may include the use of geri-gloves.
■ ROSACEA Rosacea is an inflammation of the face, involving the nose, cheeks, chin, and forehead. If the eye is involved, conjunctivitis, blepharitis, and iritis may occur. The typical presentation is one of erythema and telangiectasis with papules and pustules) frequently mistaken for acne). Nasal involvement that leads to hypertrophy is termed rhinophyma and is more commonly seen in men.	The condition occurs most frequently in individuals over the age of 30, in women and light-skinned individuals. The cause of rosacea is unknown; however, reactions to follicular mites and increased production of sebum have been implicated. The condition is cyclic and comes and goes. There have been reports of a correlation of *Helicobacter pylori* with rosacea, but no conclusive research studies were found (Parish & Witkowski, 1995).	*Pharmacologic:* Topical hydrocortisone, topical metrogel, oral tetracycline, and metronidazole are all common treatments. *Nonpharmacologic:* The clinician should consult with the physician or refer to a dermatologist for treatment of more complicated cases. Rhinophyma has also been treated with scalpel excision or skin grafts.	*Client education:* Ingestion of hot liquids, alcohol, exposure to sunlight, and stress exacerbate the symptoms. A delay or lack of treatment may result in progression of the condition.

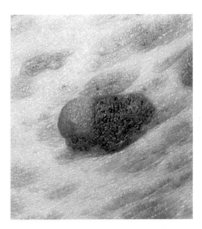

Figure 14–1. Seborrheic Keratosis. *(Source: Bondi, E., Jegasothy, B., & Lazarus, G. [1991]. Dermatology diagnosis and therapy. [p. 393]. East Norwalk: Appleton & Lange, Used with permission.)*

superfatted soap for bathing. In Mrs. Smith's case, the use of a low-dose topical steroid might have alleviated the itch–scratch cycle and subsequent iatrogenic effects.

■ DERMATOSES

XEROSIS

Xerosis, also known as asteatotic eczema, is quite common in older adults and is reported to occur in 59% to 85% of older adults (Hardy, 1996). Presentation depends on the severity of the condition, but the skin is characteristically dry and scaly. Common sites include the legs, back, and arms. In more severe cases, superficial fissuring and erythema of the epidermis known as eczema craquelè (French for "marred with cracks") occurs primarily on the lower legs (Kleinsmith & Perricone, 1989).

Age-related Changes

No single factor is currently identified as the cause of dry skin. Aging changes that are believed to contribute to dry skin are outlined in Table 14–1. Physiologically, a

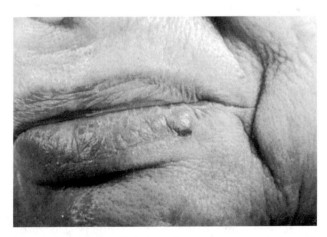

Figure 14–2. Venous lake. A dilated blood-filled channel typically seen on the lower lip. *(Source: Habif, T. P. [1996]. Clinical dermatology: A color guide to diagnosis and therapy, 3rd ed. St. Louis: Mosby-Yearbook. Used with permission.)*

TABLE 14–4. CAUSES OF PRURITUS WITHOUT RASH

Occult skin disease	Irritant contact dermatitis: soaps, fiberglass, dusts, fumes
	Allergic contact dermatitis: early posion ivy or other allergens
	Infestation: scabies, pubic lice, head lice, body lice
	Xerosis
	Urticaria
Systemic reactions to drugs or chemicals	Allergic reactions (including urticaria) ·
	Pharmacologic reaction: heparin, narcotic withdrawal, drugs causing flushing (eg, nicotinic acid)
Occult systemic disease	Diabetes mellitus, biliary obstruction, uremia, lymphoma, leukemias, polycythemia, carcinoid syndrome, hyper- and hypothyroidism
Psychogenic disorders	Delusions of parasitosis, hypervenilation, delirium tremens

Source: Adapted from Flowers, F. P., & Krusinski, P. A. (1984). *Dermatology in ambulatory and emergency medicine: A clinical guide with algorithms.* (p. 408). Chicago: Year Book Medical. Reprinted with permission.

major contribution is a loss of moisture from the stratum corneum. This creates a stiff surface that increases the identifiable scaling and cracking seen with dry skin. A reduction in sebum was once felt to be a major cause of skin dryness. However, recent investigations have identified that although sebum production does decline with age, it is not necessarily correlated with the degree of skin dryness (Dowing et al., 1989). In addition, frequent bathing, believed to be a major contributing factor in dry skin, has been refuted in a recent clinical trial (Hardy, 1996). Environmental factors that are thought to contribute to skin dryness include excessive use of soap and low relative humidity. (Franz & Kinney, 1986).

Assessment

Assessment of xerosis includes direct observation of the extent of the inflammation and a general evaluation of the client's current environment and bathing routine. A functional assessment is important to identify how the condition impacts day-to-day activities.

Clinical Management

Clinical recommendations for controlling dry skin include increasing humidity in the environment to at least 60%, lowering water temperature to between 90° and 105°F and reducing the use of irritating soaps. Superfatted soaps have been found to be less drying because they provide a film of oil on the skin's surface (Hardy, 1996). Among soaps tested in one study with older adults, Dove (Lever Brothers Company, New York, NY) was found to provide the lowest level of irritation (Frantz & Gardner, 1994a). Moisturizers in the form of creams, lotions, or ointments are applied topically to the skin to reduce the signs and symptoms of dry skin. Only products with a low alcohol content should be considered for treatment. Ointments with a petroleum base appear to be superior. These are best applied while the skin is still wet in order to trap moisture between the skin and ointment and enhance absorption of the water into the skin. Ointments with a lanolin base should be used cautiously because a high incidence of allergic reactions occurs in patients with stasis dermatitis. Bath oil has not been found to increase skin hydration and is potentially hazardous for older adults bathing alone due to the risk of falling on oily surfaces (Frantz & Gardner, 1994a).

Pharmacologic Measures. The use of topical steroids in older adults with pruritic conditions is often inappropriately instituted as a first-line treatment. Although sometimes indicated, topical steroids should not be considered benign because of their potential for local and systemic adverse reactions. Adrenal suppression has occurred as a result of potent topical corticoids, as well as milder topical agents used with occlusive-type dressings. Skin atrophy presenting as a dermatitis may occur when the steroid is discontinued. Contact sensitivity to topical steroids can occur and may complicate the original diagnosis. In general, using the least-potent steroid concentration, limiting the duration of the exposure, tapering the dosage, and using emollients following treatments are methods to reduce side effect profiles (Katz, 1995). For an excellent review of topical cortisteroids, see Habif (1990).

DERMATITIS MEDICAMENTOSA

Dermatitis medicamentosa is a reaction to a drug. It is worthy of mention for two reasons. First, almost any drug may cause skin eruptions and subsequent pruritus. Second, older adults are at increased risk for this condition because two thirds of those over the age of 65 consume on average 5 to 12 medications daily (Hume &

Owens, 1995). One study identified that 23% of skin eruptions were caused by drug ingestion in patients over the age of 60 (Beachman, 1995).

Clinical Management
Skin reactions caused by medication generally resolve after the offending agent is removed. A thorough medication history should be taken, including over-the-counter (OTC) products and previous reactions to a similar class of medication. Frequently, institutions or large pharmacies have computerized reports on the various types of interactions that may occur between medications. These may be beneficial for the clinician evaluating the potential interaction of multiple medications. The primary-care physician should be consulted to assist in review and reduction of any unnecessary medication.

Setting-specific Issues
Community dwelling elderly should be encouraged to fill all prescriptions at one pharmacy to reduce the potential of medication interactions.

········ *vignette* ················

Mr. Smith is a 65-year-old man in fairly good health. He presents with fever and erythematous target lesions across his upper torso. Medications include allopurinol, digoxin, phenytoin (Dilantin), trimethoprim–sulfamethoxazole (Septra), and hydralazine hydrochloride (Apresoline). All of Mr. Smith's medications might be causing this type of rash. Review all medications for possible drug reactions.

SEBORRHEIC DERMATITIS

Clinical Presentation

Seborrheic dermatitis is described as an inflammatory disease of the skin and may include symptoms of pruritus and erythema. It appears as a greasy scaliness, commonly affecting the scalp, face, chest, and, to a lesser extent, the intertriginous areas and the external ear canals. It often causes recurrent eye irritation, blepharitis, and eyelid redness. Although the etiology is unknown, a yeast, *Pityrosporum ovale*, has been implicated as the causative factor. Genetic and environmental factors may also influence the course of remissions and exacerbations. Seborrheic dermatitis is fairly common in the elderly, affecting 20% of the population (Goldfarb et al., 1996). It is more pronounced in patients with Parkinson's disease, as well as Parkinson's symptoms induced by neuroleptics, and has been reported to be one of the most common skin manifestations of acquired immune deficiency syndrome (AIDS) and AIDS-related complex. Interestingly, the dermatitis occurs before the presence of the AIDS symptoms (Habif, 1990).

Clinical Management

Treatment consists of frequent cleansing of the affected areas with antiseborrheic shampoo and use of mild topical steroids such as Valisone or Aristocort in category VII or VIII. In addition, ketoconazole cream may be applied daily to more difficult cases. Zinc soap and selenium lotions are helpful in maintaining remission (Habif, 1990).

CONTACT DERMATITIS

Contact dermatitis is caused by skin contact with an allergen. This type of dermatitis can occur with frequently used products such as soaps, lanolin-based emollients, and topical medication. Products that have been used over many months may still result in a reaction. The affected area is usually at the site of contact of the offending agent. Erythema followed by clear vesicles is the typical pattern. Chronic skin changes take on a more scaly appearance.

Age-related Changes

Older adults are predisposed to contact dermatitis due to a number of physiologic reasons, including the skin's reduced barrier function, inability to clear chemicals, and dry skin. A delay in hypersensitivity brought on by the irritant may make the allergic reaction difficult to diagnose.

Clinical Management

Treatment includes identification and removal of the offending agent. Topical corticosteroid therapy is used to reduce inflammation and pruritis. More complex cases are referred to a dermatologist for patch testing.

LICHEN SIMPLEX CHRONICUS

Clinical Presentation

Lichen simplex chronicus is a localized eczematous disorder (see Figure 2 of Color Plate within this chapter). The condition is extremely itchy, and it is believed that the itching leads to chronic changes in the skin. Areas most affected include the back of the wrist, neck, lower legs, forearms, and anogenital region. The plaques become thick, and prominent skin lines appear (lichenification). Factors that are believed to predispose patients to this condition include dermatitis, dry skin, and stress. Several authors

(Buckley & Rustin, 1990; Habif, 1990) report an association of lichen simplex chronicus with underlying psychiatric or personality disorder.

Assessment

If the condition occurs in the anogenital region, it should be differentiated from lichen sclerosus atrophicus. Considered a premalignant condition, lichen sclerosus presents as ivory white and atrophic and is extremely itchy (Buckley & Rustin, 1990).

Clinical Management

Dry skin should be treated as previously discussed. Nonpharmalogic measures such as the identification of stressful factors should be explored with the client. The first-line treatment is generally topical steroids. An occlusive dressing over the topical steroids may speed absorption and reduce nighttime itching. Intralesional steroids may be used in severe cases.

■ PARASITIC AND FUNGAL CONDITIONS

ANGULAR CHEILITIS

Age-related Changes

Skin around the folds of the mouth lose tone and become more prominent, generally as a result of loss of teeth and atrophy of the alveolar bone. This creates an overlap at the edges of the lips, which predisposes individuals to this condition.

Clinical Presentation

Angular cheilitis, also called perlèche or angular stomatitis, is an inflammation of the corners of the mouth (see Fig. 14–3). Patients develop maceration, *Candida* in-fections, and painful fissures, as the area is constantly moist from saliva.

Assessment

Because a deficiency in iron or B-complex vitamins may also lead to angular cheilitis, careful evaluation of the client's nutritional status is warranted. Other conditions that may contribute to the problem include seborrheic or contact dermatitis.

Clinical Management

The reasons for the endentulous condition or improperly fitting teeth should be discussed with the client. Frequently identified factors that may contribute include poorly aligned dentures, financial inability to access proper dental facilities, or impaired cognitive status. In cases involving a client who is cognitively impaired and dental interventions are not realistic, the use of barrier products such as Aquafor (Belersdorf, Norwalk, CT) applied regularly to the corners of the mouth is an alternative intervention. Topical antifungals are used to treat superimposed fungal infections and low-dose topical steroids may be used to relieve the inflammation.

INTERTRIGO

Intertrigo is a common problem in older adults. This is frequently observed in obese individuals who have poor hygiene. It typically occurs in the folds of the abdomen, under the breast, and in the groin area. Friction between the folds of skin along with moisture creates a condition in which yeast thrive.

Assessment

Candida infections often appear as white satellite pustules surrounding red, shiny

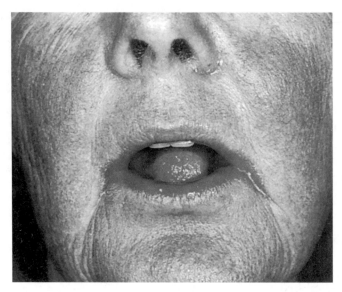

Figure 14–3. Angular cheilitis (perlechè). Skin folds at the angles of the mouth are red and eroded. *(Source: Habif, T. P. [1996]. Clinical dermatology: A color guide to diagnosis and therapy, 3rd ed. St. Louis: Mosby-Yearbook. Used with permission.)*

skin. The client frequently complaints of burning and itching. Skin erosion may occur if left untreated.

Clinical Management

Obese clients should be encouraged to lose weight. Functional limitations related to self-care should be assessed. Moist areas of skin should be dry and clean. In severe cases or for individuals with pendulous breasts, absorptive padding is required to control excessive moisture. An inexpensive method that is helpful in controlling moisture is achieved by placing two panty liners with the tape side placed back to back. The usual treatment consists of a application of an antifungal powder such as nystatin (Mycostatin) for 7 to 14 days. Psoriasis, seborrheic dermatitis, and contact dermatitis may aggravate this condition.

SCABIES

Clinical Presentation

Scabies may occur in individuals of any age group. The condition is mentioned here because of its close association with group living environments. Preexisting xerosis makes the condition difficult to diagnose. Scabies is caused by the *Sarcoptes scabies var hominis* mite. Female mites burrow beneath the skin and the reaction develops 4 to 8 weeks after infestation. Burrows of the mite can be frequently seen between the fingers, on the wrists, and in the folds of the abdomen.

Assessment

Habif (1990) describes a method to identify burrows by touching the area with a felt-tip pen and then wiping the skin clean with an alcohol wipe. The burrows absorb the ink, leaving a dark line behind. Mites are most active at night, causing sleeplessness and the potential for changes in mental status.

Clinical Management

Treatment involves eradicating the mite and treating the underlying dryness and pruritus. Topical steroids will ameliorate symptoms for a short period of time. Older adults may have few signs of the mite but may itch severely. Decreased immunity may allow the mite to survive and burrow in great numbers (Hardy, 1996).

Norwegian scabies is a form of scabies that results in crusted lesions, primarily on the hands and feet. It occurs more frequently in patients with neurologic or mental disorders such as Down syndrome and senile dementia or those on immunosuppressive drugs. The condition is characterized by gray scales and thick, crusty lesions; loss of hair; wartlike formations; and a lack of inflammation (Habif, 1990; Barnes et al., 1987).

Skin scraping to identify the mite is used to confirm the diagnosis if it is not obvious by clinical signs. The client should be instructed to wash all clothing and linens once the treatment has been administered. Individuals who have had close contact should undergo the same treatment. Pruritus following the treatment for up to several days is common. The client should be encouraged to use an emollient on a regular basis to reduce skin dryness and irritation.

A scabicide lotion is applied at bedtime from the neck down and rinsed off the following day. A bath prior to the application is not advised, because moisture actually increases the skin's permeability and absorptive properties. Lindane is still used, but it is stored in the liver and can cause convulsions with excessive use. Permethrin dermal cream 5% has demonstrated low mammalian toxicity and has demonstrated an acceptable level of treatment success (Taplin et al., 1986).

Setting-specific Issues

Environments in which a large number of individuals share common living quarters, such as nursing homes, group homes, and assisted-living environments predispose older adults to this skin problem. Roommates or direct-care providers must also receive simultaneous treatment for this condition.

.... *vignette* ....

Mrs. Harrison is an 86-year-old, severely demented woman residing in a nursing facility. The night staff have reported that the client is increasingly agitated, especially at night. The client's main diagnoses are cirrhosis of the liver, chronic obstructive pulmonary disease (COPD), and dry skin. The client was placed on topical steroids for a recent rash with no itching. The skin was thin and dry, with crusted lesions on her feet. Medications include prednisone 20 mg PO qd and theophylline 200 mg q6h. The night staff reported the client to be agitated and believed the theophylline and prednisone were causing the restlessness and insomnia. Because of the client's lung status, the medication could not be discontinued. Therefore, alprazolam (Xanax) 1 mg at bedtime for agitation was added to the drug profile. Several weeks later, staff members on the nursing wing were diagnosed with scabies, but no one else on the wing had any signs of the infestation. Dermatology was requested to inspect all of the clients with skin changes to localize the host. Mrs. Harrison's crusted foot lesions underwent skin scrapings, and millions of mites were visible under the microscope. A diagnosis of Norwegian scabies was made.

CLINICAL PEARL

Steroids can mask the symptoms of scabies. Atypical presentations are possible, especially in individuals with neurologic disorders.

BULLOUS PEMPHIGOID

Bullous pemphigoid is a blistering disease observed almost exclusively in older adults. The etiology is unknown; however, it is thought to be related to the formation of an antibody that affects the epidermal basement membrane. The disease occurs almost exclusively in the elderly with a mean age of onset of 72 years (Goldfarb et al., 1996). The disease occurs equally in both sexes. The course of the disease is described as self-limiting, with most cases having a one-year duration. Remission and exacerbations may occur throughout the course of the disease and may last as long as 5 to 6 years (Lever, 1979).

Clinical Presentation

Usual Presentation of Disease. The skin changes associated with pemphigoid include areas of erythema, pruritic plaques, and the development of vesicle fluid-filled lesions (see Figure 3 of Color Plate within this chapter). Itching may precede the course of the lesions and has

been reported to occur up to 10 months prior to the diagnosis (Beachman, 1995). The vesicles may be dense and frequently occur on the flexural aspects of the arms, legs, and abdomen. Oral lesions are reported in 25% of patients (Goldfarb et al., 1996).

Atypical Presentation of Disease. Bullous pemphigoid must be differentiated from other bullous diseases such as pemphigus vulgaris, which has a more ominous outcome. Clients whose immune systems are impaired may develop secondary infections. No clear relationship between bullous pemphigoid and malignancy exists, although some forms of internal malignancy can cause a bullous eruption.

Assessment

History/Diagnostic Studies. The client's health status is reviewed to rule out any underlying immunologic conditions. Blood work should include complete blood count (CBC), glucose, electrolytes, blood urea nitrogen (BUN), creatinine, liver function tests (LFTs), thyroid studies, and stool for occult blood. The client should be referred to a dermatologist for a skin biopsy to confirm the diagnosis.

Physical. Whereas pemphigus vulgaris primarily affects people in middle age, bullous pemphigoid is generally found in people over the age of 60. Nikolsky's sign is helpful in differentiating the two diseases. This sign is positive when traction on the lesion causes flaccid removal of the epidermis. Nikolsky's sign is positive for blistering diseases such as pemphigus vulgaris or epidermolysis bullosa and negative with pemphigoid bullous (Goldberg & Bronson, 1991).

Clinical Management

Pharmacologic Measures. The combined therapy of steroids and immunosuppressives reduces steroid side effects. The strength of the steroid is related to the extent of the disease (Habif, 1990).

Nonpharmacologic Measures. Clients with this condition require reassurance that the condition is self-limiting. Individuals may be embarrassed by the cosmetically unattractive lesions. Extremely itchy lesions or those located in areas that rub on clothing may be additionally distressful. A functional assessment, concentrating on how the disease is impacting the client's daily life is essential in the overall treatment plan. Those clients with recurring lesions may benefit from support groups or individual counseling. Clients with impaired immune systems from other health conditions should be monitored closely for signs of infection.

HERPES ZOSTER

Herpes zoster (shingles) is a viral infection caused by reactivation of the latent varicella zoster virus in the dorsal sensory ganglia. A weakened immune system is a proposed cause for reactivation. The incidence of zoster increases with age, with an estimate that an 85-year-old person has a 50% risk of an attack (Gilchrest, 1986). The prevalence of this disease in older adults has been suggested to correlate with a decline in cell immunity (Jolleys, 1989). The condition generally is not recurring, but reactivation may occur in 5% of cases. There remains no gender or race-related incidence to the disease. Demographic, seasonal, or occupational differences do not appear to affect the incidence or prevalence of the disease (Whitley, 1992).

Presentation

Usual Presentation of Disease. This disease is characterized initially by development of a tingling, burning, or itching sensation. A maculopapular-type rash occurs several days later, followed by a group of clear fluid-filled vesicles. The rash is usually located on one side of the body and follows along a dermatome. The most typical nerves associated with this condition are the ophthalmic division of the trigeminal, cervical, lumbar, sacral, or thoracic nerve. The client may complain of a general malaise, headache, or low-grade fever. Herpes zoster is reported as a self-limiting disease, with eruption of the vesicle occurring for up to 2 to 3 weeks and typical resolution of the pain associated with the lesions resolving in 2 to 4 weeks. The frequency and severity of complications increase with age. Reportedly, the main complication is postherpetic neuralgia, occurring in up to 47% of individuals over the age of 60 (Jolleys, 1989). The course of postherpetic neuralgia is somewhat variable and is reported to continue for more than a year in some patients (Goldfarb et al., 1996). The pain associated with this condition can be debilitating, especially in older individuals with previous functional limitations. Several associated incidences of depression and suicide due to the intractable pain associated with this neuralgia have been reported (Bernstein et al., 1987; Beachman, 1995).

Atypical Presentation of Disease. Lesions which form at the end of the nose may be an early marker for involvement of the ophthalmic nerve. This is termed Hutchinson's sign (Habif, 1990). Disseminating herpes occurs in immunocompromised patients and carries a mortality rate of approximately 20% if untreated (Whitley, 1992). Individuals who have never had chickenpox can develop the varicella virus after being exposed to a person with herpes zoster (Habif, 1990).

Assessment

A careful review of the client's symptoms and the pattern of the pain is essential to an early diagnosis. Because paresthesia may occur up to a week prior to the development of the vesicles, it may mimic other conditions such as cardiac or pleural disease. Individuals must be asked how much pain they are experiencing, using a standard pain scale. The pain associated with preherpetic neuralgia may be confused with angina, nerve compression, or biliary colic (Chenitz & Takano Stone, 1991).

Clinical Management

Pharmacologic Measures. Early recognition and treatment of the condition are essential. Acyclovir 800 mg orally 5 times a day for 7 to 10 days, famciclovir 500 mg three times a day for 7 days, or valacyclovir 1 mg three times daily for 7 days are currently the treatments of choice. Treatment by acyclovir within 48 hours has been reported to decrease lesion healing time and reduce pain (Goldfarb et al., 1996). Topical applications of Burrow's solution can be helpful to dry and soothe the lesions (Whitley, 1992). Habif (1990) reports the use of Betadine (povidone iodine) whirlpools as being effective in removing crusted le-

sions and reducing irritation. One study applying topical capsaicin to lesions in patients with chronic postherpetic neuralgia resulted in relief in 75% of patients. Capsaicin was applied locally four times a day for up to 1 month, with a minor side effect of a mild to moderate burning sensation reported (Bernstein et al., 1987). Narcotic therapy is commonly used to control the pain. However, close monitoring of narcotic use in older adults is warranted because of potential for iatrogenic effects such as falling, infection, confusion, and constipation. Intralesional steroids and injections of xylocaine directly into the lesions have also been used for extensive postherpetic neuralgia (Habif, 1990).

Nonpharmacologic Measures. Because of frequent dosing, an assessment of the client's ability to take medication properly is essential. This involves an evaluation of the client's mental status, dexterity, knowledge of the importance of the medication, and affordability. Depending on the assessment, the treatment regimen for medication compliance may include daily medication boxes, timed medication machines, or community support services. The pain associated with zoster can be debilitating, and older adults frequently reduce their daily activity. This loss of mobility can lead to a multitude of comorbidities. Psychologically, chronic pain may result in depression and social isolation. Likewise, pain that results in immobility may lead to pneumonia and pressure ulcers. A functional assessment to determine the extent to which the pain is impacting on daily living is key to supporting the client through the chronic pain associated with this disease.

Rehabilitation. The use of home health agencies, rehabilitative professionals, social workers, mental health professionals, and spiritual supports are important in reducing comorbidity and maintaining function in longstanding or painful cases. Individuals who are particularly frail may require a respite stay in a rehabilitative unit or a live-in companion.

.... *vignette* ....

An 85-year-old cognitively intact woman complained of left-sided rib pain and a burning feeling. She thought she might have rolled on something in the bed since she kept all kinds of objects in the bed such as glasses, pens, books, and so on. Examination revealed no shortness of breath, rash, or point of tenderness to touch. Three days later, a linear maculopapular rash occurred across her back and chest. She was treated with 800 mg acyclovir 5 times daily for 10 days. Her pain was managed with acetaminophen (Tylenol).

CLINICAL PEARL

Consider herpes zoster even without the presence of a rash. A shortened course has been demonstrated when antiviral medications are started early in the course of the disease.

■ STASIS DERMATITIS AND VENOUS ULCERATION

Venous ulcers comprise 90% of all clinical ulcers. They are fairly common in the elderly, with estimates of between 500,000 and 600,000 occurring annually in those over the age of 60. The highest incidence of occurrence is at age 70 (Elder & Greer, 1995). See Chapter 6 for a review of the diagnosis and management of peripheral vascular disease. This section will focus on the dermatologic manifestations of the disease.

CLINICAL PRESENTATION

Venous ulcerations are caused from a variety of physiologic changes. Values within the perforating veins (veins that connect the superficial to the deep venous system) fail. Continuous high pressure widens the endothelial pores of the capillary beds. Protein is released into the extracellular fluid, causing a pericapillary barrier, which interferes with the exchange of oxygen and nutrients. Clinically, the most common area for ulcer formation is the medical aspect of the lower leg. Risk factors include venous insufficiency and previous deep vein thrombosis (DVT). Patients complain that their legs are tired, tender, and feel heavy. Arthritis can also weaken the calf muscle and reduce the efficiency of the calf as a pump. Lower leg edema is described as tender, unlike the edema associated with other disease states such as cirrhosis, heart failure, or kidney disease.

Assessment

It is important to differentiate venous ulcers from those caused by arterial insufficiency and diabetic structural changes. It is not uncommon for a client to present with a mixed ulcer. A comparison of arterial, neuropathic, and venous ulcers is located in Table 14–5. Workup for the differential diagnosis is located in Table 14–6. The edema associated with venous

**TABLE 14–5.   ARTERIAL, VENOUS, AND NEUROPATHIC ULCERS OF THE LOWER
EXTREMITIES: A COMPARISON**

	Arterial	Neuropathic (Diabetes	Venous
Predisposing factors	Peripheral vascular disease (PVD) Diabetes Advanced age	Diabetic with peripheral neuropathy	Valve incompetence in perforating veins History of deep vein thrombophlebitis and thrombosis Previous history of ulcer Advanced age Obesity
Assessment	Thin, shiny, dry skin Loss of hair on ankle and foot Thickened toenails Pallor on elevation and dependent rubor Cyanosis Decreased temperature Absent or diminished pulses	Diminished or no sensation in foot Foot deformities Palpable pulses Warm foot If patient has coexisting PVD, same assessments as arterial	Firm ("brawny") edema Dilated superficial veins Dry, thin skin Evidence of healed ulcers Lipodermatosclerosis present
Location	Between toes or tips of toes Over phalangeal heads Around lateral malleolus Where subjected to trauma or rubbing of footwear	Plantar aspect of foot Over metatarsal heads Under heel	Medial aspect of lower leg and ankle May extend into malleolar area
Characteristics	Even wound margins Gangrene or necrosis Deep, pale wound bed Painful Cellulitis	Painless Even wound margins Deep Cellulitis or underlying osteomyelitis Granular tissue present unless coexisting PVD	Irregular wound margins Superficial (into dermis) Ruddy, granular tissue Usually painless Exudate usually present
Conservative treatment	Bedrest as feasible Treat any cellulitis Topical care Patient education and support	Treat cellulitis Rule out osteomyelitis Metabolic diabetic control No weight bearing Contact casting	Elevate extremity as feasible Therapeutic vascular compression Topical care: absorption dressings and

TABLE 14–5.   ARTERIAL, VENOUS, AND NEUROPATHIC ULCERS OF THE LOWER EXTREMITIES: A COMPARISON (CONT.)

	Arterial	Neuropathic (Diabetes	Venous
Conservative treatment (cont.)		Topical care Orthotics Patient education and support	debridement, as indicated Patient education and support
Surgical treatment	Revascularization Angioplasty	Aggressive debridement Revascularization if coexisting PVD indicates it	Skin grafting

Source: Adapted, with permission, from Zink, M., Rousseau, P., & Holloway, G., (1992). *Acute and chronic wounds lower extremity ulcer.* (p. 173). St. Louis: Mosby.

insufficiency may make it difficult to palpate a pulse, making the use of a portable Doppler helpful. An ankle/brachial index is a quick method for determining the extent of arterial insufficiency (see Fig. 14–4 for this procedure). In venous disease, the ankle pressure should equal or be higher than the arm pressure and the ankle/brachial index greater than one (Burton, 1993b). However, clients who report a history of arterial insufficiency, signs of claudification, or pain at rest should be considered for vascular studies. Ulcer evaluation includes direct observation of the periwound margins, evidence of granulation, induration, stasis dermatitis, and infection. Venous ulcers typically have an irregular border (see Figure 4 of Color Plate within this chapter). The limb circumference should be measured and compared with the nonaffected leg. A discussion of the client's previous activity level, ulcer treatments, and current level of pain are essential in determining how the ulcer is affecting the client's function. Pain has been demonstrated to be related to poor healing of venous leg ulcers and

should be adequately controlled to enhance compliance (Johnson, 1995). Because venous ulcers have a recurrence rate of up to 76%, the client's ability or willingness to follow the clinician's recommendations is a key factor in the healing process (Barr, 1996).

Diagnostic Studies. The Trendelenburg test, or retrograde filling test, may be used to identify incompetent valves within the communicating and saphenous systems. With the client supine, elevate one leg to 90° and manually occlude the great saphenous vein in the upper thigh. Have the client stand while continuing to occlude the vein. Assess for venous filling of the leg, which should occur distally. After 20 seconds, release the compression on the saphenous vein and watch for any sudden additional filling. Slow venous filling should continue and be complete within 35 seconds. Sudden filling of the superficial veins, with occlusion of the saphenous vein, is indicative of valvular incompetency within the saphenous vein. (Bates, 1995). Noninva-

TABLE 14–6.   DIFFERENTIAL DIAGNOSIS OF LEG ULCERS

Vascular diseases
  Arterial (hypertensive atherosclerotic, vasospastic)
  Venous (venous stasis ulcer)
  Lymphedema
Metabolic disorders
  Diabetes mellitus
  Necrobiosis lipoidica diabeticorum
  Porphyria cutanea tarda
  Gout
  Pancreatitic (pancreatitis, carcinoma)
Infections
  Bacterial (especially *Staphylococcus aureus, Streptococcus*)
  Spirochetal (syphilis)
  Fungal (deep fungal; mycetoma)
  Viral
Vasculitis
  Hypersensitivity vasculitis
  Polyarteritis
  Systemic lupus erythematosus
  Rheumatoid vasculitis
  Wegener's granulomatosis
  Lymphomatoid granulomatosis
Lymphedema
  Congenital
  Postinfectious
  Postsurgical
Drugs
  Halogens (bromide, iodide)

Ergotism
Drug-induced vasculitis
Anticoagulant necrosis (sodium warfarin, heparin)
Hematologic abnormalities
  Hypercoagulable states (Prot C, S, ATIII deficiency), lupus anticoagulant syndrome
  Sickle cell anemia
  Thalassemia
  Polycythemia vera
  Leukemia
  Dysproteinemia (cryoglobulinemia, macroglobulinemia)
Tumors
  Cutaneous (basal cell cancer, squamous cell cancer, sarcoma, malignant melanoma, Merkel cell tumor)
  Secondary (metastatic carcinoma, lymphoma)
  Kaposi's sarcoma
Miscellaneous
  Pyoderma gangrenosum
  Trauma (including factitial)
  Burns
  Pressure sores, neuropathic ulcers
  Insect bites (brown recluse spider)
  Ulcerative lichen planus
  Bullous diseases (epidermolysis bullosa)
  Sweet's syndrome
  Idiopathic

Source: Reprinted, with permission, from Burton, C. S. III. Management of chronic and problem lower extremity wounds. *Dermatol Clin, 11*(4), 1993.

sive testing such as duplex ultrasonography, photoplethysmography, and arterial Doppler studies are also useful in assessing valvular competency.

Clinical Management

The mainstay of venous ulcer treatment is the application of a local wound dressing, supported by compression of the entire extremity. Moist wound healing assists with autodebridment, collagen production, and the prevention of a dry wound crust (Barr, 1996). Compression reduces the damage associated with the leakage of fluid caused by the high pressure in the superficial veins and improves venous return. Compression is contraindicated if there is a history of DVT, arterial insufficiency, or spreading lymphatic cancer. Initially, elevating the extremity is helpful

All you'll need is a sphygmomanometer and a handheld Doppler. Follow these steps:

1. With the patient supine, take the blood pressure in both arms. Use the higher of the two systolic pressures as the brachial pressure in the ratio.
2. Place the blood pressure cuff on the patient's leg just above the malleoli. Place the Doppler probe at a 45-degree angle to the dorsalis pedis or posterior tibial artery.
3. Inflate the cuff until the Doppler signal stops. Keeping the Doppler probe over the artery, slowly deflate the cuff until the Doppler signal returns. Record the number as the ankle systolic pressure.
4. Divide the ankle systolic pressure by the higher of the two arm systolic pressures to obtain the ankle brachial index (ABI). Suppose, for example, your patient's systolic brachial pressures are 120 and 129 and her ankle systolic pressure is 65. Dividing 65 by 129 gives you an ABI of 0.5.

Interpret the results according to these guidelines:
- 0.9 to 1—normal
- 0.75 to 0.9—moderate disease
- 0.75 to 0.5—limb-threatening

Note: The ABI isn't reliable in patients with diabetes because arterial calcification causes falsely high ABIs.

Figure 14–4. How to do an ankle brachial index. *(Used with permission from the December issue of* Nursing 96, *Springhouse Corporation.)*

in reducing the venous hypertension. Generally, elevating the legs 18 cm above the heart for 2 to 4 hours during the day and at nighttime is sufficient. Bedrest poses additional risks for older clients. An alternative schedule of chair rest with leg elevation is recommended to enhance circulation. Once compression is adequate, the client should be encouraged to walk because this enhances circulation. Compression can be maintained through the use of elastic stockings, which can be custom fit to the client's legs. To improve the underlying venous pathology, the pressure should be maintained at 20 to 30 mm Hg at the ankle, with an even and gradual reduction to 10 mm Hg at the infrapetellar notch. For those individuals with arthritis, there are stocking-donning stands and sticky rubber gloves to assist in application. For severely arthritic clients or those who cannot tolerate maximum compression, there are devices termed legging orthosis. These consist of compression bands that can be removed dur-

ing bathing and at nighttime. The Duke boot has demonstrated adequate pressure for healing and consists of a hydrocolloid dressing followed by an Unna boot (impregnated zinc oxide, glycerin, and gelatin bandage) and a Coban elastic compression bandage. The use of a hydrocolloid dressing directly over the wound can reduce irritation. There are a variety of compression products on the market (see Table 14–7). Barr (1996) examined studies involving various treatment modalities for venous ulcer compression treatment and found minimal research to support Unna boot use over other compression products. Compression pumps are available for clients whose edema is particularly resistant to conventional compression. The pump is generally used for 2 to 3 hours a day and may be used to reduce edema prior to stocking application. Most of the lower leg edema associated with venous insufficiency responds poorly to diuretics. Older adults are particularly susceptible

TABLE 14–7. WOUND PRODUCTS BY MANUFACTURER/WOUND TYPE WITH CLINICAL CONSIDERATIONS

Hydrocolloids—Pressure ulcer, venous ulcers. Promotes moist healing. Should be used with caution in patients with infection, diabetes mellitus or peripheral vascular disease. Conformable but may tear fragile skin. Assists with autolytic debridement. May cause maceration of skin edges. Characteristic odor and yellow exudate is normal with dressing removal.

Product	Manufacturer
Comfeel Plus Contour Comfeel Plus Clear Comfeel Plus PRD Comfeel Plus Ulcer	Coloplast Sween 1955 West Oak Circle Marietta, GA 30062 1-800-533-0464
Cutinova Hydro	Beiersdorf-Jobst, Inc. 653 Miami St. Toledo, OH 43605 1-800-537-1063
Duoderm CGF Duoderm Border Dressing Duoderm Extra Thin	CovaTec 100 Headquarters Park Drive Skillman, NJ 08558 1-800-422-8811
Replicare Restore Restore CX	Hollister, Inc. 2000 Hollister Dr. Libertyville, IL 60048
Tegasorb Tegasorb Thin	3M Healthcare 3M Center Bldg. 275-4E-01 St Paul, MN 55144 1-800-228-3957
Ultec	Sherwood-Davis & Geck 1915 Oak St. St. Louis, MO 63103 1-800-325-7472
J&J Ulcer Dressing	Johnson & Johnson Medical, Inc. 2500 Arbrook Arlington, TX 76004 1-800-423-5170
Derm Assist Hydrocolloid	Wilshire Medical Products 11420 Mathis Ave. Dallas, TX 75234 1-800-234-8132
Intrasite	Smith and Nephew United 11775 Starkey Rd. P.O. Box 1970 Largo, FL 1-800-876-1261

Film Dressings—Used for skin tears, on blisters, over hydrocolloid dressings for additional adhesiveness, on Stage II pressure ulcers and donor sites. Avoid wounds with excessive drainage or evidence of infection. Reduces friction burn. Allows for the exchange of oxygen but not bodily fluids. Prepare surrounding skin with skin prep. Allow skin surface to dry before applying dressing.

Product	Manufacturer
ACU-Derm	Acme United Corp. 75 Kings Highway Cutoff Fairfield, CT 06430 1-800-835-2263
Bioclusive MVP Bioclusive Select	Johnson & Johnson Medical, Inc. 2500 Arbrook Arlington, TX 76004 1-800-423-5170
OpSite Transparent dressing OpSite Post-op OpSite Flexigrip	Smith and Nephew United 11775 Starkey Rd. P.O. Box 1970 Largo, FL 1-800-876-1261

Pro-Clude

P.O. Box 1970
Largo, FL
1-800-876-1261

3M Tegaderm transparent
3M Tegaderm HP
3M Tegaderm dressing with absorbent pad

3M Healthcare
3M Center Bldg. 275-4E-01
St Paul, MN 55144
1-800-228-3957

Blister film

Sherwood-Davis & Geck
1915 Oak St.
St. Louis, MO 63103
1-800-325-7472

Polyskin II
Polyskin MR

Kendall Health Care Products
15 Hampshire St.
Mansfield, MA 02048
1-800-346-7197

Foam dressings—Pressure ulcer with minimal drainage, around drainage tubes, secondary dressing for wounds with packing or over hydrocolloids for venous stasis ulcers with a lot of drainage.

Foams are conformable and may be used on body sites with hair, infected wounds, and as packing. Maceration may occur; use skin prep around wound on intact skin.

Polyderm Border

DeRoyal
200 DeBusk Lane
Powell, TN 37849
1-800-251-9864

Curofoam Hydrophilic

Kendall Health Care Products
15 Hampshire St.
Mansfield, MA 02048
1-800-346-7197

Allevyn and Allevyn wound cavity dressings

Smith and Nephew United
11775 Starkey Rd.

ConvaTec
100 Headquarters Park Drive
Skillman, NJ 08558
1-800-422-8811

LYOfoam A
LYOfoam C

Acme United Corp.
75 King Highway Cutoff
Fairfield, CT 06430
1-800-835-2263

Mitraflex Plus
Mitraflex SC

ConvaTec
100 Headquarters Park Drive
Skillman, NJ 08558
1-800-422-8811

Exudate Absorbers—May be used on pressure ulcers with heavy exudate. Helpful for use after debridement or to wick away moisture from the wound site.

May be used on infected wounds. Many may be packed directly into wound cavities. Should not be used on dry or gangrenous wounds.

Alginates—Natural fiber made of seaweed.

Use on heavily exudating wounds.

Algosteril

Johnson & Johnson Medical, Inc.
2500 Arbrook
Arlington, TX 76004
1-800-423-5170

Curbasorb

Kendall Health Care Products
15 Hampshire St.
Mansfield, MA 02048
1-800-346-7197

Kaltostat Fortex
Kaltostat Rope

ConvaTec
100 Headquarters Park Drive
Skillman, NJ 08558
1-800-422-8811

(Continues)

TABLE 14-7. WOUND PRODUCTS BY MANUFACTURER/WOUND TYPE WITH CLINICAL CONSIDERATIONS (CONT.)

Product/Wound Type	Manufacturer/Address	Clinical Considerations
Seasorb	Coloplast Sween 1955 West Oak Circle Mamarietta, GA 30062 1-800-533-0464	
Kalginate	DeRoyal Industries, Inc. 200 DeBusk Lane Powell, TN 37849 1-800-251-9864	
Dermacea	Sherwood-Davis & Geck 1915 Oak St. St. Louis, MO 63103 1-800-325-7472	
Restore Calci Care	Hollister, Inc. 2000 Hollister Dr. Libertyville, IL 60048	
Sorbsan	Dow Hickman Pharmaceuticals 10410 Corporate Drive Sugar Land, TX 77478 1-800-231-3052	
Copolymer starch dressings		Mainly used to fill dead space in deep wounds. Many absorb up to 20 times their weight in drainage. Monitor wound bed for drying properties. Fillers used in combination with other wound products such as hydrocolloids.
Debrisan beads/paste (used to fill and absorb exudate, autolytic)	Johnson & Johnson Medical, Inc. 2500 Arbrook Arlington, TX 76004 1-800-423-5170	
Bard absorptive dressing	Patient Care Division	
Comfeel paste and powder	8195 Industrial Blvd. Covington, GA 30014 1-800-526-4453 Coloplast Sween 1955 West Oak Circle Marietta, GA 30062 1-800-533-0464	
DuoDerm paste and granules	ConvaTec 100 Headquarters Park Drive Skillman, NJ 08558 1-800-422-8811	
Replicare paste	Smith and Nephew United 11775 Starkey Rd. P.O. Box 1970 Largo, FL 1-800-876-1261	
Curasalt	Kendall Health Care Products 15 Hampshire St. Mansfield, MA 02048 1-800-346-7197	
Mesalt	Molnlyckel/Scott Health Care 500 Baldwin Tower Eddystone, PA 19022 1-610-499-3362	
Hydrogels—May be used with stage II pressure ulcers, skin tears, donor sites, surgical incisions, radiation desqaumation and excoriations. May be used under hydrocolloid wound products.		Used to promote a moist healing environment. Use on lightly exudating wounds. Provides a cooling effect which may reduce pain. Requires a secondary dressing. Use enough gel so the wound does not dry out between dressings. Monitor for wound edge maceration.

Product	Manufacturer
Aquasorb Aquasorb Border	DeRoyal Industries, Inc. 200 DeBusk Lane Powell, TN 37849 1-800-251-9864
Hydrogel Derm gel gauze	Wilshire Medical Products 11420 Mathis Ave. Dallas, TX 75234 1-800-234-8132
IntraSite gel dressing	Smith and Nephew United 11775 Starkey Rd. P.O. Box 1970 Largo, FL 1-800-876-1261
Restore gel/gauze	Hollister, Inc. 2000 Hollister Dr. Libertyville, IL 60048
Second Skin	Spenco Medical Corp PO Box 2501 Waco, TX 76702 1-800-877-3626
Vigilion	C. R. Bard, Inc. Patient Care Division 8195 Industrial Blvd. Covington, GA 4453 1-800-526-4930
CaraGauze Strips Carrasyn Gel Carra-Sorb M Carrasyn V Carrasyn Spray Gel	Carrington Laboratories, Inc. 2001 Walnut Hill Lane Irvington, TX 75038 1-800-527-5216
Elasto-Gel	South West Technologies 1746 Levee Rd. Kansas City, MO 64116
Comfeel Purilon gel	Coloplast Sween 1955 West Oak Circle Marietta, GA 30014 1-800-533-0464
Normalgel	Molnlyckel/Scott Health Care 500 Baldwin Tower Eddystone, PA 19022 1-800-499-3362
Transorb Hydrogel Transorb Impregnated Pads	B. Braun Medical, Inc. 727 W. Glendale Avenue Milwaukee, WI 53209 1-800-362-3215
Restore Strip Restore Sponge	Hollister, Inc. 2000 Hollister Dr. Libertyville, IL 60048
Wound Dress	Coloplast Sween 1955 West Oak Circle Marietta, GA 30062 1-800-533-0464
Biolex	C. R. Bard, Inc. Patient Care Division 8195 Industrial Blvd. Covington, GA 30014 1-800-526-4453
Enzymatic Debriding Agents— Used to debride necrotic tissue. Use on yellow or black wounds.	Not recommended in presence of acute infection. Barrier intact skin with Vaseline prior to applying product.
Biozyme	Armour Pharmaceutical Co. 500 Arcola Rd. P. O. Box 1200 Collegeville, PA 19426-0107 1-800-727-6737

(Continues)

TABLE 14-7. WOUND PRODUCTS BY MANUFACTURER/WOUND TYPE WITH CLINICAL CONSIDERATIONS (CONT.)

Product	Manufacturer/Address	
Elase	Parke-Davis 201 Tabor Road Morris Plains, NJ 07950 1-800-223-0432	
Pan-fil Ointments	Rystan Company 47 Center Avenue P.O. Box 214 Little Falls, NJ 07424-0214 1-800-323-1603	
Collgenase/Santyl	Knoll Pharmaceutical 3000 Continental Drive North Mount Olive, NJ 07828 1-800-526-0710	
Travase	Fujisawa USA, Inc. Parkway North Center 3 Parkway North Deerfield, IL 60015-2548 1-800-727-7003	
Other debridement: Hypergel (used on black wounds)	Molnlyckel/Scott Health Care 500 Baldwin Tower Eddystone, PA 19022 1-610-499-3362	
Curafil Gel wound dressing	Kendall Health Care Products 15 Hampshire St. Mansfield, MA 02048 1-800-346-7197	
Leg Ulcer Wrap—Used for venous ulcers. Provides compression for venous insufficiency. The Unna boot is an impregnated zinc oxide, calamine product.		Apply according to product direction. Uneven application can cause uneven pressures, ulcerations, and poor healing. May be used with hydrocolloid directly over wound to avoid boot rubbing on ulcer.
Unna-Flex Elastic Unna Boot Unna-Flex Duoderm SCB	ConvaTec 100 Headquarters Park Drive Skillman, NJ 08558 1-800-422-8811	
Profore	Smith and Nephew United 11775 Starkey Rd. P.O. Box 1970 Largo, FL 1-800-876-1261	
Dyna-Flex Compression System	Johnson & Johnson Medical, Inc. 2500 Arbrook Arlington, TX 76004 1-800-423-5170	
Gelocast	Beiersdorf-Jobst, Inc. 653 Miami St. Toledo, OH 43605 1-800-537-1063	

This list is not inclusive but is representative of what is currently available for wound products. Refer to manufacturer's directions for use. No endorsement of any product in this table is intended.

to the side effects of diuretics, including dizziness, falls, incontinence, and dehydration.

Complications

Individuals with venous dermatitis are reported to be carriers of *Staphylococcus aureus,* so this type of bacteria should be considered when a cellulitis surfaces (Burton, 1993b). The efficacy of topical antibiotics in the treatment of leg ulcers has demonstrated mixed results. In general, cultures are not helpful in determining a course of treatment because the wound is generally colonized with a variety of organisms. If the colonization is impeding the granulation of the tissue, then local antibiotic treatment may help to reduce the bacterial count so that healing can occur. However, local antibiotic treatment may do more harm than good because clients with venous stasis ulcers frequently demonstrate hypersensitivity and allergic reactions to many local products. If the wound does not heal, both cultures and biopsies are warranted. (See section on pressure ulcers for culturing techniques.) Tenderness, pain, leukocytosis, fever, and nausea are indicators of infection. Appropriate antibiotic therapy includes cephalexin (Keflex) 250 mg four times a day for 10 to 14 days or dicloxacillin 250 mg four times a day for 10 to 14 days. In the presence of *Pseudomonas,* appropriate antibiotic therapy might include ciprofloxacin hydrochloride (Cipro) 500 to 750 mg twice a day for 10 to 14 days (Elder & Greer, 1995).

STASIS DERMATITIS

Clinical Presentation

Stasis dermatitis is a common occurrence in people with venous insufficiency. It is a result of an accumulation of by-products caused by the breakdown of the cells and the leakage of protein in the surrounding tissue. The result is a scaly, itchy, erythematous skin surface. Secondary skin infections can occur from the client's scratching. However, dermatitis is frequently mistaken for cellulitis. As previously discussed, local reactions are frequent in patients with venous insufficiency, especially those with stasis dermatitis. Contact dermatitis may be suspected when there are symptoms such as itching, oozing, and vesicles, or if redness appears. Lanolin and neomycin are common topical allergens in patients with venous ulcers. Cetearyl alcohol can also cause allergic reactions and is present in many paste compression bandages (Wilson et al., 1991).

Clinical Management

A reaction to topical products may occur many weeks after the first application and can even occur with the application of steroid-based preparations. Patch testing is sometimes recommended for clients with sensitivity to a variety of products. Treatment for stasis dermatitis includes corticosteroid topical for mild cases and orally for more involved cases. Saline soaks with mild steroid ointment is effective for particularly weepy areas.

■ PRESSURE ULCERS AND WOUND MANAGEMENT

There is a wealth of information discussing the prevention and treatment of pressure ulcers. However, there remains little uniformity of treatment between health-care settings. One retrospective study conducted in a long-term care facility over a period of 5 years identified 72 different ulcer treatments (Thomas, 1996). Although greatly limited by setting, this review demonstrates the lack of uniformity and standardization of treatments for pressure ulcers. The clinical practice guidelines produced by the Agency for Health Care Policy and Research (AHCPR) provide clinicians with basic information on the current state of pressure ulcer prevention, assessment, and treatment. There remains a large body of information that is yet to have been analyzed. This lack of scientific data is surprising given that 3 million people are presently affected by pressure ulcers in the United States, 60,000 die of complications each year, and the cost of healing one ulcer has been estimated to range from $5,000 to $20,000 (Thomas, 1996; Barhyte et al., 1995).

AGE-RELATED CHANGES

The prevalence rate for ulcer development in older adults is between 11.6 and 27.5%. Approximately 70% of all pressure ulcers occur in patients who are over the age of 70. For patients who reside in nursing homes, development of a pressure ulcer is a poor prognostic sign, carrying a mortality rate of 66% (Takano Stone & Chenitz, 1996). Certain medical conditions such as femoral fractures carry extremely high risks, with a reported 66% of patients developing pressure ulcers in this diagnostic category. Many of the aging changes identified in Table 14–1 are responsible for predisposing older adults to pressure ulcer formation.

CLINICAL PRESENTATION

Pressure ulcers are defined as "localized areas of tissue necrosis that develop when soft tissue is compressed between a bony prominence and an external surface" (Bryant et al., 1992). Kemp and Krouskop (1994) further elaborate that soft tissue ischemia and necrosis may occur when high pressure is maintained over a short span, as well as when low pressure is maintained for a prolonged period. Three main factors that determine whether pressure is enough to create ulcer formation include (1) intensity, (2) duration of the pressure, and (3) the tolerance of the tissue to endure the pressure. The potential for developing pressure ulcers occurs when external pressure exceeds that of the capillary arteriole pressure of 32 mm Hg. Capillary closure occurs with much less pressure in individuals with multiple risk factors. Tissue damage includes oxygen deprivation, accumulation of waste products, and a leakage of fluid into the interstitial space, with a subsequent reduction in nutrient delivery. Factors contributing to pressure ulcer development are outlined in Figure 14–5.

ASSESSMENT OVERVIEW

The complexity of treating pressure ulcers is frequently underestimated by clinicians. There is no single instrument to predict the development of a pressure ulcer. Neither has a unified method for classifying, assessing, or treating the ulcers been developed. Both the AHCPR and the Wound Ostomy and Continence Nursing Association (WOCN) have identified that the pressure ulcer care and prevention must take into account several key components. These include pressure ulcer etiol-

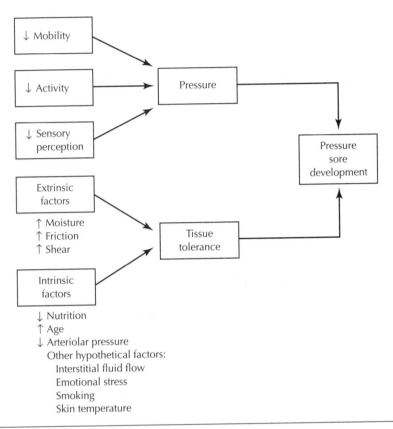

Figure 14–5. Factors Contributing to the Development of Pressure Ulcers. *(Source: Reprinted from Braden, B., & Bergstrom, N. [1987]. A conceptual schema for the study of the etiology of pressure sores. Rehabilitation Nursing, 12(1): 8, with permission of the Association of Rehabilitation Nurses, 4700 W. Lake Avenue, Glenview IL 60025-1485. Copyright © 1987.)*

ogy; valid risk and skin assessment tools; individualized skin care plans, with appropriate support surfaces and positioning techniques; and accurate documentation (Wolf, 1995). Pressure ulcers do not exist in isolation from the client's general health and functional status. A multidimensional assessment process is frequently warranted (see Table 14–8).

Risk Assessment

In many cases, pressure ulcers are preventable. Currently, it is recommended that clients who are bed- or chairbound receive further assessment for risk via a risk assessment tool. Implementation of various strategies to reduce the risk of ulcer development and close monitoring over time should be part of the treatment plan. Commonly identified risk factors are outlined in Fig. 14–5. Additional risk factors include physical and chemical restraints, malnutrition, and fecal incontinence. The level of risk is a combination of both the severity of the risk factor and the absolute number (Smith, 1995). There are a variety of risk assessment tools available in the literature. The most

TABLE 14–8.   PRESSURE ULCER ASSESSMENT GUIDELINES FOR OLDER ADULTS: A MULTIDIMENSIONAL APPROACH

Health history and physical: Review of general health status **Contributing diseases/conditions:** Diabetes, cardiovascular disease, low blood pressure, anemia, kidney disease, neurologic disorders, weight loss, alcohol use, pain, odor, infections, abnormal skin exam, prior skin breakdown **Functional assessment:** Ability to reposition, ability to complete treatment or access to home health services. Barriers to treatment real or perceived Healing goals—palliative vs. healing	**Independent risk factors:** Smoking, increased age, immobility, fever, poor nutrition, lower body weight **Review of specific laboratory values:** Complete blood count, lytes, sed rate, glucose, lymphocytic count, serum albumin **Psychosocial considerations:** Depression, cognitive status, life style/stressors, cultural/ethnic considerations, financial resources, social support

common and extensively tested scales include the Norton and the Braden Scales (See Fig. 14–6 for the Braden Scale.)

Direct Assessment

Identification of the various potential pressure sites is essential in implementing a plan for pressure relief. Pressure ulcers occur most frequently on the sacrum, ischia, great trochanter, buttocks, lateral malleoli, and heels. General guidelines for direct wound assessment are identified in Table 14–9. Direct ulcer evaluation, using a systematic format, should be conducted at least weekly. A pressure evaluation tool called the Pressure Sore Status Tool relies on multiple items for assessing wound healing (see Fig. 14–7). The tool is currently undergoing extensive evaluation by multiple nursing facilities throughout the United States (National Pressure Ulcer Assessment Panel Newsletter, vol. 5, no. 1, June 1997). A variety of methods to stage pressure ulcers have been described in the literature. The most accepted definitions as identified by AHCPR are outlined in Table 14–10. Staging wounds assists in standard-

izing the description and serves as a method to gauge treatments. A method of classification that is particularly helpful in teaching caregivers how to identify appropriate treatments by anatomical changes is staging by color. Evaluation of the wound by color can clue the clinician to multiple key factors (see Figure 5 of Color Plate within this chapter).

- Red: Healthy granulation tissue. Initiallly wound color is pink; color depth increases as layer thickens.
- Yellow: Thick, tenacious exudate ranging in color from creamy white to yellow fibrous material.
- Black: Black, gray, or brown in color; may present as a thick eschar.

Limitations to this system are obvious since there are various shades of color. Wounds that have arterial insufficiency are pale red, whereas venous insufficiency wounds are dusky ruby red. New granulation tissue is light red, whereas established tissue is beefy red. Wounds that are red and friable may indicate an underlying infection (Bates-Jensen, 1995).

	1	2	3	4
SENSORY PERCEPTION Ability to respond meaningfully to pressure-related discomfort	**1. Completely Limited:** Unresponsive (does not moan, flinch, or grasp) to painful stimuli, due to diminished level of consciousness or sedation, OR limited ability to feel pain over most of body surface.	**2. Very Limited:** Responds only to painful stimuli. Cannot communicate discomfort except by moaning or restlessness, OR has a sensory impairment which limits the ability to feel pain or discomfort over 1/2 of body.	**3. Slightly Limited:** Responds to verbal commands but cannot always communicate discomfort or need to be turned, OR has some sensory impairment which limits ability to feel pain or discomfort in 1 or 2 extremities.	**4. No Impairment:** Responds to verbal commands. Has no sensory deficit which would limit ability to feel or voice pain or discomfort.
MOISTURE Degree to which skin is exposed to moisture	**1. Constantly Moist:** Skin is kept moist almost constantly by perspiration, urine, etc. Dampness is detected every time patint is moved or turned.	**2. Moist:** Skin is often but not always moist. Linen must be changed at least once a shift.	**3. Occasionally Moist:** Skin is occasionally moist, requiring an extra linen change approximately once a day.	**4. Rarely Moist:** Skin is usually dry; linen requires changing only at routine intervals.
ACTIVITY Degree of physical activity	**1. Bedfast:** Confined to bed	**2. Chairfast:** Ability to walk severely limited or nonexistent. Cannot bear own weight and/or must be assisted into chair or wheelchair.	**3. Walks Occasionally:** Walks occasionally during day but for very short distances, with or without assistance. Spends majority of each shift in bed or chair.	**4. Walks Frequently:** Walks outside the room at least twice a day and inside room at least once every 2 hours during waking hours.
MOBILITY Ability to change and control body position	**1. Bedfast:** Does not make even slight changes in body or extremity position without assistance.	**2. Very Limited:** Makes occasional slight changes in body or extremity position but unable to make frequent or significant changes independently.	**3. Slightly Limited:** Makes frequent though slight changes in body or extremity position independently.	**4. No Limitations:** Makes major and frequent changes in position without assistance.

Figure 14-6. Braden Scale for Predicting Pressure Sore Risk

	1. Very Poor:	2. Probably Inadequate:	3. Adequate:	4. Excellent:		
NUTRITION Usual food intake pattern	Never eats a complete meal. Rarely eats more than 1/3 of any food offered. Eats 2 servings or less of protein (meat or dairy products) per day. Takes fluids poorly. Does not take a liquid dietary supplement, OR is NPO and/or maintained on clear liquids or IVs for more than 5 days.	Rarely eats a complete meal and generally eats only about 1/2 of any food offered. Protein intake includes only 3 servings of meat or dairy products per day. Occasionally will take a dietary supplement, OR receives less than optimum amount of liquid diet or tube feeding.	Eats over half of most meals. Eats a total of 4 servings of protein (meat, dairy products) each day. Occasionally will refuse a meal, but will usually take a supplement if offered, OR is on a tube feeding or TPN regimen, which probably meets most of nutritional needs.	Eats most of every meal. Never refuses a meal. Usually eats a total of 4 or more servings of meat and dairy products. Occasionally eats between meals. Does not require supplementation.		
	1. Problem:	2. Potential Problem:	3. No Apparent Problem:			
FRICTION AND SHEAR	Requires moderate to maximum assistance in moving. Complete lifting without sliding against sheets is impossible. Frequently slides down in bed or chair, requiring frequent repositioning with maximum assistance. Spacticity, contractures, or agitation leads to almost constant friction.	Moves feebly or requires minimum assistance. During a move skin probably slides to some extent against sheets, chair, restraints, or other devices. Maintains relatively good position in chair or bed most of the time but occasionally slides down.	Moves in bed and in chair independently and has sufficient muscle strength to lift up completely during move. Maintains good position in bed or chair at all times.			
						Total Score

Figure 14–6. Braden Scale for Predicting Pressure Sore Risk. (cont.) *(Source: Copyright Barbara Braden and Nancy Bergstrom, 1988.)*

TABLE 14–9.   GUIDELINES FOR DIRECT WOUND ASSESSMENT

Measurement:
Three dimensional—length × width × depth.
The wound should be assessed for evidence of tunneling, sinus tract formation, or undermining.

Measurement Tips:
If the wound is tunneling or has undermining, the clinician should measure all areas. This is best accomplished by inserting gently into the wound a gloved hand and then measuring this against a disposable measuring guide.
Dividing the ulcer in a clockwise fashion, placing 10 o'clock vertical to the client's head, will assist with standardization in measurement and description between providers.

Wound Staging:
NPUAP and AHCPR Wound Staging— Stage I-IV.
Ulcers do not progress backward through the stages of the healing process. Wounds in various stages also heal differently. Wounds that contain eschar cannot be staged until the eschar has been removed. Identifying stage I pressure ulcers is particularly difficult in clients with orthopedic devices because the skin is not visible. Skin in darkly pigmented people should be assessed by localized skin changes such as temperature, edema, or induration rather than the traditional observation of just redness.

Wound Classification by Color:
This type of staging identifies pressure ulcers as red, yellow, and black (see Figure 5 of Color Plate within this chapter).
Limitations:
Staging by color is limited because wounds may present with more than one color, and underlying structures such as tendons may be mistaken for yellow exudate. In addition, this type of assessment has not been tested for reliability and validity. The usefulness of color staging may be enhanced by identifying the percentages of each color within the wound. Color classification is most effective when used as part of an overall program of wound assessment.

Photographs:
Photographing the wound is especially helpful in settings in which there are multiple health-care providers.

The photograph will help to document the wound's progress, assist with reimbursement, and provide legal documentation and education in wound management. Informed consent is generally necessary for photographing.

Wound Characteristics:
Descriptors: inflammation, induration, ischemic tissue, granulation, epithelialization, exudate, odor. The type of exudate is generally described as serous, serosanguineous, bloody, or purulent.

Fibrinous debris, which is generally white or yellow in color, is frequently normal in healing wounds. Wound beds that are particularly pale may indicate anemia. Wound exudate in limited amounts is not necessarily detrimental and has been found to be an excellent source of fibroblast activity. The consistency of exudate depends on the type of dressing used. Drainage that is copious or contains an odor requires further assessment. Hydrocolloid dressings tend to

(Continues)

TABLE 14–9.   GUIDELINES FOR DIRECT WOUND ASSESSMENT (CONT.)

	melt down when exposed to body temperature, and the drainage may be thick yellow or slightly green, with a musty odor. However, the wound bed should appear clean after the wound is cleansed. *Pseudomonas* has a sweet odor, and anaerobic bacteria have a characteristic foul smell.
Wound Edges: Assessment Descriptors: Color, thickness, degree of attachment, tunneling, undermining.	The edges of chronic wounds may also present with thick, rolled wound margins (called epiboly). This is caused when epithelial cells are unable to migrate across the wound due to lack of moisture in the wound bed.
Surrounding Skin: Redness, warmth, induration, hardness, swelling, skin heat, pain.	Macerated tissue generally appears white in color. Erythema may be due to unrelieved pressure or as a result of irritation from dressing products and tape.

PRESSURE RELIEF

A variety of methods and products are available to prevent ulcer formation through pressure relief. Support surfaces are generally designed for reducing or relieving pressure. The main difference by strict definition is that pressure-relieving devices consistently reduce pressure below capillary closing, whereas pressure reducing devices do not. Of all prevention methods to heal wounds, the most important factor is reducing the interface pressure. The most widely accepted forms of prevention include turning at least every 2 hours, body positioning to reduce pressure on bony prominences, proper transfer techniques to reduce shearing and friction, application of barrier products to reduce moisture, and the use of pressure-reduction devices. Immobility is a prime risk factor in the development of a pressure ulcer. The lack of desire to change position because of depression, pain, excessive sedation, or impaired movement from a neurologic condition that impedes the person's ability to perceive the sensation of ulcer formation are all contributing factors. Few pressure-reduction devices have undergone extensive clinical trials, and the current literature does not identify one support surface as exceptional over another in all clinical circumstances. See Barhyte et al. (1995) for an excellent review of a standardized method for assessing mattresses. Figure 14–8 outlines a method for managing tissue load. Preventative skin programs, which have incorporated alogorithms to identify proper support surfaces, report decreased annual patient-care costs and incidences of pressure ulcer development (Wolf, 1995).

NAME:_____

Complete the rating sheet to assess pressure sore status. Evaluate each item by picking the response that best describes the wound and entering the score in the item score column for the appropriate date.

LOCATION: Anatomic site. Circle, identify right (R) or left (L) and use **"X"** to mark site on body diagrams:

_____ Sacrum & coccyx	_____ Lateral ankle	
_____ Trochanter	_____ Medial ankle	
_____ Ischial tuberosity	_____ Heel	_____ Other site

SHAPE: Overall wound pattern; assess by observing perimeter and depth.
Circle and *date* appropriate description:

_____ Irregular	_____ Linear or elongated	
_____ Round/oval	_____ Bowl/boat	
_____ Square/rectangle	_____ Butterfly	_____ Other shape

Item	Assessment	Date	Date	Date
		Score	Score	Score
1. SIZE	1 = Length × width <4 sq cm 2 = Length × width 4–16 sq cm 3 = Length × width 16.1–36 sq cm 4 = Length × width 36.1–80 sq cm 5 = Length × width >80 sq cm			
2. DEPTH	1 = Nonblanchable erythema on intact skin 2 = Partial-thickness skin loss involving epidermis &/or dermis 3 = Full-thickness skin loss involving damage or necrosis of subcutaneous tissue; may extend down to but not through underlying fascia; &/or mixed partial- & full-thickness &/or tissue layers obscured by granulation tissue 4 = Obscured by necrosis 5 = Full-thickness skin loss with extensive destruction, tissue necrosis, or damage to muscle, bone, or supporting structures			
3. EDGES	1 = Indistinct, diffuse, none clearly visible 2 = Distinct, outline clearly visible, attached, even with wound base 3 = Well defined, not attached to wound base 4 = Well defined, not attached to base, rolled under, thickened 5 = Well defined, fibrotic, scarred or hyperkeratotic			
4. UNDERMINING	1 = Undermining <2 cm in any area 2 = Undermining 2–4 cm involving <50% wound margins 3 = Undermining 2–4 cm involving >50% wound margins 4 = Undermining >4 cm in any area 5 = Tunneling &/or sinus tract formation			
5. NECROTIC TISSUE TYPE	1 = None visible 2 = White/gray nonviable tissue &/or non-adherent yellow slough 3 = Loosely adherent yellow slough 4 = Adherent, soft, black eschar 5 = Firmly adherent, hard, black eschar			
6. NECROTIC TISSUE AMOUNT	1 = None visible 2 = <25% of wound bed covered 3 = 25% to 50% of wound covered 4 = >50% and <75% of wound covered 5 = 75% to 100% of wound covered			

Figure 14–7. Pressure Sore Status Tool *(Continues)*

Item	Assessment	Date	Date	Date
		Score	**Score**	**Score**
7. EXUDATE TYPE	1 = None or bloody 2 = Serosanguineous: thin, watery, pale red/pink 3 = Serous: thin, watery, clear 4 = Purulent: thin or thick, opaque, tan/yellow 5 = Foul purulent: thick, opaque, yellow/green with odor			
8. EXUDATE AMOUNT	1 = None 2 = Scant 3 = Small 4 = Moderate 5 = Large			
9. SKIN COLOR SURROUNDING WOUND	1 = Pink or normal for ethnic group 2 = Bright red &/or blanches to touch 3 = White or gray pallor or hypopigmented 4 = Dark red or purple &/nonblanchable 5 = Black or hyperpigmented			
10. PERIPHERAL TISSUE EDEMA	1 = Minimal swelling around wound 2 = Nonpitting edema extends <4 cm around wound 3 = Nonpitting edema extends ≥4 cm around wound 4 = Pitting edema extends <4 cm around wound 5 = Crepitus &/or pitting edema extends ≥4 cm			
11. PERIPHERAL TISSUE INDURATION	1 = Minimal firmness around wound 2 = Induration <2 cm around wound 3 = Induration 2–4 cm extending <50% around wound 4 = Induration 2–4 cm extending ≥50% around wound 5 = Induration >4 cm in any area			
12. GRANULATION TISSUE	1 = Skin intact or partial-thickness wound 2 = Bright, beefy red; 75% to 100% of wound filled &/or tissue overgrowth 3 = Bright, beefy red; <75% & >25% of wound 4 = Pink &/or dull, dusky red &/or fills ≤25% of wound 5 = No granulation tissue present			
13. EPITHELIALIZATION	1 = 100% of wound covered, surface intact 2 = 75% to <100% of wound covered &/or epi- thelial tissue extends >0.5 cm into wound bed 3 = 50% to <75% of wound covered &/or epi- thelial tissue extends to <0.5 cm into wound bed 4 = 25% to <50% of wound covered 5 = <25% of wound covered			
TOTAL SCORE				
SIGNATURE				

PRESSURE SORE STATUS CONTINUUM

```
1    10    13    15    20    25    30    35    40    45    50    55    60    65
├────┼─────┼─────┼─────┼─────┼─────┼─────┼─────┼─────┼─────┼─────┼─────┼────┤
Tissue      Wound                                              Wound
health      regeneration                                       regeneration
```

Plot the total score on the Pressure Sore Status Continuum by putting an **"X"** on the line and the date beneath the line. Plot multiple scores with their dates to see at a glance regeneration or degeneration of the wound.

Figure 14–7. Pressure Sore Status Tool (cont.). *Source: Copyright 1990 Barbara Bates Jensen. Used with permission. Advances in Wound Care, July/August, 1995, Vol. 8. No. 4. NPUAP Proceedings 1995.*

TABLE 14–10.   UNIVERSAL STAGING SYSTEM FOR PRESSURE ULCERS

Stage I	Stage II	Stage III	Stage IV
Nonblanchable erythema of intact skin: the heralding lesion of skin ulceration. In individuals with darker skin, discoloration of the skin, warmth, edema, induration, and hardness may also be indicators.	Partial-thickness skin loss involving epidermis or dermis, or both. The ulcer is superficial and presents clinically as an abrasion, blister, or shallow crater.	Full-thickness skin loss involving epidermis or dermis, or both. The ulcer is superficial and presents clinically as an abrasion, blister, or shallow crater.	Full-thickness skin loss with extensive destruction, tissue necrosis, or damage to muscle, bone, or supporting structures (such as tendon and joint capsule). Undermining and sinus tracts also may be associated with stage IV pressure ulcers.

Source: Agency for Health Care Policy and Research, Clinical Practice Guidelines for Pressure Ulcers. U.S. Department of Health and Human Services.

.... *vignette* ....

Mr. Sullivan is a 68-year-old patient with multiple sclerosis (MS), who resides in a long-term care facility. He has a longstanding stage III sacral pressure ulcer. He refuses to be turned or use chair pressure-relief devices. He also maintains a poor diet, refusing nutritional supplements and additional vitamin supplementation. His care plan identifies multiple nursing measures to promote healing and reduce further skin breakdown. The nursing measures are not carried out because the client continually refuses treatment. During state inspection, the facility is cited for failure to demonstrate that they provided adequate care for Mr. Sullivan. The main justification for this deficiency is the lack of documentation of Mr. Sullivan's refusal of nursing treatment and lack of alternative treatment options provided to the patient.

Clients with chronic conditions such as pressure ulcers may use their disease process as a means of controlling their health-care treatment and may be depressed as a result of their chronic condition. In such cases, it is common to find clients and their direct-care providers at odds with the treatment plan. Educating the direct-care staff on delivering care that allows the cognitively intact client to make individual choices is essential. One method is by developing a written treatment contract that identifies a plan of care on which both parties can agree. This is especially helpful when working in long-term care facilities, where surveyors may cite the facility for failing to provide proper pressure relief even though the client is not compliant with the interdisciplinary care plan.

PAIN

The assessment of pain in clients with pressure ulcers is frequently neglected. This is compounded by the fact that pain is particularly difficult to evaluate in

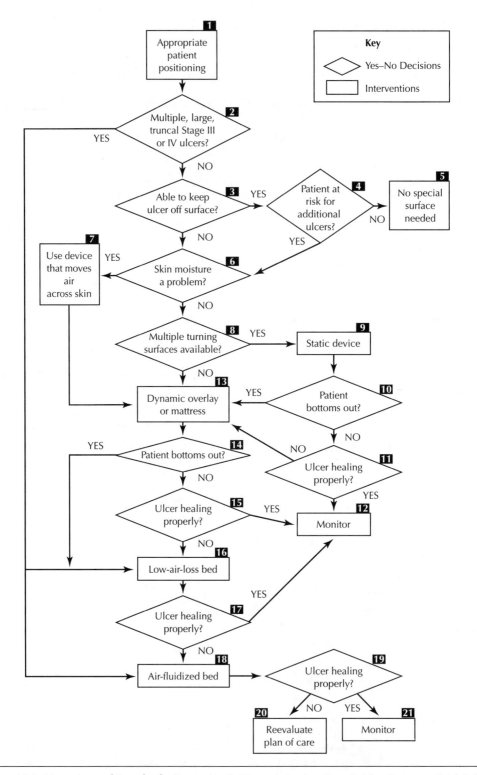

Figure 14–8. Management of tissue loads. *(Source: Used with permission from Pressure Ulcer Treatment: Quick Reference Guide for Clinicians.* Advances in Wound Care, *8[2], 22–44. Copyright © Springhouse Corporation.)*

clients who are cognitively impaired. Clinicians should routinely assess the type and severity of the pain reported by the client, using a standard pain scale. One study identified that patients with cognitive impairment had an easier time rating their pain on the Faces Pain Rating Scale (Rook, 1996). Clients who are experiencing pain will generally limit their movements, which further reduces the potential for healing. Clients who are cognitively impaired may exhibit their pain through increased episodes of agitation. Therefore, assessing for and providing pain relief as part of the overall treatment plan is essential. Pressure-relieving devices may assist with pain reduction, and dressings such as hydrogel or hydrocolloids are cooling and can reduce burning and irritation. A study by Dallam et al. (1995) concluded that patients with stage IV pressure ulcers did not necessarily have less pain then those with less extensive wounds. The study concluded that many patients may not be able to verbalize their pain, and therefore pain may go unreported.

NUTRITION

The patient's overall nutritional status is important to the healing process. For a detailed review of nutrition in the older adult, see Chapter 8. Inadequate protein remains a key factor in promoting the healing process. In patients who are severely protein deficient, soft tissue breakdown is more common because hypoproteinemia leads to edema (Bryant et al., 1992). Protein status can be assessed in a variety of ways, including a 24-hour urine, calculated for nitrogen balance, albumin, prealbumin, or transferrin. Total lymphocytic count (% of lymphocytes

× white blood count [WBC]) is also very sensitive to protein depletion, and a count less than 800 is considered a marker of malnutrition. Albumin is generally a poor marker of nutritional status for wound healing because it has a half-life of 21 days. Therefore, laboratory testing may be of limited value in detecting early protein depletion. Physiologic stress brought on by a number of factors lowers albumin even with an adequate protein store (Thomas, 1997). Prealbumin is an earlier marker of protein depletion but is rarely ordered because of the laboratory expense. Protein deficiencies may not be seen in patients who have recently reduced their protein intake and normal lab values and body weight may be maintained despite the need for protein supplementation. The use of supplemental vitamins in wound healing without the presence of known deficiency remains controversial (Thomas, 1997). Nevertheless, many older adults who are at risk for developing pressure ulcers have inadequate nutritional intake and a period of supplementation followed by reevaluation of healing appears prudent (Gambert & Gaunsing, 1980). Guidelines for the use of vitamins and protein supplementation are outlined in Table 14–11. The simplest method for assessing intake is a 3-day caloric count.

CLINICAL MANAGEMENT

Cleansing

Wounds should be cleansed with the most nontoxic product available to avoid injury to granulating tissue. Table 14–12 identifies agents that promote or delay epidermal resurfacing. The wound-cleansing product most physiologically

TABLE 14–11.   GUIDELINES FOR VITAMIN AND PROTEIN SUPPLEMENTATION FOR PRESSURE ULCERS

Vitamin C, 250 mg qd PO	Lack of vitamin C from diet or trauma reduces the ability of the wound to form new capillaries (Doughty, 1992).
Protein supplementation: Clients with pressure ulcers should receive at least 1.0 to 1.50 grams of protein per kilogram of weight a day (Thomas, 1997).	Low protein stores have been demonstrated to be a risk factor for the development of and the delayed healing ability of pressure ulcers (Thomas, 1997).
Vitamin A—The recommended dose is 20,000 to 25,000 IU for 10 days or a tid application topically.	Vitamin A helps to restore the normal inflammatory response and is therefore recommended for clients who are receiving steroid therapy (Doughty, 1992).
Zinc supplementation, 150 mg daily for a short trial; should not continue if the wound does not appear to be responding.	Zinc levels decline during injury and with chronic steroid use. Excessive zinc levels can interfere with copper absorption and have been found in animal models to decrease wound strength (Thomas, 1997).

compatible is normal saline. Although relatively inexpensive, the product frequently comes in a large container for single patient usage and must be disposed of within 48 hours in most institutional settings. There have been multiple studies demonstrating that full-strength povidone iodine, peroxide, and Dakin's solution impede fibroblast activity (Coletta, 1995). The benefit of topical antibiotics as illustrated in Table 14–13 may be due to their moist properties rather than their antimicrobial property (Goode & Thomas, 1997). There are a variety of skin cleansers available for commercial use. The rule of thumb in selection is ease of application, maintaining sterility from one patient to another, cost, and toxicity to tissue. Wound irrigations can be used to remove surface contaminants and assist with the granulating process. The recommended force is 8 pounds per square inch, which can be achieved with a 35-mL syringe and a 19-G angiocath

(Frantz & Gardner, 1994b). Some commercial products on the market also meet these criteria, reducing nursing time and equipment disposal costs.

Debriding

Debridement can be performed in several different ways, including sharp incision and mechanical, chemical, and autodebridment. Sharp debridement is generally indicated when infection is present. Surgical debridement can be associated with bacteremia. Therefore, patients with implanted devices should receive antibiotic therapy prior to debridement (Smith, 1995). Mechanical debridement includes wet-to-dry dressings, hydrotherapy, and irrigations. Wet-to-dry dressing removal can impede granulating tissue and should be used in situations in which the granulating tissue can be isolated from the necrotic tissue. In addition, wet-to-dry dressings may be painful. Hydrotherapy is effective, but care should

TABLE 14–12.   SELECTED TOPICAL AGENTS/DRESSINGS

Agent	Relative Healing Rate (%)[a,b]
Hydrocolloid (DuoDerm) (ConvaTec, Princeton, NJ)	+36
Transparent adhesive dressings	
BlisterFilm (Sherwood Medical, St. Louis, MO)	+33
Bioclusive (Johnson & Johnson, Arlington, TX)	+20
OpSite (Smith and Nephew, Largo, FL)	+18
Benzoyl peroxide (20%)	+33
Bacitracin zinc	+30
1% Silver sulfadiazine (Silvadene [Hoechst Marion Roussel, Kansas City, MO])	+28
Polymyxin B sulfate and Bacitracin zinc ointment (Polysporin [Warner Wellcome, Morris Plains, NJ])	+25
Johnson & Johnson's First Aid Cream (Arlington, TX)	+20
Neomycin sulfate powder	−5
Dakin's solution (1% sodium hypochlorite)	−6
Hydrogen peroxide (3%)	−8
Povidone iodine solution	−10
Wet-to-dry gauze	−15
Furacin (Roberts Pharmaceutical, Eatontown, NJ)	−30
Triamcinolone acetonide (0.1%)	−34

[a] Compared to untreated.

[b] Positive numbers indicate agents that *promote* epidermal resurfacing; negative numbers indicate agents that *delay* epidermal resurfacing.

Source: Reprinted with permission from Alvarez, O., Rozint, J., & Wiseman, D. (1989). Moist environment for healing: Matching the dressing to the wound. *Wounds, 1,* 35–51. Copyright © 1989, Health Management Publications, Inc., Wayne, PA.

be taken to avoid high-pressure jets. Irrigation with a waterpick has been effective in some situations, but it is often messy, with concentration of the solution's force difficult to regulate. Chemical debridement takes from several days to several weeks to work. It is not effective on thick eschar and requires that the tissue be cross-hatched. Some of the chemicals are irritating to surrounding tissue, and a barrier product such as petroleum jelly should be placed on the wound's perimeter. Chemical debriding agents are inactivated by other agents used in wound treatments, and product directions should be followed carefully

(Goode & Thomas, 1997). Autolytic debridement is the process of allowing the wound fluid to help self-digest the devitalized tissue by covering it with an occlusive-type dressing. This process should not be used if the wound is infected or if there is compromised circulation.

Dressing Selection

There is an overwhelming array of commercial dressings on the market. Consideration in dressing selection includes the ease of application, wound type, stage, overall appearance of the wound bed, pain control, and cost. The immediate goals of the wound treatment should also be reviewed in the context of the client's clinical situation (healing versus palliative care). Undermining and tunneling should be identified, and areas should be packed to fill the dead space. Packing should be performed lightly to avoid excessive pressure on capillary blood flow. Major dressing categories are outlined in Table 14–7.

Healing Process

Supportive healing environments include removing necrotic tissue, identifying and treating infections, preventing premature closure, maintaining a moist environment while reducing maceration, and maintaining an adequate body temperature to improve blood flow. Moist wounds heal faster than dry wounds. The reason for this is that epidermal cells require moisture to migrate across the surface of the wound. Wound fluid contains a number of cellular factors that are believed to be an excellent medium for fibroblastic growth (Motta, 1993). Moist wounds also heal with less scarring and decrease wound pain (Goode & Thomas, 1997). In general, the age-related changes in the phases of the healing process include a delayed initiation and slower progression. The distinct systematic phases of healing do not necessarily reach the same plateaus as in younger subject (Eaglestein, 1989). The client's overall health history should be reviewed to identify risk factors that may potentially hinder the healing process. Chronic disease or conditions that damage vessels, such as radiation, peripheral vascular disease, anemia, and diabetes, limit the availability of oxygen and nutrients. The loss of oxygen through vasoconstriction should be minimized by maintaining body warmth, reducing smoking, and treating pain. The

clinician should evaluate the therapeutic effect of beta blockers, which cause vasoconstriction, and diuretics, which cause constriction and hypovolemia, in relation to the client's overall physical condition (Stotts & Hunt, 1997).

Although wound bacterial counts with greater than 100,000 organisms affect localized healing, an exception to this is beta-hemolytic streptococcus, which can impede wound healing at colony counts less then 100,000 (Doughty, 1992). Wounds that do not heal or exhibit signs of clinical infection, such as fever, erythema, edema, or foul-smelling drainage, should be evaluated for antibiotic therapy. Older adults may not exhibit the normal fever or immune response, so fever may be absent or delayed. In general, wound cultures are not necessary. The majority of pressure ulcers are colonized with bacteria, and they do not necessarily impede wound healing. If the wound contains foul-smelling drainage, the client has a fever, or the wound is not healing, cultures may be indicated. Needle aspiration is the best method for culturing pressure ulcers because it can differentiate between skin and tissue organisms (Stotts & Hunt, 1997). Swab cultures are the most common method of obtaining a wound culture. However, their benefit is extremely limited because they evaluate only surface bacterial contamination. Wound preparation for culturing includes cleansing the wound with normal saline, avoiding pus or necrotic tissue during swabbing, and removing all prior wound preparations at least 24 hours prior to obtaining the culture (Elder & Greer, 1995). Wounds that do not heal or have uneven or suspicious-looking margins should be referred for a tissue biopsy. Very foul-smelling wounds are usually contaminated with anaerobic organisms. *Pseudomonas aeruginosa* and *Providencia* species are two organisms that are not associated with simple wound colonization. When evidence of infection exists, reducing the colony count to less than 10^5 within the wound bed can improve healing (Coletta, 1995). Topical antibiotic treatment remains controversial because of the tendency of some antibiotics to damage the granulating tissue. Topical sliver sulfadiazine and gentamicin may be effective in reducing the bacteria's growth. Metronidazole has been used in wounds containing anaerobes to reduce odor and colony count (McMullen, 1992). If instituted to reduce colony counts, topical antibiotic therapy should be limited to a 2-week trial period. The antibiotic chosen should cover gram-negative, gram-positive, and anaerobic organisms (Elder & Greer, 1995). Systemic antibiotics are not necessary to treat chronic wounds unless they are grossly infected.

Complications

Sepsis and osteomyelitis remain two of the most serious complications associated with pressure ulcers. Sepsis carries a 50% in-hospital mortality rate (Patterson & Bennett, 1995). Polymicrobial bacteremia is common and often includes gram-negative rods and anaerobes. Antibiotic therapy must be broad enough to cover anaerobic organisms, gram-negative bacilli, and gram-positive cocci, until blood cultures isolate the organism. Osteomyelitis is the presence of an infection in the bone. Wounds that do not heal or cause persistent fevers, pain, or drainage should be evaluated for osteomyelitis. The most accurate method for identifying osteomyelitis is bone biopsy. This is

not always practical, and a combination of WBC, erythrocyte sedimentation rate (ESR), and plain x-rays is reported to have a predictive value of 69% when all three are positive (Bergstrom, 1995). Although uncommon, tetanus infections do occur in deep wounds, and patients should receive prophylaxis if indicated (Coletta, 1995).

SETTING-SPECIFIC ISSUES

Pressure ulcers require an interdisciplinary approach. The primary-care physician, surgeon, nutritionist, occupational therapist, physical therapist, and social worker may be consulted for professional expertise. Education of the client and the primary caregiver regardless of setting remains the key to prevention and healing of the majority of pressure ulcers.

Community-dwelling clients who have functional limitations may not be able to provide for pressure relief independently, and attention should be paid to educating caregivers in the home setting. Referral to a home-care agency is necessary for most community-dwelling clients with pressure ulcers. Individuals who demonstrate cognitive impairment or depression or those who lack adequate social or financial supports may not be in a position to carry through with treatment recommendations. Social workers who can provide both mental health counseling and financial assessments are an important part of the team. Likewise, clients who have neurologic or musculoskeletal conditions that require extensive supine or wheelchair-bound status should be referred to an occupational or physical therapist to identify the proper seating device or rehabilitative measures to provide pressure relief.

■ HAIR

By age 50, half of the population has gray hair. The loss of color is related to a decline in the melanocytes and melanocytic activity in the hair bulb. Androgenetic alopecia is an autosomal dominant trait, dependent on androgen hormones and genetic predisposition. Hair loss is more pronounced in men and follows the typical pattern of frontal recession. Women are also affected, but the hair loss is usually more diffuse, with a slower rate and later onset. Extensive frontotemporal hair loss in women is not commonly seen, and the clinician should refer individuals with this finding for a full evaluation for a possible excessive androgen condition (Sawaya, 1997).

CLINICAL MANAGEMENT

There are a variety of cosmetic approaches to hair loss that are beyond the scope of this chapter. Hair transplantations, although expensive, are currently conducted as an alternative to hair loss. Even slight hair loss, especially in women, has been reported to result in social anxiety and a decline in psychosocial well-being (Cash et al., 1993). The clinician should explore with the client the extent to which the hair loss may be affecting overall self-esteem.

Pharmacologic Measures

There are a variety of treatments currently under investigation for the regrowth of hair. See Sawaya (1997) for a full review. The most widely known and frequently used drug is minoxidil. The usual dosage is 2% applied topically to the scalp twice a day. The medication takes up to 4 months before regrowth is observed and has not been clinically demonstrated to affect frontal hair regrowth. Rather, it is reported to provide for moderate regrowth of vertex hair in approximately 26% of patients and must be used continuously in order for hair growth to continue (Goldfarb et al., 1996).

Propecia (finasteride), a new drug developed from prostate research, has been found to be most effective in androgenic vertex thinning. Like Rogaine, the drug must be used continuously to avoid hair loss. The dosage orally is 1 mg daily. There is no report of major drug interactions. However, sexual dysfunction has been reported in a small percentage of users. The drug will significantly elevate PSA levels. A new topical antiandrogen receptor blocker under investigation is called RU5884 (Sawaya, 1997).

■ NAILS

AGE-RELATED CHANGES

Nails generally become thick and brittle with age. Toenails thicken and become more difficult to cut. The growth of the nail decreases, and longitudinal ridges are characteristic. Neglected toenails become excessively long and curved, taking on a ram-horn appearance, termed onychogryphotic.

TINEA UNGUIUM (ONYCHOMYCOSIS)

Clinical Presentation

Usual Presentation of Disease. Fungal infections are common in older adults and are frequently difficult to treat. The

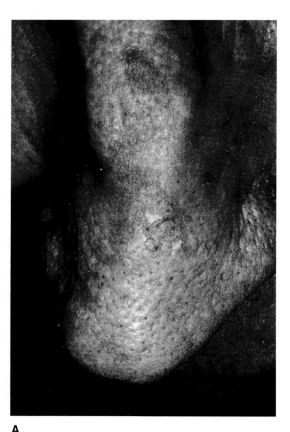

A

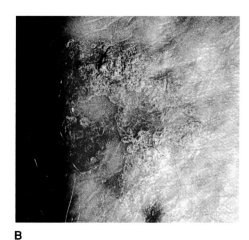

B

Figure 1 A & B. Actinic keratosis. These solitary lesions have a red base and the typical dry adherent, yellow-brown scale. *Source: Habif, T. P. (1996). Clinical Dermatology: A Color Guide to Diagnosis and Therapy, 3d ed., St. Louis: Mosby-Yearbook. Used with permission.*

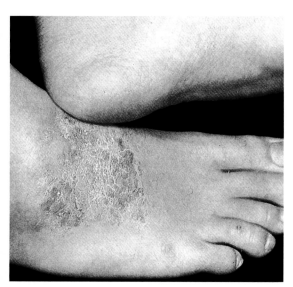

Figure 2. Lichen simplex chronicus. This localized plaque of chronic eczematous inflammation was created by rubbing with the opposite heel. *Source: Habif, T. P. (1996). Clinical Dermatology: A Color Guide to Diagnosis and Therapy, 3d ed., St. Louis: Mosby-Yearbook. Used with permission.*

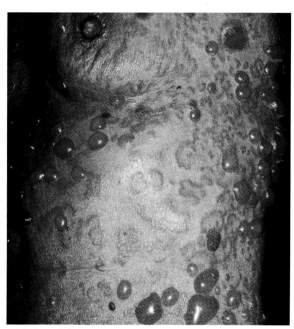

Figure 3. Bullous pemphigoid. Generalized eruption with tense blisters arising from an edematous erythematous annular base. *Source: Habif, T. P. (1996). Clinical Dermatology: A Color Guide to Diagnosis and Therapy, 3d ed., St. Louis: Mosby-Yearbook. Used with permission.*

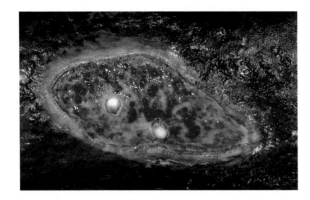

Figure 4. Typical appearance of a venous stasis ulcer and surrounding skin changes in a patient with chronic venous insufficiency. *Source: Bondi, E. E., Jegasothy, B. V., and Lazarus, G. S. (1991). Dermatology: Diagnosis and Therapy, 1st ed., Norwalk, CT: Appleton & Lange. Used with permission.*

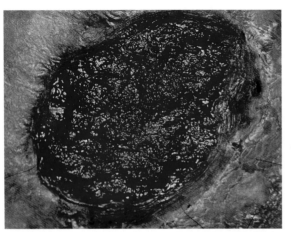

A

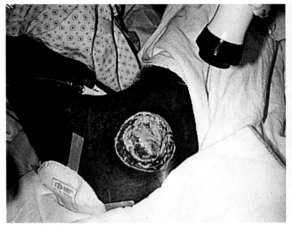

B

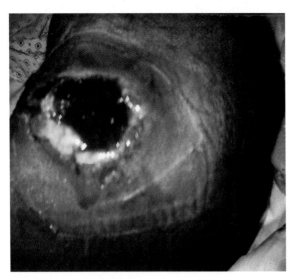

C

Figure 5. Pressure ulcers demonstrating color classification. A. Red; B. Yellow; C. Black.

appearance of infections includes yellowish longitudinal streaks, whitish yellow areas near the cuticle, and destruction of the nail plate. A fine, white, powdery substance may form under the nail bed (Langana, 1992). Tinea unguium, or onychomycosis, is a dermatophyte infection of the toenail plate and is quite common in the elderly, especially among males. Occasionally, the infection is due to *Candida*. The condition is asymptomatic but may show signs of erythema and tinea pedis. The condition should be distinguished from similar nail changes that occur as a result of normal aging.

Atypical Presentation of Disease. Psoriasis is sometimes mistaken for onychomycosis. Both conditions may be present simultaneously. A helpful diagnostic differentiation is that in psoriasis there may be pitting of the nail plate.

Clinical Management

Confirmation of the fungus should be performed by a dermatologist. Topical creams do not always penetrate the nail bed and infections are frequently recurring. Surgical removal is sometimes required (Goldfarb et al., 1996). Nail brittleness can be improved by avoiding harsh chemicals. Lactic acid 12% lotion has been shown to be effective in improving nails brittleness. See Habif (1990), for an excellent review of the treatment of nail fungus.

Pharmacologic Measures. Onychomycosis frequently recurs and is resistant to treatment. Two new classes of drugs, azoles and allylamines, have shown promising results. Table 14–13 outlines the effectivness of each drug against various conditions. The oral doses are itraconazole 200 mg or terbinafine 250 mg, used daily for 3 months. Both have demonstrated a low relapse rate (Goldfarb et al., 1996). All of these medications have significant drug interactions with such common medications as H_2 blockers, warfarin, and oral hypoglycemics (Brodell & Elewski, 1995).

Rehabilitation. The clinician should identify how nail care is obtained and by whom. Barriers to obtaining podiatry

TABLE 14–13.   EFFICACY OF SYSTEMIC ANTIFUNGAL DRUGS

	Dermatophytes	*Candida*	*Pityrosporum*
Griseofulvin	+	−	−
■ AZOLES			
Itraconazole	++	++	++
Ketoconazole	+	++	++
Fluconazole	+	++	+
■ ALLYLAMINES			
Terbinafine	++	+	−

++, Very effective, +, effective, −, not effective.
Source: Reprinted with permission Mosby-Year Book, Elewiski B. E. Clinical Pearl: Mechanisms of action of systemic antifungal agents, (1993); 28, 5 ppS28-S34.

care should be explored and health education provided on the benefits of routine nail care. Older adults may neglect their nails for a variety of reasons. Lack of flexibility or hand strength, fine tremors, and failing eyesight are common physical deficits that reduce older adults' ability to independently cut their own nails. Nails may be neglected because of financial reasons as well. Routine podiatry care billable under Medicare is limited to such conditions as diabetes mellitus and peripheral vascular disease. Long untreated nails place the older adults at risk for infections as well as changes in gait which could lead to falling. A consult to physical or occupational may be appropriate to identify methods for the client to maintain independence in foot hygiene.

.... *vignette* ....

Mrs. Keller is a 100-year-old woman living in senior housing, who experienced three falls within 1 week. Each time she was brought to the emergency room, she was found to be without injury and sent back to her apartment, only to fall again. The nurse practitioner made a home visit per request of Mrs. Keller's case manager. Mrs. Keller answered the door, walking with a walker. She displayed an obvious gait abnormality (she walked on the side of her left foot and the ball of her right). She was initially hesitant to remove her footwear because she was ashamed of the condition of her feet. She admitted that her failing eyesight and back pain made it impossible for her to care for her feet. Upon observation, the client had ingrown toenails, a callus on the heel of her right foot, and an infected bunion on her left foot. These conditions were causing an alteration in the client's gait and subsequent falls. Following treatment of these conditions, the client's falls subsided.

CLINICAL PEARL

Explore all potential reasons for falling and consider poor foot hygiene as a potential contributor to falls in older adults.

 ## CASE STUDY #1

Mrs. Jones is a 75-year-old woman admitted to a subacute-care facility on the second day post–right hip replacement. You are called by the nurse to evaluate a red area near the client's left hip.

The client is noted to have a non-blanchable stage I maroon-colored area 5 cm × 5 cm in circumference near her left ischium. She is complaining that the area feels hot and that it burns.

The client is incontinent of urine. Her coccyx has a 1/2 cm × 1/2 cm slit opening with surrounding satellite red pustules and is extremely macerated. The client is refusing most of her dietary intake secondary to nausea.

Diagnosis is as follows:

1. S/P right hip replacement
2. Diabetes mellitus
3. Osteoarthritis
4. History of recurrent pneumonia
5. Iron deficiency anemia

The social history is positive for tobacco use. The client is taking the following medications:

- Gynase prestab (10 mg/d
- Warfarin (Coumadin) 2.5 mg adjusted daily per protime
- Fesol 200 mg tid
- Oxycodone hydrochloride and acetaminophen (Percocet) 5 mg q4h for pain

Lab results reveal the following: red blood cells (RBCs), 3.29; hemoglobin, 10.3, hematocrit, 30.5; albumin, 3.0; urine routine and microscopic WBC 20, RBC 50; and blood glucose, 350.

QUESTIONS

1. Please identify appropriate interventions given the preceding information.

Mrs. Jones refuses to turn every 2 hours secondary to pain and stiffness from her osteoarthritis. Her coccyx is now a stage II yellow pressure ulcer, which continues to be aggravated by moisture from her incontinence.

2. Please list appropriate interventions for the above information.

Mrs. Jones' left ischial area looks like a very large boil, with erythema and induration surrounding the entire area.

3. Please list interventions for the above clinical situation.

Following debridement, the area is noted to progress to a stage III yellow/black pressure ulcer, and she reports increasing pain at the site.

4. Please identify appropriate interventions for the above clinical situation.

ANSWERS

1. A. Assess physical status and abnormal laboratory findings including: elevated blood glucose, anemia, urinary infection, incontinence, nausea/poor nutritional intake, level of pain, complaint of heat and burning at left ischium with nonblanchable stage I maroon-colored area, open area on coccyx with surrounding satellite red pustules and skin maceration.

   B. Rational/possible treatment interventions

   (1) Nonblanchable stage I maroon-colored skin change is a poor prognostic sign for underlying tissue death. The patient's pain and burning are the first sign of tissue ischemia. Measure the entire maroon area and obtain permission from the patient to photograph the coccyx. Com-

plete a pressure risk assessment and place the patient on a pressure reducing mattress. Relieve pressure by turning the patient every 1-2 hours. Assess all bony prominences for signs of break down.

(2) The urinary infection and incontinence are contributing to the maceration. This may contribute to soft tissue infection when there is a break in skin integrity. Culture and treat the urinary infection. Apply a barrier product to the entire coccyx area to reduce the urine contact with the skin. The satellite red pustules are a classic sign of a *Candida* infection and should be treated with a topical antifungal.

(3) The anemia and low protein intake are risk factors for the development of a pressure ulcer. Because of the patient's nausea consider a reduction in the oxycodone hydrochloride and acetaminophen and iron supplementation. For the first day following medication reduction, concentrate on increasing clear fluid intake.

(4) The elevated blood glucose may be a result of the urinary infection. Consider increasing the oral hypoglycemic until the infection is under control.

2. A. Rational/possible treatment interventions:

(1) Adequate pain control is essential in wound treatment complicance. Assess Mrs. Jones' level of pain using a pain rating scale from 1 to 10.

(2) Provide education regarding the need to turn and relieve pressure. Consult with physical therapy for alternative positioning. Provide regular ROM to reduce joint stiffness. Consider the use of plain acetaminophen 1 every 6 hours for arthritis pain.

(3) Toilet Mrs. Jones every 2 hours. If this is not possible, use soft wicking material between Mrs. Jones' legs to absorb urine and reduce exposure of skin to urine.

(4) Debride the yellow area in the pressure ulcer using an enzymatic debriding agent (see Table 14–7 for product examples)

3. Pressure areas that take on a boil appearance with erythema and induration are termed "walled-off pressure ulcers." They indicate severe injury in underlying tissue. This type of ulcer requires immediate surgical debridement and possible intravenous antibiotic therapy.

4. Increased pain in a pressure ulcer especially following deep debridement with evidence of local tissue infection is indicative of osteomyelitis. Evaluate for the presence of osteomyelitis through the following diagnostic tools: x-ray, erythrocyte sedimentation rate, and WBC.

CASE STUDY #2

Mr. Jones is an 87-year-old male presenting to the senior center wellness clinic with a 13-year-old lower leg ulcer. He reports that his ulcer has been throbbing recently and he is requesting wound-care options.

Mr. Jones lives alone in a dwelling without running water. He is grossly unkempt and dressed in filthy clothing and smells of strong body odor. His wound is covered with a soiled, saturated gauze dressing, which is secured with masking tape. His socks are filthy and full of holes, and his feet are caked with dirt.

The left foot ulcer is below the left lateral malleolus and lateral aspect of the left foot. It measures 5.5 cm × 7 cm in size. The periwound margin is macerated, but the entire area surrounding the ulcer is bright red and itchy and has scaly, thickened tissue surrounding the entire wound. The wound bed is pink, 92% granulating tissue, with minimal yellow eschar. There is a foul-smelling, tan drainage. Left dorsalis pedis and posttibial are diminished but palpable. The foot is cool to touch with dependent rubor. Edema in the lower leg, 2+, is tender to the touch.

Mr. Jones' medical history includes diabetes mellitus (DM) diet control and previous varicose vein ligation. He is a one-pack-a-day cigarette smoker. Previous wound treatments include silver sulfadiazine (Silvadene) ointment, hydrocolloid dressings, gingen green tincture, povidone iodine (Betadine), and saline dressings. He is currently being treated with lanolin ointment on the scaly areas surrounding the wound. Mr. Jones washes the wound with saline and applies whatever dressing is available. His current medications include aspirin 1 qd and furosemide (Lasix) 40 mg.

Mr. Jones reports that his meals consist of mostly canned soups and cereal. He is a strict vegetarian. During further conversations with Mr. Jones, he reveals that he is quite well off financially and it is his preference to live the way he does.

Mr. Jones agrees to blood work and a culture of his leg ulcer.

- CBC—RBC, 4.0; HCT, 40; HGB, 12; WBC, 10.2
- Blood glucose, 140
- Lytes-K, 3.0, Na, 135, Cl, 101
- Albumin, 3.0
- Culture reveals mixed flora

QUESTIONS

1. Please identify immediate interventions.

2. What might be the cause of the erythema around Mr. Jones' leg ulcer?

ANSWERS

1. Elicit from Mr. Jones his perception of his medical and social situation in relationship to his leg ulcer. Identify to what extent he is willing to accept medical interventions. Identify previous treatment options for their success and compliance. Clarify willingness to improve life style to foster healing (ie, nutrition, running water, regular ulcer care, smoking cessation). Complete a history and physical concentrating on Mr. Jones' vascular status and left foot ulceration. Mr. Jones has a number of vascular risk factors; therefore, at minimum, an ankle brachial index should be performed to rule out evidence of arterial involvement. Measure, describe, and photograph the ulcer's appearance. The culture reveals mixed flora, which is common in most chronic wounds. It generally does not require treatment unless there is evidence of systemic infection or the wound is not healing. In Mr. Jones' case it is difficult to tell what might be contributing to the lack of wound healing; therefore, local treatment and monitoring prior to instituting antibiotic therapy would be the first course of action.

2. The most likely cause of the erythema around Mr. Jones' leg ulcer is stasis dermatitis with local reaction or allergic reaction. Lanolin is frequently an offending agent for local inflammation.

■ REFERENCES

Barhyte, D. Y., McCance, L., Valenta, A., et al. (1995). Selection of a standard hospital mattress: data-based decision making. *J Wound Ostomy Cont Nurs, 22*(6), 267–270.

Barnes, L., McCallister, R. E., & Lucky A. W. (1987). Crusted Norwegian scabies. *Arch Dermatol, 123*, 95–97.

Barr, D. M. (1996). The Unna boot as a treatment for venous ulcers. *Nurse Pract, 21*(7), 55–77.

Bates, B. (1995). *A guide to physical examination and history taking*. Philadelphia: J. B. Lippincott.

Bates-Jensen, B. M. (1995). Indices to include in wound healing assessment. *Adv Wound Care, 8*(4), 28–33.

Beachman, B. E. (1995). Geriatric dermatology. In Reichel, W. (Ed.), *Care of the elderly: Clinical aspects of aging*. (pp. 416–425). Williams & Wilkins, Baltimore, MD.

Bergstrom, N. I. (1997). Strategies for preventing pressure ulcers. *Clin Geriatr Med 13*(3), 437–451.

Bernstein, J. E., Bickers, D. R., Dahl M. V., et al. (1987). Treatment of chronic post herpetic neuralgia with topical capsaicin. *J Am Acad Dermatol, 17*, 93–96.

Brodell, R. T., & Elewski, B. E. (1995). Clinical pearls: Systemic antifungal drugs and drug interactions. *J Am Acad Dermotol, 33*, 259–260.

Bryant, R. A., Shannon, M. L. Pieper, B., et al. (1992). Pressure ulcers. In Bryant, R. (Ed.), *Chronic wound care* (pp. 105–155). St. Louis: Mosby.

Buckley, M., Rustin, A. (1990). Management of irritable skin disorders in the elderly. *Br J Hosp Med, 44*, 24–29.

Burton, C. S. (1993a). Treatment of leg ulcers. *Dermatol Clin, 11*(2), 315–323.

Burton, C. S. (1993b). Management of chronic and problem lower extremity wounds. *Dermatol Clin, 11*(4), 767–773.

Chenitz, C., Takano Stone, I., Salisbury, S. A. (1991). Physical assessment of the eye, ear, nose and neck. In Chenitz, C., Takano Stone, I., & Salisbury, S. A. (Eds.). *A guide to advanced practice.* (pp. 32–39). Philadelphia: W. B. Saunders.

Coletta, E. M. (1995). Pressure ulcers practical considerations in their prevention and treatment. In Reichel, W., (Ed.). *Care of the elderly: Clinical aspects of aging.* (pp. 380–396). Williams & Wilkins, Baltimore, MD.

Dallam, L., Smith, C., Jackson, B. S., et al. (1995). Pressure ulcer pain: Assessment and quantification. *J Wound Ostomy Cont Nurs, 22*(5), 211–218.

Doughty, D. (1992). Principles of wound healing and wound management. In Bryant, R. A. (Ed.). *Chronic wound care* (pp. 31–61). St. Louis: Mosby.

Dowing, D. T., Stewart, M., Strauss, J. S. (1989). Changes in sebum secretions and the sebaceous gland. *Clin Geriatr Med, 5*(1), 109–114.

Dunn, L. B., Damesyn, M., Moore, A. A., et al. (1997). Does estrogen prevent skin aging? Results from the first national health and nutrition examination survey. *Arch Dermatol, 133,* 339–342.

Eaglestein, W. H. (1989). Wound healing and aging. *Clin Geriatr Med, 5*(1), 183–187.

Elder, D. M., & Greer, K. E. (1995). Venous disease: How to heal and prevent chronic leg ulcers. *Geriatrics, 50*(8), 30–36.

Fenske, N. A., & Lober, C. W. (1986). Structural and functional changes of normal aging skin. *J Am Acad Dermatol, 15*(4), 571–585.

Frantz, R. A., & Gardner, S. (1994a). Clinical concerns: Management of dry skin. *J Gerontol Nurs, 20*(9), 15–18.

Frantz, R. A., Gardner, S. (1994b). Elderly skin care: Principles of chronic wound care. *Journal of Gerontological Nursing, 20*(9), 35–44.

Gambert, S. R., & Gaunsing, A. R. (1980). Protein-calorie malnutrition in the elderly. *J Am Geriatr Soc, 28,* 272–275.

Gilchrest, B. A. (1986). Skin diseases in the elderly. In Calkins, E., Ford, A., & Katz, P. (Eds.). *Practice of geriatrics.* (pp. 513–522). Philadelphia: W. B. Saunders.

Goldberg, S. H., & Bronson, D. (1991). Blistering diseases: Diagnostic help for primary care physicians. *Postgrad Med, 89*(2), 159–162.

Goldfarb, M., Ellis, C. N., & Voorhees, J. (1996). Dermatologic diseases and problems. In Cassel, C. K., Cohen, H. J., et al. (Eds.). *Geriatric medicine* (pp. 667–680). New York: Springer.

Goode, P. S., & Thomas, D. T. (1997). Pressure ulcers: Local wound care. *Clin Geriatr Med, 13*(3), 543–552.

Grove, G. L. (1989). Physiologic changes in older skin. *Clin Geriatr Med, 5*(1), 115–125.

Habif, T. (1990). *Clinical dermatology,* C. V. Mosby.

Hardy, M. A. (1996). What can you do about your patient's dry skin. *J Gerontol Nurs, 22*(5), 10–18.

Holdiness, M. (1988). On the classification of the sign of Leser–Trélat. *J Am Acad Dermatol, 19*(4), 754–757.

Hume, A. L., & Owens, N. J. (1995). Drugs in the elderly. In Reichel, W. (Ed.). *Care of the elderly* (pp. 41–64). Williams & Wilkins'. Baltimore, MD.

Johnson, M. (1995). Healing determinents in older people with leg ulcers. *Res Nurs Health, 18*(5), 393–403.

Jolleys, J. (1989). Treatment of shingles and post-herpetic neuralgia. *British American Journal, 298* (June), 1537–1538.

Katz, H. (1995). Topical corticosteroids. *Dermatol Clin, 13*(4), 805–815.

Kemp, M. G., & Krouskop, T. A. (1994). Pressure ulcers: Reducing incidence and severity by managing pressure. *J Gerontol Nurs, 20*(9), 27–34.

Kleinsmith, D., & Perricone, N. (1989). Common skin problems in the elderly. *Clin Geriatr Med, 5*(1), 189–211.

Kligman, L. H. (1986). Photoaging: Manifestations, prevention and treatment. *Dermatol Clin, 4*(3), 517–528.

Kligman A. M., & Graham, J. A. (1989). The psychology of appearance in the elderly. *Clin Geriatr Med, 5*(1), 213–221.

Kurban, R. S., & Kurban, A. K. (1993). Common skin disorders of aging: Diagnosis and treatment. *Geriatrics, 48*(4), p. 30–42.

Langana, F. L. (1992). Dermotological pedal manisfestations in the elderly. *Topics in Geriatric Rehabilitation, 7*(3), 14–23.

Lever, W. F. (1979). Pemphigus and pemphigoid. *J Am Acad Dermatol, 1,* p, 2–31.

Lin, A. N., Carter, D., & Balin, A. (1989). Non melanoma skin cancers in the elderly. *Clin Geriatr Med, 5*(1), 161–170.

McMullen, D. (1992). Topical metronidazole. Part II: Clinical use in malodorous ulcerating skin lesions. *Ostomy/Wound management, 38*(3), 42–47.

Motta, G. J. (1993). Dressed for success: How moisture-retentive dressings promote healing. *Nursing 93,* December, 26–33.

Parish, L. C., & Witkowski, J. A. (1995). Acne rosacea and *Helicobacter pylori* bethrothed. *Int J Dermatol, 34*(4), 236–237.

Patterson, J. A., & Bennett R. G. (1995). Prevention and treatment of pressure sores. *J Am Geriatr Soc, 43,* 919–927.

Rook, J. L. (1996). Wound care pain management. *Adv Wound Care, 9*(6), 24–31.

Sawaya, M. E. (1997). Clinical updates in hair. *Dermatol Clin, 15*(1), 37–43.

Stotts, N. A., & Hunt, T. K. (1997). Managing bacterial colonization and infection. *Clin Geriatr Med, 13*(3), 565–573.

Shelley, W. B., & Shelley, E. D. (1982). The ten major problems of aging skin. *Geriatrics, 37*(9), 107–113.

Smith, D. M. (1995). Pressure ulcers in the nursing home. *Am Coll Phys, 123,* 433–442.

Stotts, N. (1990). Seeing red and black. The three-color concept of wound care. *Nursing 90,* February, 59–61.

Stone Tankano, J. (1991). Pressure sores. In Chenitz, C., Tankano Stone, I., & Salisbury, S. A. (Eds.). *A guide to advanced practice.* (pp. 247–265). Philadelphia: W. B. Saunders.

Taplin, D., Meinking, T. L., Porcelain, S. L., et al. (1986). Permethrin 5% dermal cream: A new treatment for scabies. *J Am Acad Dermatol, 15,* 995–1001.

Thomas, D. R. (1997). The role of nutrition in prevention and healing of pressure ulcers. *Clin Geriatr Med, 13*(3), 497–511.

Thomas, D. R. (1996). Pressure ulcers. In Cassel, C. K., Cohen, H. J., Larson, E. B. et al. (Eds.). *Geriatric medicine* (pp. 767–785). New York: Springer.

Weiss, J. S., Ellis, C. N., Headington, J. T., et al. (1988). Topical tretinoin improves photoaged skin: A double-blind vehicle controlled study. *JAMA, 259,*(4), 527–532.

Whitley, R. J. (1992). Therapeutic approaches to varicella-zoster virus infection. *J Infect Dis, 166*(Suppl. 1), s51–s57.

Wilson, C. L., Cameron, J., Powell, S. M., Cherry, G., & Ryan, T. J. (1991). High incidence of contact dermatitis in leg-ulcer patients—implications for management. *Clin Exp Dermatol, 16,* 250–253.

Wolf, J. G. (1995). Selection of appropriate support services. *J Wound Ostomy Cont Nurs, 22*(6), 259–262.

15

PSYCHOSOCIAL ISSUES

Debbora Sutherland • Victoria L. Bourque Sklar

■ INTRODUCTION

Nurses and certified nursing assistants (CNAs) in a long-term care facility were presented with the following situation:

vignette

Mr. Brent came to live at the home just before Christmas. He has lived here for 4 months. He has lost 20 pounds and cannot sleep more than a few hours at a time. During the day, he complains of having no energy. He said, "My life is worth nothing." He simply wants to be alone and refuses all assistance. He has been talking less and less and spending more time in his room in bed. When staff try to assist him, he hits them or spits at them.

When the nursing staff were asked what they suspected was the problem, the various responses included: "He's sick," "He's got a urinary tract infection," and "He's demented."

Finally, a CNA with personal experience suggested that the problem might be depression.

This chapter will review some of the major psychosocial issues with which older clients may present. The majority of older adults will cope with age-related changes in healthy and effective ways. However, a significant number of the clients that advanced practice gerontologic nurses encounter will experience some sort of psychic distress. Some will develop symptoms of depression or anxiety in response to stressful events. Others may present with psychotic symptoms. Personality changes may occur that will present unique challenges. There will also be a group of older adults that may have been diagnosed with psychiatric disorders in younger adulthood that they will carry into old age.

At times, psychiatric illness is hard to differentiate from several other common problems in older clients, such as substance abuse, medication side effects, dementia, and delirium. It is important that the advanced practice gerontologic nurse recognize psychiatric problems and know how to intervene.

■ GRIEF AND LOSS

vignette

Mrs. Herman is a 69-year-old white female living in elderly congregate housing. She moved from Florida to be near her only son and his wife after the death of her husband of 50 years. He died of a heart attack following elective surgery. Mrs. Herman feels that the hospital was at fault for his death. She is angry and bitter about this.

Mrs. Herman presented at the Senior Wellness Program with concerns about her health, including high blood pressure, shortness of breath, insomnia, and low back pain. She felt that her son did not take her health problems seriously and did not spend enough time with her. She expected more support from him after she moved to be closer to him, leaving behind her home and her friends. She is lonely and overwhelmed by the responsibility of paying her bills, shopping, and driving. She was very concerned about her income, which was significantly reduced after the death of her husband. Her husband had balanced the budget when he was alive. He also did most of the driving. She felt that she had no one to talk to and that her son was tired of hearing her talk about her husband and his death. She was anxious about her ability to cope and felt that she needed to find ways to keep busy and meet new people.

AGE-RELATED CHANGES

Mrs. Herman experienced many of the losses common to older people: widowed at age 69 with many years of life to look forward to; loss of income; relocation following a crisis, with the loss of friends and familiar activities; and increased health problems, without access to familiar health-care providers. She had not spent adequate time to grieve the loss of her husband when she moved far from her home and friends of many years, thereby experiencing more loss. She also had to give up her 12-year-old dog when she moved, and she missed caring for him. She felt that she had no one to talk to and no one to care for. She was all alone.

Kastenbaum (1981) reported that the process of grieving in older individuals is often much more complex than in younger individuals because multiple losses are experienced so close together in time that there is no time to resolve one loss before the next occurs, resulting in "bereavement overload."

A comprehensive review of theoretic perspectives on response to significant loss may be found in *Bereavement, Reactions, Consequences and Care* (Osterweis et al., 1984). However, most twentieth century theorists agree on a general course of grieving.

CLINICAL PRESENTATION

The presentation of the stages and signs and symptoms of grieving are listed in Table 15–1.

RISK FACTORS

Factors that may result in a more intensive or difficult bereavement include:

TABLE 15–1.   STAGES OF GRIEVING

Phases of Grieving	Emotional Expressions	Somatic Expressions	Resolution
Phase 1—From time of event, lasts several weeks	Shock and disbelief Emotional numbness Cognitive confusion Intense anxiety Significant mood fluctuations	Sleeplessness Loss of appetite Vague muscular aches and pains Shortness of breath Chest pain	Increase in visits to primary-care provider, with focus on somatic problems and requests for medications to relieve symptoms
Phase 2—From 4th to 6th week to one year	Sadness Anger Guilt Relief and other strong emotions surface Emotional lability	Physical symptoms Frequent crying Chronic sleep disturbance Depression Poor appetite Decreased energy Fatigue Loss of interest in usual activities Difficulty paying attention and concentrating	Searching for the deceased Auditory and visual hallucinations of the deceased The sense of the presence of the deceased Searching for the meaning of the death Review of the meaning of the death
Phase 3—At least one additional year or may not be completed	Gradual disengagement of psychic energy from the deceased and reinvestment in other persons and activities	Somatic, cognitive, and behavioral symptoms abate Loneliness diminishes	Development of new relationships or old relationships are strengthened New skills are learned to function in new role

1. Age of the survivor—most studies have found older bereaved adapt better than the young
2. Gender of the survivor—males are at higher risk of mortality than females
3. Mode of death—violent or unexpected deaths, particularly suicide, present higher risks to the survivor
4. Presence of significant depression shortly following the death
5. Poor self-esteem, preexisting insecurity, and dependency
6. Prior relationship satisfaction, with ambivalent or very positive relationships leading to more severe depression
7. Poor health
8. Substance abuse
9. Multiple life stressors
10. Lack of adequate social support
11. Lack of belief in a power greater than oneself

Bereaved persons are at risk of increased drinking, drug abuse, major depression, and anxiety disorders, including posttraumatic stress disorder (Osterweis et al., 1984; Zisook & Schuchter, 1994). Some people are affected so severely by grief that they may die or commit suicide. Others acknowledge the loss but manage to go on with their lives. Still others face the challenges of grieving and develop increased feelings of pride and self-reliance when they learn to handle responsibilities they were previously unable to cope with.

Uncomplicated bereavement is associated with frequent physician visits, self-perceived poor health, disrupted work performance, and disturbed social adjustment. When grief responses and preoccupation with the deceased interfere with function and are accompanied by dysphoria lasting beyond the first year, dysfunctional grieving needs to be evaluated.

CLINICAL PEARL

Chronic grief is difficult to identify in older people because losses have occurred long ago.

ROLE OF THE ADVANCED PRACTICE REGISTERED NURSE IN BEREAVEMENT CARE

The Advanced Practice Registered Nurse (APRN) has the opportunity to assess and facilitate grief resolution in the bereaved. At the time of loss, the bereaved person needs support from a member of the health-care team who provided care to his or her loved one and with whom a therapeutic relationship has been estab-

lished. The person sought out for support may be the APRN at the Senior Wellness Program, the APRN in the primary-care physician's office, the APRN who facilitates the Bereavement Support Group in the community, the APRN who provided care to his or her loved one in the long-term care facility, or the APRN to whom he or she is referred in the community. Staff nurses also need to be able to intervene appropriately with the dying and the bereaved, and it is the role of the APRN to educate and role model appropriate interventions to the staff nurse (Glass, 1993).

The most important function of the APRN is to be there, to care, to listen, and to share the silence.

CLINICAL PEARL

The less we say, the better.

There is no right or wrong way to grieve. Although the meaning of death varies markedly across cultures, as do norms for displaying grief, Cowles (1996) found no particular differences in the individual intrapersonal experience of grief that can be attributed to cultural heritage or ethnicity alone. Hence, the APRN can encourage individuals of any culture to share memories, reminisce about the deceased, and call the deceased by name. By offering permission to grieve, cry, and be angry, sad, hurt, and relieved, the APRN can be a valuable source of support.

Most proposed treatments prescribe prolonged attention to the subjective emotional aspects of the loss (Raphael et al., 1993). However, Bonanno et al.

(1995) found that emotional avoidance during bereavement may serve adaptive functions in regulating the emotional pain of loss, thereby allowing the person to maintain a high level of functioning.

CLINICAL PEARL

Each person grieves in his or her own way.

Let the grieving person set the pace. Help him or her to take care of unfinished business. Tell him or her that writing letters, journaling, and talking to the deceased may be helpful in resolving any feelings of regret for what he or she has or has not said and done. Help with closure when the grieving person asks and is ready. Attending wakes, funerals, and memorials will help the individual accept that death has really occurred.

Bereaved people need support long after the funeral is over. Often, during the second phase of grieving, family and friends have tired of hearing about the loss and pressure their loved ones to get over it and get on with life. During this time, APRNs can be very helpful by providing emotional support, particularly during holidays, birthdays, and anniversaries, which may always be difficult for the bereaved, particularly during the first few years following the death. Healing rituals such as visiting the grave with flowers, letters, candles, giving a gift to the hospital or nursing home on the deceased one's birthday, planting a tree or rosebush, and writing memories of the loved one can comfort the bereaved as these rituals ensure that their loved one is remembered and cared for.

vignette

Mrs. Herman was able to accept the support offered at the Senior Wellness Program. She chose weekly supportive counseling sessions during which she reviewed the circumstances surrounding the death of her husband many times. She was able to write a letter to him expressing her feelings. She requested information on ways to keep busy and accepted recommendations that helped her structure her days. Gradually, she was able to taper, then discontinue, counseling visits. She relapsed on the anniversary of her husband's death, presenting once again with multiple somatic concerns that slowly dissipated with supportive counseling. She was treated with nortriptyline, but her primary-care physician did not believe that it helped and discontinued the medicine. She made new friends, became involved in the political activities of her housing complex, and went to the coffee shop to visit with the manager every day, Monday through Friday. She continues to present once or twice a year with vague somatic complaints, always around the holidays or the anniversary of her husband's death. Each time she comes, she needs a decreased number of visits before she is ready to terminate counseling.

■ DEPRESSION

Depression is the most common psychiatric disorder in the older adult population: 20% to 40% of Americans over age 60 suffer from depression or depressed symptoms (Valente, 1994). The highest rates are found among clients who are medically ill or in long-term care. Depression is one of the most misdiagnosed, underdiagnosed, and undertreated illnesses experienced by older individuals. Barriers to care include avoidance secondary to the stigma attached to mental illness, subtle forms of ageism on the part of the older adults themselves, and providers who attribute symptoms to expected outcomes of physical illness or the normal changes associated with aging (Lipowski, 1990). Cultural differences also act as a barrier to receiving treatment. In many cultures, it is more acceptable to admit to physical symptoms than to signs of mental illness.

AGE-RELATED CHANGES

Decreased concentrations of dopamine, norepinephrine, serotonin, and acetylcholine occur with aging and may be major factors in depression among older clients. Elevated cortisol, sodium, and monoamine oxidase (MAO) levels may also be etiologic factors. A significant number of older people have no resources as the result of multiple losses. The impact of loss on the elderly is greater because, unlike the young, older adults do not have losses offset by gains or opportunities. As people encounter losses and other negative stresses at various transitional points in later years, it is important to consider the potentially negative consequences of eliminating one of their most essential resources—the social network (Thompson, 1996). The availability of social support is a significant determinant of both physical and mental health in older adults. Those who lack social support fare significantly worse in recovery from illness, duration of hospitalization, and discharge home (Ryan & Austin, 1989).

CLINICAL PRESENTATION

Usual Presentation

Changes in appetite, insomnia or hypersomnia, criticism of others, envy of others, social withdrawal, loss of motivation, constipation, rumination about problems, pessimism, guilt feelings, loss of self-esteem, decreased sense of lifelong accomplishments, feelings of helplessness, hostility, agitation, aggression, and anxiety are all symptoms frequently seen in the depressed older adult. Refer to the *Diagnostic and Statistical Manual of Mental Disorders,* 4th ed. (DSM-IV), for complete criteria for affective disorders (American Psychaitric Asociation [APA], 1994).

Atypical Presentation

The older client may deny the presence of depressed mood and instead present with vague somatic complaints such as headache, backache, joint pains, gastrointestinal (GI) distress, decreased energy, and complaints of memory or concentration disturbances (Cooper et al., 1994). In a large community sample of people over the age of 50, those who denied feeling sad or dysphoric, but who reported other symptoms associated with major depression, were found to be at increased risk for death and functional impairment after a 13-year follow-up interval (Gallo et al., 1997).

Onset and duration are particularly important in making the differential diagnosis of depression. One must distinguish between depression and uncomplicated bereavement. Symptoms requiring further evaluation for depression include suicidal ideation, marked functional impairment, psychomotor retardation, and/or morbid preoccupation with worthlessness.

RISK FACTORS

Risk factors for geriatric depression include female gender; divorced or separated marital status in men; married status in women; low socioeconomic level; recent adverse and unexpected life events; and severe impairment in health, resulting in disability (Alexopoulos, 1996).

ASSESSMENT

Depression may result from medical illness, medications, or psychiatric syndromes. Diagnosis is further complicated by coexisting conditions or altered presentation in older clients. In 30% of depressed elderly people, the depression stems from a treatable illness. A number of neurologic, endocrine, metabolic, and nutritional disorders are frequently characterized by depressive manifestations. Older clients who are most likely to become depressed are those with Alzheimer's (40% to 50%) or Parkinson's (40%) dementia, cancer, myocardial infarction (MI), chronic obstructive pulmonary disease (COPD), stroke (particularly left brain), as well as those in pain or undergoing dialysis. Thyroid disorders, particularly hypothroidism, may mimic the presentation of a major depression.

Iatrogenic depression must be considered in older persons using multiple medications. Medications that may precipitate depression in clients include antihypertensives, neuroleptics, minor tranquilizers, digitalis, antiparkinsonian agents, antineoplastic drugs, corticosteroids, anticonvulsants, hormones, and nonsteroidal anti-inflammatory drugs (NSAIDs). Alcohol can also cause depressive episodes.

Late-onset depression is associated with a lower frequency of family history of depression and tends to be less severe than lifelong depression that lasts into old age (Gurland, 1992). However, it is more persistent, complicated, and difficult to treat, with a higher frequency of cognitive impairment, cerebral atrophy, deep white matter changes, recurrences, medical comorbidity, and mortality (National Institutes of Health [NIH], 1991).

Several standard depression scales (eg, the Beck Depression Inventory, the Zung Self-Rating Depression Scale, and the Hamilton Depression Rating Scale) have been shown to be as appropriate for use in elderly populations as they are in the general adult population. A 15-item self-test geared specifically for older adults is the short form of the Geriatric Depression Scale (GDS) in Appendix C of this text. The GDS is useful for identification of depressive symptoms in the elderly because of its simplicity and focus on symptoms that are more significant in the older person. However, depression expressed primarily as somatic preoccupation will be missed if the GDS is used as the only assessment tool. Depression scales should not be used solely as the method of diagnosis of depression.

GERIATRIC DELUSIONAL DEPRESSION

Although unlikely to reside in the community, between 20% and 45% of hospitalized older depressives have accompanying delusions. Delusional depression requires the presence of a false fixed belief that develops during an episode of major depression. Delusional clients provide elaborate justifications and details to support their beliefs. It is important to distinguish between delusional depression and cognitive impairment. The delusions present with a delusional depression are sustained and organized, whereas the delusions found in dementia are typically transient and reactive. Geriatric delusional depression is associated with increased mortality and a poorer prognosis (Meyers, 1992).

GERIATRIC MANIA

Little research has been done in this area; however, clinical experience suggests geriatric persons presenting with mania are a heterogeneous group; some have had recurrent episodes of mania from an early age, while others developed mania with or without depression late in life. Clients with unipolar depression may change polarity with increased age. The possibility of psychiatric comorbidity, particularly dementia, must be considered. Severe mania can be life threatening through the effects of lack of sleep, poor nutrition, and noncompliance with medical treatment. Suicide is associated with bipolar disorders and advanced age. It is uncertain whether the incidence or intensity of manic episodes increases, decreases, or remains the same with aging.

.... *vignette* ....

Mrs. Freeman was a 76-year-old white female, living alone in an apartment in a three-family home in the city. She was newly diagnosed with bipolar disorder, and treatment with valproic acid was initiated by her psychiatrist. She spoke rapidly, nonstop, shifting from one concern to another without completely finishing her thoughts. She had multiple concerns about her health, her apartment, her medications, and her shoes. It was very difficult to follow what she was trying to say. She slept 2 to 3 hours a night and was always on the go. She could not slow down or focus on one subject at a time. A month after starting valproic acid, she was able to focus on one concern at a time, to finish her thoughts, and to sleep 7 hours at night.

▪ SUICIDE

AGE-RELATED CHANGES

The rate of suicide is higher in older adults than in any other age group. In fact, the suicide rate in those 80 to 84 years of age is twice that of younger individuals (NIH, 1992). The suicide rate of older men is seven times that of older women. Older clients are the least likely to divulge suicidal thoughts, as they do not share feelings easily.

RISK FACTORS

Risk factors for suicide include bereavement, hopelessness, worthlessness, and giving away personal or prized possessions. Most suicide victims do not want to die but see suicide as a solution to a problem (eg, life-threatening or chronic disease, loneliness).

CLINICAL PEARL

Treat all suicide messages seriously, even when the person jokes or says he or she does not mean it.

ASSESSMENT

Assess lethality of method and likelihood of rescue. Pay particular attention to depressed, potentially suicidal individuals when their depression begins to lift because they have energy to make and carry out a plan. If community dwelling, refer to the crisis intervention center or emergency room for immediate admission if at high risk with a realistic and lethal plan. Instill hope by informing them that treatment is effective 85% of the time with medications and/or psychotherapy.

CLINICAL PEARL

A history of two or more previous attempts is the highest predictor of future attempts.

If not at immediate risk and amenable to therapy, assess nonverbal cues, delirium, symptoms of depression, personal history, and history of substance abuse. Speak with the family, but be aware that there may be hidden agendas or different opinions on what is in the best interest of the client. At highest risk is the older, white, single, alcoholic male, living alone, with no friends, who has attempted suicide in the past.

CLINICAL MANAGEMENT

The goals of treatment for depression include eliminating symptoms of depression; reducing the risk of relapse and recurrence; increasing quality of life; improving functional status; and decreasing health costs, morbidity, and mortality.

The three major categories of treatment for depression are psychosocial therapies, psychopharmacology, and electroconvulsive therapy (ECT).

Psychosocial Therapies

Psychotherapy is important in treating depressed older adults. Psychotherapies, including cognitive–behavioral, interpersonal, and psychodynamic psychotherapies, have been found effective in treating mild to moderate depression (Reynolds et al., 1994). Individual psychotherapy that is structured, goal oriented, and time limited is believed the most effective for the older client (Gomez & Gomez, 1993). Insight-oriented psychotherapy; life review; and cognitive, group, and family therapies should be provided by mental health professionals.

Therapies of value to the depressed older client that may be provided by advanced practice nurses not certified in mental health include music and dance, reminiscence, art, and activity therapies. Self-care methods include exercise, time spent in the sunshine, and healthy dietary habits.

Pharmacotherapies

Because of changes having to do with detoxification and elimination of drugs in older clients, special precautions must be taken. Concomitant physical illness and the interactions of antidepressant drugs with medications for the treatment of systemic diseases require low initial doses, careful titration, and gradual increases to achieve therapeutic effectiveness (Buschmann et al., 1995). See Table 15–2 for a list of antidepressant medications.

TABLE 15–2. ANTIDEPRESSANT MEDICATIONS

Generic Name	Brand Name	Class	Geriatric Dose
Amitriptyline	Elavil	TCA	30–100 mg
Amoxapine	Asendin	Heterocyclic	50–150 mg
Bupropion	Wellbutrin	Aminoketone	75–150 mg
Desipramine*	Norpramin	TCA	20–100 mg
Doxepin	Sinequan	TCA	30–150 mg
Fluoxetine	Prozac	SSRI	5–20 mg
Fluvoxamine	Luvox	SSRI	25–150 mg
Dextroamphetamine	Dexedrine	Stimulant	2.5–30 mg
Imipramine	Tofranil	TCA	30–100 mg
Isocarboxazid	Marplan	MAOI	5–15 mg
Methylphenidate	Ritalin	Stimulant	5–40 mg
Nefazadone	Serzone	Phenylpiperazine	100–400 mg
Nortriptyline*	Pamelor	TCA	10–50 mg
Paroxetine*	Paxil	SSRI	10–20 mg
Phenelzine	Nardil	MAOI	15 mg
Protriptyline	Vivactil	TCA	10–20 mg
Sertraline*	Zoloft	SSRI	50 mg
Tranylcypromine	Parnate	MAOI	10–20 mg
Trazodone	Desyrel	Triazolopyridine	50–150 mg
Trimipramine	Surmontil	TCA	25–150 mg
Venlafaxine	Effexor	Phenylethylamine	37.5–150 mg
Hypericum	St. John's Wort	Natural extract	300 mg tid

* Recommended for older adults.
TCA, tricyclic antidepressant; SSRI, selective serotonin reuptake inhibitor; MAOI monoamine oxidase inhibitor.
Information adapted from Frierson et al. (1991), Harrer & Sommer (1994), and Lesseig (1996).

CLINICAL PEARL

Physiologic aging changes affect absorption, distribution, metabolism, and excretion and may potentiate the effect of medications or cause toxic side effects.

Although findings have been contradictory on the efficacy of selective serotonin reuptake inhibitors (SSRIs) in the older depressed client, they are currently being utilized as first-line treatment for depression in older adults due to their low side effect profile and decreased incidence of cognitive dysfunction. Common side effects include nausea, tremor, anxiety, headaches, sweating, insomnia or somnolence, and impaired sexual function. Many of the side effects are transient and will completely resolve within 3 weeks of the initiation of therapy. Selective serotonin reuptake inhibitors are suitable for once-a-day dosing, therefore enhancing potential compliance.

Unlike tricyclic antidepressants (TCAs), SSRIs have a very low rate of cardiac adverse effects and remarkable safety in overdose. Selective serotonin reuptake inhibitors can inhibit the activities of certain P_{450} enzymes. As a result, drug interactions with SSRIs are an important source of potential morbidity, as there are many drugs that may interact and new interactions are still being discovered (Sheline et al., 1997). The most critical of these interactions are the life-threatening ventricular arrhythmias which can occur when terfenadine or astemizole are combined with fluvoxamine or nefazadone (Sheline et al., 1997). Serotonergic syndrome, characterized by hypertension, GI distress, sweating, hyperthermia, and death, can occur when an SSRI is combined with a monoamine oxidase inhibitor (MAOI), tryptophan, lithium, or carbamazepine.

Although there is ample evidence that TCAs are effective in the treatment of depression in the elderly, older adults often cannot tolerate the side effects of a full therapeutic dose of a TCA. Side effects include sedation, weight gain, orthostatic hypotension, potentiation of central nervous system (CNS) drugs, blurred vision, dry mouth, memory impairment, constipation, and urinary retention. They are contraindicated for those with cardiac arrhythmias or cardiac conditions because they are cardiotonic (Lube, 1990). Of the TCAs, nortriptyline and desipramine have fewer side effects and are recommended for use in the older adult. However, another problem is the high rate of noncompliance because of side effects experienced at therapeutic doses.

Contrary to widespread clinical opinion, the use of MAOIs, especially phenelzine, has been found to be safe and effective in older adults, but they have not been widely used for treatment of geriatric depression (NIH, 1991) due to dietary and drug–drug interactions. However, MAOIs are not cardiotoxic and may be indicated for clients with cardiac arrhythmias (Gomez & Gomez, 1993).

Significant antidepressant response occurs later in older adults than in young adults. Therefore, clients must be informed that it may take as long as 6 to 12 weeks before they feel the full effect of the antidepressant.

A total of 1592 patients have been studied in 25 double-blind controlled studies (15 compared to placebo, 10 compared to antidepressant drugs) investigating the efficacy of St. John's Wort extract, standardized to contain 0.3% hypericum, three times a day in treating mild to moderate depression. St. John's Wort extract was effective in 65% to 80% of subjects with mild to moderate depression and virtually free of side effects at the standard dosage of 300 mg PO three times a day. Results from a second very large study involving 3250 patients conducted in Germany indicated a 50% reduction in frequency and intensity of depressive symptomatology with clinically insignificant frequency and severity of side effects (*Am J Natur Med*, 1995; Harrer & Sommer, 1994). The authors were very clear that St. John's Wort is *not* appropriate for the treatment of severe depression, defined as depressions associated with psychotic symptoms, depressions with serious risk of suicide, and depressions with such severe vegetative symptoms that family or professional life is disrupted.

Medically ill depressed individuals may have difficulty with traditional antidepressant medications, because of the side effect profile, the delayed onset of action and the drug–drug interactions. Psychostimulants, methylphenidate, and dextroamphetamine are safe and effective treatments for depression in the ill older client. Beneficial effects are generally seen within 36 hours, and habituation, contrary to general opinion, is not a problem. Some studies suggest that dextroamphetamine is more beneficial for the treatment of major depression and methylphenidate is more effective in the treatment of adjustment disorder with depressed mood (Frierson et al., 1991). Relapse during treatment, as well as after discontinuation of the medication, is much more common with methylphenidate than with dextroamphetamine. Improvement is noted in all neurovegetative signs of depression, including insomnia and anorexia. Major side effects are tachyarrhythmias and increased anxiety in people with agitated depression. The medication is usually discontinued without withdrawal symptoms or relapse after 90 days.

Geriatric mania can be precipitated by treatment with antidepressant therapy. Lithium salts are the drug of choice for mania in the older client (Young, 1992). Age-related changes require the use of lower lithium doses to achieve therapeutic effect. About one half to two thirds of the dose required for younger individuals is usually sufficient for older adults. Older adults show high lithium plasma levels at relatively low doses because of age-related reduction in renal clearance. Although controlled studies are lacking, it has been suggested that lithium plasma levels of 0.3 to 0.6 mEq/L are clinically effective in older adults. Acute toxicity, including delirium, can occur at plasma levels less than 1.5 mEq/L in elderly clients. Clients with Parkinson's disease and those receiving neuroleptics are prone to lithium-induced delirium. Salt depletion caused by vomiting or diarrhea, thiazide diuretics, NSAIDs, and an-

giotensin-converting enzyme (ACE) inhibitors may raise lithium levels and lead to toxicity (Alexopoulos, 1996). Valproic acid, carbamazepine, and clonazepam are used for lithium-refractory or -intolerant bipolar patients. These medications are also used for impulse control.

Delusional depression is treated with a combination of antidepressant and antipsychotic medications. Treatment solely with an antidepressant can cause an increase in psychotic symptomatology.

Clients who do not respond fully to one or two medication trials or are suicidal, psychotic, bipolar, or in need of formal psychotherapy should be referred to psychiatric/mental health specialists (Lesseig, 1996).

Adequate duration of antidepressant therapy is necessary for successful treatment. Continuation of treatment at full therapeutic dose should extend a minimum of 6 to 12 months following resolution of symptoms in order to be effective (NIH, 1992). Longer treatment is required for those with recurrent episodes.

Electroconvulsive Therapy

Although ECT is the most effective treatment available for more severe major depressions (Scovern & Kilmann, 1980) due to its safety and rapid onset of action, it is generally underused or unavailable (NIH, 1991). In the presence of self-destructive behavior, such as a suicide attempt or refusal to eat, as well as for those suffering from major depression with melancholia and especially major depression with psychotic symptoms associated with agitation or withdrawal, ECT is the treatment of choice.

Cardiovascular effects including premature ventricular contractions, ventricular arrhythmias, and transient systolic hypertension are of most concern, although monitoring during treatment usually precludes permanent problems. Brief confusion and amnesia are common following treatments; however, a small number of patients do suffer from prolonged memory deficits.

Without prophylactic intervention after treatment, relapse exceeds 50% in the year after a course of ECT. In some clients, weekly or monthly maintenance treatments may be necessary. Others respond well to antidepressant or lithium maintenance therapy.

Treatment of depression with ECT is costly and requires a referral to a psychiatrist. See Benbow's (1991) review on the role of ECT in the treatment of depression in old age for more information.

ROLE OF THE APRN IN TREATING GERIATRIC DEPRESSION

As an APRN assessing geriatric depression, always recommend nonpharmcologic measures to combat depressive symptomatology. The role of the APRN lends itself to the development of one-to-one therapeutic relationships with clients. First-line drugs, such as an SSRI, nortriptyline, desipramine, and St. John's Wort, should be prescribed whenever quality of life and/or functioning can be improved *and* the individual agrees to try medication. The person always has the right to refuse treatment unless declared gravely disabled or a danger to self and/or others. The decision to commit a person for a period of observation is made by a physician. Once the observation period is up, the decision for any further involuntary commitment is made by a judge.

■ ANXIETY

Because they often resemble physical illness, anxiety symptoms can be very difficult to diagnose. When anxiety and depression occur together, it can also be very difficult to diagnose because many of the symptoms of both disorders are the same. Although they are difficult to diagnose, Sheikh (1995) suggests that when all of the anxiety diagnoses are considered as a group, anxiety disorders are the most prevalent psychiatric conditions in the older adult.

AGE-RELATED CHANGES

Symptoms of anxiety disorders typically begin earlier in life. However, it is possible for an older adult with no prior history of anxiety symptoms to develop them. Anxiety symptoms in older adults are very similar in presentation to those in younger adults, though phobic anxiety is considered to be more common in the elderly (Pasnau & Bystritsky, 1990). Sheikh (1996a) has also observed that in the case of late-onset panic disorder, there may be fewer panic symptoms, less avoidance, and lower scores on somatization measures in older adults. Salzman (1990) suggests that pure anxiety disorders are rare in older adults and that anxiety symptoms in older clients are often seen in combination with symptoms of depression, physical illness, and cognitive disorders.

There are many possible contributing factors to the presence of anxiety symptoms in late life. These include feelings of loneliness, uselessness, and worthlessness; the stress of trying to cope with multiple losses; fears of isolation and/or death; chronic health problems; decreased sensory functioning; decreased general functioning; and financial concerns (Smith et al., 1995).

CLINICAL PRESENTATION

The most common anxiety disorders found in older adults are panic disorder (with or without agoraphobia), social phobia, specific phobia, generalized anxiety disorder, posttraumatic stress disorder, obsessive–compulsive disorder, anxiety disorders caused by a general medical condition, anxiety and agitation associ-

ated with dementia, and anxiety disorders caused by substance abuse (Sheikh & Salzman, 1995). The latter two disorders are discussed in Chapters 3 and 16, respectively. Table 15–3 provides a review of anxiety disorders and their symptoms. For a more complete review of anxiety disorders and related symptoms, see the DSM-IV (APA, 1994).

ASSESSMENT

Very often, anxiety is manifested through multiple complaints of a psychologic and physiologic nature. Some of the more

TABLE 15–3.   ANXIETY DISORDERS*

Disorder	Symptoms
Panic disorder	Panic attacks, which are characterized by the following: shortness of breath, palpitations, diaphoresis, shaking, choking sensations, gastrointestinal discomfort, fear of going crazy, fear of having a heart attack, and/or fear of dying.
Specific or social phobias	Persistent fear when exposed to a specific stimulus (eg, heights, snakes) or a fear of humiliating oneself in social situations. Exposure to or anticipation of exposure to the stimulus or situation produces anxiety and/or panic symptoms.
Obsessive–compulsive disorder	Obsessions (persistent thoughts or impulses) and/or compulsions (eg, handwashing, checking, counting). Obsessions cause an increase in anxiety symptoms, and compulsions are an attempt by the individual to decrease this anxiety.
Posttraumatic stress disorder	Caused by exposure to a traumatic event and characterized by the following: recurrent thoughts of the event, nightmares about the trauma, illusions, hallucinations, flashbacks, intense anxiety, inability to recall all or parts of the trauma, sleep disturbance, anger, irritability, exaggerated startle response, and/or difficulty concentrating.
Generalized anxiety disorder	Restlessness, easily fatigued, difficulty concentrating, irritability, muscle tension, sleep disturbance, and/or increased distress.
Anxiety disorder due to a general medical condition	Anxiety, panic attacks, obsession, and/or compulsions in the presence of a general medical condition.

* Although anxiety disorders are found in individuals of all ages, these are the disorders most likely to be found in the elderly.
Source: Adapted from American Psychiatric Association (1994). *Diagnostic and statistical manual of mental disorders* (4th ed.). Washington, DC: American Psychiatric Association.

common psychologic complaints are nervousness, tension, worry, irritability, dread, and difficulty concentrating, while common physiologic complaints are of restlessness, shortness of breath, palpitations, dyspnea on exertion, heartburn, nausea, vomiting, insomnia, choking sensations, and tremors (Smith et al., 1995). When assessing anxiety symptoms, it is important to take a careful history to determine if the client has any previously diagnosed psychiatric and/or medical conditions. There are many medical conditions that can imitate anxiety symptoms. These include cardiovascular conditions (eg, angina pectoris, MI, cardiac arrhythmias); pulmonary disorders (eg, COPD, pulmonary embolism, pneumonia, hypoxia); neurologic illnesses (eg, temporal-lobe epilepsy, movement disorders, CNS infections or masses); and endocrine disorders (eg, hypoglycemia, hyperthyroidism) (Sheikh, 1992, 1996a). In addition, pain can be a significant cause of anxiety in older clients (Pasnau & Bystritsky, 1990). When indicated, the appropriate diagnostic tests can help rule out a physiologic basis for anxiety.

Pseudoephedrine (found in many over-the-counter [OTC] preparations), caffeine, neuroleptics, thyroid replacement treatments, steroids, and antidepressants are all examples of drugs that can cause an individual to present with anxiety symptoms (Sheikh, 1996a; Smith et al., 1995; Salzman, 1992). It is also important to consider the possibility of withdrawal from alcohol, anxiolytics, or other substances. In addition, depression can sometimes be accompanied by a significant amount of anxiety.

Along with gathering data about psychiatric and medical history and symptoms, it is important to take a social history. This will not only help to determine any significant social stressors, but will help the APRN gain information about social supports, which will be very useful in planning strategies for the treatment and management of anxiety.

CLINICAL MANAGEMENT

Anxiety is a normal emotion. It occurs in each of us on a daily basis. Often, our anxiety about a certain event can motivate us to prepare for the event (eg, an upcoming final exam) and once the event has passed our anxiety decreases. This type of anxiety needs no treatment other than to prepare for the event and perhaps the support of family and friends. Anxiety of this sort also responds well to relaxation or stress-reduction exercises such as deep breathing, meditation, getting a massage, taking a walk, or taking a hot bath. Anxiety disorders often respond well to relaxation exercises and psychotherapy, but at times medication is needed to help relieve symptoms. Sometimes, treatment with medication is a temporary measure, and at other times symptoms are severe enough that medication is required on an ongoing basis. In trying to determine the appropriate treatment for the anxious older client, it is important to assess the impact of the anxiety symptoms on the social and emotional functioning as well as on the physical status of the individual (Salzman, 1992).

Psychotherapies

Cognitive-behavior therapy has been shown to be effective in the treatment of anxiety disorders (Sheikh, 1996). This type of therapy works by teaching clients to change the way they think and behave which helps to change the way they feel. It can be effective alone or when used in combination with medication. As in the treatment of depression, psychotherapy for those with anxiety disorders should be done by mental health professionals.

Pharmacotherapies

Benzodiazepines are the most frequently prescribed anxiolytic in any age group including the elderly (Sheikh, 1996a). Of concern with the use of benzodiazepines is the increased risk of side effects in older adults. These include sedation, lethargy, ataxia, depression, paradoxic reactions, confusion, memory problems, cognitive impairment, and weakness (Salzman, 1990, 1992). The use of benzodiazepines must be monitored closely to avoid potential problems with tolerance, dependence, abuse, and toxicity (Young & Meyers, 1996). For this reason, it is often recommended that benzodiazepines be used cautiously and for a time-limited basis (Young & Meyers, 1996; Sheikh, 1996a). Benzodiazepines with a short half-life, such as lorazepam and oxazepam, are preferred, as they are less likely to produce cumulative effects. However, there are some disadvantages to short-acting benzodiazepines, including the occurrence of withdrawal symptoms that can mimic episodes of increased anxiety (Smith et al., 1995). Benzodiazepines are effective for the treatment of anxiety disorders as well as for anxiety associated with depression. Alprazolam and clonazepam are both used in the treatment of panic disorder and are effective in blocking acute panic symptoms (Salzman, 1992). Sheikh (1996a) reports that in the preliminary analysis of a study of panic disorder in patients aged 55 and over, alprazolam, an

intermediate half-life agent, was found to be more effective in blocking panic attacks when compared with placebo.

Typical daily dosages for the commonly used benzodiazepines in the older adult are as follows: alprazolam, 0.25 to 0.75 mg; clonazepam, 0.5 to 1.5 mg; lorazepam, 0.5 to 2 mg; oxazepam, 10 to 30 mg (Semla et al., 1997).

Of the SSRIs, paroxetine is approved for the treatment of panic disorder. The recommended daily dose is 40 mg (Semla et al., 1997), though as with all medications prescribed for the elderly, one should "start low and go slow." Initiating treatment at 10 mg a day for 1 to 2 weeks and increasing in increments of 10 mg at a time can help to decrease the potential for adverse effects, which can help improve compliance. Common side effects include nausea, diarrhea, ataxia, and tremor. Because they are often well tolerated in the elderly and because they do not lead to dependence, SSRIs are a good choice for this population.

Unfortunately, there are some disadvantages to the use of SSRIs. Because they are relatively new, they are more expensive than other medications used in the treatment of anxiety (Laraia, 1995). Another disadvantage is that they take so long to work that in cases of severe anxiety or panic, it may be necessary to augment with benzodiazepines initially and then taper and discontinue once the response to the SSRI has been determined.

Selective serotonin reuptake inhibitors are also useful in the treatment of obsessive–compulsive disorder. Fluoxetine has been approved for treatment of this disorder. The recommended dose is not more than 80 mg daily (Semla et al., 1997). As with paroxetine, it is recommended that the starting dose for the elderly is 10 mg daily. This can gradually be increased by 10-mg increments until the optimum dose is reached.

Sertraline is also effective in the treatment of anxiety disorders. The starting dose for the elderly is 25 mg daily and can be increased by increments of 25 mg until the desired effect is achieved. The dosage range for sertraline is typically 75 to 100 mg daily, though in some cases doses as high as 200 mg may be needed (Semla et al., 1997).

Buspirone may be effective for the long-term treatment of anxiety in the elderly, but it is important to remember that it can take 3 to 4 weeks before the desired effect is obtained, and it may be necessary to combine it with a short-acting benzodiazepine in the interim (Sheikh, 1992). It is considered to be a safer alternative to benzodiazepines. The recommended dose is 20 to 30 mg daily, though doses as high as 60 mg daily may be necessary (Semla et al., 1997). In clinical practice, the use of buspirone has been somewhat disappointing for the treatment of anxiety disorders. It does seem to be effective in some individuals with symptoms of anxiety or agitation related to dementia.

Tricyclic antidepressants can also be useful in treating anxiety disorders but should be used cautiously, as they tend to cause undesirable side effects. The tricyclics most often recommended for treatment of anxiety are imipramine and clomipramine, but, unfortunately, they are also more likely than nortriptyline and desipramine (which have not been proven to be useful in the treatment of anxiety) to cause adverse effects (Sheikh, 1996a).

Neuroleptic medications are not commonly used in the treatment of anxiety disorders but may be useful in the treatment of posttraumatic stress disorder if there are psychotic symptoms present. They are also indicated for treatment of the anxiety and agitation associated with dementia, which is discussed in Chapter 3.

ROLE OF THE APRN IN TREATING ANXIETY

The APRN is often in a unique position to be able to assess for the presence of anxiety symptoms that masquerade as medical problems or that are a result of a known medical illness. Anxiety symptoms that are mild may be able to be treated with nonpharmacologic methods such as deep breathing and relaxation exercises. *The Relaxation & Stress Reduction Workbook*, 4th ed. (Davis et al., 1995) provides easy-to-follow techniques, many of which can be effectively used with the elderly.

Anxiety symptoms that do not respond to nonpharmcologic interventions may respond to medication. If a trial of a benzodiazepine, an SSRI, or buspirone is ineffective, or if the anxiety symptoms are severe, a referral to a mental health professional should be made.

■ SCHIZOPHRENIA

AGING CHANGES

Schizophrenia in older adults was previously classified into two different categories: the chronic early-onset schizophrenic who had reached old age and the late-onset schizophrenic. Both were considered to be essentially the same disorder except that the symptoms did not appear until after the age of 45 in the late-onset category. The DSM-IV no longer makes this age distinction (APA, 1994).

Jeste et al. (1996) observed that bizarre delusions which are persecutory in nature, auditory hallucinations, and depression are commonly seen in late-onset schizophrenia.

Although very little is known about the long-term course of early-onset schizophrenia, it is believed that approximately one third of patients will experience a remission or will be left with only mild symptoms. It is also believed that the positive symptoms decrease in severity over time, while the negative symptoms tend to persist and may even increase in severity (Jeste et al., 1996; Kaplan et al., 1994). In a review of the literature on the outcomes of schizophrenia into later life, Cohen (1990) found that, in the studies he reviewed, both positive and negative symptoms tended to decrease in severity and that social involvement and coping tended to improve with age. In addition, he notes that whereas older schizophrenics do tend to exhibit cognitive impairments, the deficits are not consistent with the typical presentation of someone with Alzheimer's dementia.

CLINICAL PRESENTATION

Schizophrenia is commonly thought of as being characterized by the presence of delusions and hallucinations. Although it is true that at least one of these symptoms is commonly seen in individuals with this disorder, they do not have to be present for a diagnosis to be made. Other symptoms of schizophrenia include disorganized speech, grossly disorganized or catatonic behavior, and disturbances in social and/or occupational functioning (APA, 1994).

Symptoms are often referred to as either positive or negative. Chesla (1996) defines positive symptoms as those that represent an excess or distortion of normal functioning and negative symptoms as those that represent a deficit in functioning. Positive symptoms include hallucinations, bizarre behavior, loose associations, and increased speech. Negative symptoms can resemble symptoms of depression and include lack of motivation, poor grooming, social withdrawal, flattening or blunting of affect, poverty of speech or speech content, anhedonia, cognitive defects, and attention deficits (Kaplan et al., 1994).

For further information on criteria for the diagnosis of schizophrenia and other psychotic disorders, see the DSM-IV (APA, 1994). In addition, Kaplan et al.'s *Synopsis of Psychiatry*, 7th ed. (1994) provides an excellent review of schizophrenia. Chesla's chapter in Wilson and Kneisl's *Psychiatric Nursing*, 5th ed. (1996) provides a review of schizophrenia as well as nursing interventions that can be used with schizophrenic clients.

ASSESSMENT

When psychotic symptoms are present in older clients, it is important to rule out organic illness first. There are a number of disorders associated with secondary psychosis in older adults, including disorders of the thyroid; hypoglycemia; Parkinson's disease; Alzheimer's, Pick's, and vascular dementias; hydrocephalus; viral encephalitis; neurosyphilis; deficiencies of thiamine, niacin, vitamin B_{12}, and folate; toxic effects of medications; systemic lupus erythematosus (SLE); hyponatremia; and delirium (Jeste et al., 1996).

It is important to remember that the older adult will be more sensitive to neuroleptic medications because of changes in absorption, metabolism, drug distribution, and excretion that occur with aging (Tran-Johnson et al., 1992).

SCHIZOAFFECTIVE DISORDER

Schizoaffective disorder is characterized by the presence of a mood disorder in addition to the symptoms of hallucinations, delusions, disorganization, and/or the negative symptoms of schizophrenia. The classifications of schizoaffective disorder are either depressive or bipolar type. The DSM-IV (1994) provides a more thorough definition of this disorder. Schizoaffective disorder is not as prevalent as schizophrenia and has a slightly better prognosis than schizophrenia, but the prognosis is worse than in mood disorders (Chesla, 1996).

CLINICAL MANAGEMENT

Psychotic symptoms are treated with neuroleptic medications. Thioridazine and haloperidol have been two of the most commonly used neuroleptic agents in the elderly (Tran-Johnson et al., 1992). However, newer agents such as risperidone and olanzapine are being considered first in the treatment of psychosis due to claims of fewer side effects.

Studies on the effect of risperidone in the elderly are limited, though some have found it to be effective in the treatment of psychosis. In a study of 11 elderly patients diagnosed with either schizophrenia, schizoaffective disorder, bipolar disorder, or senile dementia, Madhusoodanan et al. (1995) found

risperidone to be effective in reducing both positive and negative symptoms of schizophrenia. The side effect that led to discontinuation of this medication was hypotension, and this was found to be present more commonly in those patients with preexisting cardiac disease. They concluded that despite this finding, risperidone was found to be safe and effective for use with the elderly due to its minimal side effect profile. Unlike other neuroleptics, risperidone rarely causes anticholinergic, extrapyramidal, or sedative effects and has a low incidence of tardive dyskinesia. The authors recommended starting doses of 0.5 mg PO twice a day that can be slowly titrated in increments of 0.5 mg weekly. Dosages of 4 to 8 mg are recommended, though doses higher than 6 mg daily may increase the chance of extrapyramidal side effects (Semla et al., 1997).

Traditional neuroleptics continue to be used in the treatment of schizophrenia in older adults. One of these agents might be used if there is a history of a positive response and it was well tolerated. Recommended starting doses are haloperidol 0.5 mg to 2 mg/d and thioridazine 10 mg to 50 mg/d. These doses can be titrated gradually until the desired effect is achieved or the side effects become intolerable (Tran-Johnson et al., 1992). Once the desired effect has been achieved, the dose may be able to be decreased with the goal to maintain the individual on the lowest possible dose while maintaining symptom control.

If trials of risperidone, olanzapine, haloperidol, and/or thioridazine are ineffective or if the symptoms are severe, a referral to a psychiatric clinical specialist or a psychiatrist is recommended. It is not uncommon for individuals with psychotic disorders to be nonadherent to medications. For this reason, supportive counseling can be very helpful.

CLINICAL PEARL

It is not always possible to completely eliminate all psychotic symptoms with antipsychotic medication. Decreasing symptoms to the point of not interfering with daily functioning may be an acceptable goal for some clients.

ROLE OF THE APRN IN THE MANAGEMENT OF SCHIZOPHRENIA

One of the most important roles of the APRN in managing a client on a neuroleptic medication is to monitor for side effects. Even if there are no side effects initially, they can develop over time. The Abnormal Involuntary Movement Scale (AIMS) examination is the most commonly used tool for evaluating the presence of neuroleptic-induced side effects. Munetz and Benjamin (1988) give an excellent explanation of how to conduct an AIMS exam, as well as how to score the exam. AIMS exams should ideally be conducted prior to the initiation of a neuroleptic medication and repeated every 6 months. Most institutions have a form that they use for these examinations, and they should remain a permanent part of the client's medical record.

Because of the potential for irre-

versible side effects, it is important to review the reason for initiation of the medication as well as the possible side effects with the client and his or her family or significant support persons. It is also important to document this discussion in the client's medical record.

It is very important for the APRN to monitor for potential side effects of neuroleptic medications because of their possible severity. Potential side effects include anticholinergic effects, hypotension or orthostatic hypotension, sedation, photosensitivity, and extrapyramidal side effects. Extrapyramidal side effects can involve acute dystonic reactions, which are typically seen as severe or bizarre muscle contractions of the face, neck, and/or back and can also include laryngeal spasm (Trigoboff, 1996). These symptoms tend to occur at higher doses, although swallowing difficulties are not uncommon in older clients even at low doses. Symptoms can be relieved with benztropine or diphenhydramine and can be administered intramuscularly for severe presentations.

Other potential extrapyramidal side effects include parkinsonian syndrome, akathisia, and tardive dyskinesia. Trigoboff (1996) gives the following descriptions of these adverse effects:

1. Parkinsonian syndrome is caused by the dopamine blockade effect of neuroleptic medications, and it is characterized by the presence of masklike facies, resting tremor, shuffling gait, and rigidity of posture with slow voluntary movements.
2. Akathisia is motor restlessness that is often expressed by pacing, shift-

ing weight from one foot to the other, or by the inability to sit or stand still.

3. Tardive dyskinesia is characterized by involuntary movements of the face, tongue, and mouth; choreiform movements of the upper extremeties; slow, writhing contractions of the arms and legs; and tense tonic contractions of the neck and back. This is an irreversible condition that often appears or worsens after a dose reduction or discontinuation of the medication.

In a study designed to assess the functional status of older persons with schizophrenia, Krach (1993) found that akathisia was often misdiagnosed as anxiety, agitation, or an exacerbation of psychiatric symptoms. This led to an increase in the neuroleptic medication, which in turn resulted in worsening of the akathisia. Akinesia, a feeling of being slowed down or sluggish, should lead to an assessment for changes in gait and upper body movement, characterized by slowed, stiff movements, increased muscle tone, and cogwheel rigidity. An important observation was that patients tended to complain more of restlessness (akathisia) than rigidity.

Detzer and Huston (1986) offer the following suggestions for working with schizophrenic clients: try to minimize anxiety to help decrease the chances of exacerbating psychotic symptoms; speak directly and to the point; do not engage in a discussion of the client's delusions, but do offer reassurance; and be firm without being threatening.

■ DIFFICULT PERSONALITIES

Individuals with difficult personalities can present many unique challenges to the advanced practice nurse in any setting. In general, personality is thought to remain stable throughout the life span (Ebersole & Hess, 1990; Friedman, 1993; Fogel & Sadavoy, 1996). However, it is not clear whether personality disorders change in older adults, although one thing remains true: An individual with a difficult personality can be one of the most difficult people to treat. For more detailed explanations of individual personality disorders, see the DSM-IV (APA, 1994).

AGE-RELATED CHANGES

In a review of the literature, Kroessler (1990) concluded that the stress of normal aging may change a variety of preexisting behaviors as well as produce new ones; personality seems to remain stable as we age; healthy personality traits remain as durable as unhealthy traits; and the elderly are not immune to personality disorders. Rosowsky & Gurian (1992) state that severe personality disorders in older adults are probably far more prevalent than has been reported. One reason for this underreporting may be that clinicians may fail to recognize such behavior in older adults as lifelong pathologic traits and mistake it for a normal reaction to aging. Clinicians are more likely to diagnose major mental illnesses (ie, depression, anxiety) that often occur along with a personality disorder, and miss the underlying personality disorder. The presence of cognitive impairment and lack of history further complicates the process of accurately diagnosing a personality disorder in the older adult (Agronin, 1994).

CLINICAL PRESENTATION

Sadavoy (1987) describes the behavioral syndrome of clients with character disorders as such:

> These are the patients who are unreasonably demanding and overly sensitive to criticism or disappointment. Their personal relationships are unstable and they cause others to feel burdened. Their emotional reactions are intense, impulsive, and labile, especially with respect to rage and depression. Crisis and stress are often badly handled and may lead to severe breakdown, suicidal impulsivity, or other forms of self-destructiveness. While severe symptoms may appear intermittently, the core pathology has been present throughout life and does not diminish with aging, although its manifestations may change.

He goes on to state that there are three major pathways that predominate symptom expression in the older adult with a character disorder. The first is that interactional patterns with family members, friends, and caregivers are expressed as clinging, depressive panic, or angry entitlement. The second is a that there is a heavy focus on somatic concerns in which the body is used as a way to communicate needs and there is a subsequent overreliance on health-care systems. The final way that older adults may express their symptoms is through depressive withdrawal in order to express feelings of hopelessness and defeat when faced with crises of old age.

CLINICAL MANAGEMENT

An understanding of how symptoms may be expressed is helpful in planning for the care of an older adult with a difficult personality. One of the greatest challenges for the advanced practice nurse is to determine which symptoms are the result of true physical illness versus manifestations of the underlying personality disorder. Often, if an individual has been identified to have a difficult personality, physical illness may be missed. Proper treatment of physical illness may also help decrease behaviors associated with personality disorders. A concurrent psychiatric disorder can lead to an increase in somatic symptoms, neediness, or other difficult behaviors. Treatment of underlying symptoms of depression or anxiety may help lessen those of the personality disorder, though this will certainly not alleviate all of the symptoms.

A sudden change in personality must be evaluated to rule out any underlying medical condition that could be the cause. Possible causes would include Parkinson's disease, dementia, stroke, or systemic illness (Holroyd & Rabins, 1994).

Psychotropic medications are not indicated in the treatment of personality disorders unless there is underlying depression or anxiety disorder. Management of these illnesses has been described previously. At times, an older adult with a personality disorder may have symptoms of delusions with or without paranoia to the extent that it interferes with functioning. Neuroleptic medications can sometimes be helpful in these instances. Usually, an antipsychotic that also has anxiolytic properties with a low side effect profile (ie, perphenazine, thioridazine, or risperidone) may be the best choice (Fogel & Sadavoy, 1996). Dosages should be started low and gradually titrated as needed.

ROLE OF THE APRN IN THE MANAGEMENT OF DIFFICULT PERSONALITIES

The APRN is often one of many care providers servicing a client with a difficult personality. This is especially true in long-term care facilities or home-care agencies in which the APRN is requested by the staff to help manage an older adult with a difficult personality. Regardless of the setting, there are some interventions that can be applied that may make the management of these clients successful. Fogel and Sadavoy (1996) recommend that it is crucial to establish a relationship with the client that allows for the regulation of interpersonal distance and affective expression in such a way that it provides the client with both comfort and stability. Being able to identify and work within the framework of the strengths, deficits, and defenses of personality-disordered clients is also an important aspect of their management (Rosowsky & Gurian, 1992). Sadavoy (1987) suggests that there are four goals of treatment for older adults with personality disorders. These include containing and limiting disturbing or destructive behaviors; establishing a working alliance between the client, caregivers, and family; developing a cohesive team approach with the client; and reducing the client's reliance on early pathologic behaviors by dissipating inner tension, altering interpersonal stressors, and, when possible, changing or modifying defense mechanisms.

When working with a client who has a character disorder, it is important for all team members to be consistent in their approach to him or her. This can be particularly difficult in a long-term care setting where multiple staff may have very different approaches to the client, resulting in confusion for an individual who is already in a state of emotional turmoil. It can also provide a particularly manipulative client with a wealth of situations in which to try to exert control and wreak havoc on a unit. The role of the APRN in this situation would be to identify the problem, provide education to the staff about personality disorders, and help them to formulate a plan of care to help deal with problem behaviors. It will be very important to stress the need and reasons for consistent follow-through. In addition, it is necessary to share the plan, including interventions and rationales, with the client. Often, a written contract can be helpful and the client can be given a copy to keep. Campbell and Poole's chapter in Wilson and Kneisl's *Psychiatric Nursing,* 5th ed. (1996) outlines specific nursing interventions for different personality disorders.

■ CONCLUSION

This chapter reviewed some of the major psychosocial problems encountered in working with older adults. Because diagnosis of these problems may be very difficult, it is important for advanced practice gerontologic nurses to have a basic understanding of the effects of psychosocial issues on older individuals. The role of the advanced practice gerontologic nurse is to diagnose and manage acute and chronic medical conditions of older clients. Assessment of the individual should include a discussion of any psychosocial problems, including any past psychiatric history and treatment, as well as identification of support systems. Management of medical conditions should include their impact on the emotional well-being of the individual. In addition, the advanced practice gerontologic nurse is in a position to assess the impact of mental health on a client's physical status and functioning.

Other responsibilities of the APRN include referral and collaboration with medical and specialty clinics; supportive counseling, referral, and collaboration with appropriate mental health providers (see Table 15–4); medication management; performing annual physical examinations; episodic care as needs arise; and ordering and evaluating laboratory results and other clinical data. The APRN should also be available to assist with illness prevention and health maintenance activities such as immunizations, weight loss, exercise, smoking cessation, alcohol reduction and/or cessation, grief counseling, and stress management.

In this current era of managed care, the role of advanced practice gerontologic nurses will continue to expand. Advanced practice registered nurses will be called upon more and more to provide primary care in a variety of settings. It is important to be aware of the stigma of mental illness that continues to exist despite efforts of public education to reduce it. This stigma is exhibited in the differences in reimbursement provided

TABLE 15–4.   REFERRAL SOURCES

Referrals	Areas of Expertise	Reimbursement
Clergyperson	Spiritual counseling Grief counseling Family problems	No
Social worker	Assessment and diagnosis Psychotherapy Marital/family therapy	Yes
Psychologist	Assessment and diagnosis Neuropsychologic testing Psychologic testing Psychotherapy	Yes
Psychiatric clinical nurse	Assessment and diagnosis Psychotherapy Medication management	Yes
Psychiatrist	Assessment and diagnosis Psychotherapy Medication management Electroconvulsive therapy Involuntary commitment Competency evaluation	Yes

by Medicare for medical care (80%) when compared to the reimbursement provided for psychiatric care (50%). It is also found in access to care, as shown by the advent of the minimum data set, which selectively discriminates against those with mental illness who may be as functionally impaired (or more so) as those with a medical illness. Advanced practice gerontologic nurses need to advocate for legislation as well as public education to abolish this stigma against psychiatric illness and its inherent inequities.

vignette

Mrs. Bowman is an 82-year-old woman with a long history of bipolar disorder who for many years was maintained on a dose of 150 mg of lithium bid. She reported having visual hallucinations that consisted of seeing black, wiry things coming out of the light and out of her hair when she looked in the mirror. Her urologist had put her on an OTC antihistamine for urinary incontinence, and this was stopped by the psychiatrist who suspected a possible delirium due to the anticholinergic effects of the antihistamine. However, the symptoms did not improve and in fact got worse. Mrs. Bowman became more irritable, more pressured in her speech, and also had some difficulty sleeping. Her visual hallucinations got worse despite the addition of haloperidol (Haldol). Her lithium level was 0.9, which was higher than her usual level of 0.4 to 0.5. Her blood urea nitrogen (BUN) and creatinine were at the high end of normal, which was also higher than usual for Mrs. Bowman. When she started to become more confused and forgetful, lithium

toxicity was suspected. Lithium was stopped and valproic acid was started, but she became more manic and confused. She did not remember the names of her therapist or her psychiatrist. She had difficulty remembering the name of the apartment building she had lived in for many years, and she was not oriented to the date. She was hospitalized on a geropsychiatric unit, where the valproic acid was discontinued and lithium was restarted. A diagnosis of dementia was given. Upon discharge, Mrs. Bowman was transferred to a skilled nursing facility. Her confusion continued, and it was noted that her lithium levels were still up in the 0.8 to 0.9 range. Her psychiatrist adjusted her dose, and she presently receives lithium 150 mg qd on Monday, Tuesday, Wednesday, Friday, and Saturday. Her level is 0.3 to 0.4, her confusion has cleared, and she is fully oriented and independent in all of her activities of daily living.

vignette

Mrs. Stone is a 72-year-old with a history of paranoid schizophrenia that was first diagnosed when she was in her 20s. She has had several in-patient hospitalizations, but for the past 5 years she has been able to be treated on an outpatient basis. In the past, Mrs. Stone would require hospitalization for noncompliance with her medications that would lead to an increase in her paranoia and auditory hallucinations. She would become more threatening and hostile, though she never actually became physically abusive. These were the symptoms she exhibited that led to her last psychiatric hospitalization 5 years ago. Because of her long history of noncompliance with medications, her psychiatrist on the inpatient unit decided that she might be better treated with haloperidol decanoate (Haldol LA).

On discharge from the hospital, she was transferred to the intermediate unit of a long-term care facility and attended a partial hospital program. After several months, she was able to relocate to a group home and eventually to a home for the aged, where she lives in a one-room apartment with a nurse on staff from 7 A.M. to 3 P.M. She no longer attends the partial hospital program and has the opportunity to attend activities in the facility where she resides though most often she prefers to keep to herself.

She receives Haldol LA every 3 weeks. This is administered by visiting nurses. She sees an APRN every 2 months for medication visits. Mrs. Stone continues to experience auditory hallucinations but has a good understanding of the fact that they increase when she becomes anxious and she recognizes that by going somewhere (like her quiet apartment) to decrease her stimulation, this helps to decrease the voices. Although Mrs. Stone may not be able to return to a totally independent living situation, decanoate medication has allowed her much more independence than she might otherwise have.

 ## CASE STUDY #1

Mr. Patrick was a 75-year-old white Irish-American male admitted to the geropsychiatric unit. He had a long history of alcohol abuse, but had never actually been diagnosed as an alcoholic. He had retired from his job as a factory worker at the age of 70 and spent most of his afternoons socializing with other retired factory workers at the neighborhood bar. The bar had closed about a year ago. Mr. Patrick had become increasingly withdrawn, refusing to get out of bed or dress himself. Six months ago, his wife had him admitted to a long-term care facility where he deteriorated further to the point where he refused to eat, drink, or talk, and, finally, he became incontinent of urine and stool.

QUESTIONS

1. What signs and symptoms does Mr. Patrick exhibit?

2. What aging changes has he experienced?

3. What risk factors are present in Mr. Patrick?

4. What assessment tools might be helpful in evaluating him?

5. What diagnoses would you consider for him?

6. What would be the most appropriate treatment for Mr. Patrick? Why?

ANSWERS

1. Increasing withdrawal; refusal to get out of bed, dress, or talk; incontinence of urine and stool.

2. Losses, including retirement and loss of his social support system from the bar.

3. History of alcohol abuse, elderly, white male, social isolation.

4. Mini-Mental State Exam (MMSE); geriatric depression scale (GDS); history and physical; urinalysis; bloodwork, including B_{12}, folate, and thyroid functions; and computed tomography (CT) scan.

5. His diagnosis was depression.

6. ECT because of his complete vegetative state.

 ## CASE STUDY #2

Miss Kramer is an 80-year-old single woman, living in an elderly complex. She is fiercely independent and needs to be in complete control of her life at all times. She is blind in her left eye (since 1925), has 1/4 vision in her right eye, and was diagnosed with macular degeneration in 1992. She wears bilateral hearing aids. Her medical history includes gastrectomy and colostomy, cholecystectomy, hemorrhoidectomy, removal of benign tumor from left breast, throat polyps, colitis, hypertension, congestive heart failure (CHF), severe arthritis and osteoporosis with multiple compression fractures, and a fractured left hip. She has been hospitalized three times this year with pneumonia and has required rehabilitation in a long-term care facility following each hospitalization. She was very dissatisfied with her care and treatment in each of two long-term care facilities. She lost two brothers this year, one after a long battle with Alzheimer's disease, and the other, suddenly, of a heart attack. She feels responsible for his death, as she involved him in a major family conflict and feels the stress of this conflict led to his death. She has been giving away her prized possessions and is preparing for her death. She has even purchased the gown she wants to wear when she is buried. She is very irritable, has significant intermittent memory deficits and word-finding difficulties, and has given up all previous activities she enjoyed. She complains of back pain, shortness of breath, diarrhea, lack of appetite, and problems sleeping. Medications include dipyridamole (Persantine) 20 mg PO bid, potassium chloride (K-Dur) 20 mEq PO bid, furosemide (Lasix) 80 mg PO qd, diphenoxylate hydrochloride with atropine sulfate (Lomotil) prn, propoxyphene napsylate with acetaminophen (Darvocet N) 100 PO q4h prn, temazepam (Restoril) 15 mg PO hs, calcium 600 mg 2 tabs PO qd, calcitriol (Rocaltrol) 0.25 mg once a week, and diclofenac sodium (Voltaren) 50 mg PO bid pc.

QUESTIONS

1. What psychosocial factors may contribute to Miss Kramer's problem?
2. Does she have any medical problems that would contribute to psychosocial difficulties? If so, what are they?
3. What losses has she experienced?
4. Does she take any medication that might affect her adversely? If so, what are they, and how might they affect her?

You learn that she takes multiple medications, including herbal remedies and supplements. You also learn that Miss Kramer takes her medications as she thinks she needs them and there are times when she either overuses or underuses prescribed medications. In addition, because of her fiercely independent nature, you learn that you can never *tell* her what to do.

5. How might you assess Miss Kramer's medication use?
6. How will you intervene if you suspect she has been misusing medications?
7. What diagnosis might you consider for her?

ANSWERS

1. Never married; fierce independence; need for control; rehabilitation in long-term care facilities after hospitalizations.
2. Sensory impairment, including blindness and deafness; history of gastrectomy and colostomy; electrolyte imbalance; CHF; pneumonia; pain due to arthritis and osteoporosis.
3. Sight, hearing, health and mobility, independence and control, death of two brothers.
4. Lasix and K-Dur: fluid loss, dehydration, and electrolyte imbalance; Lomotil: constipation; Darvocet N: constipation, confusion; Restoril: confusion, sedation, and falls; Voltaren: constipation, kidney function, ulcers; calcium: constipation.
5. Ask her to show you what she takes if you see her in her home or ask her to bring in all of her medications if you see her in an office setting.
6. Explain the appropriate use of her medications and what the adverse effects are.
7. Depression.

■ REFERENCES

Agronin, M. E. (1994). Personality disorders in the elderly: An overview. *J Geriatr Psych, 27*(2), 151–191.

Alexopoulos, G. S. (1996). Sadavoy, J., Lazarus, L. W., Jarvik, L. F., & Grossberg, G. T. (Eds.). *Comprehensive review of geriatric psychiatry II* (2nd ed.). (pp. 563–572). Washington, DC: American Psychiatric Press.

American Psychiatric Association (1994). *Diagnostic and statistical manual of mental disorders* (4th ed). Washington, DC: American Psychiatric Association.

Benbow, S. M. (1991). ECT in late life. Special issue: Affective disorders in old age. *Int J Geriatr Psych, 6*(6), 401–406.

Bonanno, G. A., Keltner, D., Holen, A., & Horowitz, M. J. (1995). When avoiding unpleasant emotions might not be such a bad thing: Verbal-autonomic response dissociation and midlife conjugal bereavement. *J Personality and Soc Psychol, 69*(5), 975–989.

Campbell, J. B. & Poole, N. K. (1996). Clients with personality disorders. In Wilson, H. S., & Kneisl, C. R. (Eds.). *Psychiatric nursing* (5th ed.). (pp. 470–522). Menlo Park, CA: Addison-Wesley Nursing.

Chesla, C. A. (1996). Clients with schizophrenia and other psychotic disorders. In Wilson, H. S., & Kneisl, C. R. (Eds.), *Psychiatric nursing* (5th ed.). (pp. 297–322). Menlo Park, CA: Addison-Wesley Nursing.

Cohen, C. I. (1990). Outcome of schizophrenia into later life: An overview. *Gerontologist, 30*(6), 790–797.

Cooper, J. W., Gordon, N., Radovich, C., & Siegel, A. P. (1994). The recognition and management of depression in the long-term care institution. Publication of the Eli Lilly Co. Nov, 1–14. New York: NCM.

Cowles, K. V. (1996). Cultural perspectives of grief: An expanded concept analysis. *J Ad Nurs, 23*, 287–294.

Davis, M., Robbins Eshelman, E., & McKay, M. (1995). *The relaxation and stress reduction workbook* (4th ed.). Oakland, CA: New Harbinger Publications.

Detzer, E., & Huston, L. (1986). When schizophrenia complicates med/surg care. *RN*, January, 51–53.

Ebersole, P., & Hess, P. (1990). *Toward healthy aging: Human needs and nursing response* (3rd ed.) (pp. 38–39). St. Louis, MO: C. V. Mosby.

Fogel, B. S. & Sadavoy, J. (1996). Somatoform and personality disorders. In Sadavoy, J., Lazarus, L. W., Jarvik, L. F., & Grossberg, G. T. (Eds.). *Comprehensive review of geriatric psychiatry II* (2nd ed.). (pp. 637–658). Washington, DC: American Psychiatric Press.

Friedman, R. S. (1993). When the patient intrudes on the treatment: The aging of personality types in medical management. *J Geriatr Psych, 26*(2), 149–177.

Frierson, R. L., Wey, J. J., & Tableu, J. B. (1991). Psychostimulants for depression in the medically ill. *AFP, 43*(1), 163–167.

Glass, B. C. (1993). The role of the nurse in advanced practice in bereavement care. *Clin Nurse Spec, 7*(2), 62–66.

Gomez, G. E., & Gomez, E. A. (1993). Depression in the elderly. *J Psychosoc Nurs and Mental Health Services, 31*(5), 28–33.

Gurland, B. (1992). The impact of depression on quality of life of the elderly. *Clin Geriatr Med, 8*(2), 377–386.

Harrer, G., & Sommer, H. (1994). Treatment of mild/moderate depression with hypericum. *Phytomedicine, 1*, 3–8.

Holroyd, S. & Rabins, P. V. (1994). Personality disorders. In Hazzard, W. R., Bierman, E. L., Blass, J. P., et al. (Eds.). *Principles of geriatric medicine and gerontology* (3rd ed.). (pp. 1131–1136). New York: McGraw-Hill.

Jeste, D. V., Harris, M. J., & Paulsen, J. S. (1996). Psychoses. In Sadavoy, J., Lazarus, L. W., Jarvik, L. F., & Grossberg, G. T. (Eds.). *Comprehensive review of geriatric psychiatry II* (2nd ed.). (pp. 593–614). Washington, DC: American Psychiatric Press.

Kaplan, H. I., Sadock, B. J., & Grebb, J. A. (1994). Schizophrenia. In Kaplan, H. I.,

Sadock, B. J., & Grebb, J. A. (Eds.). *Kaplan and Sadock's synopsis of psychiatry* (7th ed.). (pp. 457–486). Baltimore, MD: Williams & Wilkins.

Kastenbaum, R. J. (1981). *Death, society, and human experience* (2nd ed.). St. Louis, MO: C. V. Mosby.

Krach, P. (1993). Nursing implications: Functional status of older persons with schizophrenia. *J Gerontol Nurs, 19*(8), 21–27.

Kroessler, D. (1990). Personality disorder in the elderly. *Hosp Commun Psych, 41*(12), 1325–1329.

Laraia, M. (1995). Panic. *ADV Nurse Pract,* December, 24–29.

Lesseig, D. Z. (1996). Primary care diagnosis and pharmacologic treatment of depression in adults. *Nurse Practitioner, 21*(10), 72–84.

Lipowski, Z. J. (1990). Somatization and depression. *Psychosomatics, 31,* 13–21.

Lube, E. A. (1990). Psychotropic drugs. In Hogstel, M. O. (Ed.). *Geropsychiatric nursing,* (pp. 110–176). St. Louis, MO: C. V. Mosby.

Madhusoodanan, M. D., Brenner, R., Araujo, L., & Abaza, A. (1995). Efficacy of risperidone treatment for psychoses associated with schizophrenia, schizoaffective disorder, bipolar disorder, or senile dementia in 11 geriatric patients: A case series. *J Clin Psych, 56*(11), 514–518.

Meyers, B. S. (1992). Geriatric delusional depression. *Clin Geriatr Med,* 8, 299–308.

Munetz, M. R. & Benjamin, S. (1988). How to examine patients using the abnormal involuntary movement scale. *Hosp Commun Psych, 39*(11), 1172–1177.

National Institutes of Health Consensus Development Panel on Depression in Late Life. (1992). Diagnosis and treatment of depression in late life. *JAMA, 268,* 1018–1024.

National Institutes of Health Consensus Development Conference Statement on Diagnosis and Treatment of Depression in Late Life. (1991). Nov 4–6, *9*(3), 1–27.

Osterweis, M., Solomon, F., & Green, M. (Eds.). (1984). *Bereavement: Reactions, consequences and care.* Washington, DC: National Academy Press.

Pasnau, R. O. & Bystritsky, A. (1990). Importance of treating anxiety in the elderly ill patient. *Psych Med, 8*(3), 163–173.

Raphael, B., Middleton, W., Martinek, N., & Misso, V. (1993). Counseling and therapy of the bereaved. In Stroebe, M. S., Stroebe, W., & Hansson, R. (Eds). *Handbook of bereavement.* (pp. 427–453). Cambridge, UK: Cambridge University Press, 427–453.

Reynolds, C. F. III, Small, G. W., Stein, E. M., & Tesi, L. (1994). When depression strikes the elderly patient. *Patient Care,* February 28, 85–102.

Rosowsky, E. & Gurian, B. (1992). Impact of borderline personality disorder in late life on systems of care. *Hospital and Community Psychiatry, 43*(4), 386–389.

Ryan, M. C., Austin, A. G. (1989). Social supports and social networks in the aged. *Image: Journal of Nursing Scholarship, 21,* 176–180.

Sadavoy, J. (1987). Character disorders in the elderly: An overview. In Sadavoy, J., & Leszcz, M. (Eds.). *Treating the elderly with psychotherapy: The scope for change in later life.* (pp. 175–229). Madison, CT: International Universities Press.

Salzman, C. (1990). Anxiety in the elderly: Treatment strategies. *J Clin Psych, 51*(10) (Suppl.), 18–21.

Salzman, C. (1992). Treatment of anxiety. In Salzman, C. (Ed.). *Clinical geriatric psychopharmacology* (2nd ed.). (pp. 189–212). Baltimore, MD: Williams & Wilkins.

Scovern, A. W. & Killmann, P. R. (1980). Status of ECT: Review of the outcome literature. *Psychological Bulletin, 87* 260–303.

Semla, T. P., Beizer, J. L., & Higbee, M. D. (1997). *Geriatric dosage handbook.* Hudson, OH: Lexi-Comp.

Sheikh, J. I. (1992). Anxiety disorders and their treatment. *Clin Geriatr Med, 8*(2), 411–425.

Sheikh, J. I. (1996a). Anxiety disorders. In Sadavoy, J., Lazarus, L. W., Jarvik, L. F., & Grossberg, G. T. (Eds.). *Comprehensive review of geriatric psychiatry II* (2nd ed.). (pp. 614–636). Washington, DC: American Psychiatric Press.

Sheikh, J. I. & Salzman, C. (1995). Anxiety in the elderly. Course and treatment. *Psych Clin North Am, 18*(4), 871–883.

Sheline, Y. I., Freedland, K. E., & Carney, R. M. (1997). How safe are serotonin reuptake inhibitors for depression in patients with coronary heart disease? *Am J Med,* 102: 54–59.

Smith, S. L., Sherrill, K. A., & Colenda, C. C. (1995). Assessing and treating anxiety in elderly persons. *Psychiatric Services, 46*(1), 36–42.

St. John's wort vs. tricyclic antidepressants. *Am J Natur Med, 2*(3), 8–17.

Thompson, L. W. (1996). Cognitive-behavior therapy and treatment for late-life depression. *J Clin Psych,* 57(Suppl. 5), 29–37.

Tran-Johnson, T. K., Krull, A. J., & Jeste, D. V. (1992). Late life schizophrenia and its treatment: Pharmacologic issues in older schizophrenic patients. *Clin Geriatr Med,* 8(2), 401–409.

Trigoboff, E. (1996). Psychopharmacology. In Wilson, H. S., & Kneisl, C. R. (Eds.). *Psychiatric nursing* (5th ed.). (pp. 776–815). Menlo Park, CA: Addison-Wesley Nursing.

Valente, S. M. (1994). Recognizing depression in the elderly. *Am J Nursing, 94*(12), 19–24.

Young, R. (1992). Geriatric mania. *Clin Geriatr Med, 8*(2), May, 387–399.

Young, R. C. & Meyers, B. S. (1996), Psychopharmacology. In Sadavoy, J., Lazarus, L. W., Jarvik, L. F., & Grossberg, G. T. (Eds.). *Comprehensive review of geriatric psychiatry II* (2nd ed.). (pp. 755–817). Washington, DC: American Psychiatric Press.

Zisook, S., & Schuchter, S. R. (1994). Grief and bereavement. In Sadavoy, J., Lazarus, L. W., Jarvik, L. F. & Grossberg, J. T. (Eds.). *Comprehensive review of geriatric psychiatry II* (2nd ed.) pp. 529–562. Washington, DC: American Psychiatric Press.

16

SUBSTANCE ABUSE ISSUES

Melissa Gorecki-Scavetta

■ INTRODUCTION

Substance abuse in the older adult has received increased recognition in literature over the past decade. Diagnosis, intervention, and treatment of this problem in the aging population, however, remains inherently complex.

■ DEFINING THE PROBLEM

Epidemiologic statistics concerning the incidence and prevalence of geriatric substance abuse vary greatly and are dependent on a number of research variables. Broad definitions encompassing "older adult" and "substance abuse," screening tools utilized, and treatment setting all have some effect on research and statistical outcomes. Current literature, however, consistently cites lack of recognition as leading to underreporting and subsequently underdiagnosis and

treatment of substance abuse within the elderly population.

Issues involving recognition and underreporting often begin with societal myths regarding the aging process, which health-care practitioners may bring to clinical practice. Many believe that older adults simply do not abuse substances intentionally. Thus, indicators of abuse or dependence are not adequately pursued. Issues of abuse are also frequently clouded by very real medical and/or drug complications, resulting in underdiagnosis of substance abuse as a primary problem (Thibault & Maly, 1993; McInnes, 1994).

Elderly adults influenced by the effects of alcohol or drugs may present a very different clinical picture from their younger cohorts. Problems of abuse may appear as subtle somaticisms or florid states of confusion, making accurate assessment and diagnosis difficult. When established patterns of abuse are recognized, clients are sometimes viewed as inappropriate to treat due to advanced age, complicating physiologic factors, or potential nonresponsiveness to treatment (Thibault & Maly, 1993).

Substance abuse in the older adult population is a prevalent and treatable condition, requiring a heightened sense of awareness on the part of the healthcare practitioner.

INCIDENCE AND PREVALENCE

Alcohol is the most frequently and intentionally abused substance by elderly patients (Thibault & Maly, 1993). Community-based statistics indicate the prevalence of alcoholism in men aged 50 through 60 at approximately 5% to 15%, and in women, 1% to 5% (Atkinson, 1984; King et al., 1994).

Among older adults in institutionalized settings, the prevalence is estimated much higher at 15% to 20% (Thibault & Maly, 1994); some studies have indicated a rate as high as 60% (Atkinson, 1984; Solomon, 1994; Szwabo, 1993).

While the population over age 60 constitutes approximately 12% of the current U.S. population, they account for 25% of all prescriptions written (King et al., 1994). The use of more medication than is clinically indicated creates a special set of problems for the geriatric patient. While all medications have a potential for misuse and/or abuse, if utilized outside of established pharmaceutical guidelines, many potentially addictive and dependency-forming drugs are prescribed for older adults. The development of a dependency problem in the older adult increases the risk of accidents, general illeffects, and withdrawal syndrome.

Older adults experience minor health problems (eg, constipation, diarrhea, gastric reflux, arthritis, pain) at a greater rate than younger adults and purchase a variety of nonprescriptive preparations to combat these problems. A 1978 survey indicated the daily use of over-the-counter (OTC) medications in people over age 60 at 69% (Szwabo, 1993). While recent literature suggests a more limited use of nonprescriptive medications by the elderly (Eckian, 1985), the likelihood of misuse/abuse, adverse reactions, and drug–drug interactions with prescriptive medications and/or alcohol are potentially problematic and deserving of attention.

Although the use of illicit substances can occur in older adults, the incidence is considerably lower than that of the current younger cohort. It should be noted that this may change as the "baby boom" generation (born 1946 through 1964) ages because of prior exposure to and use of illicit drugs in that group (Thibault & Maly, 1994).

CAUSATIVE FACTORS

The causes of substance abuse are almost always multifactorial. These causative factors may include biochemical predisposition, family history, learned abuse patterns, psychologic dependence, personality, socialization, exposure, comorbidity with mental illness, and stress associated with the realities of daily living.

Substance abuse in the geriatric client may be new in onset or of a longstanding, chronic nature. The psychosocial issues of aging that may contribute to substance abuse may include health difficulties, issues of bereavement or loss (eg, spouse/loved ones, financial status, independence, retirement, changes in living environment), feelings of anxiety, depression, guilt, loneliness, hopelessness, and isolation.

Although some older adults consciously abuse substances, others begin this practice in an insidious and unintentional way. It may involve a drink every night to help "relax" or an OTC preparation nightly to aid sleep. Often, it is related to the prescribing practices of health-care practitioners (Finch, 1993; Montamat & Cusack, 1992). When a client seeks help for a medical or emotional problem, we tend to validate complaints with a prescription (Lipton & Lee, 1988). Failure to recognize underlying psychosocial issues, underestimating the intricacies of aging physiology and pharmacokinetics, or fearing confrontation of an abuse problem can create unnecessary polypharmacy and potential substance abuse or dependence.

DIAGNOSIS

Diagnostic clarification is important in differentiating true substance abuse or dependence from the sequelae associated with polypharmacy, adverse drug reactions, and unintentional misuse (Finch, 1993).

Polypharmacy

Polypharmacy is commonly defined as the use of more medication than is clinically indicated or needed by an individual (Montamat & Cusack, 1992). The term *polypharmacy* usually refers to medication combinations that are prescriptive in nature. Polypharmacy in the elderly contributes to an increase in adverse drug reactions and drug–drug interactions secondary to the presence of multiple medications, often further com-

plicated by underlying disease states associated with aging (Montamat & Cusack, 1992).

Adverse Drug Reactions

Adverse drug reactions are the undesirable effects of a drug when taken at the recommended or usual dosage (Lipton & Lee, 1988). Adverse reactions may be predictable or common but relatively benign (eg, constipation or dry mouth). They also may be unpredictable and/or harmful, such as allergic reactions or anaphylaxis (Lipton & Lee, 1988). Adverse reactions can occur with a single medication or with combinations of medications (Lipton & Lee, 1988).

Misuse

Misuse of a substance occurs when it is taken for a purpose for which it was not intended or taken in dosages, frequencies, or combinations other than recommended (Finch, 1992). Misuse may be intentional or unintentional. Common examples of intentional misuse may include: purposeful overuse or underuse of a medication for a variety of causes; taking someone else's medication; using combinations of medications despite side effects or drug–drug warnings; or knowingly using a medication to treat a problem for which it is not indicated (Finch, 1993; Montamat & Cusack, 1992). Unintentional misuse usually arises secondary to misunderstanding or issues of cognitive dysfunction, for example, misreading instructions or labels, mixing up pills or dispensing times, forgetting to take medications, or taking medications for unintended uses due to confusion surrounding the reason for use (Finch, 1993; Montamat & Cusack, 1992). Circumstances that lead to decreased access

TABLE 16–1.   CRITERIA FOR DIAGNOSIS OF SUBSTANCE ABUSE AS ESTABLISHED BY DSM-IV

1. Recurrent substance abuse resulting in a failure to fulfill major role obligations at work, school, or home
2. Recurrent substance use in situations in which it is physically hazardous
3. Recurrent substance abuse–related legal problems
4. Continued substance use despite having persistent or recurrent social or interpersonal problems caused or exacerbated by the effects of the substance

The above criteria may not have ever met the criteria for substance dependence.

Source: Modified from American Psychiatric Association (1994). *Diagnostic and statistical manual of mental disorders* (4th ed.). Washington, DC: American Psychiatric Association. Reprinted with permission.

to medications (finances, transportation) may also contribute to underuse of medications.

Abuse

The *Diagnostic and Statistical Manual of Mental Disorders* (DSM-IV) defines *substance abuse* as "a maladaptive pattern of substance use manifested by recurrent and significant consequences related to the repeated use of substances." Further diagnostic criteria include at least one of

the factors (see Table 16–1) occurring within a 12-month period (American Psychiatric Association [APA], 1994).

Dependence

The DSM-IV defines *substance dependence* as "a cluster of cognitive, behavioral, and physiological symptoms indicating that the individual continues use of the substance despite significant substance-related problems. There is a pattern of repeated self-administration that usually

TABLE 16–2.   CRITERIA FOR DIAGNOSIS OF SUBSTANCE DEPENDENCE AS ESTABLISHED BY DSM-IV

1. Tolerance, as defined by a need for markedly increased amounts of a substance to achieve intoxication or desired effect or markedly diminished effect with continued use of the same amount of substance
2. Withdrawal, as characterized by withdrawal syndrome for the substance or the same substance is taken to relieve or avoid withdrawal symptoms
3. Use of a substance in larger amounts or over a longer period than intended
4. A persistent desire or unsuccessful efforts to cut down or control substance use
5. Spending a great deal of time in activities necessary to obtain the substance or recover from its effects
6. Giving up or reducing important social, occupational, or recreational activities because of substance use
7. Continued substance use despite knowledge of having a persistent or recurrent physical or psychologic problem that is likely to have been caused or exacerbated by the substance

Source: Modified from American Psychiatric Association (1994). *Diagnostic and statistical manual of mental disorders* (4th ed.). Washington, DC: American Psychiatric Association. Reprinted with permission.

results in tolerance, withdrawal, and compulsive drug-taking behavior." The salient difference between substance abuse and dependence is the development of tolerance, physiologic dependence, and withdrawal syndrome. Individuals displaying criteria consistent with substance abuse are diagnosed as substance dependent if they have ever previously been diagnosed or met the criteria of dependence. Further diagnostic criteria of substance dependence include at least three factors (see Table 16–2) at anytime during a 12-month period (APA, 1994).

It is important to note that some studies challenge the efficacy of using the DSM-IV to diagnose older adults. Criteria associated with social and occupational functioning may not be pertinent. The older adult is less likely than the younger cohort to experience the legal consequences of abuse or dependence, which involve driving and work-related issues. They are often retired or widowed, making assessment of dysfunction in work expectations and relationships difficult (King et al., 1994).

■ AGE-RELATED CHANGES

The biologic changes of aging affect the older adult's response to alcohol and drugs. This is related to altered pharmacokinetics and pharmacodynamics.

ABSORPTION

While a decrease in gastrointestinal (GI) function exists in the elderly (ie, decreased acid secretion, blood flow, peristalsis), little evidence exists to suggest that absorption of substances is significantly altered (Lipton & Lee, 1988; McCormack & O'Malley, 1986).

METABOLISM

Once absorbed, alcohol and drugs are carried via the bloodstream to the liver, where most metabolism occurs (Lipton & Lee, 1988). Liver function tends to decline with age secondary to decreased blood flow and liver mass. Genetic, environmental, and physical factors, as well as enzyme systems and concomitant drug use, may also alter liver function (Lipton & Lee, 1988; McCormack & O'Malley, 1986). When the liver is unable to process or extract alcohol and drugs, more of the substance remains in circulation, creating increased availability and effect (Lipton & Lee, 1988).

DISTRIBUTION

Distribution refers to the process by which metabolites, the by-products of metabolism, are distributed to cells throughout the body (McCormack & O'Malley, 1986). Distribution is related to body composition or body fat, lean mass, and water volume (McCormack & O'Malley, 1986). Generally speaking, the percentage of lean mass and water volume decreases and body fat increases with age. Decreased lean mass and water volume means that alcohol and water-soluble drugs may have increased plasma or blood levels secondary to a decrease of volume distribution (Lipton & Lee, 1988; McCormack & O'Malley, 1986). An increase in body fat means fat- or lipid-soluble drugs may have lower plasma or blood levels due to an increase of volume distribution (Lipton & Lee, 1988; McCormack & O'Malley, 1986).

EXCRETION

Following distribution, substances are cleared or excreted through the kidneys. Renal function declines with age secondary to a decline in the glomerular filtration rate or filtering capacity (Lipton & Lee, 1988; McCormack & O'Malley, 1986). This means renally excreted drugs have a decreased rate of elimination and potentially longer half-life (Lipton & Lee, 1988; McCormack & O'Malley, 1986).

■ ALCOHOLISM

The use of alcohol to the point of abuse or dependence may become apparent to the health-care practitioner through recognition of the signs and symptoms of acute intoxication, subtle behavioral changes or indicators of abuse, physiologic effects related to long-term use, or withdrawal/abstinence syndrome.

The following discussion focuses on the diagnostic classifications of alcohol abuse and dependence, which are indicative of an intentional use of alcohol despite psychosocial and physical ramifications.

CLINICAL PRESENTATION

Usual Presentation of Disease

More often than not, alcoholism in the older adult manifests itself with subtle physiologic, psychologic, and behavioral characteristics.

Common physiologic presentations may include residual smell of alcohol; facial flushing; swollen or reddened eyes; hand tremor; dehydration; malnourishment; vague somaticisms or complaints of "not feeling well"; difficulties with sleep; sexual dysfunction; poor concentration and attention; evidence of increased "accidents" with bruising, lacerations, or fractures; and the onset of any

number of biological effects (O'Neil, 1995) (see Table 16–3). Great care should be taken in determining whether these physiologic effects are related to aging pathophysiology versus a true alcohol problem.

Although the onset of alcohol dependence in later life does occur, it is more often associated with a lifelong pattern. The most important diagnostic criteria in differentiating alcohol dependence from abuse are the presence of tolerance and a history of physical withdrawal with cessation of use.

Tolerance is the metabolic or pharmacodynamic occurrence in which more alcohol is gradually required to achieve the same intoxicating effect. Individuals with elevated tolerance may display significant blood alcohol levels with few symptoms of intoxication or abuse. However, the evidence of general organ dysfunction is more prevalent. Neurologic complications such as delirium, seizure, and Wernicke–Korsakoff syndrome also increase in incidence (Maisto et al., 1991).

Alcohol withdrawal or abstinence syndrome occurs when alcohol-dependent individuals experience a drop in their normally high blood alcohol level. A form of central nervous system (CNS) excitability follows in which symptomatology progresses and worsens if the dependence goes untreated (Blum, 1994; Maisto et al., 1991). The effects of alcohol withdrawal are delineated by stages (mild, moderate, severe) and are based on the degree of dependence (amount of alcohol consumed), severity of withdrawal symptoms, and general physical health (see Table 16–4). Recovery from withdrawal for the generally healthy adult occurs within 5 to 7 days. The re-

TABLE 16–3.   POTENTIAL PHYSIOLOGIC EFFECTS OF ALCOHOL ABUSE AND DEPENDENCE

Body Temperature
↓ Core temperature

Cardiovascular
Arrhythmia
Hypertension
Coronary artery disease
Congestive heart failure
Cardiomyopathy
Stroke

Gastrointestinal
Reflux/heartburn
Esophageal varices
Gastritis
Ulcerations
Hemorrhage
Vomiting
Diarrhea
Anorexia/weight loss

Genitourinary
↑ Urination
Sexual dysfunction
Renal failure

Pancreas
Pancreatitis
Diabetes

Liver
Fatty liver
Cirrhosis
Hepatitis
Ascites
Hepatomegaly
Hypertension

Metabolic
Thiamine, vitamin B_{12}, and folic acid deficiencies
↓ Immunity and ↑ infections
↑Cholesterol
Dehydration
Malnutrition

Respiratory
Pneumonia
Tuberculosis

Neurologic
Delirium
Psychosis
Seizure
Ataxia
Tremor
Dementia
Wernicke–Korsakoff syndrome

covery period for the elderly client is frequently longer, with some literature indicating a recovery period as long as 30 days (Blum, 1984). Statistics surrounding mortality from alcohol withdrawal in the younger cohort vary from 12% to 20%. Statistics pertaining to the older adult are unavailable, but presumably higher.

Psychologically, the comorbidity of anxiety disorders and depression in alcoholism are high. Elderly clients often present with low self-esteem and symptomatology consistent with major depression, such as feelings of sadness, hopelessness, inadequacy, shame, isolation, withdrawal, loneliness, amotivation, or

suicidal ideation (O'Neil, 1995). Questions related to suspected abuse may be met with a variety of responses, such as denial, rationalization, or sometimes grateful acknowledgment (Szwabo, 1993).

Behavioral indications of alcoholism in the older adult may include a sudden change in appearance (eg, disheveled or improper dress), personality change, client or familial reports of increased social discord (eg, spouse, children, friends, neighbors), frequently missed appointments or an increase in office visits with apparent somaticisms, and an acknowledgment of noncompliance with

TABLE 16–4.   POTENTIAL PHYSIOLOGIC EFFECTS OF ALCOHOL WITHDRAWAL

Mild *(6–8 h after cessation)*	Moderate *(12–72 h after cessation)*	Severe *(72+ h after cessation)*
Weakness	Hallucinations (visual	↑ Disorientation
Anxiety	or auditory)	Restlessness
Tremors	Seizures	Agitation
Diaphoresis	Disorientation	Panic
Headache	Delusions	Severe diaphoresis
Nausea		Fever
↑ Heart rate		Delirium tremens
Hypertnesion		Vivid auditory, visual, or tactile
↑ Respiratory rate		hallucinations
Insomnia		

medications secondary to fears associated with potential alcohol–drug interactions (O'Neil, 1995).

CLINICAL PEARL

Alcoholism is a primary disease process and needs to be treated as such.

Atypical Presentation of Disease

The presentation of alcoholism in the elderly patient may be typical, but often preexisting health problems are magnified or complicated by the effects of alcohol (Thibault & Maly, 1993). Older adults may not identify themselves as having developed an unhealthy pattern of alcohol use. They do not always meet all DSM-IV criteria associated with alcohol abuse and dependence, and instances of misuse may not be adequately identified or addressed.

ASSESSMENT

History

The identification of an alcohol problem is best verified by client or family, if possible. Knowledge concerning current drinking patterns (eg, amount and length of time of consumption), history of abuse or dependence, psychosocial stressors, available support systems, and prior treatment are helpful in assisting with diagnostic clarification and directing appropriate treatment.

Two alcohol screening tools commonly utilized in assessing alcoholism are the Michigan Alcohol Screening Test (MAST) (see Table 16–5) and the CAGE (see Table 16–6), both of which display a relatively high degree of specificity in the general population (Mayfield et al., 1974; Selzer, 1971). Data concerning the specificity of use in the elderly population, however, are unclear (King et al., 1994). Assessing for falls or "accidents," driving mishaps, sleep disturbance, and general dysfunction may be more useful.

TABLE 16–5.   MICHIGAN ALCOHOLISM SCREENING TEST (MAST)

Yes	No		Questions
☐	☐	0	1. Do you enjoy a drink now and then?
☐	■	2	2. Do you feel you are a normal drinker?
■	☐	2	3. Have you ever awakened the morning after some drinking the night before and found that you could not remember a part of the evening before?
■	☐	1	4. Does your wife (or parents) ever worry or complain about your drinking?
☐	■	2	5. Can you stop drinking without a struggle after one or two drinks?
■	☐	1	6. Do you ever feel guility about your drinking?
☐	■	2	7. Do friends and relatives think you are a normal drinker?
☐	■	2	8. Are you always able to stop drinking when you want to?
■	☐	5	9. Have you ever attended a meeting of Alcoholics Anonymous (AA)?
■	☐	1	10. Have you gotten into fights when drinking?
■	☐	2	11. Has your drinking ever created problems with you and your wife?
■	☐	2	12. Has your wife (or other family member) ever gone to anyone for help about your drinking?
■	☐	2	13. Have you ever lost friends or girlfriends because of your drinking?
■	☐	2	14. Have you ever gotten into trouble at work because of drinking?
■	☐	2	15. Have you ever lost a job because of drinking?
■	☐	2	16. Have you ever neglected your obligations, your family, or your work for 2 or more days because you were drinking?
■	☐	1	17. Do you ever drink in the morning?
■	☐	2	18. Have you ever been told you have liver trouble? Cirrhosis?
■	☐		19. Have you ever had delirium tremens (DTs), severe shaking, heard voices, or seen things that weren't there after heavy drinking?
■	☐	5	20. Have you ever gone to anyone for help about your drinking?
■	☐	5	21. Have you ever been in a hospital because of drinking?
☐	☐	0	22. Have you ever been a patient in a psychiatric hospital or on a psychiatric ward of a general hospital?
☐	☐	0	23. a. Have you ever been seen at a psychiatric or mental health clinic, or gone to any doctor, social worker, or clergyman for help with an emotional problem?
■	☐	2	b. Was drinking part of the problem?
■	☐	2	24. Have you ever been arrested, even for a few hours, because of drunk behavior?
■	☐	2	25. Have you ever been arrested for drunk driving?

Darkened responses are indicative of a positive alcoholic response. A score of three points or less is considered nonalcoholic, a score of four points is suggestive of alcoholism, and a score of five or more points indicates alcoholism.

Source: Adapted from Selzer, M. L. (1971). The Michigan Alcohol Screening Test: The quest for a new diagnostic instrument. *Am J Psych, 2,* 1653–1658. Reprinted with permission.

TABLE 16–6.   CAGE SCREENING QUESTIONNAIRE

1. Have you ever felt you should *cut down* on your drinking?
2. Have people *annoyed* you by criticizing your drinking?
3. Have you ever felt bad or *guilty* about your drinking?
4. Have you ever had a drink first thing in the morning to steady your nerves or get rid of a hangover (*eye opener*)?

A positive response to any of the above indicates the need for further assessment of an alcohol abuse or dependency problem.
Source: From Mayfield, D. G., McLeod, G., and Hall, P. (1974). The CAGE questionnaire: Validation of a new alcoholism screening instrument. *Am J Psych, 131,* 1121–1123. Reprinted with permission.

Physical Examination

Indications of alcoholism are not always accompanied by biologic organ changes. See prior discussion and Table 16–3 for assessment of possible physiologic manifestations. Assess appearance, hydration, nutritional status, mental status, and affect and mood. Facial flushing; swollen, reddened eyes; telangiectasis; hand tremor; and bruises or lacerations are not diagnostic but should be noted as part of the total presentation.

Diagnostic Studies

Laboratory abnormalities in the geriatric client are often related to underlying physiologic problems or altered pharmacokinetics, unrelated to alcohol. However, a general laboratory workup is advisable to assist in the assessment/recognition of physiologic illness that may have been caused or exacerbated by alcohol use. Laboratory studies related to liver, kidney, metabolic, and pancreatic function are important, as well as complete blood count (CBC). Blood alcohol levels fluctuate, according to alcohol consumption and metabolic absorption (Maisto et al., 1991). Although helpful in recognizing an abusive pattern, blood alcohol level alone is not a predictor of tolerance or dependence.

Diagnostically, an electrocardiogram (ECG) is always prudent, especially in instances of concomitant cardiovascular disease or dependency in which the likelihood of withdrawal exists. Electroencephalograms (EEGs), computed tomography (CT scan) and magnetic resonance imaging (MRI) may also be of assistance when changes in cognition or evidence of trauma (eg, falls/fractures/accidents) are present.

CLINICAL MANAGEMENT

Pharmacologic Measures

The pharmacologic management of alcoholism in the general, healthy, younger adult client is complex at best. Alcohol withdrawal carries a significant risk of mortality and requires ongoing skillful assessment and treatment. Inpatient hospitalization provides this management, as well as an examination of further treatment options, such as preventative pharmacologic and nonpharmacologic intervention. Referral for treatment should occur when an abusive pattern or physiologic dependence on alcohol is recognized.

Nonpharmacologic Measures

Alcoholism is a chronic disease process that requires treatment as a primary illness in the geriatric client. Identified symptoms of abuse or dependence should be addressed by the health-care practitioner in a direct, nonjudgmental manner, stressing the seriousness of the physiologic effects of alcohol use and its potentiating effects concerning existing age-related health problems and medication use. Underlying psychosocial stressors of later life that may contribute to use should be examined, as well as the comorbidity of mental illness. Older adults who attribute alcohol use to chronic pain or discomfort associated with disorders such as arthritis, neuropathy, and cardiac or respiratory difficulties require special consideration and reassurance that they "won't be left in pain." A multidisciplinary approach in which there is consistent contact with the treating specialist is helpful in monitoring the recovery process and allaying clients' fears. Pain clinics provide pharmacologic and nonpharmacologic alternatives to pain reduction and can be greatly helpful in these circumstances.

The ultimate goal of alcohol treatment is abstinence. However, abstinence is not possible for some clients, and relapse is common. The life stressors that contribute to one's drinking often remain after treatment. When faced with the same stressors again, the alcoholic client may feel overwhelmed or inadequate to manage these recurrent stressors and return to a pattern of drinking. Early intervention or reengagement in treatment is important in relapse to prevent a return to the consequences of prior use. Geriatric clients with a significant history of alcohol dependence and relapse should be encouraged to participate in ongoing treatment. If the physiologic consequences of long-term alcohol

use become evident, such as repeated injuries secondary to "accidents," malnutrition, dehydration, cirrhosis, hemorrhage, or the onset of alcohol-related dementia, attention to the client's overall health and safety is warranted. The institution of a health-care guardian is sometimes necessary in instances in which danger to oneself or others is likely to occur secondary to issues of chronic use.

Client Education

Older adults who have developed alcoholism as a new problem should receive the benefits of a structured alcohol program to assist in providing education concerning the alcohol disease process, impact on physical and emotional well-being of self and significant others, identification of "triggers" or potential stressors, and coping skills to aid in the prevention of relapse. Older adults with a history of chronic alcoholism may have received prior treatment and believe that they already possess the needed tools to remain alcohol free. Substance abuse programs may differ in philosophy and approach, depending on theoretical basis. Assessment of prior treatment efforts and available personal support systems are important in developing a treatment plan.

Rehabilitation

Successful rehabilitation or treatment of alcoholism in the older adult is based on individual willingness/acceptance of the disease, as well as available personal and community support systems. Available treatment options may include, in varying combinations, structured hospital or alcohol/drug treatment programs, Alcoholics Anonymous (AA), individual and family therapies, halfway houses, assisted living environments, and home health-care programs.

Many elderly exhibit concomitant mental illness, such as depression, anxiety, or mild dementia, and physical problems requiring rehabilitation and nursing assistance. This is sometimes incompatible with generalized substance abuse programs. Some alcohol/drug programs have developed specialized "geriatric" programs or tracks and are able to negotiate these problems. Psychiatric partial hospital and medical day care settings may also be beneficial in attending to concomitant illness while managing alcoholism as a primary problem.

Older adults with severe problems of repeated relapse, limited support systems, and/or physiologic illness (age or alcohol related) may benefit from a more structured living environment. Halfway houses, homes for the aged, and intermediate or skilled nursing facilities can sometimes provide the necessary physical assistance and supportive environment needed for recovery. However, the concomitant need to remain in active treatment remains. Facilities vary in their ability to provide monitoring of a primary alcohol problem, though some willingly work collaboratively with area programs.

Alcoholics Anonymous is a voluntary recovery program based on a 12-step approach, which stresses abstinence and endorses group support and spirituality as guiding principles to maintain sobriety. Alcoholics Anonymous has assisted over one million people in alcohol recovery and possesses a large membership. This is often beneficial to older clients, as sponsors are available and important to isolated elderly (Thibault & Maly, 1993). Several meetings may be available at varying times in the same geographic area, making compliance easier.

Caregiver Issues

Alcoholism affects not only the individual but the entire family system. Because family therapy is an integral part of treatment, and family willingness to participate should also be assessed. Many specialized alcohol programs offer family therapy as part of their curriculum. If not, this therapy may be sought through outpatient office settings.

Al-Anon, similar to Alcoholics Anonymous, is a support group available to the family members of alcoholics and is also helpful.

■ PRESCRIPTION DRUG USE

Prescription drugs possess numerous beneficial and appropriate uses. The increased prevalence of prescription medication use in the older adult population appears unavoidable, on some level, due to the increased presence of disease states that frequently accompany aging. Attention to medication side effects, drug interactions, issues of polypharmacy, and sound assessment skills related to aging pathophysiology are of paramount importance in the practice of geriatric health care. Balancing these issues will always require a sense of increased awareness of the part of geriatric practitioners.

All prescription medications are abusable and carry the potential of adverse sequelae if utilized as such. However, few medications possess psychoactive properties which often lead to abuse and dependency.

The categories of medications that possess mood-altering or psychoactive qualities include antidepressants, neuroleptics, stimulants, benzodiazepines, opioids, and barbiturates. The medications from the benzodiazepine, opioid, and barbituate categories create a greater likelihood of tolerance, cross-addiction, and physical dependence (Maisto et al., 1991). Similar to alcohol, medications from these three categories produce CNS effects, which some people find attractive. These effects may include a general feeling of well-being, relaxation, increased self-confidence, dysinhibition, or euphoria. Unlike alcohol, prescription medications may provide a false sense of security, contributing to abuse, as they are prescribed or given by a licensed health-care practitioner.

The development of an abusive pattern or dependency from medications with CNS effects has serious consequences for the elderly client. Ill effects, such as decreased motor coordination, poor concentration/attention, tremor, increased anxiety, seizures, depression of heart rate, blood pressure, and respiratory function, as well as symptoms of withdrawal, contribute to accidents, overdose, and fatalities.

Regardless of the causative factors contributing to an abusive pattern, increased awareness of the signs of abuse associated with these medication classifications, withdrawal secondary to physical dependency, and awareness surrounding prescribing practices are all important factors in the treatment of the older adult population.

CLINICAL PRESENTATION

Usual Presentation

The typical symptoms of prescription drug abuse in the elderly frequently become evident through the recognition of adverse effects associated with overuse, the development of tolerance or cross-tolerance, and/or withdrawal due to physical dependence. Behavioral indicators are usually subtle in presentation and are indicative of the insidious nature in which many substance abuse problems develop for the older adult. However, more blatant symptoms of drug-seeking behavior do occur, similar to the younger drug-abusing cohort.

Benzodiazepines are one of the more commonly prescribed medication classifications possessing psychoactive properties (Atkinson, 1984; Finch, 1993). Barbiturates, opioids, and their derivatives are used to a lesser degree (Jaroszewski, 1997) but are deserving of some discussion. Older adults are often plagued by issues of chronic pain in which the use of these medication categories may be indicated.

Benzodiazepines (see Table 16–7) are often used in the treatment of disorders

TABLE 16–7. COMMONLY PRESCRIBED BENZODIAZEPINES

Alprazolam (Xanax)

Chlordiazepoxide (Librium)

Clonazepam (Klonopin)

Clorazepate (Tranxene)

Diazepam (Valium)

Estazolam (Prosom)

Flurazepam (Dalmane)

Lorazepam (Ativan)

Oxazepam (Serax)

Temazepam (Restoril)

Triazolam (Halcion)

Generic names (Trade names).
List not all inclusive.

such as insomnia, anxiety, panic, depression, and withdrawal from alcohol. Benzodiazepine tolerance tends to develop slowly, and higher doses are generally required for tolerance to occur (Maisto et al., 1991). However, they possess a relatively long half-life, and withdrawal symptoms often do not become evident for longer periods of time (Marks, 1985). Ill effects or adverse drug reactions may occur with the single dosing of a medication, but overuse or misuse may heighten the likelihood of undesirable sequelae in the older adult (Maisto et al., 1991). Table 16–8 illustrates potential adverse reactions often associated with benzodiazepines.

Barbiturates and opioids may be used as analgesics for the purpose of pain control due to chronic conditions or secondary to surgical intervention, or for seizure control. Shorter acting barbiturates and opioids may also be used in the detoxification of individuals who have developed a physiologic dependence on

medications from these pharmaceutical classifications (Maisto et al., 1991). Both barbiturates and opioids possess the potential to create tolerance and, subsequently, dependence quite rapidly. It is primarily because of these effects that their use has declined in recent years (Maisto et al., 1991; Wartenberg, 1987).

In addition to the problems created by adverse drug reactions associated with prescription medications (ie, benzodiazepines, barbiturates, opioids, and their derivatives), the development of tolerance and dependence has the potential to create an even greater concern—physiologic withdrawal. Whereas mild withdrawal syndrome is not necessarily a life-threatening condition in the younger cohort, withdrawal effects involving cardiovascular and respiratory function in the presence of underlying disease states present a greater risk for the older adult, contributing to fatalities.

Tolerance refers to the occurrence of a diminished effect with a particular med-

TABLE 16–8. POTENTIAL ADVERSE REACTIONS AND WITHDRAWAL SYNDROME OF BENZODIAZEPINES

Adverse Reactions	Withdrawal Syndrome
Slurred speech	Restlessness
Sedation	Irritability
Ataxia	Increased anxiety
Disinhibition/euphoria	Tremor
Decreased concentration/attention	Confusion
Delirium	Diaphoresis
	Nausea/vomiting
	Insomnia
	Increased heart rate
	Hypertension
	Paranoia
	Hallucinations (auditory and visual)
	Seizures

ication, as the body becomes accustomed or less sensitive to it (Blum, 1984). Dependence indicates the development of physiologic need in which the body experiences symptoms of withdrawal if the drug is discontinued (Blum, 1984).

Cross-tolerance and cross-dependence can occur between individual medications within a particular class of drugs (Maisto et al., 1991). They can also occur between medications from seemingly different classifications that act at similar receptor sites in the body (Maisto et al., 1991). For example, an individual who has used a particular benzodiazepine for the purpose of sleep over a period of time may experience a diminished effect or tolerance. Switching or changing medications within the same classification has little effect on the sleep problem, as they are chemically similar and act similarly in the body. This same individual may also experience a decreased effect with other medication classifications, such as barbiturates or opioids, as they also operate at similar receptor sites with some of the same CNS effects (Blum, 1984; Maisto et al., 1991). The presence of cross-tolerance and cross-dependence is the underlying etiology for using alternate medication classifications in instances of withdrawal (Blum, 1984; Maisto et al., 1991). For instance, benzodiazepines are commonly used in the client experiencing alcohol withdrawal due to the similarity of CNS effects.

The symptoms of drug tolerance, dependence, and withdrawal are often difficult to predict. To some degree, it is based on individual pathophysiology and pharmacokinetics. Withdrawal symptoms depend on the length of time an individual has taken a drug, the dosage, drug half-life, and rate of taper. Clients with a

history of substance abuse are more likely to develop recurring problems with cross-tolerance and cross-dependence.

The phenomenon of "rebound anxiety," associated with benzodiazepines, warrants mention in assessing issues of dependency and withdrawal. Anxiety, the primary disorder for which benzodiazepines are prescribed, can be a recurring syndrome (Marks, 1985). Symptoms of benzodiazepine withdrawal (see Table 16–8), such as restlessness, irritability, increased anxiety, tremor, diaphoresis, and so forth, may actually be a recurrence of the preexisting anxiety disorder, affecting treatment management.

Common behavioral indicators of prescription drug abuse are listed in Table 16–9. Assessment of the causative factors contributing to abuse, such as psychosocial issues of aging, physical discomfort due to underlying disease states, and the onset of mental illness (eg, depression) should be closely examined, in addition to the presence of a tolerant or dependent state (Finch, 1993).

Atypical Presentation

Atypical presentations of prescription drug abuse in the older adult are frequently more of an issue of underrecognition. Elderly adults do not fit the stereotypical presentation of younger drug-abusing cohorts, and are less likely to be identified (Atkinson, 1984; Juergens, 1994). The symptoms associated with adverse drug reactions and withdrawal syndrome sometimes mimic those of underlying disease states. For example, an older adult with an established history of cardiac disease, who presents with slurred speech, drowsiness, and gait incoordination, is likely to be viewed as experiencing a cerebrovascular accident

TABLE 16–9. BEHAVIORAL INDICATORS OF PRESCRIPTION DRUG ABUSE

Evidence of adverse effects associated with medication overuse (eg, sedation, slurred speech, gait changes, personality change)

Dishonesty associated with amount of medication use or frequency/early medication refills

The presence of tolerance or need for increased medication dosing

Evidence of "doctor shopping" or prescriptions from multiple physicians

Repeated losing of prescriptions or pills (eg, accidentally throwing away or spilling medications)

Calling for refills after hours

Frequent emergency room visits

Strong preference for a particular drug (eg, "allergic" to others, "nothing else" works)

Sophisticated knowledge of drugs

Incongruence between severity of the complaint and the physical presentation

Source: Modified from Finch, J. (1993). Prescriptin drug abuse. *Primary Care, 20,* 236. Used with permission.

(CVA). The possibility that he or she may be misusing or experiencing the early signs of withdrawal associated with his nightly sleeping pill may not be in the forefront of the practitioner's thinking.

ASSESSMENT

History

The evidence of a prescription drug abuse problem should be corroborated with the client and family, if possible. Knowledge of recent medication use, amount, and duration provides some assistance in formulating treatment in situations in which withdrawal is likely. Assessment of factors contributing to abuse, such as altered cognition, prior history of substance abuse and/or treatment, recent psychosocial stressors, and available support systems to assist with future prevention are all an important part of history taking (Finch, 1993).

Physical Examination

The physical sequelae associated with prescription drug abuse vary and are de-

pendent on the properties of the individual medication used, as well as pathophysiology, pharmacokinetics, and underlying disease states. The reader is referred to the previous discussion and is encouraged to utilize supervising physicians, hospital guidelines/protocols, and pharmaceutical reference guides for remaining questions.

Diagnostic Studies

A number of laboratory methodologies exist to assist in detecting the presence of psychoactive medications and illicit substances and are often used in acute circumstances of overdose and/or withdrawal. However, in most instances, older adults or available support systems are able to confirm the suspected medication of use/abuse. Diagnostic testing, such as ECGs, are helpful in instances of prescription drug abuse or dependence, in which cardiovascular or respiratory function may be affected. Additionally, EEGs, CT scans, MRIs may be indicated where changes in cognition or instances of trauma exist.

CLINICAL MANAGEMENT

Pharmacologic Measures

Adverse reactions to prescription medications are frequently eliminated by simply lowering the dose of medication or discontinuing it. However, older adults who have developed a dependency on prescription drugs, in which withdrawal syndrome is likely, frequently require hospitalization for skilled monitoring. Geriatric health-care practitioners should seek referral for detoxification and/or treatment for these clients on the recognition of symptomatology consistent with tolerance or dependence.

In cases in which the ongoing need for potentially addictive medications is substantiated and deemed appropriate, clients should be cautioned/reminded not to abruptly stop these treatments.

When initiating the use of prescription drugs with an abuse or dependency potential, health-care practitioners should maintain clear indications for use (Finch, 1993; Montamat & Cusack, 1992). Using medications with a shorter half-life, beginning with small doses, and

> ### CLINICAL PEARL
>
> When prescribing medications for the elderly, remember "start low, go slow."

> ### CLINICAL PEARL
>
> Use caution with prescription medications possessing CNS effects in clients with a history of alcoholism, as they may precipitate relapse.

titrating doses slowly are important practices in preventing the development of tolerance and dependence (Finch, 1993; Thibault & Maly, 1993).

Nonpharmacologic Measures

The development of a problem with prescription drugs in the older adults is often a blend of client *and* health-care practitioner-related factors.

In clinical practice, the misuse of medications by the elderly is more common than the actual presence of a deliberate abusive pattern (Finch, 1993). Table 16–10 illustrates common patient-related factors contributing to misuse. Concerns regarding prescription medication use may be met by any variety of patient responses. However, health-care practitioner concerns are usually well received if presented in an empathic manner, stressing the ill effects of adverse drug reactions and addiction potential. There is no replacement for solid assessment skills and accurate history taking. Attempt to clarify the reasons surrounding misuse, whether physiologic, emotional, or psychosocial in nature. Utilize specialists of alternate health-care disciplines to assist in addressing these issues, for example, pain clinics for issues of chronic pain; psychiatry for underlying issues of depression, anxiety, and age-related psychosocial dynamics; and home health-care agencies in instances in which complex medication regimens exist to assist with further medication teaching.

Practitioner-related factors contributing to prescription drug use problems are frequently related to prescribing practices. Literature surrounding these practices is well documented; potential contributory factors are shown in Table 16–10 (Montamat & Cusack, 1992).

TABLE 16–10.   POTENTIAL CAUSES OF PRESCRIPTION DRUG ABUSE AND POLYPHARMACY

■ **PATIENT-RELATED FACTORS**

Expectation of physician to prescribe medication

Inadequate reporting of current medications

Failure to complain about symptoms, especially if related to medication

Use of multiple, automatic refills without visiting physician

Hoarding prior medications

Use of multiple pharmacies or multiple physicians

Borrowing medications from family members or friends

Self-medication with over-the-counter drugs

Impaired cognition or vision

Economic factors such as high drug costs

■ **PRACTITIONER-RELATED FACTORS**

Presuming that patients expect prescription of medication

Drug treatment of symptoms without sufficient clinical evaluation

Treating conditions without setting goals of therapy

Communicating instructions in unclear, complex, or incomplete manner

Failure to review medications and their possible adverse effects at regular intervals

Use of automatic refills without adequate follow-up

Lack of knowledge of geriatric clinical pharmacology, leading to inappropriate prescribing
    practices

Inadequate supervision of medication in long-term care

Failure to simplify drug regimens as often as possible

Source: Modified from Montamat, S. C., & Cusack, B. (1992). Overcoming problems with polypharmacy and drug misuse in the elderly. *Clin Geriatr Med, 8,* 150. Used with permission.

Client Education

Information pertaining to the ongoing treatment of elderly adults who have developed an abusive pattern or addiction to prescription medications is poorly defined. Suggested client education and treatment strategies are similar to those of alcoholism (Finlayson, 1984). Older adults who have developed a later-life prescription drug abuse or dependency problem as defined by the DSM-IV may benefit from a drug treatment program. Treatment that stresses the impact of prescription drugs on physical and overall emotional well-being, as well as the identification of potential stressors contributing to abuse, may be of assistance in preventing relapse.

Rehabilitation

The issues surrounding rehabilitation from prescription drug abuse in the elderly client are also similar to those of alcoholism. (See the Rehabilitation section under Alcoholism for information pertaining to treatment setting options.)

Alcoholics Anonymous, founded to assist in the recovery of alcoholism, may have some efficacy, according to literature, for those individuals with prescription drug abuse problems as well. Narcotics Anonymous is a similar program, encompassing individuals with addictions to all mood-altering substances.

Caregiver Issues

The presence of a support system is important in the recovery of any substance abuse problem. In relation to the geriatric population, this is frequently the primary caregiver. The availability and willingness of the primary caregiver, whether family, friend, or neighbor, is an integral part of treatment in defining the need for supplemental community or institutional supports. Some families are able to maximize resources to assist in issues such as ensuring medication compliance, providing transportation to healthcare appointments, and so on. Others are not in a geographic, financial, or time-related position to provide help. Family dynamics are complex. In instances in which ongoing issues of substance abuse are present, family members may feel helpless or as if they "can't do anymore." Intermediate or skilled nursing facilities, rest homes or homes for the aged, home health-care agencies, day-care programs, and health-care guardians/conservators are available options to supplement treatment support.

■ NONPRESCRIPTION DRUG USE

Nonprescription or OTC medications are a controversial form of self-help treatment. Literature related to OTC medica-

tions is reflective of a dichotomy concerning the appropriateness and effectiveness of use. In reference to the current aging population, OTC use appears to be an integral part of managing self-limiting health problems.

For many elderly, nonprescription medications are a time-saving and cost-effective measure. Older adults, who are often restricted by financial issues, may find OTC medications less expensive than prescription medications (Lipton & Lee, 1988). The additional time and cost of a visit to the family practitioner and the transportation to get to appointments also weighs into the financial equation. At least one recent survey indicates safe and effective response with OTC medications in the geriatric population, along with a high degree of expressed satisfaction with use (Eckian, 1985).

In contrast, some literature questions the efficacy and safety of use. While all nonprescription preparations must meet standards through the U.S. Food and Drug Administration (FDA), it does not eliminate the problems of adverse drug reactions, drug–drug interactions, misuse, or abuse. Table 16–11 illustrates some of the more commonly utilized OTC drug groups and potential adverse effects.

Geriatric health-care practitioners should routinely assess for the use of OTC medications in elderly clients. The causative factors contributing to misuse and abuse of nonprescription medications are the same as those previously discussed within the Alcoholism and Prescription Drug Use sections of this chapter. Elderly clients frequently do not associate OTC preparations as medications the practitioner may be interested

TABLE 16–11. MAJOR OVER-THE-COUNTER DRUG GROUPS, THEIR USES, AND ADVERSE EFFECTS

Drug Group	Found in OTC Drugs Used for:	OTC-Induced Medical Problems
Analgesics (aspirin, acetaminophen)	Headache Arthritis Sedation	Gastrointestinal bleeding Metabolic problems Delirium Nephropathy
Phenolphthalein and others	Laxatives	Metabolic problems Malabsorption Osteomalacia Abdominal pain
Antihistaminics	Sedation	Central anticholinergic syndrome
Anticholinergics	Cold/allergy Diarrhea	Drug interactions
Sympathomimetics	Cold/allergy	Drug interactions Vascular disease
Alcohol	Cough syrups Other tonics	Intoxication Alcoholism
Caffeine	Many OTC drugs, beverages	Anxiety Cardiac arrhythmias Gastric disease Osteoporosis
Nicotine	Tobacco	Oral/lung cancers Osteoporosis Emphysema Muscle weakness

Modified from Kofoed, L. L. (1984). Abuse and misuse of over-the-counter drugs by the elderly. In Atkinson, R. M. (Ed.), Alcohol and drug abuse in old age. (p. 53). Washington, DC: American Psychiatric Press. With permission.

in (Montamat & Cusack, 1992). Request that clients bring in *all* of their medications to appointments regularly (Thibault & Maly, 1993).

CLINICAL PEARL

Remember to counsel clients with a known history of substance abuse concerning the addictive potential of some OTC medications.

CASE STUDY #1

Mrs. Armstrong is a 70-year-old divorced female who was assigned to your caseload this morning on a general medical–surgical floor within a large urban hospital. She was transferred to your floor from the emergency room the evening prior, where she was admitted after being found by neighbors in her apartment building disheveled, confused, wandering, and smelling of alcohol. Informal information indicates that her living conditions were unkempt/unclean. On admission to the emergency room, she was found to have a blood alcohol level of 0.14. Laboratory studies also indicated mild elevation in gamma-glutamyl transaminase (GGT) and low red blood cells (RBCs). She was tremulous and her sensorium continued to fluctuate during her stay in the emergency room. She also vomited a small amount of "coffee ground" emesis and was incontinent of urine twice. She was diagnosed with acute alcohol intoxication and admitted for further workup of possible GI bleeding or esophageal varices. This morning, you find her slightly tremulous and mildly confused concerning the prior evening's events; however, she is otherwise well oriented. She reports a "headache and stomach upset." You note that she appears frail and of less-than-ideal body weight. Mrs. Armstrong states, "I received some bad news yesterday and I guess I drank too much. I am absolutely humiliated and want to go home. Will I be able to leave today?" With further assessment, you find that she has a history of prior alcohol treatment twice, and was able to sustain a significant length of sobriety until the last few months. She reports a series of recent psychosocial stressors coupled with problems associated with sleep, poor appetite, and motivation. Mrs. Armstrong believes that she already "knows enough about alcoholism" and is not in need of treatment.

QUESTIONS

1. What physiologic symptoms presented are likely to be related to a diagnosis of alcohol dependence?

2. What behavioral/psychologic indicators are present that may further support a diagnosis of alcohol dependence?

3. Would you refer Mrs. Armstrong for treatment? If yes, based on your knowledge of your own local resources, where would you send her?

ANSWERS

1. Elevated GGT, low RBC's, vomiting, urinary frequency, possible GI bleeding or esophageal varices, less-than-ideal body weight, and poor appetite. The presence of an elevated blood alcohol level is indicative of an abusive pattern, but not a sole indicator of tolerance or dependence. However, Mrs. Armstrong's prior admission for alcohol treatment is consistent with the DSM-IV criteria associated with alcohol dependence.

2. Mrs. Armstrong's disheveled personal appearance and home prior to hospital admission, poor coping/relapse associated with recent psychologic stressors, and feelings of "humiliation" are all behavioral indicators of alcoholism. Sleep disturbance, poor appetite, and recent lack of motivation may indicate an underlying mental illness or depression.

3. Yes! Regardless of her age, prior treatment experience, and extended length of sobriety, Mrs. Armstrong should be encouraged to reenter some form of alcohol treatment. The treatment program you choose will depend largely on resources available to you in your community. In Mrs. Armstrong's case, an alcohol treatment program that is able to address possible underlying mental illness or a psychiatric partial hospital program with an alcohol track may work well.

 CASE STUDY #2

Mr. Boyd is a 66-year-old single male who presents as a self-referral to the suburban general medical office where you are currently employed as a geriatric health-care practitioner. He begins his interview with you by stating, "No one seems to be able to help me." He indicates a longstanding history of difficulties with "anxiety," for which he has been treated by a number of local internists and mental health professionals over the past 15 years. Mr. Boyd describes feeling "lonely and anxious," and he spends most of his days lying in bed sleeping or watching television. He finds such tasks as fixing himself meals or attending to issues of hygiene cumbersome. A brief physical exam is found to be within normal limits pending laboratory blood work. He appears well nourished and well groomed. He has been diagnosed with hypertension, which is stable on a current low dose of an antihypertensive. His blood pressure in your office is 124/78. Mr. Boyd later indicates that he has been taking "some old medication" that he has in his possession. You learn he has been taking approximately 5 to 7 mg of alprazolam (Xanax) a day. While this dose is more than prescribed for him in the past, per his admission, he states: "It helps me feel better when I take more. The dose isn't a problem, is it?" He requests a refill on his Xanax. You discuss your concerns surrounding his current dose and possible need for substance abuse treatment. He is willing to participate in treatment, but comments, "I'm not going to see any of the quacks in this area. I've already seen them all."

QUESTIONS

1. What behavioral indicators are present that suggest a prescription drug abuse problem?

2. Is Mr. Boyd's prescription drug abuse intentional or unintentional?

3. What are the concomitant signs of an underlying major depression?

ANSWERS

1. Mr. Boyd's explanation, "No one seems to be able to help me," and reports of "loneliness and anxiety" are consistent with feelings of despair and isolation. Further behavioral indicators of prescription drug abuse are present in his hoarding of old medication, knowingly taking more medication than is indicated, and "doctor shopping."

2. Both. It is clear that Mr. Boyd is knowingly taking more medication than is previously or currently indicated. However, he is anxious, distressed, and verbalizes unclear guidelines surrounding his alprazolam use (ie, "The dose isn't a problem, is it?").

3. Symptomatology consistent with major depression may include his generalized anxiety state, verbalized feelings of loneliness, increased sleep, and lack of motivation (eg, increased time in bed, verbalized difficulties attending to nutritional status and hygiene).

▪ REFERENCES

American Psychiatric Association. (1994). *Diagnostic and statistical manual of mental disorders* (4th ed.). Washington, DC: American Psychiatric Association.

Atkinson, R. M. (1984). Substance use and abuse in late life. In Atkinson, R. M. (Ed.). *Alcohol and drug abuse in old age.* (pp. 2–21). Washington, DC: American Psychiatric Press.

Blum, K. (1984). *Handbook of abusable drugs.* New York: Gardner Press.

Eckian, A. G. (1985). Self medication with over-the-counter drugs. In Moore, S. R., & Tal, T. W. (Eds.). *Geriatric drug use—clinical and social perspectives.* (pp. 39–46). New York: Pergamon Press.

Finch, J. (1993). Prescription drug abuse. *Primary Care, 20,* 231–239.

Finlayson, R. E. (1984). Prescription drug abuse in older persons. In Atkinson, R. M. (Ed.). *Alcohol and drug abuse in old age.* (pp. 62–70). Washington, DC: American Psychiatric Press.

Jaroszewski, E. (1997). Drug abuse. In Rakel, R. E. (Ed.). *Conn's current therapy.* (pp. 142–147). Philadelphia: W. B. Saunders.

Juergens, S. M. (1994). Prescription drug dependence among elderly persons. *Mayo Clin Proc, 69,* 1215–1217.

King, C. J., Van Hasselt, V. B., Segal, D. L., & Hersen, M. (1994). Diagnosis and assessment of substance abuse in older adults: Current strategies and issues. *Addictive Behaviors, 19,* 41–55.

Lipton, J. L., & Lee, P. R. (1988). *Drugs and the elderly.* Stanford, CA: Stanford University Press.

Maisto, S. A., Galizio, M., & Connors, J. G. (1991). *Drug abuse and misuse.* Chicago: The Dryden Press.

Marks, J. (1985). *The benzodiazepines—use, overuse, misuse, abuse* (2nd ed.). Boston: MTP Press Limited.

Mayfield, D. G., McLeod, G., & Hall, P. (1974). The CAGE questionnaire: Validation of a new alcoholism screening instrument. *Am J Psych, 131,* 1121–1123.

McCormack, P., & O'Malley, K. (1986). Biological and medical aspects of drug treatment in the elderly. In Dunkle, R. E., Petot, G. J., & Ford, A. B. (Eds.). *Food, drugs and aging* (pp. 19–27). New York: Springer.

McInnes, E., & Powell, J. (1994). Drug and alcohol referrals: Are elderly substance abuse diagnoses and referrals being missed? *BMJ, 308,* 444–446.

Montamat, S. C., & Cusack, B. (1992). Overcoming problems with polypharmacy and drug misuse in the elderly. *Clin Geriatr Med, 8,* 143–158.

O'Neil, C. (1995). Identifying alcohol dependence in women. *ADV Nurse Pract,* 43–46.

Selzer, M. L. (1971). The Michigan Alcoholism Screening Test: The quest for a new diagnostic instrument. *Am J Psych, 127,* 1653–1658.

Solomon, K., Manepalli, J., Ireland, G. A., & Mahon, G. M. (1993). Alcoholism and prescription drug abuse in the elderly: St. Louis University grand rounds. *J Am Geriatr Soc, 41,* 57–69.

Szwabo, P. A. (1993). Substance abuse in older women. *Clin Geriatr Med, 9,* 197–208.

Thibault, J. M., & Maly, R. C. (1993). Recognition and treatment of substance abuse in the elderly. *Primary Care, 20,* 155–165.

Wartenberg, A. (1987). The opiates and opiate abuse. In Herrington, R. E., Jacobson, G. R., & Benzer, D. G. (Eds.). *Alcohol and drug abuse handbook.* (pp. 19–53). St. Louis, MO: Warren H. Green.

17

NEGLECT AND ABUSE ISSUES

Ann Marie DiLoreto

■ INTRODUCTION

Although the concept of elder abuse has been known to man since the beginning of time, it is only since the late 1970s that elder abuse literature and research has been documented as a medical, social, and psychosocial problem. The purpose of this chapter is to provide information for the advanced practice nurse (APN) to identify and intervene appropriately in elder abuse cases.

Abuse in the elderly is as difficult to identify as it is to prove. Many victims will not admit to being abused by family and/or caregivers. Noted injuries are downplayed or hidden from the health-care professional. The client is often ashamed of the abuse by his or her "loved ones," and therefore the problem remains hidden. The literature review finds that almost anyone can be a victim of some kind of abuse or neglect: physical, emotional, or financial. Accordingly, the potential abuser can be anyone in

contact with the elderly (eg, family, friend, spouse, caregiver, stranger).

The definition of elder abuse varies, depending on the author's orientation or viewpoint. In some literature, elder abuse has been referred to as *elder mistreatment*. Aravanis et al. (1994) uses the term elder mistreatment as a broader statement that implies "violation of any legal or human rights. These rights promote self-respect and dignity." They propose: "Physical abuse shall mean acts of violence, resulting in pain, injury, impairment or diseases of an elderly person."

Abuse includes intentional infliction of physical or sexual injury or assault. Sexual abuse is considered a form of physical abuse. Ramsey-Klowsnik (1991) indicates that behaviors such as molesting, with kissing and provocative touching, and oral/vaginal/anal rape with penis, fingers, or objects are abusive. Sexual harassment and threatening to perform sexual acts are also termed abusive.

Physical neglect (Aravanis et al., 1994) involves the failure to provide "goods or services needed for functioning, or to avoid harm." This may include withholding maintenance care, including hygiene and food, as well as failure to provide physical aids and safety measures.

Psychologic abuse (Aravanis et al., 1994) is "the behavior that causes mental anguish in the client." This may include verbal threats and berating, as well as infantilizing and isolating the client from others.

Psychologic neglect (Aravanis et al., 1994) involves "the failure to provide the elderly client with social stimulation." This may include social isolation by leaving the client alone, ignoring the client, or refusing outside interaction.

Financial/material abuse (Aravanis et al., 1994) involves the "misuse of the elderly client's resources for the gain of another." Financial/material neglect (Aravanis et al., 1994) involves "failure to use funds/resources needed to maintain or restore the client's health or well being."

The cultural and societal norms of the 1990s place additional stress on the client, as well as the caregiver. Family values have changed radically since the 1940s and 1950s. An industrial society finds more women in the workplace for a longer time span of their lives. More women are single due to widowhood or divorce. Families have less support, or have disjointed help and support due to the caregiver's schedule. The elderly may be seen as old, burdensome, and easy prey for abuse. Old age and dependency are not cherished values in today's society. The caregiver may be neglectful, or provide lip service by doing the least possible for the client, with little warmth or empathy. Care may be mediocre at best, especially if the caregiver views the situation as long term or futile.

Society views the family unit as sacrosanct. A family should be nurturing, caring, and protective of all family members. It is difficult to "see" or to "recognize" elder abuse in an outwardly supportive family unit. What happens behind closed doors may not be privy to others, leading to a decrease in the detection of abuse.

"Ageism" also influences the detection of abuse. Clients' revelations may be passed off as "confusion" and "forgetfulness," and thus may not be addressed by providers/family members. The client is therefore denied his or her full rights as a human being due to "old age."

■ AGE-RELATED CHANGES

Growing old brings about anatomic as well as physiologic changes in the body. Erickson (1963) looks at the elder years as achieving integrity versus despair as the developmental milestone. As clients review their lives, they need to see their lives as having meaning and purpose, as well as being fulfilling, and providing a sense of satisfaction and contentment in later life. If clients see their lives as meaningless, they will face later life with feelings of despair, hopelessness, and futility.

Growing old successfully requires the client to make adaptations and set goals to master age-related changes. Elderly clients need the support and caring of others to work through adaptations and goals. Goals/adaptations include reevaluating self-concept and self-worth, as well as reestablishing an identity in an aging body. Additional goals include conserving energy and resources, feeling safe in their environment, and keeping active and in contact with family and friends.

Elderly persons who have difficulties with these developmental tasks may be lonely, depressed, and negative in their outlook on life. This negative outlook can radiate to caregivers, who in turn become frustrated with not being able to help or with being rejected by the elderly client.

■ RISK FACTORS

Fulmer and O'Malley (1987) identify several risk factors that are common in elder abuse and neglect situations. The most common factors include a substance abuse history or mental illness in the client and/or caregiver. Abusive behavior by the caregiver in the past is a risk factor for future abuse. Financal dependency of the caretaker on the client sets the stage for abuse, as the caregiver is frustrated but knows that he or she could not survive without the client.

Additional factors indicated by Fulmer and O'Malley (1987) include lack of a support system in the environment of the client who is chronically ill, dependent, or impaired. The client may have few alternatives and minimal contacts for support and care other than the present caregiver. If the needs of the client exceed the caregiver's abilities, the caregiver is unable to cope and loses control. Widowed women who are very old and in ill health are at the greatest risk for being abused.

Considering the above factors, caregiver–elder interactions occur in an environment filled with stressors. Usually, the interactions are in balance, but should one side of the scale change (ie, an increase in stress), the balance is upset, resulting in an abusive response. The unbalancing stressor can occur in the client's or caregiver's world. Stressors on the client's side include exacerbation of illness or disease, leading to an increase in dependency. Stressors in the caregiver include family problems, loss of income or, an increased dependency on substances. This unbalancing situation can occur with random frequency and intensity or daily. The situation could be the incident that begins abusive behavior or reactivates a long history of abuse on both sides.

Stressors identified by Kosberg (1988) include substance abuse, physical illness, mental problems, economic hardship, marital problems, lack of supports, and changes in the household (eg, someone moving in or out). All of these affect the caregiver–elder interactive process.

■ CLINICAL PRESENTATION OF ABUSE

USUAL PRESENTATION

Clients rarely tell providers they are being abused or taken advantage of. The reasons for nondisclosure include embarrassment, fear of further abuse, or a resignation/acceptance of the abusive situation. Resignation usually occurs if the abuse has been going on for a long period of time. Some elderly may be impaired physically and cognitively, and thus are unable to relate their plight accurately, if at all. Others blame themselves and, therefore, do not report abusive behavior. They blame themselves for their incontinence, immobility, their son's alcohol abuse, and so on. Telling someone about the abuse may put them in a worse situation (ie, nursing home placement or further abuse).

The elderly client may present with vague complaints and with an increase in the frequency of physician visits. The vague complaints may be due to the client's unwillingness to disclose the abuse and the abuser. Although unwilling, he or she may recognize the need for care and support, and hope the provider does also.

Frequent physician visits may be due to lack of compliance with follow-up appointments and treatments, leading to increasing illness. Frequency in visits may also indicate a crisis situation in the family in which the elderly may be severely injured and need acute care.

ATYPICAL PRESENTATION

Atypically, the client may report the abuse and ask for help.

ASSESSMENT

Early recognition of symptoms of abuse can lead to prevention of other types of abuse, as well as ongoing exacerbation of present abuse. Being knowledgeable about the client and his or her situation can help in early detection.

CLINICAL PEARL

Listen with ears and eyes. Words answer the questions, but the tone of voice, word choice, facial expression, and content say so much more. Observe for eye contact, posture, and presentation, as well as gestures used by the client.

Evaluation of the client in view of the present environment is important, as different data will be observed in a home setting versus the emergency room. Identify where the client is being seen and why the client is being seen today. Try to find out what is and what was going on in the client's life, leading him or her to be seen. Document all disclosures/observations of the client.

CLINICAL PEARL

Abuse does not exist in a vacuum. One abusive behavior can lead to another. Abusive behaviors overlap (eg, sexual and/or financial abuse can lead to emotional abuse).

A good assessment is based on establishing a working relationship with the client. It is helpful if the client knows the practitioner and has had a positive relationship in the past. This may allow the client to relate more honestly what is happening. Questioning should be concrete, concise, and nonthreatening. It is important to consider the client's educational level, as well as cultural issues that can impact on the client's willingness to share feelings with nonfamily. Document and preserve any and all evidence of abuse.

CLINICAL PEARL

The assessment/examination of the client should be done privately, away from the caregiver.

▪ PHYSICAL ABUSE/NEGLECT

PHYSICAL ABUSE

Assessment

Observe the client's overall appearance for cleanliness of body and clothing, as well as appropriate clothing. Observe the body, fingernails, and hair for cleanliness. Observe for odors, as well as skin hydration, turgor, and edema, which may indicate inadequate fluid intake. Look for bruising (ie, various stages and patterns of ecchymoses over the body and limbs). Observe the body for cuts, welts, lacerations, and bite marks. Observe the placement of burns and welts to determine if they were inflicted by the client or others. Cigarette burns may indicate a lack of supervision while smoking, deliberate attention-seeking behavior, or the client's wish to end his or her life. Burns from hot liquids may indicate a lack of supervision in the home while the client is preparing meals or bathing, or the behavior of an angry caregiver. Burnlike marks or excoriation about the ankles or wrists may indicate the use of a restraint and the client's struggle to free him- or herself.

Observe the body for the presence and stage of an open decubiti, which may indicate constant bedrest without position changes. Observe the genital/rectal area for redness and excoriation due to prolonged skin contact with urine/stool. Observe the skin folds and scalp for infestation with lice or scabies.

The head and neck should be inspected for cuts and abrasions from falls. Look for hand marks, indicating a slap. Check the neck area for bruising or hand marks, indicating an attempt at choking. Check for loose or missing teeth, or nasal problems due to a punch or a blow to the face. Observe for abnormal hair loss or scalp bleeding, indicating hair pulling as an abusive behavior. Question the client regarding recent falls and injuries to the head.

CLINICAL PEARL

When asking about falls, phrase the question as, "When was the last time you fell?" This may alleviate fear of admitting a fall or its consequences.

Observe the extremities for functional abilities, range of motion, and painful movement of the joints. Look at the condition of the skin and toenails for adequate care of the lower extremities. Long, jagged toenails, corns, calluses, dirt between the toes, and flaky skin are often signs of self- or caregiver neglect.

Ask the client about his or her diet and the method of obtaining food and meals. A 24-hour recall of dietary intake is often helpful if the client is not impaired in short-term memory. Clients may have family/friends who shop for them, but at a great cost, both financially and emotionally. They may decline the offer of someone shopping for them and starve themselves. Others may be forced to eat foods they cannot eat or do not like in a nursing home or home setting; thus, they refuse meals and become malnourished and dehydrated. If you are visiting a client in his or her home, accept any offer of food or drink to assess the availability of food and the client's ability to prepare it. If the client offers to show you around the kitchen, accept and note what foods are around.

Observe for sleep/rest disturbances (eg, circles under the eyes, listlessness, lack of energy).

Assess for diarrhea or constipation due to poor nutrition (ie, improper foods and fluids or medication intake). Observe for bleeding in the rectal/vaginal area and evaluate to rule out sexual abuse or trauma. Check the skin in the perineal area for signs of trauma or excoriation due to incontinence or poor toileting habits. Also observe for rashes indicating venereal diseases.

PHYSICAL NEGLECT

This term encompasses the failure of the caregiver to provide adequate care or services needed for the client's highest level of functioning.

The client may be unsure of medication names/doses and may not be in control of medication administration. Many elderly depend on others to provide the right medication. Questioning the client regarding proper dosing is important. The client and caregiver may be forgetful and unaware of when the last dose was given, leading to possible over- or underdosing. Limited finances can lead to infrequent dosing or total stoppage of medication. Alcohol usage should be investigated. Sleepless, noisy clients may be given a drink to calm them, thus leading to a drug interaction or a fall.

Assess for physical neglect, characterized by withholding of care needed for the client's well-being. This care may encompass supervision of care in the home, keeping regular appointments with health-care professionals, or providing assistive devices (eg, eyeglasses, hearing aids, canes) for optimal functioning.

Bourland (1990) states that neglect is the intentional or unintentional withholding of activities that are required for activities of daily living (ADL) (ie, shopping, cooking, cleaning) or for the avoidance of physical harm and mental suffering.

Intentional neglect is the deliberate withholding of care/services to retaliate for previous problems or grievances, or to gain monetary reimbursement. Unintentional neglect results from the caregiver's lack of knowledge of resources. The caregiver may be overwhelmed with his or her own problems and unable to provide care for the client, or may be ignorant of available support services in the community.

Assessment
Observe for: malnourishment, unclean clothing, rash due to incontinence, dehydration, frequent falls, burns, or injuries due to lack of supervision or care. Observe that necessary devices needed by the client are present and workable.

Diagnostic Studies
Lab tests provide an adjunct in the detection of physical, sexual, and medical abuse/neglect. X-rays may detect new or old fractures. Blood work may be ordered to screen for infection, dehydration, malnutrition, sexually transmitted disease, or medication toxicity. Blood counts, blood coagulability, and toxicology screens for alcohol/drugs may also be indicated.

■ SEXUAL ABUSE

ASSESSMENT

Observe for walking difficulties, and bleeding, drainage, or bruising of the perineal/rectal area. Note any blood stains on the client's underwear. Inquire about perineal itching or difficulties voiding. Questions regarding menopause or sexual history may encourage the client to share present abusive situations. Ask if the client is being forced to tolerate sexual touching and/or kissing, or being asked to do so to another.

■ PSYCHOLOGIC/EMOTIONAL ABUSE/NEGLECT

Psychologic abuse is less overt and more difficult to detect and assess. Threats and verbal barrage may be used to coerce the elderly into compliance and submission.

ASSESSMENT

Observation of the client–caregiver interaction can give clues to communication style and the relationship. Ask the client if he or she is subjected to threats, yelling, harshness, and/or harassment from caregivers. The client may be more willing to share such incidents if the caregiver is not a relative. The client may present with vague complaints because psychologic abuse is often so overwhelming that it is unexplainable. Aravanis (1994) indicates that clients who are psychologically abused react with resignation, fear, depression, crying, mental confusion, and ambivalence. Behaviors such as poor eye contact, blunted affect, isolation, and poor interactions need further investigation. Sengstock and Steiner (1996) indicate that feelings of helplessness, depressed mood, loss of interest, and hopelessness are not part of the normal aging process. These symptoms may indi-

cate emotional distress, such as abuse or depression.

A client's verbalization of being "bad" and a burden to others may also indicate psychologic abuse. Assess the client–caregiver relationship by learning about the types of activities the client is dependent on the caregiver to provide. Sengstock and Steiner (1996) indicate that the relationship and interactive style between client and caregiver is important.

Withdrawal, anxiety, fears, and feelings of humiliation are signs of a negative relationship. Threats of abandonment and/or nursing home placement are abusive. The client's mistrust of others, or extreme pain/anxiety or panic with hands-on care, may also indicate abuse (Sengstock & Steiner, 1996).

Positive signs include two-way communication, mutual consultation in day-to-day life, and displays of affection (ie, gentleness, touching and hugging between client and caregiver).

DIAGNOSTIC STUDIES

Mental status exams, as well as depression rating scales, can be used to identify the symptoms and diagnose depression. Neuropsychologic testing to determine psychologic functioning may be helpful as an adjunct in diagnosing abuse and depression.

■ FINANCIAL/MATERIAL ABUSE/NEGLECT

Material abuse is the misuse of the elder client's funds, services, or belongings for the benefit of others and to the detriment of the client. The literature refers to financial abuse as exploitation.

ASSESSMENT

Careful questioning and listening can uncover financial abuse. Questions surrounding the control of the client's finances and property can provide information to the clinician. Financial abuse is common among family members who know how much money the elder client has and how to get at it. In a home situation, the APN should observe for deprived conditions (eg, inadequate heat, furnishings, cleanliness).

Brickman and Adelman (1988) suggest the following as indicators of financial abuse: "Sudden inability to pay bills, unexplained withdrawal from the bank, great variance between the client's lifestyle and assets, as well as new, unexplained interest by family members in the elder's money/wealth."

CLINICAL PEARL

Thorough documentation of abusive situations helps to provide baseline data for future assessments, allows the APN to use information in the future, and communicates to clients that they are being listened to.

▪ PREVENTION

Abuse and neglect of the elderly may have dire consequences for them in the short and long term. Advanced practice nurses can help to minimize the abuse by assisting the elderly to deal with their present situations. Assisting clients to de-

velop positive coping skills and adapt to their environment, as well as educating them about utilizing appropriate resources, can help to decrease stress and increase safety and recognize abusive situations.

Helping elderly clients to adapt to their environment includes teaching them the use of assistive devices, sensory aids, and, possibly, medications usage. These interventions may make clients more mobile, more functional, and less vulnerable to environmental changes and stressors.

▪ CLINICAL MANAGEMENT

Elder abuse is difficult to identify but more difficult to prove. The clinician must have a good knowledge of elder abuse and the laws pertaining to abuse in the state where he or she is practicing. Identification of the problem by the clinician does not lead to resolution of the problem. The client must recognize the behavior as abusive and want it to stop. Management depends on the client's acceptance or rejection of the intervention(s), as well as the client's competency to make that decision. The term *intervention* is used to describe any and all behaviors/actions to remove the client, change the abusive situation, and keep the client safe.

All 50 states have protective agencies involved in helping to identify and intervene for the abused, neglected, and exploited elderly, as well as to determine the need for services. The reauthorization of the Older Americans Act in 1992 has allowed federal funding to be used to prevent elder abuse and neglect through these agencies. Mandatory reporters include physicians, residents, interns, administrators, nursing aides, dentists, osteopaths, social workers, physical therapists, registered nurses, medical examiners, clergy, optometrists, and pharmacists.

To initiate an intervention, interview the client alone. This approach may allow the client an opportunity to disclose more accurate information. Reassure the client of your intention in questioning him or her. Attempt to determine whether the abuse is chronic, acute, or intergenerational. Share with the client your observations and concerns, and ask for validation. The client needs to know what your action will be. Once the client is removed from the situation, it is also important to share your observations and your intended actions with the abuser. It is important to protect the client from retaliation by the abuser during this period. Allow the client to participate in the management of this situation as tolerated.

The client has the right to self-determination and autonomy. The client should have input in the intervention and can accept or reject it. If the client is not competent to decide for him- or herself, the courts will be involved to protect the client. The incompetent client in danger needs to be removed from the situation immediately. Treatment of medical conditions induced by abuse or neglect (as well as counseling about the abuse) is important to stabilize the client. Allow the client to express his/her feelings and fears in a nonthreatening environment. Do not judge or attempt to place blame. Active listening and validation of feelings is important. Help the client to understand the options available and what is involved with each option.

COLLABORATION

A community social worker, physician, family members, and others in contact with the client should be involved in both identification and interventions. Information and observations, as well as input into the intervention, are needed from everyone involved with the client to protect and prevent further abuse.

The Client in Imminent Danger

Based on the previously described assessment, the client in imminent danger will need crisis intervention. The goal is to remove the client from danger and begin stabilization of the client emotionally and physically. The APN may be involved in assisting with removal and stabilization. Meeting with the client to identify needs, as well as a plan for the future, is important. Intervention may involve moving the client out of the home, at least temporarily, until a safe plan can be established. The client may seek temporary alternative housing/placement to protect him- or herself and to de-escalate the situation. If the client wishes to return home and will accept services, the APN can make contact or coordinate referrals with adult protective services as mandated in the state.

Appropriate interventions in this situation may include a court order to keep the abuser away, a full investigation by the state's protective agency, and ongoing monitoring of the situation by the protective agency. Both the client and the abuser will need ongoing counseling/therapy to work through their feelings. The client may need services from a nursing agency, day-care program, or home-care program to meet his or her basic needs.

If the client refuses to be removed from the home and refuses services, his or her decision-making ability and/or competence will need to be evaluated. (See Chapter 18 for more information.) If competency needs to be determined, a court hearing can be scheduled.

The court will determine the issue of competency and the need for services to be put in place to keep the client safe. If the client is deemed competent and he or she wishes to return to the abusive situation, the provider, as well as the protective agency, will need to continue to offer services and keep close contact with the client. Support services can be offered to the client on an ongoing basis.

The Client in No Imminent Danger

If there is a suspicion of abuse and the client is not in immediate danger, the clinician should continue to assess needs and support the client. Counseling and education of the client is important. The clinician continues to negotiate goals and inform the client of services available. Services include case management, counseling services for the client and the abuser, and treatment services. The investigation of alternative methods of caregiving are helpful. These include day-care programs, home care, and assisted living programs, among others. Referrals to a psychotherapist for both the client and caregiver (for individual or joint counseling) may be reasonable interventions. The identification of caregiver support groups may be helpful to support stressed caregivers.

Education in the use of and assistance with obtaining self-care devices for the client's home are also helpful (eg, canes, walkers, wheelchairs, safety call devices, and grab bars). Involving an occupational/physical therapist to assess the client's safety, as well as to ease caregiving, is important. Encouraging the client to socialize with others in senior centers and church groups is helpful to decrease feelings of isolation and raise self-esteem and socialization. It is imperative to have ongoing monitoring and follow-up of the client.

If the client declines the above and is incompetent, the court again will be asked to determine follow-up care and needed services. If the client is competent and refuses services, the provider needs to maintain contact in a supportive, nonthreatening way and notify the protective agency of the refusal. The protective agency will attempt to make ongoing visits and assessments, as permitted by the client.

CLIENT EDUCATION

Supportive psychotherapy may be educational, as well as therapeutic. It allows the client to examine the situation and to identify what he or she can expect or achieve. Competent clients and families of incompetent clients will need to begin to think for themselves and use their abilities to make good decisions. Support and education should be directed to assist the client to raise his or her self-esteem and allow him or her to function at the highest level of psychosocial well-being. Empowerment of the abused elderly will help to decrease their dependency. Education of the client regarding factors that can lead to an escalation in violence is also important. Education about the incidence of elder abuse and the tendency for it to increase in severity and frequency as time goes by is helpful.

Development and review of a safety plan is important. Educate clients in strategies to use if violence reoccurs. Written information regarding numbers to call (eg, a friend or 911) will be helpful in a stressful situation. Education should be provided regarding available options, such as counseling to assist in making changes in their lives, as well as community agencies that can be helpful. Once contact is made and an abusive situation is identified, it is important for the APN to be involved and available so that intervention can be implemented at the client's request.

WORKING WITH FAMILIES/CAREGIVERS

Working with families/caregivers who are the abusers is important in order to break the cycle of abusive behaviors. Caregivers may be under tremendous stress and overburdened with care responsibilities for a dependent family member. Referral to a psychotherapist may be helpful to assist in allowing the family members to work out their problems, individually or as a group. Additional referrals to home-care agencies that can provide training in caregiving, as well as information on aging, stress, anger management, and resources, would be helpful to caregivers.

Information that may also be beneficial to families/caregivers includes names/locations of support groups, adaptive devices to help with care in the home, and incontinence products. Psychotherapist referrals for caregivers/clients may be helpful, especially in working out family issues. Other agencies helpful to families/caregivers include adult protective agencies and long-term care ombudsmen, Medicaid fraud units, area agencies on aging, mental health services, and financial/legal services.

SETTING-SPECIFIC ISSUES

Institutions

The symptoms of physical, emotional, and sexual abuse and neglect are similar, regardless of care setting.

Recent research focuses on the care provider in nursing homes, homes for the aged, and home-care agencies. Despite their presence on the front line—providing physical and psychosocial care to the vulnerable, dependent elderly—care providers are predominantly assistants or aides with minimal training/education around elder-care issues. Care is often provided under stressful working conditions, such as staff shortages, inadequate direct supervision, or scarcity of resources. The caregiver may also be the target of abuse from the client and his or her visiting family.

Studies have attempted to identify why some paid caregivers are abusive and others in similar situations are not. Pillemer and Moore (1989) found that workers who had low job satisfaction and their own stresses were more likely to abuse clients and treat them like children.

Although elder abuse does occur in institutions, there are safeguards in place to prevent or detect it rapidly. Institutions have to maintain licensure to care for the elderly. An accusation/incident of abuse requires a full investigation by state authorities. Administrators in institutions readily replace abusive workers. Proactively, administrators should focus on creating resources to support the caregiver. Importantly, the caregiver needs education and training in recognizing the types of abuse, as well as ways to deal with the abusive behavior of the client.

Caregivers also need to know that if problems occur, they will be able to state those problems and feel that they are being heard. It is when the caregiver feels unsupported and in trouble that the abu-sive behavior becomes a reality. Additional acknowledgment and rewarding of competent caregivers is important. Staff might profit from a break room to which they can go if pressure mounts. Support groups for staff and easy access to administration can help to deal effectively with the issues of client care.

CASE STUDY #1

Mr. Carmen is an 85-year-old, Spanish/English-speaking male, who was found by the police, wandering outside in the snow at 9 P.M. on a cold January night. He was dressed in jeans and a thin jacket, but was not wearing underwear, socks, or shoes. Mr. Carmen was cooperative but could not provide data as to why and how he was found in a nearby town.

He was admitted to the emergency room for evaluation. His Mini-Mental State Exam, in English and Spanish, was 10/30. He was disorganized and incoherent at times. Medically, he was found to be dehydrated and malnourished, as well as anemic. He had severe frostbite on the toes of his left foot. He was admitted to the geriatric service for a full assessment.

Attempts were made to reach his next of kin by phone and registered letter. No one was found. After a 2-week search, the police department notified the hospital that a missing person's report had been filed. They referred the person filing the report to the hospital. A woman who identified herself as Rosa, a friend, came to see Mr. Carmen. She stated that she took care of Mr. Carmen, but she had gone away for 2 weeks, leaving him on his own. She requested the keys to his apartment, as well as authorization to go into the apartment. She stated that she would cash Mr. Carmen's checks and buy food for him.

The team reviewed this case, and a psychiatric diagnosis of vascular dementia with delusions was made. A computed tomography (CT) scan of the head supported this diagnosis. The team did not allow Mr. Carmen to give up his keys or sign an authorization. Because of his cognitive limitations, the team elected to file for conservatorship of person and estate. Nursing home placement was found in a dementia unit, where both staff and clients spoke English and Spanish.

QUESTIONS

1. What types of suspected abuse and/or neglect can be identified in this case?
2. Would Mr. Carmen be at risk if discharged back into the community?

ANSWERS

1. Physical abuse/neglect would be suspected, due to Mr. Carmen's poor health and medical problems that need attention. Financial abuse/neglect is also a possibility, due to the friend's check cashing and buying only food. When in the community, Rosa infrequently followed up with him to determine if he could obtain food because of his decreased access to a store and/or a decreased ability to communicate?

2. He is at increased risk for physical neglect and financial abuse, unless the situation changes.

 ## CASE STUDY #2

Mrs. Kendall is a 72-year-old female who lives at home with her 76-year-old husband. She was admitted to the emergency room (ER) and then to the geriatric unit for evaluation and workup for dementia. The visiting nurse had found the patient wandering about the house, wearing only a T-shirt. She was smoking a cigarette while wandering in the kitchen, and her facial expression was "blank." There were cigarette butts and ashes all over the kitchen and living room floors. Per the visiting nurse, Mrs. Kendall has become progressively more confused and disorganized over the past 2 weeks. She has been increasingly assaultive and aggressive, biting and hitting her husband, who is her primary caregiver. The nurse reports a significant decrease in appetite, sleep, and ADL abilities, to the point of minimal functioning. These symptoms represent a significant decline from her baseline cognitive and functional status over the past 5 days.

Mr. Kendall returned home about one-half hour after the nurse arrived. Mrs. Kendall's internist had prescribed lorazepam (Ativan) 0.25 mg tid to decrease restlessness and agitation. Mr. Kendall has given his wife three to five pills per day due to her restlessness. He does not believe in spending money for "junk drugs." He believed that the prescribed dosage of Ativan did not help, so he increased it.

The nurse spent approximately 30 minutes with Mr. Kendall in an attempt to get him to allow his wife to be transferred to the ER for evaluation by her internist. He has refused to permit help in the home to assist with Mrs. Kendall's care or home management. He became angry and threatened to kill everyone if anyone attempted to touch his wife. The nurse called the local police and ambulance to assist with transporting Mrs. Kendall to the ER. She was admitted to the geriatric service for evaluation.

Mr. Kendall constantly begged to take his wife home, stating "I'm a good man. I can't live without mommy. Please let me take her home." Much time was spent in supportive counseling of Mr. Kendall, explaining his wife's illness and her present needs. It was determined that Mr. Kendall needed more follow-up and support around his own memory problems and accepting his wife's hospitalization. The Kendalls have one

daughter, who has refused to become involved in her parents' problems. The daughter reports that Mr. Kendall refuses company and will not allow visitors in the home.

Discussion at a multidisciplinary team meeting included a plan to place Mrs. Kendall in a nursing home. Because of her dementing process, she needed a structured, safe environment. Her husband refused to allow placement, but he did agree to 24-hour supervised care in the home with the help of outside supports. A referral was made to the visiting nurse for ongoing support and evaluation in the home. Upon discharge, a referral was made to protective services in the town where the Kendalls reside. A referral was made for Mr. Kendall to be evaluated by his internist.

QUESTIONS

1. What are the risk factors for potential abuse in this situation?
2. Identify the abuse, or potential abuse, situations.

ANSWERS

1. The risk factors include Mrs. Kendall's dementia and her dependency on her husband. Mr. Kendall has difficulty caring for his wife but is unable/unwilling to allow help.

2. Potential abuse situation: physical neglect and abuse, emotional neglect.

■ REFERENCES

Aravanis, S. C., Adelman, R. D., Breckman, R., et al. (1994). Diagnostic and treatment guidelines on elder abuse and neglect. American Medical Association: Sec. 94-677.

Bourland, M. D. (1990). Elder abuse from definition to prevention. *Postgrad Med, 87*(3), 139–44.

Brickman, R. S., & Adelman, R. D. (1988). *Strategies for helping victims of elder mistreatment.* London: Sage Press.

Erickson, E. H. (1963). *Childhood and society* (2nd ed.). New York: Norton Press.

Fulmer, T., & O'Malley, T. A. (1987). *Inadequate care of the elderly: A health care prespective on abuse and neglect.* New York: Springer.

Kosberg, J. I. (1988). Preventing elder abuse. Identification of high risk factors prior to placement decisions. *Gerontologist, 28,* 43–50.

Pillemer, K., & Moore, D. (1989). Abuse of patients in nursing homes: Findings from a survey of staff. *Gerontologist, 29,* 314–320.

Ramsey-Klowsnik, H. (1991). Elder sexual abuse. Preliminary findings. *J Elder Abuse and Neglect, 3,* 73–90.

Sengstock, M. C., & Steiner, S. C. (1996). Assessing non-physical abuse. In Baumhover, L. A., & Beal, S. C. (Eds.). *Abuse, neglect and exploitation of older persons: Strategies for assessment and intervention.* Baltimore: Health Professionals Press.

18

ETHICAL ISSUES

Leslie Walker • Terrie Wetle

■ INTRODUCTION

Advanced practice gerontologic nurses are presented with a range of ethical challenges in caring for older adults across the health-care continuum. The primary nurse on the caregiving team frequently has an opportunity to become most familiar with the client. The nurse–client relationship engenders a sense of mutual trust, placing the nurse squarely on the front line of interaction between the client and the health-care system. The transmission of information to clients and families is a central role for a primary nurse, who assists clients and surrogates in making a variety of decisions regarding medical treatment, living arrangements, and coordination of community-based services. It is important to note that physical and cognitive impairments, ageism, and fragmentation of services may place older adults at increased "ethical risk" in the many decisions surrounding health care, requiring particu-

lar support and attention from the health-care professional (Wetle, 1988).

These substantial responsibilities to clients and to the workplace must be fulfilled in a manner that is consonant with the nurse's own professional ethical values. Ethical concerns may arise in the many varied settings of nursing practice: in community settings, where individual safety and autonomy must be carefully balanced (Agich, 1990; Collopy et al., 1990); in the acute hospital, where the level of patient participation in treatment decisions must be appropriately determined; and in nursing homes, where the right of individual residents must be weighed against those of the broader "community" or residents in the facility (Wetle et al., 1988). This chapter will (1) provide an overview of core ethical concepts relevant to advance practice gerontologic nursing; (2) identify specific practice settings in which ethical dilemmas typically arise for the advanced practice nurse (APN), and (3) apply key principles in each of the respective delivery settings using a case-based approach, with discussion of opportunities and constraints for ethics-based decision making in each setting.

■ CORE ETHICAL CONCEPTS IN GERONTOLOGIC NURSING

A number of fundamental ethical principles may be drawn upon to establish a framework for providing ethically appropriate nursing care. This section will define core principles of bioethics and discuss how each concept relates to the practice of gerontologic nursing (Beauchamp & Childress, 1989). Patient-based principles include autonomy, decisional capacity, substituted judgment, and best-interest standards. Ethical principles most relevant to health-care professionals include beneficence, nonmaleficence, and paternalism. Responsibilities for advance care planning are also discussed.

PATIENT-BASED PRINCIPLES

Autonomy
The principle of self-determination is a central tenet for many societal and individual values espoused in Western cultures. With respect to health care, this value is expressed in a strong commitment and respect for the notion of client autonomy. Autonomy refers to the right of the individual to hold views, make decisions, and take voluntary actions based on personal preferences and beliefs. This principle also serves as the basis for the legal requirement of informed consent to treatment. Informed consent is a formal process by which an individual capable of making decisions is provided information about his or her medical condition, treatment alternatives, and the risks and benefits of each course of action, in order to allow the client to freely give permission for or refuse medical treatment.

It is critical to note that individual autonomy may be expressed at two distinct levels: agency (the freedom to decide among all options) and action (the freedom to carry out the course of action chosen) (Gadow, 1980). In an ideal world, clients would be provided all information required to execute a fully informed choice among all possible options. In reality, however, there are a number of confounding factors that may preclude the client's actually executing an independent action. The notion of a "web of influence" has been described by Agich (1990). The strands of this web include financial and caregiver resources, health-care delivery system factors, and individual preferences and competencies. The older adult may be excluded from the decision-making process because of assumptions (correct or not) about his or her ability to meaningfully participate in such decisions.

Direct Versus Delegated Autonomy. Autonomy has also been further delineated by Collopy (1988). The distinction with the most important implications for practice is the concept of direct versus delegated autonomy. Direct autonomy refers to decisions and actions made and expressed by the individual. Delegated autonomy occurs when the individual chooses to assign decision-making authority to a surrogate or proxy. The client's preference for direct or delegated autonomy determines which individual will receive relevant information and make decisions. Honoring a preference for delegated autonomy may be difficult for the nurse, who must consider and balance the client's right to be informed with his or her expressed desire to have such decisions made by someone else.

Competent Versus Incapacitated Autonomy. Competent versus incapacitated autonomy focuses on the decisional capacity (ability or competence to make decisions) of the individual, an area in which there has been a growing interest in recent years. Both legal and medical systems make an assumption that each client is competent to participate in treatment decisions until otherwise determined. It is important to note that "incompetence" is a legal designation, which should be used only upon formal determination by a court. In the majority of circumstances, the nurse is concerned with the client's cognitive and emotional capacity to understand and appreciate the nature and potential consequences of a health-care decision, and therefore to participate in decision making and to provide meaningful informed consent.

Despite substantial effort to develop accurate, reliable, statistically validated instruments to assess capacity, the complex nature of capacity may impede accurate assessment (Janofsky et al., 1992; Silberfeld et al., 1993). The element of capacity that complicates evaluation is that capacity is rarely absolute and, in fact, is decision-specific, meaning that different levels of capacity are required, depending on the potential consequences of the decision. Therefore, capacity should be evaluated by a "sliding scale" approach (Schwartz & Blank, 1986). In addition, capacity often fluctuates over time, even over the course of a day, rendering an "absolute" determination of capacity impossible for some individual clients (Appelbaum & Grisso, 1988; Drano, 1985; Kapp & Mossman, 1996; Lo, 1990; McCullough, 1984).

Other Dimensions of Autonomy. There are three other dimensions of autonomy described by Collopy (1988). Authentic versus inauthentic autonomy is a differentiation that requires exploration of whether the individual's stated preference is consistent with his or her broader personal values and health beliefs. Immediate versus long-term autonomy acknowledges that decisions made in the present have the potential to have an impact on expression of autonomous wishes in future circumstances. Finally, Collopy distinguishes between autonomy as a negative versus a positive right. Conceptualized as a negative right, autonomy demands freedom from unwanted or inappropriate interference. Viewed as a positive right, an individual's autonomous action reflects the effective support of both caregivers and systems and results in identification and enhancement of choices.

Issues of autonomy are especially complex when caring for older persons who may have a compromised ability to express autonomous preferences. Further, active involvement of multiple family members as surrogates may challenge the nurse to facilitate discussion among interested parties in order to ensure representation of the client's autonomous wishes in the process.

Substituted Judgment

For those who are so impaired as to be unable to participate in treatment decisions, a hierarchy of standards should be used in the decision process. Most preferable are advance directives, provided by the individual while capable, which declare preferences regarding future medical treatment. Advance directives include both instructional directives (informal letters or written statements, or legal documents such as living wills that explicitly describe treatment wishes) and proxy directives (appointments of surrogate decision makers).

Because only 10% to 25% of the adult population report having completed an advance directive (Teno et al., 1994; Elpern et al., 1993), the health-care team most often relies on family, friends, or other caregivers to provide information regarding the older adult's past statements or behaviors that might indicate what his or her preferences would be in the current circumstances. This history of the client's prior expressed preferences, values, and life style when competent is then used to make a substituted judgment regarding the appropriate course of action to take currently. Substituted judgment requires the surrogate decision maker to draw upon clear evidence of what the client would have wanted in these circumstances were he or she still able to make decisions.

Best Interest

In the absence of clear evidence of an incompetent older adult's previous desires, surrogate decision makers should be guided by what is in the client's best interest. The principle of best interest seeks treatment choices that maximize potential benefit while minimizing burdens and risks of treatment. Best-interest decisions are not as desirable as substituted judgments from an ethics perspective because they disregard individual au-

tonomy and are subject to disagreement regarding the "true" best interest of the client. In some cases, the appointment of a guardian to participate in treatment decisions on behalf of the incapacitated individual may be necessary when a surrogate has not been previously identified. Advanced practice nurses who are assisting surrogate decision makers can be helpful by distinguishing between substituted judgment and best interest and urging decisions based on the former if possible: "Did you and your mother ever discuss what she would want done in these circumstances?" as compared to "What do *you* think is the best for your mother?"

APN-BASED CONSIDERATIONS

Beneficence and Nonmaleficence

In addition to the ethical principles closely associated with client rights and responsibilities, there are additional ethical concepts that guide the health-care professional's actions and accordingly affect individual client autonomy. Beneficence, a primary human value, involves acts that do good for others or promote their welfare. Just as the notion of autonomy supports individual rights in health care, the principle of beneficence is central to codes of ethics in the helping professions. Related to beneficence is the concept of nonmaleficence, an obligation to do no harm. This notion is embodied in the direction of the Hippocratic oath to "first, do no harm" and requires the health professional to carefully assess all risks of an intervention. These concepts are reflected in the American Nurses Association's *Code for*

Nurses (1976), which states: "The nurse's primary commitment is to the client's care and safety."

Duties to beneficence may be complicated by acts that are paternalistic in nature. Paternalism involves one or more individuals making decisions on behalf of the client. Two distinct types of paternalism have been defined, each with very different ethical implications. The first, "weak" paternalism, refers to making decisions for another who is unable to make decisions for him- or herself due to cognitive impairment or mental illness (Thomasma, 1983; Perry & Applegate, 1985). Acts of this nature may be ethically justified by the principles of beneficence and the honoring of the client's wishes in accordance with the decision-making hierarchy previously described. The second type, "strong" paternalism, refers to the usurping of decision making from an individual who *is* capable of making decisions, and this type of paternalism is rarely justified from an ethical perspective.

RESPONSIBILITIES FOR ADVANCE CARE PLANNING

The promotion of patient self-determination in medical decision making has received considerable attention over the past decade, particularly as it relates to end-of-life care. This interest has been expressed at the federal level by the passage of the Patient Self-Determination Act (PSDA) of 1990 and at the state level by substantial statutory and case law supporting the use of advance directives (Cantor, 1993). The PSDA is a social policy that creates an obligation for health-care providers to address issues of end-of-life decision making with clients,

emphasizing the client's right to self-determination in making treatment decisions. The PSDA reflects a heightened awareness by Congress of the need to recognize individual rights and preferences in the provision of health care in institutional environments and to enhance client autonomy in medical decision making. The law mandates that, effective December 1, 1991, residents of nursing homes and other health-care facilities must be informed in writing of their existing rights under state law to make health-care decisions, as well as their option to execute advance directives. The law also requires health-care facilities receiving Medicare and Medicaid reimbursement to prepare policies that allow individuals to exercise these rights, and to document in the client's medical record whether the individual has a formal advance directive. Finally, the PSDA requires that providers train their staff and educate the community about advance directives (Omnibus Budget Reconciliation Act [OBRA], 1990).

Efforts to provide meaningful enhancement of client self-determination generally, and the use of advance directives specifically, require accurate assessment of the individual's capacity to participate in discussions of this nature. However, in addition to the challenges noted earlier, both methodologic and procedural difficulties in assessing the capacity of individuals to participate in formulation of advance directives persist (Bradley et al., 1997; Kapp & Mossman, 1996; Lo, 1990; Mezey et al., 1994; Silberfeld et al., 1993; Walker & Blechner, 1995). Although there are numerous validated quantitative scales for determining cognitive function, the development of instruments that assess decisional capacities to participate in discussions around advance care planning has just begun (Mezey et al., Folstein et al., 1975; Pfeiffer, 1975; Kahn et al., 1960).

Procedural impediments to thoughtful determinations about individual abilities to engage in advance care planning derive from the nature of typical encounters with health-care delivery systems (Walker & Blechner, 1995; Mezey et al., 1994). In most cases, admission to a hospital or nursing home is an interaction crowded with bureaucratic procedures involving financial, logistic, and medical issues. Moreover, this may often be a period marked by fear and anxiety. The procedures involving the PSDA may be conducted by a clerical staff person, such as an admitting clerk, who may not be skilled at providing information about or discussing advance directives.

▪ SETTING-SPECIFIC ISSUES

In this section, key concepts will be explored in vignettes that illustrate ethical issues in a variety of settings.

HOME-BASED SERVICES

vignette

Mrs. Brown is an 83-year-old widow with a history of hypertension, diabetes, and a hip fracture 2 years previously. She is housebound due to limited mobility, and her visiting nurse has observed weight loss and failure to take medications as prescribed. The visiting nurse has also noted that Mrs. Brown seems less cheerful and interactive, and she suspects that

Mrs. Brown is skipping meals. The house is in disarray, and the refrigerator contents frequently include spoiled items and food not recommended for Mrs. Brown's diabetic diet. Although Mrs. Brown lives alone, her daughter drops in to shop and run errands.

The visiting nurse is concerned with the apparent worsening of Mrs. Brown's condition and discusses an alternative living arrangement. Mrs. Brown refuses, indicating that she is jut fine where she is. The daughter agrees, saying that her mother spent 2 months in a nursing home, rehabilitating from her broken hip, and "it almost killed her . . . I promised her I would never put her in a place like that again."

Evaluating Risk and Client Preference

Several ethical considerations come into play in the delivery of home care to older adults. Certainly, respect for the individual's autonomous decisions and preferences is a key factor. In this case, Mrs. Brown has made a clear statement as to her preference to stay at home, and this preference is supported by a family caregiver. However, another consideration in this case is beneficence, as expressed by a professional obligation to protect the client's safety. Moreover, an argument could be made that balances the potential for long-term autonomy (restoring the client's health and optimum function) against short-term autonomy (respecting the client's expressed preference to stay at home). It is also possible that an acute health condition may be clouding the client's cognitive function and causing excess disability. For Mrs. Brown, careful attention to assessment for depression, as well as attention to diet and medication management, may restore her to prior levels of better function. Such an intervention may require encouraging Mrs. Brown to submit to additional evaluation and treatment, and may necessitate enlisting the aid of family members to implement the plan.

Role of Family Members

Also of ethical relevance is the nature and scope of family involvement in home care. Dilemmas arise when interests of individual family members conflict. For example, the desire of a hospitalized older adult to be discharged to her daughter's home may conflict with the preferences and interests of the daughter or her spouse. Changing dependency relationships also challenge accustomed family relationships and "ways of doing family business." When there are unclear or inconsistent views about responsibilities of one generation to another, feelings of guilt or abandonment may result. Confusion regarding intergenerational expectations exists at both the public and the family level. Such confusion may cause resentment or anger and may raise problems in arranging care in the community that involves integration of formal and informal supports.

Individual Autonomy Versus Safety

Safety is a major concern in home-based care of frail or cognitively impaired older persons. Evaluation of risk is subjective and inextricably linked to the individual client. Research has shown that factors beyond the facts of the individual case have strong influences on the decisions of case managers and home-care nurses regarding whether the older adult should remain at home (Clemens & Hayes, 1997). These factors include how well the nurse or other case manager knows the client, the social class/status of the client, and the nature of family relationships surrounding the client. Although protection of clients is certainly an important aspect of home-based care, safety is frequently used as a "trump card" to inappropriately override autonomous decisions of older clients. These issues require careful thinking, clear communication, and effort to disentangle the intertwined aspects of complex cases.

ACUTE HOSPITAL SETTINGS

.... *vignette* ....

Mr. Ramsey is an 87-year-old man who was admitted emergently to the hospital. He has a history of an aortic aneurysm (found by ultrasound) and is complaining of severe and increasing abdominal pain. There is no underlying disease. Mr. Ramsey has severe dementia, which impacts on his decisional capacity to participate in the treatment decision at hand. His wife is fully competent and has not left Mr. Ramsey's side since the admission. The health-care team explains to Mrs. Ramsey that the aneurysm has enlarged significantly and is at risk of dissecting unless a surgical repair is made. Mrs. Ramsey is advised that the surgery is a highly invasive and risky procedure for a patient in Mr. Ramsey's condition, but that if he survives the surgery he could be expected to recover with a several-month stay in the rehab unit of a nearby nursing home. She is also informed that not repairing the aorta has a high risk of morbidity and mortality. Mrs. Ramsey adamantly refuses the surgery, claiming that she and her husband have always promised each other never to allow the other to be sent to a nursing home.

Concerned about the possibility that this single factor may be disproportionately influencing Mrs. Ramsey from fully considering the risks and benefits of the procedure, the team meets with the son and daughter. Mrs. Ramsey has developed the strongest rapport with Ms. Sanders, the charge nurse, who emerges as the key facilitator in the discussions with the family. Ms. Sanders inquires at length about Mr. Ramsey's prior statements about living in a nursing home, and asks whether the family believe his convictions would hold even if it were planned as a temporary stay in a subacute rehab unit. The son thought that his father might have been open to such an arrangement; however, the daughter and wife maintained their position that this action would be in direct conflict with Mr. Ramsey's heartfelt wishes. As there is no written advance directive, the wife is asked to make a substituted judgment based on evidence of her husband's prior wishes, and decides to refuse the procedure. The nurse speaks to the son and daughter in order to ensure that they understand the consequences of their decision. The team is conflicted, as they are unsure about the clarity and relevance of the evidence of Mr. Ramsey's prior wishes. The family ultimately agrees to the surgery and consents to a short rehabilitative nursing home stay, in keeping with Mr. Ramsey's wishes.

Surrogate Decision Making

This case illustrates a number of the difficult ethical considerations that may arise during the course of an acute hospitalization. Perhaps the most central concern is

the balancing of individual autonomy with the health-care team's beneficent, but conflicting, interests. The fact that Mr. Ramsey had no formal advance directive is actually quite common. When the client is unable to participate in decision making, in the absence of formal documentation of treatment wishes or a health-care proxy, the health-care team proceeds in accordance with a surrogate decision maker hierarchy. In this case, the nurse and physician consulted Mrs. Ramsey immediately to inform her of her husband's condition and treatment options. The health-care team was uncomfortable, believing that the family did not truly understand the prognosis; nor were Mr. Ramsey's prior feelings about nursing home placement clear.

Effective Communication of Risks and Benefits

Ms. Sanders acted as the liaison between the family and the team, communicating both the family's concerns and the team's position about the possibility of successful treatment. The issue of what constitutes clear and convincing evidence is a highly complex one; both the health professionals and the surrogate have essential perspectives. The health professional must ensure that all pertinent information regarding the decision is presented clearly to the surrogate so that prior expressions of preferences may be appropriately interpreted in the context of the decision at hand.

NURSING HOMES

······· *vignette* ·······

Mrs. Thomas is an 82-year-old widow with four children. She has been a resident of a nursing home for almost 1 year, having lived with her oldest daughter for 4 years prior. Mrs. Thomas had moderate cognitive impairment, poor vision, and a weak gait. Although she has a walker, she rarely uses it. She has fallen twice in the past month but has had no injuries. The facility's director of nursing developed and implemented the facility's restraint-free policy over 2 years ago, which calls for extensive documentation in those cases in which a physical restraint is deemed necessary. Mrs. Thomas has become occasionally combative, having struck Mr. White, another resident, while trying to pass him in the hall. Mr. White's son is insisting that Mrs. Thomas be prevented from hitting his father again and demands a conference with facility administration. He insists that the facility promise that his father will not be hit again and, in the absence of such assurance, states he will remove his father from the nursing home and file a complaint with the health department.

Balancing Individual and Communal Rights and Responsibilities

This case illustrates several key ethical considerations that may arise in communal living environments such as nursing homes. Perhaps most obvious is the balancing of individual residents' rights with the rights of the others living in the facility. Both Mrs. Thomas and Mr. White have a right, pursuant to federal and state regulations, to "the highest practicable physical, mental and psychosocial well-being" (OBRA, 1987, 1990). Neither Mrs. Thomas nor her daughter are concerned about the potential injury associated with a fall and have acknowledged this risk as a "cost" of Mrs. Thomas' living without a physical restraint. Yet Mr.

White has an equally explicit right to safety in his home. The question as to how to balance these two sets of rights is difficult: When does the encroachment on the rights of one resident justify constraints on another? That is, what is a fair distribution of benefits and costs? Creative caregivers might approach this particular case with alternatives in mind, applying the concepts of individualized care in order to identify strategies to address Mrs. Thomas' aggressive behavior without using restraints. In applying the conceptualization of autonomy as a positive right, the caregivers would seek all possible means to enhance Mrs. Thomas' quality of life through the protection of her autonomy. However, Mr. White's privacy must be equally valued, requiring a just course of action that allocates benefits and burdens fairly. This negotiation is perhaps among the most challenging in the nursing home setting. Finally, it should be observed that the staff have conflicting reactions toward Mr. White's family, which the nurse is quite likely to be involved in mediating. The importance of appropriate supportive mechanisms for exploration and discussion of ethical dilemmas in this setting has been noted (Walker & Blechner, 1995; Mezey et al., 1994).

It is generally recognized that older adults in nursing homes are at demonstrably increased risk for inappropriate treatment and inadequate decision-making processes. Nursing home residents in particular are at increased risk for being inappropriately excluded from healthcare decisions (Bradley et al., 1997; Wetle et al., 1988). The very nature of nursing homes may reinforce negative feelings of dependence and encourage learned helplessness. Moreover, the limited involvement of physicians in institutional care makes it unlikely that the client and physician will have the opportunity to develop a trusting relationship (Besdine, 1983; Wetle, 1988). Older persons are especially vulnerable to being left out of discussions due to frailty, advanced age, prevalence of dementia, and biased practice patterns.

Defining Justice in Congregate Settings

The concept of justice is also relevant to issues of autonomy in congregate settings. Just distribution of liberty maximizes freedom among all individuals, while also ensuring that the least advantaged benefit most. While individual residents in nursing homes are clearly entitled to both liberty and privacy, these rights must be balanced continuallly with the responsibilities and rights of the community.

MANAGED-CARE ENVIRONMENTS

vignette

Miss Green is a 79-year-old retired school teacher who suffered a stroke while gardening. After a short hospitalization, she was briefly sent to a nursing home and then to her home with a limited number of home health visits for rehabilitation. The visiting nurse is concerned that Miss Green would benefit from more rehabilitation visits, but the health maintenance organization (HMO) case manager cites company policy that sets guidelines for the number of such visits.

Representing Patient Interests

Managed-care environments provide special opportunities as well as concerns for nurses caring for older persons. Opportunities for improved geriatric care arise from centralized records, abilities to share information and coordinate care across the full range of providers, and, in some cases, access to services not usually covered in the fee-for-service system. In some cases, HMOs and other managed-care organizations have expanded on information sharing with older clients, improved management of medications across providers, and widened the availability of preventive health interventions. However, some managed-care organizations have achieved efficiencies by limiting access to certain types of care.

In the case presented above, the nurse is caught between the conflicting values of beneficence and best interest on one side and the rules and guidelines governing the provision of care in this organization on the other. This circumstance could be framed as a justice argument, in that the managed-care organization is making an effort to efficiently provide care to a *population* of clients, whereas the nurse in this case is primarily concerned with the well-being of an individual client. The most appropriate course of action in a circumstance such as this is for the nurse: (1) to use existing practice guidelines and the community standard on state-of-the-art care to make an argument for the client's well-being, and (2) to fully understand and use the rules of the organization to the advantage of the client. The questions of measurement of quality of care in such settings, as well as the most appropriate practice guidelines, are still being debated.

■ CONCLUSIONS

As key members of the health-care team, nurses have a compelling ethical obligation to act in the best interests of those who are entrusted to their care. In addition, nurses are bound by their professional code of ethics to both protect clients and advocate for enhancement of their autonomy. These complex, interrelated obligations require the careful balancing of burdens and benefits of interventions. Considerations should be based on knowledge of best-practice concepts and careful assessment of the long-term implications of actions.

Nurses have a particularly important role in decisions regarding care of older adults, particularly those who are frail and of diminished capacity to participate in treatment decisions. The nurse frequently has the opportunity through care contacts to establish a closer relationship with the client and family than may other members of the care team. Consequently, the nurse may be entrusted with information and have the ability to make observations not available to other members of the team. Elements of trust and availability may place the nurse in the key position of "translating" communications: (1) between family members and the client, and (2) from the client and family members to the physician and other members of the care team. A clear understanding of the ethical issues and values associated with caring for this population will serve the nurse well and improve quality of care to older clients.

■ KEY CONCEPTS

- Autonomy (the right of an individual to make decisions for oneself) is a fundamental ethical premise in health care.
- Older people are at increased ethical risk for a number of reasons, including ageism, physical and cognitive impairments, and fragmentation of services.
- Nurses must balance the client's right to autonomy with professional obligations of beneficence and nonmaleficence.
- Structures and formal mechanisms (such as resources, ethics committees, education and training programs) support nurses to appropriately address ethical dilemmas they face in providing care across the continuum.
- There are external and system influences that affect individual autonomy (financing, gaps in continuum).

■ WHERE TO GO FOR FURTHER INFORMATION

American Bar Association
Commission on Legal Problems of
  Elderly
1800 M Street NW
Washington, DC 20036

Midwest Bioethics Center
410 Archibald, Suite 106
Kansas City, MO 64111
(816) 756-2713

National Reference Center for
  Bioethics Literature
Kennedy Institute of Ethics
Georgetown University
Washington, DC 20057
(202) 687-3885

Office of Public Information
The Hastings Center
255 Elm Road
Briarcliff Manor, NY 10510
(914) 762-8500

■ REFERENCES

Agich G. I. (1990). Reassessing autonomy in long-term care. *Hasting Center Report,* November/December, 12–17.

American Nurses Association. (1976). *The code for nurses.* Kansas City, MO: American Nurses Association.

Appelbaum, P. S., & Grisso, T. (1988). Assessing patients' capacities to consent to treatment. *N Engl J Med, 319,* 1635–1638.

Beauchamp, T. L., & Childress, J. F. (1989). *Principles of biomedical ethics* (3rd ed.). New York: Oxford University Press.

Besdine, R. (1983). Decisions to withhold treatment from nursing home residents. *J Am Geriatr Soc, 31*(10), 602–606.

Bradley, E., Walker, L., Blechner, B., & Wetle, T. (1997). Assessing capacity to participate in discussions of advance directives in nursing homes: Findings from a study of the Patient Self Determination Act. *J Am Geriatr Soc, 45,* 79–83.

Cantor, N. (1993). *Advance directives and the pursuit of death with dignity.* Bloomington: Indiana University Press.

Clemens, E., Hayes, H. (1997). Assessing and balancing elder risk, safety and autonomy: Decision making practice of health care professionals. *HHC Svcs Qtly, 16*(2), 3–20.

Collopy, B. J., Dubler, N., Zuckerman, C. (1990). The ethics of home care. Autonomy and accommodation. *Hastings Center Report,* March/April, 1–16.

Collopy, B. (1988). Autonomy in long term care: Some crucial distinctions. *Gerontologist, 28*(Suppl.), 10–17.

Drano, J. F. (1985). The many faces of competency. *Hastings Center Report, 4,* 17–21.

Elpern, E., Yellen, S., & Burton, L. (1993). A preliminary investigation of opinions and behaviors regarding advance directives for medical car. *Am J Crit Care, 2,* 161–167.

Folstein, M., Folstein, S., & McHugh, P. (1975). Mini-mental state: A practical method for grading the cognitive state of patients for the clinician. *J Psych Res, 12,* 189–198.

Gadow, S. (1980). Medicine, ethics, and the elderly. *Gerontologist, 20*(6), 680.

Janofsky, J., McCarthy, R., & Folstein, M. (1992). The Hopkins Competency Assessment Test: A brief method for evaluating patients' capacity to give informed consent. *Hosp Comm Psych, 43,* 132–136.

Kahn, R., Goldfarb, A., Pollack, M., & Peck, A. (1960). Brief objective measures for the determination of mental status in the aged. *Am J Psych, 117,* 326–328.

Kapp, M., & Mossman, D. (1996). Measuring capacity: Cautions on the construction of a "capacimeter." *Psych Pub Pol Law, 2*(1), 73–95.

Lo, B. (1990). Assessing decision-making capacity. *Law, Medicine, & Ethics, 18,* 193–203.

McCullough, L. (1984). Medical care for elderly patients of diminished competency: An ethical analysis. *J Am Geriatr Soc, 32,* 150–153.

Mezey, M., Mitty, E., Ramsey, G. (1997). Assesment of decision-making capacity: Nursing's role. *J Gerontological Nursing, 23(3),* 28–35.

Mezey, M., Ramsey, G., & Mitty, E. (1994). Making the PSDA work for the elderly. *Generations, 18,* 13–18.

Omnibus Budget Reconciliation Act of 1987. P.L. 100-203. Subtitle C. The Nursing Home Reform Act. 42 U.S.C. 1395i-

3(a)–(h) (Medicare); 139r(a)–(h) (Medicaid).

Omnibus Budget Reconciliation Act of 1990. P.L. 101-508, Sections 4206 and 4571 (Medicare and Medicaid, respectively), 42 U.S.C. Section 1395(a)(1)(Q), 1395mm (c)(8), 1395cc(f), 1396a(a)(57),(58), 1396a(w).

Perry, C. B., & Applegate, W. B. (1985). Medical paternalism and patient self determination. *J Am Geriatr Soc, 33*(5), 353–359.

Pfeiffer, E. (1975). A short portable mental status questionnaire for the assessment of organic brain deficit in elderly patients. *J Am Geriatr Soc, 23,* 433–441.

Schwartz, H. I., & Blank, K. (1986). Shifting competency during hospitalization: A model for informed consent decisions. *Hosp Comm Psych, 37,* 1256–1260.

Silberfeld, M., Nash, C., & Singer, S. (1993). Capacity to complete an advance directive. *J Am Geriatr Soc, 41,* 1141–1143.

Teno, J., Lynn, J., & Phillips, R. (1994). Do formal advance directives affect resuscitation decisions and the use of resources for seriously ill patients. *J Clin Ethics, 5,* 23–30.

Thomasma, D. C. (1983). Beyond paternalism and patient autonomy: A model of physician conscience for the physician and patient relationship. *Ann Intern Med, 86,* 243–248.

Walker, L., & Blechner, B. (1995). Ongoing implementation of the Patient Self-Determination Act in nursing homes. *Generations, 12,* 73–77.

Wetle, T. (1988). Ethical issues. In Rowe, J. W., & Besdine, R. W. (Eds.). *Geriatric medicine.* (pp. 75–88). Boston: Little, Brown.

Wetle, T., Levkoff, S., Cwikel, J., & Rosen, A. (1988). Nursing home resident participation in medical decisions: Perceptions and preferences. *Gerontologist, 28,* 32–38.

FOLSTEIN MINI-MENTAL STATE EXAM

One Point for Each Correct Response:	Score	Possible Points
ORIENTATION:		
Day	_____	1
Date	_____	1
Month	_____	1
Year	_____	1
Season	_____	1
Place	_____	1
Floor	_____	1
Town/City	_____	1
State	_____	1
Country	_____	1

REGISTRATION:
Name three objects. Ask the patient to repeat all three objects.

One point for each correct answer.	_____	3

(*Repeat the three objects until the patient can repeat all three; they will be asked for later.)

ATTENTION/CALCULATION:
Serial sevens
($100 - 7 = 93/93 - 7 = 86/86 - 7 =$

$79/79 - 7 = 72/72 - 7 = 65$)—(stop after five answers)
OR
Spell the word "WORLD" backwards
(D-L-R-O-W) _____ 5

RECALL:
Ask the patient to recall the three objects learned above.

One point for each correct answer.	_____	3

LANGUAGE:
Point to two familiar objects (watch and pencil or pen).
Ask the patient to name them as you point.

One point for each correct answer.	_____	2
Have the patient repeat: "No ifs, ands, or buts."	_____	1

Have the patient follow a three-step command: "Take this piece of paper in your right hand.
Fold the paper in half. Place the paper on the floor." _____   3

Have the patient read and obey the following: "CLOSE YOUR EYES." _____   1

(*Write in large letters.)

(*If the patient is illiterate, subtract this point from the total possible score.)

Have the patient write a sentence of his/her choice. _____   1

(*Must have a subject and an object and make sense.)

(*If the patient is illiterate, subtract this point from the total possible score.)

Have the patient copy these intersecting pentagons. _____   1

COPY THESE	DRAW HERE

TOTAL SCORE _____ out of 30

(*Normal score is above 23, unless the total possible score has been adjusted for an illiterate patient.)

INSTRUCTIONS

ORIENTATION

Ask for the date. Then ask specifically for the parts omitted (eg., "Can you also tell me what season it is?"). (1 point for each correct) Ask in turn, "Can you tell me the name of this hospital?" (town, county, etc.). (1 point for each correct)

REGISTRATION

Ask the patient if you may test his/her memory. Then say the names of three unrelated objects, clearly and slowly, about one second for each. After you have said all three, ask him/her to repeat them. This first repetition determines his/her score (0–3), but keep saying them until he/she can repeat all three, up to six trials. If he/she does not eventually learn all three, recall cannot be meaningfully tested.

ATTENTION AND CALCULATION*

Ask the patient to begin with 100 and count backward by 7. Stop after five subtractions (93, 86, 79, 72, 65). Score the total number of correct answers. If the patient cannot or will not perform this task, ask him/her to spell the word "world" backwards.

RECALL

Ask the patient if he/she can recall the three words you previously asked him/her to remember. Score 0–3.

LANGUAGE

Naming
Show the patient a wristwatch and ask him/her what it is. Repeat for a pencil. Score 0–2.

Repetition
Ask the patient to repeat the sentence "No ifs, ands, or buts" after you. Allow only one trial. Score 0 or 1.

Three-stage Command
Give the patient a piece of plain blank paper and repeat the command. Score 1 point for each part correctly executed.

Reading
On a blank piece of paper, print the words "CLOSE YOUR EYES" in letters large enough for the patient to see clearly. Ask him/her to read it and do what it says. Score 1 point only if he/she actually closes his/her eyes.*

Writing
Give the patient a blank piece of paper and ask him/her to write a sentence for you. Do not dictate a sentence. It is to be written spontaneously. It must contain a subject and a verb and be sensible. Correct grammar and punctuation are not necessary.*

Copy
On a clean piece of paper, draw intersecting pentagons, each side about one inch, and ask him/her to copy it exactly as it is. All 10 angles must be present, and two must intersect to form a 4-sided figure to score 1 point. Tremor and rotation are ignored.*

Estimate
Estimate the patient's level of sensorium along a continuum, from alert on the left to coma on the right.

SCORING

Maximum Score	Score	
		Orientation
5	( )	What is the (year) (season) (date) (month)?
5	( )	Where are we: (state) (country) (town) (hospital)?

Maximum Score	Score	
		Registration
3	( )	Name three objects: 1 second each to say. Then ask the patient all three after you have said them. Give 1 point for each correct answer. Then repeat them until he/she learns all three. Count trials and record.
		Attention and Calculation
5	( )	Serial 7s. 1 point for each correct. Stop after five answers. Alternatively, spell "world" backwards. The score is the number of letters in correct order (eg, dlrow = 5, dlorw = 3).
		Recall
3	( )	Ask for three objects repeated

9 ( )

above. Give 1 point for each correct.

Language

Name a pencil and a watch. (2 points) Repeat the following: "No ifs, ands, or buts." (1 point) Follow a three-stage command: "Take a paper in your right hand, fold it in half, and put it on the floor. (3 points) Read and obey the following: "CLOSE YOUR EYES." (1 point) Write a sentence. (1 point) Copy design. (1 point)

Total score _____

Assess level of consciousness along a continuum: (Alert—Drowsy—Stupor—Coma)

*Lack of formal education may invalidate the use of this test. It is important to know the extent of formal education, and the ability to read and write.

Also, a hearing impairment may make the use of the word "world" difficult. Substitution of another familiar five-letter word such as "today" is acceptable. Hearing loss often impairs a persons ability to accurately repeat "no ifs, ands, or buts." If hearing loss is profound, the results of the test are generally unreliable. Similarly, poor eyesight can also invalidate the results of the test.

Source: Folstein, M. F., Folstein, S. E., & McHugh, P. R. (1975). Mini-Mental State: A practical method for grading the cognitive state of patients for the clinician. *J Psychiatr Res, 12,* 189–198, Oxford: Elsevier Science Ltd. Reprinted with permission.

PHYSICAL SELF-MAINTENANCE SCALE

	Score	% Correct	% Error
A. Toilet		66	3.8
1. Cares for self at toilet completely, no incontinence.	1		
2. Needs to be reminded, or needs help in cleaning self, or has rare (weekly at most) accidents.	0		
3. Soiling or wetting while asleep more than once a week.	0		
4. Soiling or wetting while awake more than once a week.	0		
5. No control of bowels or bladder.	0		
B. Feeding		77	3.8
1. Eats without assistance.	1		
2. Eats with minor assistance at meal times and/or with special preparation of food, or help in cleaning up after meals.	0		
3. Feeds self with moderate assistance and is untidy.	0		
4. Requires extensive assistance for all meals.	0		
5. Does not feed self at all and resists efforts of others to feed him.	0		
C. Dressing		56	4.2
1. Dresses, undresses, and selects clothes from own wardrobe.	1		
2. Dresses and undresses self, with minor assistance.	0		
3. Needs moderate assistance in dressing or selection of clothes.	0		
4. Needs major assistance in dressing, but co-operates with efforts of others to help.	0		
5. Completely unable to dress self and resists efforts of others to help.	0		
Rep. ± .96		N ± 265	
D. Grooming (neatness, hair, nails, hands, face, clothing)		42	9.4
1. Always neatly dressed, well-groomed, without assistance.	1		
2. Grooms self adequately with occasional minor assistance, eg, shaving.	0		

PHYSICAL SELF-MAINTENANCE SCALE (CONT.)

	Score	% Correct	% Error
3. Needs moderate and regular assistance or supervision in grooming.	0		
4. Needs total grooming care, but can remain well groomed after help from others.	0		
5. Actively negates all efforts of others to maintain grooming.	0		
E. Physical Ambulation	27	7.9	
1. Goes about grounds or city.	1		
2. Ambulates within residence or about one block distant.	0		
3. Ambulates with assistance of (check one) a ( ) another person, b ( ) railing, c ( ) cane, d ( ) walker, e ( ) wheelchair. 1__Gets in and out without help. 2__Needs help in getting in and out.			
4. Sits unsupported in chair or wheelchair, but cannot propel self without help.	0		
5. Bedridden more than half the time.	0		
F. Bathing		43	4.2
1. Bathes self (tub, shower, sponge bath) without help.	1		
2. Bathes self with help in getting in and out of tub.	0		
3. Washes face and hands only, but cannot bathe rest of body.	0		
4. Does not wash self but is cooperative with those who bathe him.	0		
5. Does not try to wash self and resists efforts to keep him clean.	0		
Rep. = .96		N = 265	

INSTRUMENTAL ACTIVITIES OF DAILY LIVING SCALE

Score	Male % Correct	% Error		Score	Female % Correct	% Error
	64	5.2	A. Ability to use telephone		68	4.8
1			1. Operates telephone on own initiative —looks up and dials numbers, etc.	1		
1			2. Dials a few well-known numbers.	1		
1			3. Answers telephone but does not dial.	1		
0			4. Does not use telephone at all.	0		
	15	5.2	B. Shopping		15	3.0
			1. Takes care of all shoppings needs independently.	1		
0			2. Shops independently for small purchases.	0		
0			3. Needs to be accompanied on any shopping trip.	0		
0			4. Completely unable to shop.	0		
			C. Food preparation		20	2.4
			1. Plans, prepares, and serves adequate meals independently.	1		
			2. Prepares adequate meals if supplied with ingredients.	0		
			3. Heats and serves prepared meals, or prepares meals but does not maitain adequate diet.	0		
			4. Needs to have meals prepared and served.	0		
			D. Housekeeping		51	7.1
			1. Maintains house alone or with occasional assistance (eg, "heavy work–domestic help").			
			2. Performs light daily tasks such as dishwashing, bedmaking.	1		
			3. Performs light daily tasks but cannot maintain acceptable level of cleanliness.	1		
			4. Needs help with all home maintenance tasks.	1		
			5. Does not participate in any housekeeping tasks.	0		

Rep. = .96   N = 97   Rep. = .93   N = 168

INSTRUMENTAL ACTIVITIES OF DAILY LIVING SCALE (CONT.)

Score	Male % Correct	% Error		Score	Female % Correct	% Error
			E. Laundry		41	6.0
			1. Does personal laundry completely.	1		
			2. Launders small items—rinses socks, stockings, etc.	1		
			3. All laundry must be done by others.	0		
	27	4.1	F. Mode of transportation		30	10.0
1			1. Travels independently on public transportation or drives own car.	1		
1			2. Arranges own travel via taxi, but does not otherwise use public transportation.	1		
0			3. Travels on public transportation when assisted or accompanied by another.	1		
0			4. Travel limited to taxi or automobile with assistance of another.	0		
0			5. Does not travel at all.	0		
	35	4.1	G. Responsibility for own medications		38	9.5
1			1. Is responsible for taking medication in correct dosages at correct time.	1		
0			2. Takes responsibility if medication is prepared in advance in separate dosages.	0		
0			3. Is not capable of dispensing own medication.	0		
	54	5.2	H. Ability to handle finances		52	10.0
1			1. Manages financial matters independently (budgets, writes checks, pays rent, bills, goes to bank), collects and keeps track of income.	1		
1			2. Manages day-to-day purchases, but needs help with banking, major purchases, etc.	1		
0			3. Incapable of handling money.	0		

Rep. = .96   N = 97   Rep. = .93   N = 168

Used with permission from Lawton, M. P., and Brody, E. M. (1969). Assessment of older people. *Gerontologist, 9*, 3, 180–181. Copyright © The Gerontological Society of America.

C

GERIATRIC DEPRESSION SCALE

1. Are you basically satisfied with your life? (no)
2. Have you dropped many of your activities and interests? (yes)
3. Do you feel that your life is empty? (yes)
4. Do you often get bored? (yes)
5. Are you hopeful about the future? (no)
6. Are you bothered by thoughts that you just cannot get out of your head? (yes)
7. Are you in good spirits most of the time? (no)
8. Are you afraid that something bad is going to happen to you? (yes)
9. Do you feel happy most of the time? (no)
10. Do you often feel helpless? (yes)
11. Do you often get restless and fidgety? (yes)
12. Do you prefer to stay home rather than go out and do new things? (yes)
13. Do you frequently worry about the future? (yes)
14. Do you feel that you have more problems with memory than most? (yes)
15. Do you think it is wonderful to be alive now? (no)
16. Do you often feel downhearted and blue? (yes)
17. Do you feel pretty worthless the way you are now? (yes)
18. Do you worry a lot about the past? (yes)
19. Do you find life very exciting? (no)
20. Is it hard for you to get started on new projects? (yes)
21. Do you feel full of energy? (no)
22. Do you feel that your situation is hopeless? (yes)
23. Do you think that most persons are better off then you are? (yes)
24. Do you frequently get upset over little things? (yes)
25. Do you frequently feel like crying? (yes)
26. Do you have trouble concentrating? (yes)
27. Do you enjoy getting up in the morning? (no)
28. Do you prefer to avoid social gatherings? (yes)
29. Is it easy for you to make decisions? (no)
30. Is your mind as clear as it used to be? (no)

Score one point for each response that matches the yes or no answer after the question.

Source: Adapted with permission from Yesavage, J. A., & Brink, T. L. (1983). Development and validation of a geriatric depression screening scale: A preliminary report, *J Psychiatr Res, 17,* 41. Copyright © 1983, Pergamon Journals Ltd.

D

MENTAL STATUS ASSESSMENT TOOL

CLINICAL HISTORY

Name:_____/_____
　　　　　　　　Last　　　　　　　　　　　　First
Date:_____/_____/_____　　Time:_____ [AM] [PM]
　　　Mo　　Day　　Yr

Evaluation Site:_____　　**Informant(s)**　**Date(s)**
Examiner(s):_____　　　Patient　　[] _____
　　　　　　　　　　　　　　　　　Spouse　　[] _____
　　　　　　　　　　　　　　　　　Child　　　[] _____
　　　　　　　　　　　　　　　　　Parent　　[] _____
　　　　　　　　　　　　　　　　　Nonrelative　[] _____

1. PROBLEM—Chief complaint. Narrative description (comment on patient insight)
CC:

Date of onset:　When were mental abilities completely normal: _____/_____/_____
　　　　　　　　　　　　　　　　　　　　　　　　　　　　　Mo　　Day　　Yr
Was the change associated with any event?_____

What were the first problems noticed? Briefly describe:
　[] Memory
　[] Speech
　[] Writing
　[] Reasoning
　[] Sense of direction
　[] Use of objects　　　　[] Socializing
　[] Personality　　　　　[] Occupation/Housework
　[] Other:_____

Type of onset:
   [] Abrupt (days)
   [] Gradual (weeks–months)
   [] Very gradual/insidious (years)

Course of symptoms:
   [] Steady decline
   [] Stepwise decline
   [] Fluctuating
   [] Improving
   [] Stable
   [] Other

Percent
Function   50%
Remaining

100%

0%
Onset   Time
(Months/Years)

Pace of change:
   [] Increasing
   [] Decreasing
   [] Constant

When did symptoms begin to interfere with normal/usual activities? _____

What activities were first affected? _____

   No - Yes
   [] - [] Onset and Course: Typical of AD?

2. HISTORY OF PRESENT ILLNESS: Current Function
   No - Yes
   [] - [] ORIENTATION—Temporal—Problem with?
   [] - [] Date
   [] - [] Time of day
   [] - [] Year (season)
   [] - [] Other:

   [] - [] MEMORY—Problem with?
   [] - [] Current events
   [] - [] Day-to-day events
   [] - [] Misplace objects
   [] - [] Dependent on written list
   [] - [] Forget appointments
   [] - [] Problem learning new things
   [] - [] Repeat stories, dwelling in past
   [] - [] Recalling old things
   [] - [] Family events (birthdays, etc.)
   [] - [] Difficulty with names
   [] - [] Confusion regarding alive or dead

   [] - [] THINKING—Difficulty with?
   [] - [] Job duties at work
   [] - [] Financial matters (balancing checkbook, paying bills)

[] - [] Poor judgment/decisions (business, handling money, trusting of strangers)
[] - [] Illogical behavior/actions
[] - [] Change in leisure activities (hobbies, music, games, puzzles, social outings)

[] - [] SPEAKING/READING/WRITING—Problem?
[] - [] Word-finding problem
[] - [] Change in quantity of language output
[] - [] Trouble understanding speech
[] - [] Deterioration in self-expression
[] - [] Trouble reading
[] - [] Deterioration in writing ability

2. HISTORY OF PRESENT ILLNESS: Current Function:
   No - Yes
   [] - [] SENSE OF DIRECTION—Problem?
   [] - [] Loss of direction in community
   [] - [] Disoriented in home
   [] - [] Trouble orienting clothes

   [] - [] DEPRESSIVE SYMPTOMATOLOGY
   [] - [] Depression history
   [] - [] Recently?
   [] - [] Seems depressed (sad, life not worth living, worries, helplessness, etc.)
   [] - [] Worthlessness/guilt
   [] - [] Any discussion of suicide
   [] - [] Frequent somatic complaints (aches, pains, vague symptoms, no apparent explanation)
   [] - [] Sleep disorder
   [] - [] Appetite disturbance

   [] - [] ACTIVITY CHANGES (energy, initiation, attention, inhibition)
   [] - [] Lacks interest—usual activities
   [] - [] Tends to sit unless pushed
   [] - [] Cannot concentrate
   [] - [] Leaves tasks unfinished
   [] - [] Does not initiate purposeful activity

   [] - [] OTHER BEHAVIORS
   [] - [] Paranoid (accuses others of lying or stealing, etc.)
   [] - [] Fearful or nervous (restless, pacing, worries about insignificant matters)
   [] - [] Loss of confidence, defers to others
   [] - [] Irritable (easily enraged, abusive)
   [] - [] Behavior driven (highly energetic, needs little sleep, talks incessantly)
   [] - [] Mood swings (over short period of time)
   [] - [] Emotional incontinence (inappropriate laughing or crying)
   [] - [] Interpersonal behavior is impolite, inappropriate, embarrassing, disinhibited

[] - [] Assaultive, aggressive (physical/verbal attack, breaks things, yells, etc.)

No - Yes Does patient have trouble with

[] - [] Repetitive actions, sorting, pacing, wandering, muttering, hyperkinetic
[] - [] Hallucinations, delusions, personality change, hoarding, other
[] - [] Sexual change
[] - [] Change in pain tolerance
[] - [] Do you have a theory about the cause of these changes (dementia)?
     (Who reports)

PERFORMANCE:	Does/No impairment			Reported by:	[] Self
	Does/Problem				[] Caregiver
		Quit/Unable			[] Other:
			Never Did	Who helps, what services are in place?	
ADL					
Bathing	[]	[]	[]	[]	_____
Dressing	[]	[]	[]	[]	_____
Toileting	[]	[]	[]	[]	_____
Transfers	[]	[]	[]	[]	_____
Continence	[]	[]	[]	[]	_____
Feeding	[]	[]	[]	[]	_____
Grooming	[]	[]	[]	[]	_____
Walking	[]	[]	[]	[]	Past vs. now _____
IADL					
Medicine	[]	[]	[]	[]	_____
Meal prep	[]	[]	[]	[]	_____
Housework	[]	[]	[]	[]	_____
Laundry	[]	[]	[]	[]	_____
Telephone	[]	[]	[]	[]	_____
Money man- agement	[]	[]	[]	[]	_____
Travel	[]	[]	[]	[]	_____
Shopping	[]	[]	[]	[]	_____

No - Yes

[] - [] SAFETY—Concerns/Problems
[] - [] Wandering
[] - [] Kitchen
[] - [] Driving
[] - [] Other:

3. ASSOCIATED CONDITIONS: Is there a history of:

No - Yes Describe:

[] - [] Stroke
[] - [] Transient ischemic attack, other (including amaurosis fugax)
[] - [] Focal neurologic symptoms

[] - [] Hypertension history
[] - [] Ischemic heart disease
[] - [] Valvular heart disease (rheumatic fever, subacute bacterial endocarditis, etc.)
[] - [] Arrhythmia
[] - [] Congestive heart failure
[] - [] Other heart disease
[] - [] High cholesterol or lipids, other:
[] - [] Ever smoke
      Max packs/day_____ Age start_____ Quit_____
[] - [] Problems breathing
[] - [] ETOH: Important contributing factor to cognitive decline?
      - Past life pattern:
      - Record onset, amount, type, DWI, etc.
      - Recent/present intake
      - Record the amount, type, last drink
[] - [] Any withdrawal history (blackouts, shakes, DTs)?
[] - [] Loss of consciousness
[] - [] Seizures
[] - [] Fainting
[] - [] History of coma or cardiac arrest
[] - [] Anesthesia complication (hypotension, postop confusion, other)
[] - [] Head injury (boxing history, concussion)
[] - [] History of meningitis
[] - [] Encephalitis
[] - [] Syphilis
[] - [] Parkinson's disease
      [] Tremor
      [] Walk slow or shuffling
      [] Difficulty arising from bed/chair
      [] Handwriting shaky or small
      [] Other:
[] - [] Huntington's disease
[] - [] Family history of Huntington's disease
[] - [] Headaches
[] - [] Facial numbness or weakness
[] - [] Change/Loss of smell or taste
[] - [] Swallowing difficulty
[] - [] Dizziness, vertigo
[] - [] Walking difficulty/falling
[] - [] Balance problems
[] - [] Weakness
[] - [] Clumsiness/Incoordination
[] - [] Numbness or dysesthesia
[] - [] Visual problems (diplopia, visual fields, etc.)

[] - [] Eyeglasses
[] - [] Glaucoma
[] - [] Cataracts
[] - [] Hearing problems (including tinnitus)
[] - [] Hearing aid
[] - [] AIDS or HIV exposure/risk (see transfusion history)
[] - [] Lyme disease
[] - [] Toxic exposure (chemicals, fumes, etc.)

[] - [] OTHER PSYCHIATRIC HISTORY
    [] Early growth/development
    [] Mental retardation
    [] History of manic depressive illness
    [] Schizophrenia
    [] Any psychiatric treatment
    [] Hospitalization
    [] Electroconvulsive therapy
    [] Outpatient treatment
    [] Other
[] - [] Thyroid disease history
[] - [] Diabetes or hypoglycemia
[] - [] Anemia (pernicious, etc.)
[] - [] Tuberculosis (? skin test)

4. OTHER
  No - Yes: Describe:
  [] - [] Dietary change (adequate?, vitamins)
  [] - [] Weight change   Usual wt:_____, date:_____
  [] - [] Fatigue
  [] - [] Fever, sweats
  [] - [] Skin rashes
  [] - [] Cancer history
  [] - [] Inflammatory disease (lupus, rheumatoid arthritis, etc.)
  [] - [] Abdominal (pain, nausea, vomiting, ulcers, indigestion, stomach problems, jaundice/hepatitis/liver disease, abnormal bowel movements, other)
  [] - [] Genitourinary (trouble urinating, frequency, hesitancy, prostate problems, kidney disease, etc.)
  [] - [] Incontinence of bladder or bowel
      Elaborate:
  [] - [] Vaginal bleeding, spotting, discharge
  [] - [] Lumps in breast, last mammogram:
  [] - [] Any operations
  [] - [] Any transfusions (esp. 1978–1985—HIV)
  [] - [] Any hospitalizations (other)

PRIOR WORKUP for present complaints: Check if DONE
- [] Neurologic examination
- [] Neuropsychiatric examination
- [] Psychiatric examination
- [] Blood tests
- [] X-rays
- [] CT scan of head
- [] EEG
- [] Lumbar puncture
- [] MRI of head
- [] SPECT scan
- [] Other; describe _____

Medications:
No - Yes:
[] - [] Confirmed with bag check?

Potential Offending Agent?

Check	Agent	Dose	Start	Stop
[]	1_____	_____	___/___/___	___/___/___
[]	2_____	_____	___/___/___	___/___/___
[]	3_____	_____	___/___/___	___/___/___
[]	4_____	_____	___/___/___	___/___/___
[]	5_____	_____	___/___/___	___/___/___
[]	6_____	_____	___/___/___	___/___/___
[]	7_____	_____	___/___/___	___/___/___
[]	8_____	_____	___/___/___	___/___/___
[]	9_____	_____	___/___/___	___/___/___
[]	10_____	_____	___/___/___	___/___/___
[]	11_____	_____	___/___/___	___/___/___
[]	12_____	_____	___/___/___	___/___/___
[]	13_____	_____	___/___/___	___/___/___
[]	14_____	_____	___/___/___	___/___/___
[]	15_____	_____	___/___/___	___/___/___
[]	16_____	_____	___/___/___	___/___/___

_____ # How many medications do you think are contributing to the cognitive problems?

Allergies

Agent	Nature of reaction/date, etc.
_____	_____
_____	_____
_____	_____

No - Yes:
[] - [] "Allergy" to iodinated intravenous contrast dye?

5. FAMILY HISTORY:

	Dementia? No - Yes	Age Onset	Alive? No - Yes	Cause of Death
Mother	[ ] - [ ]	_____	[ ] - [ ]	_____
Father	[ ] - [ ]	_____	[ ] - [ ]	_____

Siblings Gender	Dementia? No - Yes	Age Onset	Alive? No - Yes	Health Status/Cause of Death
[M] [F]	[ ] - [ ]	_____	[ ] - [ ]	_____
[M] [F]	[ ] - [ ]	_____	[ ] - [ ]	_____
[M] [F]	[ ] - [ ]	_____	[ ] - [ ]	_____
[M] [F]	[ ] - [ ]	_____	[ ] - [ ]	_____
[M] [F]	[ ] - [ ]	_____	[ ] - [ ]	_____
[M] [F]	[ ] - [ ]	_____	[ ] - [ ]	_____
[M] [F]	[ ] - [ ]	_____	[ ] - [ ]	_____

Children Gender	Dementia? No - Yes	Age Onset	Alive? No - Yes	Health Status/Cause of Death
[M] [F]	[ ] - [ ]	_____	[ ] - [ ]	_____
[M] [F]	[ ] - [ ]	_____	[ ] - [ ]	_____
[M] [F]	[ ] - [ ]	_____	[ ] - [ ]	_____
[M] [F]	[ ] - [ ]	_____	[ ] - [ ]	_____
[M] [F]	[ ] - [ ]	_____	[ ] - [ ]	_____
[M] [F]	[ ] - [ ]	_____	[ ] - [ ]	_____
[M] [F]	[ ] - [ ]	_____	[ ] - [ ]	

                                                          No - Yes

Any other family members with memory
   problems (or became senile)?   [ ] - [ ]
Any inherited diseases?   [ ] - [ ]
Any family history of psychiatric disease?   [ ] - [ ]
Any family history of neurologic disease?   [ ] - [ ]
Any family history of Down syndrome, mongolism, mental retardation, leukemia,
   lymphoma, Hodgkin's, myeloma?
Any significant problems other than already discussed: _____

DELIRIUM ASSESSMENT TOOLS

DIGIT SPAN

Circle maximum number completed correctly, forward and backward.

Digits Forward	Score	Digits Backward	Score
6-4-3-9	4	2-8-3	3
7-2-8-6	4	4-1-5	3
4-2-7-3-1	5	3-2-7-9	4
7-5-8-3-6	5	4-9-6-8	4
6-1-9-4-7-3	6	1-5-2-8-6	5
3-9-2-4-8-7	6	6-1-8-4-3	5

MONTHS OF YEAR

Dec	Nov	Oct	Sep	Aug
Jul	Jun	May	Apr	Mar
Feb	Jan			

DAYS OF WEEK

Sat	Fri	Thu	Wed	Tue
Mon	Sun			

Count backward from 20 to 1.

Add 1 + 3 and keep adding 3 to your answer.

AUDITORY VIGILANCE

Ask patient to tap whenever "A" is heard as you read one per second:

L T P E A O A I C T D A L A A
A N I A B F S A M R Z E O A D

F

QUICKIE NEURO EVALUATION

	Normal/ Intact	Abnormal/ Impaired
Level of Consciousness (awake, alert, aware)		
Mental Status (oriented × 3)		

Cranial Nerves:

I Olfactory
Have patient smell familiar substances
(ie, tobacco, coffee). _____ _____

II Optic
Use Snellen chart, fundoscopic exam, visual
field testing. _____ _____

III Ocolomotor
PERLA = Pupils equal, reactive to light
and accommodate. _____ _____

III Oculomotor ⎫
IV Trochlear ⎬ (EOM. Test as a unit for
VI Abducens ⎭ eye movement.) _____ _____

V Trigeminal
Test sensation on face. Test corneal reflexes. _____ _____

VII Facial
Have patient smile, frown, wrinkle forehead,
hold eyes closed. _____ _____

VII Facial ⎫
IX Glossopharyngeal ⎬ (Test as a unit for taste.)
Have patient taste familiar substances (ie, sugar,
salt, lemon). _____ _____

VIII Auditory/Acoustic
Use audiometer, or whisper test. Test for
lateralization. Test for conduction. _____ _____

X Vagus   _____   _____
   Test gag reflex. Test swallowing.
   Have patient say "ahhhh" to test symmetry of
   vocal cord movement.
XI Accessory   _____   _____
   Have patient shrug shoulders and turn head to
   side against resistance.
XII Hypoglossal   _____   _____
   Have patient stick tongue out.

Muscle Strength: Test muscle groups for strength during flexion/extension/abduc-
           tion/adduction. Grade as follows:

           5 Full strength against resistance
           4 Unable to hold against resis-
              tance
           3 Able to move against gravity
           2 Able to move when gravity is
              eliminated
           1 Contraction of the muscle can
              be palpated
           0 No contraction of the muscle
   Also observe for symmetry of strength.

   Upper Extremities:
       Have patient hold arm in a flexed position.   R____L____
       Have patient hold arm in an extended position. R____L____
       Have patient squeeze your hands tightly.   R____L____

   Lower Extremities:
       Have patient hold leg in an extended position.   R____L____
       Have patient hold leg in a flexed position.   R____L____
       Have patient press his/her feet against your
          hands.   R____L____

Cerebellar Function
       Observe gait   _____   _____
       Coordination   _____   _____
       (Observe finger to nose movements, heel to
       shin movements, rapid alternating movements.)
       Balance   _____   _____
       (Observe tandem walking: heel to toe, shallow
       knee bends, hopping on one foot.)
       Romberg   _____   _____

Sensory Function: Test all body surfaces for the following:
       Superficial pain: Test with pinprick vs. dull touch.

Light touch:	Test with a cotton ball or a soft touch.
Vibration:	Test with a tuning fork against bony prominences.
Stereognosis:	Test for recognition of familiar objects in the hands.
Proprioception:	Test for recognition of the direction of movement of the extremities, fingers, and toes.

Observe for symmetry of sensory recognition.

Hands	R____L____
Upper extremities	R____L____
Chest	R____L____
Back	R____L____
Lower extremities	R____L____
Feet	R____L____
Sacral segments (around the anus)	_____ _____

Skeletal Reflexes: Grade as follows:

Hyperactive/clonus	+ + + +
Brisker than normal	+ + +
Normal/average	+ +
Decreased	+
Absent	0

Biceps	R____L____
Triceps	R____L____
Brachioradialis	R____L____
Abdomen	R____L____
Patella	R____L____
Achilles	R____L____
Plantar	R____L____
Babinski	R____L____
Anal wink	_____

GUIDED CASE STUDIES

GUIDED CASE STUDY #1

Mr. Sinclair is an 83-year-old man who comes to an outpatient geriatric clinic with a complaint of periodic pounding noises in his head that sound like footsteps and are associated with people moving things around in his basement. Police and family members have been called to investigate and have found nothing to substantiate Mr. Sinclair's complaints. His daughter reports a change in her father's behavior, beginning 6 months ago. First, he was reluctant to socialize, and then he began accusing people of stealing things. Within the past 2 weeks, Mr. Sinclair told his daughter that his father and former boss were appearing at the foot of his bed at night. Mr. Sinclair has no prior psychiatric history.

QUESTIONS

1. What is your initial impression of Mr Sinclair's condition? Which features are consistent with dementia? delirium? depression? other psychiatric illness? How will you differentiate? What is your plan?

2. What will you focus on in your history and physical exam? What additional workup will you do?

Sigifnicant findings during the visit include the following:

- History and physical findings: hypertension, orthostasis (40-point systolic drop in blood pressure on standing); diabetes (fasting blood sugar of 182); urinary incontinence, hypothyroidism, hearing and visual impairments
- Meds: NPH (neutral protamine Hagedorn) insulin 70 units SC

qam, regular insulin 30 units SC qam, furosemide (Lasix) 40 mg PO qd, levothyroxine sodium (Synthroid) 0.085 mg PO qam, amitriptyline (Elavil) 50 mg PO qhs, enalapril maleate (Vasotec) 10 mg PO tid

- Labs: blood urea nitrogen (BUN) 45.4 (reference range 17–45), creatinine 2.2 (range 0.8–1.2), sodium 129 (range 135–145), chloride 94 (range 100–108), urinalysis: 3+ bacteria, many white blood cells, 2+ albumin

- Mental status screen: Score of 20/30 on Folstein Mini-Mental State Exam, with deficits noted in orientation, attention, short-term recall, and ability to follow commands

- Computed tomography scan: mild atrophy

3. Based on the above findings, what recommendations would you make as you collaborate with Mr. Sinclair's physician?

4. What will you focus on in follow-up visits?

Mr. Sinclair received antibiotic therapy for his urinary tract infection (UTI), his amitriptyline and furosemide were discontinued, and his blood pressure was brought under better control. He received a hearing evaluation and hearing aid, as well as an ophthalmology consult. Visiting nurses began to assess his ability to draw up and administer insulin independently and to monitor his own blood glucose. The nurse clinical specialist initiated a voiding log and a behavior diary to further assess any ongoing problems. One month later, a follow-up visit revealed improvement in orientation, memory, and concentration. Labwork was within normal limits. Auditory and visual hallucinations had stopped. Urinary incontinence persisted, and additional assessment and interventions were initiated to deal with this problem.

ANSWERS

1. The relatively acute onset of Mr. Sinclair's problems favor an acute versus a chronic process. Auditory and visual hallucinations and paranoia are consistent with delirium, although they may also be present in psychiatric disorders or dementia. The absence of prior psychiatric disorders is notable. The most important intervention at this time is to assess for reversible causes of cognitive impairment.

2. History should focus on acuity of onset of symptoms; fluctuation over time; and the nature of mental status changes, with specific inquiries regarding perceptual disturbances, change in attention span, mood, sleep pattern, and daily activities. A complete medical and psychiatric history should be sought, and all medicines used or recently stopped should be assessed. Any change in level of consciousness should be determined and a formal mental status screen administered.

Physical exam should seek metabolic, cardiac, or neurologic problems and/or signs of occult infection or malignancy. Labwork should include complete blood count with differential, chemistries, BUN, creatinine, liver function tests, folate, B$_{12}$, rapid plasma reagin (RPR), urinalysis, and stool for occult blood.

3. (a) Obtain a urine culture and treat UTI. Follow-up urinalysis 1 week after treatment. Assess for benign prostatic hypertrophy and urinary retention. Perform incontinence assessment and treat or refer as indicated.

    (b) Discontinue Lasix and hydrate. Monitor fluid balance, electrolytes, renal function, and blood sugar.

    (c) Adjust antihypertensive medicines. Be aware of the potential adverse effect of beta blockers, methyldopa, and diuretics on cognitive impairment.

    (d) Assess rationale for amitriptyline use. If possible, taper and discontinue. The high anticholinergic side effects and propensity toward sedation and orthostatic hypotension seen with amitriptyline greatly increase the likelihood of delirium.

    (e) Refer for hearing and vision evaluations and treatment.

    (f) Assess the client's accuracy and ability to draw up and administer his own insulin effectively and manage his own medication regimen (refer for home visit).

    (g) On follow-up visits, reassess mental status, lab values, hallucinations and paranoia, urinary symptoms, evidence of depression, orthostatic blood pressure, and fluid balance. If symptoms do not improve, consider psychiatric referral and/or further medical and neuropsychiatric testing.

GUIDED CASE STUDY #2

Mrs. Moore is an 84-year-old woman with a history of Alzheimer's disease, atrial fibrillation, and hypertension. She lives in assisted housing, has a companion 3 days per week and attends an adult day program 2 days per week. She is independent in all activities of daily living (ADL) but needs some assistance with instrumental activities such as shopping, cooking, and cleaning. She joins in group activities and games at the day center and is described by the staff as "cheerful and quick witted." She takes pride in her talent for ballroom dancing. Her cardiac status is stable.

QUESTIONS

1. What risk factors for delirium does Mrs. Moore possess?

Over the next 3 weeks, Mrs. Moore's physical, cognitive, and behavioral status changes. She is diagnosed with a large right pleural effusion that is tapped (1200 cc), which recurred 8 days later. She is hospitalized for a malignancy workup, which is negative. She is diagnosed with congestive heart failure (CHF) and started on furosemide (Lasix). While in the hospital, she experiences changed behavior and is described as "mean and uncooperative." She spits out food and continuously climbs out of bed. On returning home with a 24-hour companion, she has fluctuating periods of disorientation during which she neither recognizes her niece, a previously well-known family member, nor her home. She exhibits intermittent clouding of consciousness whereby she seems oblivious to the presence of others and does not respond to verbal input. At other times, she speaks jibberish and paces around the room frantically. She has periods during which she is lucid and acts appropriately.

2. What are the possible explanations for Mrs. Moore's change in behavior and cognition?

3. Is her condition consistent with delirium or dementia?

The companion is counseled regarding behavioral strategies, which include reorientation, encouraging ambulation (and dancing if desired), cueing for ADL and providing reassurance during periods of anxiety. After 1 week, the companion's hours are decreased to 8 hours per day. The provision of a safe, supportive, routinized environment eliminated the need for psychoactive medications. Twenty days after hospitalization, Mrs. Moore is able to return to her usual activities at the day program.

4. Why did Mrs. Moore's delirium take so long to clear even after her CHF was treated?

ANSWERS

1. (a) Dementia (preexisting brain impairment or injury)

   (b) Atrial fibrillation and hypertension (may contribute to hypoperfusion, embolism, cerebrovascular impairment)

2. She has had a recent exacerbation of a medical illness (CHF), has been relocated to a strange place (hospital), has had a change in her usual daily routine, has been restricted from her usual coping strategies (movement and socializing), and has been started on a new medicine. These factors, in combination with her preexisting dementia, increase the likelihood and severity of a delirium.

3. The acute onset of the change in function, cognition, and behavior; the

impaired level of consciousness; the fluctuation in cognitive impairment with lucid intervals; the disturbance in thinking and speech; and the disturbances of the sleep/wake cycle, orientation, and memory are all consistent with delirium.

4. Delirium, although acute in onset, is variable in its resolution. It may clear rapidly in response to treatment or it may linger for days, weeks, or occasionally months, especially in older adults with preexisting brain disease.

GUIDED CASE STUDY #3

Mr. Bowen is an 85-year-old white man, committed, against his will, to a psychiatric hospital following a suicide attempt after the death of his wife from a sudden heart attack. Mr. Bowen and his wife had an argument during which he left home in anger. He returned home to find her dead on the kitchen floor. He immediately stabbed himself and was found lying in his kitchen, unconscious and bleeding profusely, by his son who happened to stop by that day. During his hospitalization, Mr. Bowen frequently spoke of his feeling that there was nothing worth living for and of his desire to join his wife. He was maintained on one-to-one observation in a semiprivate room across from the nurses' station for 3 months. He refused to sign a no-suicide contract. Eventually, the one-to-one observation was reduced to 15-minute checks. He remained quiet and seclusive but would attend group activities on the unit. He was allowed to go home on a day pass for the first time 5 months after his admission, although the nursing staff verbalized concern for his safety, as he planned to go home alone for the day. He was found attempting to hang himself in his garage by his son and brought back to the hospital where he was again placed on one-to-one observation for a week, then reduced to 15-minute checks. He was eventually allowed a second pass for Easter Sunday with his children. He returned to the hospital, though his roommate was not scheduled to return until the following day. At 2 o'clock the following morning, during a 15-minute check, Mr. Bowen was found hanging from tightly knotted bed sheets in his room. The sheets were knotted so tightly, it took 20 minutes to cut them off. Three days later, he died in the intensive care unit.

QUESTIONS

1. What feeling prompted Mr. Bowen to attempt suicide?

2. What factors would concern you about his safety if he were allowed home on a pass?

3. What was the major risk factor in this man for a completed suicide?

4. What other risk factors should you be concerned about?

5. What would happen if Mr. Bowen refused to sign into the hospital voluntarily?

ANSWERS

1. Severe guilt, despair, hopelessness, desire to join his wife.

2. Refusal to sign a no-suicide contract, plan to go home alone, continued statements that he wanted to join his wife and that he had nothing to live for.

3. Two previous suicide attempts.

4. He is an elderly white male, recently widowed, feels hopeless, and has methods of committing suicide available to him.

5. There would be a commitment procedure that would be handled through the probate court to determine whether he could continue to be held involuntarily in the hospital.

 ## GUIDED CASE STUDY #4

Mr. Jobe is a 75-year-old man who lives alone in an apartment and has few social contacts. He has a history of insulin-dependent diabetes (adult onset) and a mild cerebrovascular accident. He has a history of repeated trips to the emergency room with complaints of gastrointestinal (GI) distress or concerns about his blood sugar. He also makes repeated calls to his primary-care physician, sometimes as many as 10 calls each day. He has undergone extensive medical workups that have all been negative, and his physician considers his medical condition to be stable. However, Mr. Jobe has difficulty accepting this because he feels so certain that he has cancer or some other illness that his doctor has missed.

Mr. Jobe denies sleep disturbance, and his appetite has been good. He is aware that he feels very irritable and impatient at times. He is uncomfortable in new situations and tends to spend most of his time alone in his apartment worrying about his health. He does go to the supermarket or out for a meal on occasion. He describes the following symptoms: shortness of breath; GI distress, with either constipation or diarrhea; worry that he is experiencing a change in bowel habits and therefore has cancer; palpitations; lightheadedness; and fear of dying.

At the time he was seen for evaluation, Mr. Jobe was taking alprazolam (Xanax) 1 mg tid and trazodone (Desyrel) 50 mg qam and 100 mg qhs. He reported that his present psychotropic medications were started by his former psychiatrist and he did not want to try any other medications because he was afraid he would have side effects. He was referred to a psychiatric practice where he was seen by an advanced practice nurse (APN) for evaluation of his anxiety symptoms and his medications.

Mr. Jobe was very anxious much of the time. If he worried about his blood sugar being too low or his bowel function, he would call the APN who was his therapist for reassurance. Gradually, he began to accept that when he became anxious, he would worry about his health and make repeated calls to his health-care providers. He also became aware that if he got out of his apartment even for a walk, he would feel better. However, he had difficulty following through with activities that involved a new social situation even though he reported feeling very lonely. He found that he became more anxious in these situations. He also had difficulty following through with relaxation exer-

cises such as deep breathing and found that sometimes trying to do this caused him even more anxiety.

Eventually, he consented to some changes in his medication. The first thing that was done was to replace the alprazolam with clonazepam (Klonopin). This was gradually added as the alprazolam was tapered and discontinued. The eventual clonazepam dose was 1 mg tid, and Mr. Jobe was able to tolerate this with no adverse effects. It helped to some degree, but he continued to have much anxiety and to make several phone calls a day to his therapist or his physician. He had agreed to a change in his alprazolam because clonazepam was a similar agent. However, both his therapist and his psychiatrist felt that a selective serotonin reuptake inhibitor (SSRI) would better treat his anxiety than the trazodone. Mr. Jobe continued to be reluctant to try a new medication, but eventually agreed because he was also starting to feel depressed and discouraged.

Paroxetine (Paxil) was the SSRI that was chosen for Mr. Jobe. Typically, in a person his age, the starting dose would have been 10 mg qd, but because of the concern that his fear of side effects would interfere with his ability to comply with this medication, his psychiatrist started him on a dose of 10 mg qod. He was continued at the starting dose for a period of 2 weeks. He did not experience any side effects, so the dose was increased to 10 mg qd for another 2 weeks and then increased to 20 mg qd. He stayed at this dose for several more weeks, but eventually needed to be increased to a dose of 40 mg qd. The trazodone was tapered and discontinued once he stabilized on the paroxetine. Eventually, the clonazepam was tapered to a daily dose of 0.5 mg bid.

Mr. Jobe continues to experience periods of increased anxiety, but he has been much improved with his present medications. He is now able to work on using deep breathing to help him to relax. He has met a friend in his apartment complex and the two of them have become active in the local senior citizens group. He calls his physician or therapist only on rare occasions. He no longer feels depressed, and his sense of humor has returned to the point that he can even joke about his symptoms.

QUESTIONS

1. What diagnoses would you consider for Mr. Jobe?
2. What might be the rationale for the use of clonazepam for Mr. Jobe?
3. What symptoms associated with anxiety and panic disorder does Mr. Jobe experience?
4. What symptoms associated with depression does Mr. Jobe exhibit?

ANSWERS

1. Panic disorder, depression.
2. It is effective for use in panic disorder, and Mr. Jobe's anxiety is severe enough to consider a longer-acting benzodiazepine. In addition, the alprazolam had not been effective in controlling his symptoms, so a change in medications was indicated.
3. Repeated trips to the emergency room with concerns about his health despite stable medical status and negative workup, increased calls to his health-care providers, shortness of breath, fear of dying, GI symptoms, palpitations, lightheadedness, irritability, and impatience.
4. Irritability, impatience, withdrawal from social situations, depressed mood, constipation, and rumination about problems.

GUIDED CASE STUDY #5

Ms. Randall is an 85-year-old single woman, living in an elderly housing complex. She has been living in the building for 15 years. She has been followed by a community health agency for the past 4 to 5 years, following gallbladder surgery. She is basically in good physical health. She has no living relatives and is unwilling to allow anyone to assist her with managing her affairs.

Ms. Randall has an eccentric personality. She has no known history of psychiatric diagnosis. She has consistently refused to visit any physician. She is very angry most of the time and, at times, rageful and yelling at providers and others. She frequently argues with other tenants and uses racial slurs in her conversations about them. She has much difficulty listening to reason and distorts reality most of the time. She refuses to have a phone, TV, or radio because of deafness. She does wear a hearing aid when she leaves the apartment, but otherwise keeps it in a drawer.

She has a companion who takes her shopping, banking, and so forth for about 3 hours twice a week. She has a case manager who visits her every 2 weeks. Most of the time during these visits, she verbalizes delusional and paranoid thoughts. She reports hearing noises during the night and smelling garbage being put down the toilet in her apartment. The caseworker has had a psychiatrist make a home visit; she recommended perphenazine (Trilafon), 2 mg at bedtime, and follow-up visits. She deemed Ms. Randall competent, with a paranoid delusional disorder.

Ms. Randall refused to take the Trilafon, as well as any other medication, including over-the-counter vitamins or stool softeners. She remains suspicious, paranoid, and rejecting of help. She refuses any attempt to improve her situation (ie, a phone with an apparatus for the hearing impaired, newspapers or magazines, or furniture for her apartment). She frequently states, "I don't know why people think they know what is right for me. I don't want any help or handouts."

Boundary issues are a problem with Ms. Randall. She believes in telling people what she thinks of them; often, it is not flattering. She continues to live in a situation that is mediocre at best, with minimal therapeutic supports. The caseworker has seen ants and cockroaches in Ms. Randall's apartment. She becomes hysterical when told about them, yelling, "I'm a clean person, it's those others who have bugs, not me."

Ms. Randall refuses to visit a doctor and also rejects suggestions to attend a local day program to increase her socialization. Much time is spent by the caseworker allowing Ms. Randall to relate her past life events.

QUESTION

1. What are the safety issues in this situation?

ANSWER

1. The client is at risk for physical injury or abuse by others in the apartment building. The fact that she has no phone and no hearing aid increases her vulnerability during a fire or an emergency in the building. She is also at risk for emotional neglect due to limited interactions with her caseworker and companion; the rest of her time is spent alone, ruminating on her delusional thoughts.

 ## GUIDED CASE STUDY #6

Mr. Ward is a 72-year-old male with a history of mitral valve replacement and atrial fibrillation, which is treated with digoxin. He is brought to the emergency room by ambulance. He is accompanied by his wife and daughter, who report that he got up to go to the bathroom and fell; his eyes have been open and he seems aware that they are there, but he has not spoken to them. On physical examination in the emergency room, Mr. Ward is found to have a flaccid left hemiplegia. A diagnosis of cerebrovascular accident (CVA) is made.

QUESTIONS

1. Certain risk factors and progression of onset are known to be identified with stroke types. Based on the limited history available, Mr. Ward's stroke has probably been caused by:
   (a) hemorrhage
   (b) thrombosis
   (c) embolus
2. What diagnostic studies would you expect to be a part of Mr. Ward's workup?
   (a) complete blood count (CBC) with differential, prothrombin time/partial thromboplastin time (PT/PTT), chemistry panel
   (b) computed tomography (CT) scan

of the head with and without contrast

(c) x-ray of the skull and head

(d) electrocardiogram (ECG)

3. What medications would you expect to be prescribed to Mr. Ward to decrease the possibility of future embolic events?

(a) antihypertensives

(b) anticoagulants

(c) immunoglobulins

(d) hormone treatment

ANSWERS

1. (c). Atrial fibrillation, cardiac valve disease, and abrupt onset are all factors associated with CVAs of embolic origin.

2. (a), (b), (d). The CBC is important to assess baseline hematologic function. The PT/PTT are drawn to establish coagulatory status. The chemistry panel assesses system function, including renal function with blood urea nitrogen (BUN) and creatinine, which is necessary prior to CT scan. A CT scan should be done on every stroke client as soon as possible. The CT scan will differentiate between hemorrhage and infarct. The findings on the CT scan will confirm the findings of the physical examination. There is a high correlation between cerebral infarction and cardiac abnormalities—over one third of persons with CVAs will show ECG abnormalities at some time within the first 24 hours.

3. (b). If no hemorrhage is evident on CT scan or magnetic resonance imaging (MRI), anticoagulation—initially with heparin, and later with warfarin—should be prescribed to prevent further emboli.

 ## GUIDED CASE STUDY #7

Mrs. Barker is a 56-year-old female who presents to the clinic with complaints of a tremor in her left hand, which she reports seems to increase when she is tired or stressed. Mrs. Barker is still employed and says that she believes she is slower at using the computer and filing; however, when she rushes, her tremor increases. She also reports that friends and co-workers have recently been complaining that she is not talking loud enough. A preliminary diagnosis of Parkinson's disease is made.

QUESTIONS

1. The diagnosis of Parkinson's disease is made by:

(a) history and presentation of symptoms

(b) computed tomography (CT) scan

(c) biochemical abnormalities as

screening markers

(d) magnetic resonance imaging (MRI)

(e) physical exam

2. The primary medications for treatment of Parkinson's disease include or stimulate the release of:

(a) methylphenidate

(b) levodopa

(c) dopamine

(d) phenyltriazine

(e) lithium carbonate

3. In time, Mrs. Barker may experience which of the following?

(a) loss of balance and falls

(b) rigidity and cogwheeling

(c) bradykinesia

(d) constipation

(e) difficulty swallowing

(f) all of the above

ANSWERS

1. (a), (e). Although biochemical abnormalities as markers for diagnosis of Parkinson's disease are being studied, none have been verified as diagnostically useful. A diagnosis of Parkinson's disease requires that two or more symptoms are documented on physical exam for at least 6 months, and on three or more consecutive examinations. An MRI or CT scan may be used to identify other neurologic diseases that cause movement disorders, such as stroke or tumor.

2. (b), (c). Replenishing the dopamine stores in the brain is the goal of treatment for Parkinson's disease. Since dopamine cannot cross the blood–brain barrier, therapy consists of administering levodopa (its metabolic precursor), which can cross the blood–brain barrier, or attempting to stimulate the release of dopamine from the substantia nigra.

3. (f). Parkinson's disease is an idiopathic degenerative process of the pigmented dopaminergic neurons, which is caused by an interruption or reduction of neurotransmission of dopamines in the substantia nigra. This dysfunction of the dopaminergic system results in a progressive worsening of the above symptoms.

 ## GUIDED CASE STUDY #8

Mrs. Abbott is an 83-year-old resident of a long-term care facility. Her history includes right cerebrovascular accident (CVA), hypertension (HTN), congestive heart failure (CHF), type 2 diabetes mellitus (DM), and bipolar disorder. Her medications are felodipine, acetylsalicylic acid (ASA), digoxin, lithium, and enalapril. Her diabetes is diet controlled. Mrs. Abbott is a very quiet individual and would prefer reading to more social activities. She ambulates with a cane. For the previous week, it has been reported by the nursing staff that the client is "just not herself." She is quieter, bordering on withdrawal, disoriented to place, and her appetite is decreased. She is evaluated by the practitioner after reportedly falling to the floor while on her way to the bathroom. The assessment of her includes flat affect, disorientation to time and place, hypotension, tachycardia, afebrile, lungs clear to bases, abdomen within normal limits, decreased muscle strength of left upper and lower extremities secondary to CVA, deep tendon reflexes 1+ bilaterally, and a Folstein Mini-Mental State Exam score of 18/30 (previously 23/30).

QUESTION

1. What diagnostic studies should be ordered?

ANSWER

1. The following are ordered for initial workup: orthostatic vital signs, pulse oximetry, electrolytes, urinalysis, urine culture and sensitivities, fingerstick blood glucose bid for 3 days (uncontrolled diabetes), lithium, and thyroid-stimulating hormone (TSH). The results indicated no orthostatic changes; pulse ox, 94%; fingerstick glucose, 80 and 112 for 1 day; urinalysis and urine C & S, negative; lithium level, normal; blood urea nitrogen (BUN), 28 mg/dL; creatinine, 1.2 mg/dL; sodium, 140 mmol/L; potassium, 4.6 mmol/dL; chloride, 113 mmol/dL; CO_2, 24 mmol/dL; TSH, 20.6 $\mu IU/mL$. Mrs. Abbott required additional PO intake, as she was dehydrated. Her TSH level elevation required further evaluation; a thyroid function test battery was ordered. These results were TSH, 18.28 $\mu IU/mL$; total T_4, 5.4 $\mu g/dL$; and T uptake, 103 units. The only elevation was the TSH level. The most likely reason for this elevation is the lithium medication, which causes an increase in TSH but not necessarily hypothyroidism. The client's lithium was discontinued and valproic acid (Depakote) was initiated. Within 2 weeks, the client was noted to have improved balance, appetite, and orientation. Thyroid-stimulating hormone levels at 6 and 10 weeks were 5.57 $\mu IU/mL$ and 3.68 $\mu IU/mL$.

GUIDED CASE STUDY #9

Mrs. Murray is a 66-year-old woman who presented to a family practice office with a 2-week history of tiredness. She was experiencing decreased appetite, muscle weakness, lightheadedness, left-sided sore throat for 1 week, and a "funny taste" in her mouth that had persisted for the past year. Yesterday, she had a spell of dizziness and lightheadedness after eating a good breakfast. She also complains of being more tired and slightly short of breath after climbing stairs. Her past medical history is significant for treatment of Lyme disease 1 year ago, hypertension for which she takes Vasotec (enalapril maleate) 5 mg qd, hypothroidism for which she takes Synthroid (levothyroxine) 0.15 mg qd, and

depression for which she takes Prozac (fluoxetine hydrochloride). She was recently seen by her dentist for "mouth soreness" and was started on baking soda rinses. Her grandson visited recently and was diagnosed with mononucleosis upon return home.

Mrs. Murray appears in no acute distress. Head, eye, ear, nose, and throat (HEENT) exam was unremarkable, with the exception of slight erythema in the posterior pharynx. Her neck was supple, without adenopathy. The lungs were clear bilaterally. Heart sounds were regular, with a I/VI systolic murmur over th left upper sternal border. The abdomen was soft without organomegaly. She was unable to percieve vibration bilaterally in her lower extremities.

QUESTIONS

1. What laboratory studies would you request?
2. Describe the type of anemia and possible causes.

ANSWERS

1. Lab results were received 2 days after the initial visit:
   - Chemistries: all within normal limits
   - LFTs: LDH 10,637 U/L (normal: 313–618)
     AST 122 U/L (normal 7–56)
     Alkaline phosphatase, gamma-glutamyl transpeptidase (GGT), and total bilirubin within normal limits
   - Thyroid studies: within normal limits
   - WBC: 3.1×10^3
   - RBC: 1.46 million
   - Platelets: 62,000 cu/mm

- Hg: 6.2 g
- HCT: 17

2. Mrs. Murray was admitted to the hospital to rule out the following potential diagnoses: blood dyscrasia, leukemia, connective tissue disease, hepatitis, endocarditis, and pernicious anemia. Labs were repeated and an echocardiogram, abdominal CT (to rule out mass), LDH isoenzymes, B_{12} level, Schilling's test, and bone marrow aspiration were performed. She received one unit of packed red cells. She was diagnosed with pernicious anemia and left the hospital after B_{12} therapy was initiated. After 1 week, she stated, "I feel like my old self!"

GUIDED CASE STUDY #10

Mrs. Simpson is a 62-year-old white female who was recently widowed when her husband died from myocardial infarction. She works part time for an insurance company and has three grown children. She presents to her physician with facial edema and shortness of breath. Over the past 3 years, she has been treated by her primary-care physician for chronic obstructive pulmenary disease (COPD).

During the exam, Mrs. Simpson states that her weight has been stable. She has had a cough with some shortness of breath associated with COPD, but has recently noticed swelling in her face, especially around the eyes. She admits to drinking a glass of wine daily for the past 20 years. She has a long history of cigarette smoking, which includes one to two packs per day for 35 years.

QUESTIONS

1. Certain risk factors have been identified for lung cancer. Based on Mrs. Simpson's limited history, which risk factors could point to a diagnosis of lung cancer?
   (a) smoking
   (b) alcohol intake
   (c) family history

2. Although Mrs. Simpson did not experience all of the following signs and symptoms, which are typically associated with lung cancer?
   (a) hemoptysis
   (b) wheezing
   (c) cough
   (d) weight loss
   (e) dyspnea

3. The signs and symptoms of lung cancer depend on the location of the tumor, its local or regional spread, and

the presence or absence of metastatic growth. Mrs. Simpson presents with facial edema, which may indicate local or regional spread of disease. Which tests might you expect as part of Mrs. Simpson's workup?

(a) complete blood count (CBC), chemistry panel, liver function test (LFT)

(b) computed tomographic (CT) scan of chest and upper abdomen

(c) magnetic resonance imaging (MRI) of the chest

(d) fiberoptic bronchoscopy

(e) lung tomograms

(f) fine-needle aspiration (FNA)

ANSWERS

1. (a) Yes. Because smoking has been directly linked to lung cancer, it is important to elicit information regarding smoking habits. During the history taking and physical examination, one should ask about the age at which smoking began, the number of cigarettes smoked, the duration of smoking, and the type of cigarettes smoked.

   (b) No. Oral cancer and cancer of the throat, esophagus, larynx, and liver occur more frequently in heavy drinkers of alcohol, especially when they also smoke cigarettes or chew tobacco.

   (c) Optional. A genetic predisposition has been suggested as a risk factor for lung cancer but is inconclusive.

2. (a) Yes. Blood-streaked sputum is a frequently reported symptom.

   (b) No. Wheezing is sometimes caused by airway obstruction from the tumor. It is often diagnosed during clinical examination but is an infrequent complaint.

   (c) Yes. Coughing, usually persistent, is a symptom, and the cough can be productive.

   (d) Yes. Weight loss is a clinical characteristic of lung cancer and is also an important prognostic factor.

   (e) Yes Chronic, increasing shortness of breath is often associated with the diagnosis.

3. (a) Yes. The first two tests are important for assessing baseline hematologic and systemic function, and abnormal liver enzymes may indicate liver metastasis.

   (b) Yes. Computed tomography scans can confirm an abnormality seen on chest x-ray and can detect any spread to the mediastinum. The scan should include the upper abdomen to image the liver and adrenal glands, which are frequent sites of metastasis.

   (c) No. This procedure does not add information already obtained from CT scan.

   (d) Optional. It is a definitive test for a diagnosis of lung cancer but is commonly ordered after CT scan and blood test results are available.

   (e) No. Computed tomography scans have replaced this procedure.

(f) Yes. If the lung lesion is peripheral and accessible by CT-guided biopsy, FNA may be attempted first for a definitive diagnosis. Because it does not require local anesthesia or sedation, this procedure is less invasive and uncomfortable than is bronchoscopy.

Mrs. Simpson was diagnosed with stage III lung cancer in the right upper lobe, involving the chest wall, great vessels, and brachial plexus. The tumor response to radiation therapy and chemotherapy (cisplatin and vinblastine) is moderate.

BRIEF CASE STUDIES

 ## CASE STUDY #1

Mrs. Archer is an 84-year-old woman who was seen in consultation for anorexia and weight loss (she weighs 68 lb). Initial workup for sources of weight loss (thyroid disease, malignancy, diabetes, etc.) was negative. A swallowing study was within normal limits. No signs of dementia were found.

Further exploration of the client's history with the family revealed a description of the client as a "controlling individual." She had previously fixated on weight control and had always been thin but not to this extreme. She had not eaten for 4 months despite her husband's and family's encouragement. She was eventually diagnosed with anorexia nervosa.

Teaching Points

- Eating disorders can appear in old age.
- Anorexia is frequently a symptom of occult physical illness (see Chapters 7 and 8) but may also represent psychiatric or emotional disturbances such as depression, delirium, dementia, psychosis, or, in this case, an eating disorder.

CASE STUDY #2

Mr. Lawrence is a 94-year-old man who lives alone in the community. He is functionally independent. His past medical history includes chronic obstructive pulmonary disease (COPD), congestive heart failure (CHF), two myocardial infarctions (MIs), "difficult personality," and insulin-dependent diabetes mellitus (IDDM).

Mr. Lawrence has had 10 falls within 2 days (without apparent injury). His previous fall history was approximately one fall per year. He denies any other complaints except for "weakness." His blood sugar is 148. He is afebrile and his lungs are clear, with good phonation and tactile fremitus (baseline for this client was diminished fremitus and breath sounds due to COPD). He has no cough, no egophony, and no bronchophony. Neuro exam was within normal limits except for a positive Romberg and an unsteady gait. A score of 30/30 was obtained on the Folstein Mini-Mental State Exam. A chest x-ray revealed bilateral pneumonia.

Teaching Points

- Sudden falls in a previously infrequent faller may be an early presentation of physical illness.
- Expected signs and symptoms of pneumonia are frequently absent in the elderly (no fever, shortness of breath, congestion, cough).
- Normal breath sounds and voice sounds in a client whose baseline is diminished may actually signify increased transmission and consolidation.

CASE STUDY #3

Mr. Brewer is an 85-year-old man who lives at home with his wife, both post-cerebrovascular accident (CVA). He walks with a quad cane and is normally continent if he leaves enough time to get to the bathroom. Today, he reveals new-onset urinary incontinence and reports "dribbling" and constantly being wet for 5 days. He reports difficulty emptying his bladder and starting the stream of urine (a new problem).

He denies any new medication use. During the advanced practice nurse's visit, he was observed reaching into the chair cushion. He pulled out a container of Afrin nasal spray and used it, stating he has had a cold for about a week. He also acknowledged using Comtrex cold medicine.

Teaching Points

- A new onset of urinary incontinence can be related to medication use.
- Patients often discount over-the-counter medications when reporting their medication regimen and need to be asked specifically about these agents.
- Anticholinergic meds may contribute to incontinence either directly, by decreasing bladder contractility, or indirectly, by causing bowel impaction, with resultant overflow incontinence (see Chapter 9).
- Always review a complete medication list when seeing residents of facilities. Community dwelling elders should be encouraged to bring all of their medications to each office visit.

CASE STUDY #4

Mr. Dannelli is a 92-year-old man of Italian descent who lives alone on the first floor of a three-family home. He is cognitively and functionally healthy. He reports a new onset of urgency and urinary incontinence. He is reluctant to report symptoms due to a fear of nursing home placement. He states, "I'm getting old." The problem was discovered during a home visit by the advanced practice nurse, who finds the client drying multiple pairs of underpants on his portable clothesline in his bathroom. He is afebrile. He denies frequency or dysuria. He has no history of urinary tract infections (UTIs). He does have a history of benign prostatic hypertrophy. Urine dipstick is positive for infection, and the client is treated. Symptoms resolve within 24 hours of treatment.

Teaching Points

- Follow-up is needed in this case to find out why this client has developed a UTI; prostate size may have increased due to benign prostatic hypertrophy or malignancy.
- UTIs without dysuria, frequency, or fever are common in older adults.
- Urinary incontinence is a major presenting sign of UTIs in the elderly.
- Elders often underreport treatable conditions because of a misconception that the symptom is a normal part of aging, lack of recognition of the problem as treatable, or fear that caregivers will view symptoms as an indication of increased dependancy or inability to live alone.

CASE STUDY #5

Mrs. Roland is a 94-year-old woman who lives in an apartment. She chooses to have an around-the-clock aide/companion, but she is independent in all activities of daily living. Her medical diagnoses include hiatal hernia, urge incontinence, constipation, osteoarthritis, and depression. Her medications include: cisapride (Propulsid) 1 PO tid, famotidine (Pepcid) 20 mg bid, oxybutynin 5 mg qhs, bisacodyl (Dulcolax) tabs 2 PO qhs, lactulose 30 cc bid prn, oxaprozin (Daypro) 600 mg bid, acetaminophen with codeine (Tylenol #3) 1 PO q4h prn (taken occasionally), and sertraline hydrochloride (Zoloft) 25 mg PO qam (started 2 days ago).

Mrs. Roland is very hard of hearing, despite bilateral hearing aids, and is also legally blind. She has a minor problem with short-term memory, which has gradually progressed over the past 2 years. You have been asked by Mrs. Roland's daughter to visit her mother and establish a therapeutic relationship for ongoing support.

When the advanced practice nurse (APN) meets Mrs. Roland for the first time, the aide/companion tells you she has not been herself for the past several days. She is confused, has been unable to sleep for 4 nights, and thinks her aide is her mother. She believes her daughter is an imposter.

Mrs. Roland was seen by her physician 2 days ago, who drew some blood but found nothing abnormal on physical exam. He started Mrs. Roland on Zoloft 25 mg qam, diagnosing her with depression. The APN finds her to be distractible, with poor concentration. Mrs. Roland falls asleep during conversations and scores a 7/30 on the Folstein Mini-Mental State Exam. She is wearing an old hearing aid because her new ones are in for repair. Two days later, Mrs. Roland is hospitalized with severe anemia, an upper gastrointestinal (GI) bleed and acute gastritis related to nonsteroidal anti-inflammatory drug (NSAID) use. After a delirious hospital course, she returned home and resumed her baseline functioning. Her Folstein score at this time was 24/29, and she was once again independent in all activities.

Teaching Points

- Delirium is often missed in a client with early dementia.
- NSAIDs are often associated with GI bleeding in geriatric clients.
- Frail elders can recover from delirium and resume baseline function.
- A baseline mental status exam is critical when a client is well so that comparisons can be made in the event of later changes.

CASE STUDY #6

Mrs. Johnson is a 92-year-old white female resident of an intermediate-care facility. She has moderate dementia but has remained continent of bowel and bladder. She experiences a sudden onset of urinary and fecal incontinence, which the nursing staff attribute to a progression of her dementia.

Upon exam, she is found to have not had a formed bowel movement for 6 days. A large fecal impaction is removed, followed by a Fleet enema.

Bladder and bowel continence are subsequently restored.

Teaching Points
- Do not attribute sudden changes incontinence to declining mental status in a demented client.
- Persons with dementia are at high risk for reversible causes of incontinence.
- Fecal impaction is a common cause of urinary and fecal incontinence in older adults.

CASE STUDY #7

Mrs. Thompson is an 81-year-old woman brought to the clinic by her son, who is concerned that she may have dementia. She moved from her apartment in another state to live with her son about 3 months ago, due to a decreased ability to care for herself. She was exhibiting signs of forgetfulness, decreased concentration, decreased interest in her surroundings, and falls (three falls in 1 month). She was reluctant to come to the clinic due to her beliefs as a practicing Christian Scientist. On examination, she had a Folstein Mini-Mental State score of 21/30. Of note on physical exam was a 5-lb weight loss in 1 month, hung-up deep tendon reflexes, decreased hearing, hypoactive bowel sounds, and proximal muscle weakness.

Labwork showed a thyroid-stimulating hormone (TSH) level of 18 (normal 2–10) and a thyroxine (T_4) level of 1.2 (normal 4–11). She agreed to treatment with levothyroxine sodium (Synthroid) 0.0125 mg in spite of her religious beliefs. Within 3 months, her mental status had objectively improved (Folstein score of 30/30), and she and her son reported normal cognition and increased concentration and motivation. Mrs. Thompson was able to return to independent living in her home state.

Teaching Points
- Slow dose replacement is necessary to avoid stress on the cardiac system. (The usual adult dose of levothyroxine may result in tachycardia and congestive heart failure in the older adult.)

- Hypothyroidism often presents atypically in older adults, with mental status changes, weight loss (not gain), and falls.

 CASE STUDY #8

Mrs. Powers was an 84-year-old woman who lived alone in her suburban home. She was mildly demented but able to carry out activities of daily living and most instrumental activities of daily living independently. She had a history of osteoarthritis and chronic obstructive pulmonary disease (COPD). She smoked one pack of cigarettes a day for 50 years. She complained of bony pain, increasing in intensity and duration. This was thought to be due to osteoarthritis. She also had a constant, productive cough, which was attributed to smoking and COPD. She demonstrated a change in mental status (becoming confused about who delivered her paper), which was attributed to a progression in her dementia. A short time later, she set her kitchen on fire, which resulted in her admission to the hospital, where she was diagnosed with lung cancer that had metastasized to the bone and brain. She died 2 weeks later.

Teaching Point
- Subtle signs and symptoms of a malignancy may be incorrectly attributed to chronic disease (by the client and the practitioner).

 CASE STUDY #9

Mr. Woods lived alone in a three-story Victorian home. His only living relative was a niece who lived miles away and maintained phone contact. Because of her concerns about her uncle, she established a financial conservator and arranged for case management services. A referral was made for advanced practice nursing visits for the purpose of assessment and care management.

Attempts to visit Mr. Woods failed for many weeks. He was believed to be at home but would not answer the door when the clinician arrived despite prior telephone contact. The nurse met with his neighbors at the request of the case manager. They visited Mr. Wood daily, bringing him an evening meal and helping with shopping. They were concerned about Mr. Woods' increasing dependence and asked for help on his behalf. They agreed to introduce the nurse clinician to Mr. Woods and were hopeful she could convince him to bathe.

The first visit with the neighbors and case manager revealed a friendly, extremely guarded older man, who apeared physically robust, had a steady gait, and could climb stairs without difficulty. The house was cold, dark, dirty, and filled with old newspapers. Mr. Woods clearly expressed displeasure and distrust when the nurse took his blood pressure and attempted any physical exam or health interview. He quickly denied any physical symptoms, memory problems, or difficulties maintaining his home. He proudly stated that he had not seen a doctor in 60 years! He was socially appropriate but used frequent cliches to respond to questions. He told the nurse he was careful about conserving oil when asked about the temperature in the house.

The nurse recommended basic safety measures such as smoke alarms (the client was a cigar smoker), household lighting, and repair of the client's broken front steps. These interventions were carried out in conjunction with the case manager and the financial conservator.

On the nurse's next visit, Mr. Woods would not answer the door. On the third visit, the nurse was allowed in. Over the course of the next several visits, the nurse did not perform any hands-on physical examination nor any "intrusive" interviewing. Conversation was kept on a social level to build rapport and learn more about the client's life experiences and frame of reference. He related colorful, detailed accounts of important events in his distant past. His short-term memory and new learning were significantly impaired.

As trust and rapport grew, Mr. Woods gave the nurse a tour of his entire home and began to acknowledge some problems in daily management, such as remembering barber appointments and preparing meals. He had bragged about how full his cupboards were (stocked with many canned goods by neighbors), but direct observation revealed that he could not find a can opener, and if a manual or electric opener was provided, he could not recall how to use them.

He allowed Meals-on-Wheels as the first of many subsequent community supports. As he began to see that these supports decreased his daily strain and facilitated independent living, he allowed further intervention. As all members of the team continued to work on rapport and trust, Mr. Woods gradually received homemaker services; a companion who took him to the barber and local ball games; a physician visit, which included workup for cognitive impairment; and a home health aide to assist with bathing. The physician visit was agreed to by the client because of his wish to have his hearing evaluated and improved. Approximately 2 years after the initial visit, Mr. Woods agreed to move to an assisted-living environment.

Teaching Points

- None of the positive outcomes in this case would have been achieved without firmly establishing trust and rapport, respecting client's boundaries and nonverbal messages to "back off"; this type of helping relationship may take a long time to establish; goals need to be small and the pace slow.
- It is helpful to use established, trusted relationships to facilitate interventions (such as neighbors in this case).
- Interventions that the client views as helpful and not overly intrusive (eg, fixing stairs) help to build trust and facilitate later, more personal interventions such as bathing assistance.
- Home visits, casual conversation, direct observation, and functional assessment may reveal safety hazards and subtle clues to cognitive impairment (use of cliches, inability to use can opener).
- Caring for clients with dementia often requires the ethically challenging task of balancing safety with autonomy and dignity.

CASE STUDY #10

Mrs. Gray is a 78-year-old woman with dementia, who is being relocated to a nursing home from her own home by her family due to decreased ability to care for herself, wandering, and disorientation.

As she arrived at the nursing home unit, she cried out, "Where am I and does my daughter know where I am?" She was agitated but responded well to being told she was at a nursing center and her daughter knew of her whereabouts. After a few minutes, she again cried out, "Where am I and does my daughter know where I am?"

The nursing staff assessed that this client responded well to information and could process it, but could not retain it for more than 1 minute. An attempt was made to write the information down on paper, but she was unable to read and understand. (This was confirmed by testing the portion of the Folstein that asks the client to read "close your eyes." She could read the letters but could not form the words or follow the command.) The clinician suggested that the daughter make a cassette tape, which was to be played with headphones. When the client became agitated, she heard her daughter on tape saying, "Mom, this is Mary. I love you. I know you're at the nursing center. I'll be visiting you soon. Bye." This message was played at 1-minute intervals and was needed for approximately 2 weeks while the resident settled into her new environment.

Teaching Points

- Assess the cause of agitation and assess cognitive abilities so that the appropriate level of intervention can be implemented.
- Use the Folstein Mini-Mental State Exam as an adjunct to client assessment and care planning.
- Use creativity and brainstorming to expand interventions.

CASE STUDY #11

Mrs. Keller is an 87-year-old woman with stage 2 Alzheimer's dementia, who resides in a nursing care facility. She walks around the facility and knows her whereabouts, but often repeats stories and has a difficult time remembering the date and people's names. She wears a hearing aid and glasses.

Over the course of a few days, Mrs. Keller's behavior changes. She falls three times and displays an inability to dress and feed herself. She cannot find her room and becomes suddenly incontinent of urine.

The staff recognize this change from her baseline cognitive and functional status. She is assessed and found to have coarse crackles on respiration, dullness in the right lung base, egophony, bronchophony, and whispered pectoriloquy in the right lung base. She is diagnosed with pneumonia and a fractured right hip from one of her falls and is transferred to the hospital.

She is combative at the hospital emergency room. She thrashes about, screaming for her granddaughter. Her hearing aids were left behind at the nursing home (because they were lost during the last hospital admission). Because of her behavior, Mrs. Keller was medicated with 2 mg of diazepam (Valium) IM, which led to 6 hours of sedation. Her granddaughter arrived and shared that in the past when her grandmother became agitated, she would rub her back and talk to her, which had a calming effect.

The granddaughter could not spend the night, so the staff attempted to replicate her intervention by having the granddaughter read a story into a tape recorder. Later that night when Mrs. Keller awoke and began to cry out, the nurse put a stethoscope in her ears, with the diaphragm of the stethoscope on the tape recorder. She rubbed Mrs. Keller's back as she listened to the tape of her granddaughter's voice. This immediately calmed Mrs. Keller and allowed her to relax, thereby avoiding physical and chemical restraints. This intervention was used repeatedly until her delirium cleared and she returned to the nursing facility.

Teaching Points

- Demented persons often become delirious during a physical ailment.
- Illness often presents atypically (delirium and falls as a symptom of pneumonia).
- Inquiring about previous successful interventions for challenging behaviors can save lots of work.
- Trying to replicate successful interventions in new settings requires creativity.
- The overall goal is to minimize physical and chemical restraints.

 ## CASE STUDY #12

Mr. Parker has stage 2 Alzheimer's disease and lives with his wife. He has recently stopped showering despite his wife's commands to do so, which she interprets as purposeful stubbornness.

Mr. Parker is unable to understand the abstract concepts involved in the message, "Go take a shower so you can go to day care." He becomes agitated when his wife approaches to assist him with hygienic care.

The advanced practice nurse assesses Mr. Parker's mental status, using the Folstein Mini-Mental State Exam, and finds that he can no longer follow a three-step command. The nurse demonstrates to Mrs. Parker an approach using one-step commands. At the time of the bath, she says to Mr. Parker, "Follow me" (as she walks into the bedroom), "sit down," "take off your shoes," "take off your socks," and so on. After Mr. Parker is undressed, she uses the same techniques to have him sit down on the toilet in the bathroom, which is covered with a towel. She hands him a washcloth and says, "Wash your face," followed by "rinse your face" and "dry your face." This continues until he has completed an entire sponge bath. Sponge baths were used throughout the winter. Mr. Parker agreed to shower in the summer months, using the same one-step command technique.

Teaching Points

- Advanced practice nurses provide important resources for caregivers of persons with dementia.
- Formal cognitive testing can detect changing abilities as well as assist the nurse in planning appropriate interventions.
- Bathing is a complex and fear-producing procedure that frequently causes resistance and requires creative strategies.

CASE STUDY #13

Miss Robinson is an 87-year-old woman with a diagnosis of schizophrenia, stabilized on haloperidol (Haldol) 0.5 mg PO bid for several years. She begins displaying signs of increasing paranoia, stating that people are looking at her through the walls with scopes. She has no physical complaints. Her paranoia continues to escalate and intensify.

Two weeks later, she experiences new-onset "indigestion," with mild pain in the epigastric area radiating to the interscapular area in the back. She reports immediate relief with Maalox. The pain returns 1 hour later, at which time she knocks on her neighbor's door stating that she does not feel well. She is brought to the emergency room, where she dies of a ruptured abdominal aortic aneurysm.

Teaching Points

- Exacerbations of preexisting psychiatric conditions can be early warning signs of impending physical illness.
- A physical cause of psychiatric symptoms should always be sought.
- Serious abdominal conditions can present atypically, with minor discomfort, absence of classic symptoms, and cognitive changes.

CASE STUDY #14

Mrs. Akers reports to the advanced practice nurse (APN) that items are being stolen from her room in the nursing home. Security is notified and Mrs. Akers is reassured. Over time, the complaints become more frequent and increasingly bizarre (strangers are stealing underwear from under her pillows). The APN performs a comprehensive assessment. She finds Mrs. Akers to be in excellent health, as she was 6 months prior during her yearly physical. The Folstein Mini-Mental State Exam is administered, and Mrs. Akers scores a 29/30 on the tool. She loses one point because she is unable to draw the intersecting pentagons. She has no neurologic or musculoskeletal impairments that might prevent her from doing so. Mrs. Akers is eventually referred for more in-depth neuropsychiatric test-ing, which suggests an organic defect. A computed tomography (CT) scan subsequently reveals a tumor in the frontal lobe of her brain.

Teaching Points

- Although a 29/30 is a "normal" score on the Folstein, it is important to assess not only the score, but the nature of the deficits and their correlation to client function.
- Comprehensive baseline assessment of physical and cognitive function provides solid information against which to compare follow-up problem-focused assessments.
- Paranoia may be a symptom of psychiatric illness or dementia but is frequently a herald of physical illness and delirium and warrants a thorough search for pathology.

CASE STUDY #15

Mr. Todd is an 81-year-old man who is hospitalized for an exacerbation of manic depressive illness on an inpatient psychiatric unit. He also has a history of mild dementia. His admission Folstein score is 21/30. His behavior was erratic during the few weeks prior to admission. He refused to go to day care and refused all personal care. During his first evening on the unit, he began complaining of indigestion and was treated with Maalox, with minimal relief. He became acutely disoriented, stating that it was time to go to work. He became restless and agitated. A Folstein score of 8/30 was obtained.

An electrocardiogram (ECG) and blood work ordered stat revealed a massive myocardial infarction (MI).

Teaching Points

- Older adults frequently present without the classic signs of an MI.
- The presence of delirium in a mildly demented individual may be the hallmark of serious illness.

CASE STUDY #16A

Dr. Green is a 102-year-old retired surgeon who lives in an apartment with around-the-clock services. His vision is deteriorating due to cataracts, and he is faced with making a decision about cataract surgery. After consultation with the advanced practice nurse, he decides to have lens implants when and if the time comes that he can no longer enjoy his baseball games on TV.

Teaching Points

- See below.

CASE STUDY #16B

Mr. Alden experiences increasing dyspnea on exertion and progressive deterioration in cardiac function, resulting in ischemia at rest. He is diagnosed with severe heart block, and a pacemaker is recommended. He refuses, stating "I'm 84 years old . . . I've lived a good life . . . I don't want to prolong it." He received information from the advanced practice nurse (APN), the physician, and the cardiologist regarding the risks and benefits of the procedure. Despite his previously healthy condition and his family's concern, he continued to refuse the procedure. The APN respected his right to informed consent.

One day, he mentioned that he missed bowling with his friends. The APN discussed this with him in light of his symptoms and the proposed treatment. Mr. Alden decided to have the pacemaker put in to restore function. He returned to his bowling league and celebrated his 85th birthday.

Teaching Points

- Older adults often view their health status from a "functional" viewpoint.

- Information about the functional impact of various procedures may assist with decision making.
- Autonomy and decision-making ability must be respected in the competent, decision-capable client, while providing sufficient information for informed consent.

 ## CASE STUDY #17

Mr. Kiley is an 89-year-old man who was brought to the emergency room by his 88-year-old wife because of mental status changes. He had played golf earlier in the day, followed by dinner in a restaurant. He started acting "strangely" at dinner. He was disoriented, did not know where he was, and did not recognize his wife. He had no complaints of feeling poorly.

He was found to have a ruptured gallbladder and septicemia. After emergency surgery and a prolonged recovery, he returned to his previous level of independent function.

Teaching Points
- Absence of expected symptoms (fever, pain, rebound tenderness) does not mean absence of disease.
- A chest x-ray is often warranted to rule out pneumonia in a client with a complaint of abdominal pain.
- Acute mental status changes may originate in a gastrointestinal source (peritonitis, fecal impaction).

 ## CASE STUDY #18

Mr. Duncan is an 83-year-old man who resides on a dementia care unit in a long-term care facility. His medical diagnoses include Alzheimer's dementia, peripheral vascular disease, hypothyroidism, chronic obstructive pulmonary disease, depression, history of transient ischemic attacks and phlebitis, and chronic renal insufficiency. His medications include levothyroxine sodium (Synthroid), oxazepam (Serax) bid, albuterol (Proventil) PO, Ventolin and Atrovent inhalers, and milk of magnesia.

His baseline Folstein was 11/30, and baseline behavior and function consisted of appropriate toileting, some self-care, and ability to follow directions and ask appropriate questions.

In July, despite negative x-rays of his hip and pelvis, Mr. Duncan complained of back and hip pain. Ibuprofen (Motrin) 600 mg bid was prescribed to relieve discomfort. Three days later, Mr. Duncan "took a swing at" another resident. The next day, he began to exhibit impaired gait, inability to wash himself, decreased function in all areas, and inappropriate behavior such as urinating in front of the nurses' station. Five days after this he fell, and nurses' notes described his behavior as "erratic."

The advanced practice nurse was consulted the day after the fall. Motrin was held pending lab studies. Labs revealed hypernatremia, dehydration, and acute renal failure superimposed on chronic renal insufficiency. Mr. Duncan was hospitalized. When he returned to the long-term care facility, he was fatigued, dyspneic on minimal exertion, had an unsteady gait, and required total assistance with activities of daily living.

Teaching Points

- Acute illnesses often result in functional loses which may become permanent if a rehabilitative approach is not used.
- Nonsteroidal anti-inflammatory drugs pose a risk of acute renal failure in clients with a history of renal disease. Milk of magnesia is contraindicated in persons with poor renal function.
- A sudden change in behavior in a client with dementia should be considered a possible hallmark of acute illness, and appropriate assessment should be carried out.

CASE STUDY #19

Mrs. Shaw was newly admitted to a nursing home unit. She had fallen at home and fractured her left hip. While in the hospital emergency room undergoing evaluation, she experienced sustained angina. She was admitted to the cardiac care unit, where a myocardial infarction was ruled out. She was considered a poor surgical risk, and her hip fracture was treated conservatively. She was discharged to the nursing home for follow-up care.

Mrs. Shaw was highly anxious on admission and remained so for many weeks. She complained frequently about her care and caregivers, accusing them of not caring whether she lived or died. She rang her call bell frequently and complained of constant pain despite three dose increases of her acetaminophen with codeine (Tylenol #3). She increased her demands and complaints and shouted "Just let me die," which some staff members attributed to an attempt at "manipulative" behavior. Her granddaughter and sister, who had at first visited daily, began to decrease their visits as Mrs. Shaw responded with tears, guilt, and ultimately anger.

The nurse practitioner was asked to see Mrs. Shaw to consult on pain management and behavioral difficulties. As the interview progressed, Mrs. Shaw tearfully related her feelings of isolation and loneliness since her husband's death 5 years before. She stated, "He was my world." She also related events surrounding her fall, which included lying on the floor for 5 hours until being found by a neighbor. Her granddaughter was in the process of selling her home. During this discussion, Mrs. Shaw was distractible and frequently stared at an empty space in the room. When asked what she saw there, she said, "A beautiful antique chair." Specific questioning revealed that Mrs. Shaw

had also been seeing bugs in her room and bed. A tapering of codeine dose led to gradual resolution of her delirium. Around-the-clock Tylenol for breakthrough pain and heat therapy as an adjunct was initiated. Depression assessment continued, using the Yesavage Geriatric Depression Scale (Appendix C) and clinical interview, which confirmed the nurse practitioner's suspicion of clinically significant depression. Psychiatric referral and treatment was begun.

As her depression improved, Mrs. Shaw became less "demanding, manipulative," and critical. She began to participate in self-care and rehabilitation and began to establish a positive relationship with the staff and some other residents.

Teaching Points

- Depression, pain, and delirium contribute to "difficult" behavior.
- Depression may present atypically.
- Labeling difficult behavior precludes a search for meaningful contributors.
- Appreciate the multiple losses experienced by the elderly (especially new nursing home residents).

CASE STUDY #20

Mr. Sloan presented to the clinic with a complaint of explosive vomiting three times in the past 24 hours. He also reported being unsteady on his feet and needing to hold onto the wall or rail to walk. He denied fever, chills, nausea, change in bowel habits, laxative use, or abdominal pain. He denied recent falls. His only medications were allopurinol and ramipril (Altace). Physical assessment was significant for hyperactive reflexes and positive Babinski on the left side. Bilateral cataracts obscured the optic disks. Cerebellar ataxia was present. A Folstein Mini-Mental State Exam revealed a five-point deficit from a baseline exam done during his last routine physical 6 months prior.

Further questioning revealed that Mr. Sloan had in fact fallen approximately 3 to 4 weeks prior and had hit his head on a bureau. He was referred to the physician, and a computed tomography (CT) scan revealed a moderate subdural hematoma.

Teaching Points

- Symptoms of a subdural hematoma may not be in evidence for days or weeks due to the cerebral atrophy of normal aging.
- Careful history taking and comprehensive physical examination are often necessary to elicit important findings in the older client.

CASE STUDY #21

Mrs. Walker is an 85-year-old woman who lives alone in a senior citizen housing complex. She has two cats. Her only living relative is a niece who lives 2 hours away.

She is in the mild to moderate stages of multi-infarct dementia. She displays deficits in time orientation and short-term memory. She has been a diabetic for 5 years, controlled with insulin. She often forgets or neglects to inject herself with her prescribed dose of 30 units of 70/30 insulin each morning and runs blood sugars of 250 to 350 with a glycosylated hemoglobin of 11.5. She often states that she is depressed and has nothing to live for except her cats.

She has cataract surgery, which results in an increased ability to see and an increased interest in life. She begins going out more and taking long walks. The advanced practice nurse visits and finds Mrs. Walker to be hallucinating, not recognizing the nurse or her surroundings. A fingerstick blood sugar reveals a level of 135. After a snack, her blood sugar increases to 189 and her mental status returns to baseline.

Teaching Points

- Older adults can become hypoglycemic at "normal" blood sugars if their baseline blood sugar is high.
- Delirium is often the only sign of hypothyroidism in an older adult.
- Functional changes (increased or decreased function) must be considered as a subtle indication of potential thyroid disorder.
- Sensory improvement can have positive effects on mood and outlook on life.
- Noncompliant diabetics who begin to follow prescribed regimens more carefully may become hypoglycemic and require an adjustment in their insulin dose.

INDEX

A

Abdominal pain, 210, 211*f*, 212*t*–214*t*
Absorption of substances, 509
Abuse, substance, 508
  See also Substance abuse issues
Abuse and neglect
  assessment, 532
  case studies, 540–542
  defining, 529–530
  financial/material, 535–536
  management, clinical, 536–540
  physical abuse, 533–534
  presentation, clinical, 531–532
  prevention, 536
  psychologic/emotional, 535
  risk factors, 531
  sexual abuse, 534–535
Acarbose, 363*t*, 364
Acetaminophen, 84, 105, 144, 407, 410
Acid suppressive medications, 204*t*
Acoustic neuroma, 100
Acrochordons, 423*t*
Actifed, 275*t*
Actinic keratosis, 424*t*
Activities of daily living (ADL)
  cerebrovascular accident, 316–317
  chronic obstructive pulmonary disease, 121
  congestive heart failure, 184
  instrumental, 21, 22*t*, 67, 184, 333, 565–566
  malnutrition, 226
  neurologic system, 312
  rheumatoid arthritis, 291
  screening and early detection, 21, 22*t*
  See also Exercise
Acute angle-closure glaucoma, 95
Acute gastritis, 208–209
Acute gastroenteritis, 214*t*
Acute gout, 287
Acute gout arthritis, 286
Acute labyrinthitis, 324*t*
Acute mesenteric artery ischemia, 214*t*

Acute respiratory diseases
  bronchitis, 143–145
  influenza, 143
  pneumonia, infectious, 145–150
  tuberculosis, 150–153
Acute situational anxiety, 41
Acute unilateral hearing loss, 102–103
Acyclovir, 436
Adaptin, 84
Adjuvant analgesics, 415, 416
Adrenal insufficiency, 372
Adrenergic inhibiting agents, 181*t*
Adrenocorticotropic hormone (ACTH), 287
Adverse drug reactions, 507–509
Aerobid, 135
Afrin, 275*t*
Afterload, 185*t*
Ageism, 530
Agency for Health Care Policy and Research (AHCPR), 448, 450
AIDS (acquired immune deficiency syndrome), 243, 430
Akathisia, 492–493
Akineton, 321
Albumin, 226, 228, 241, 242
Albuterol, 137, 138*t*, 139*t*
Alcohol, treatment/use issues around
  alcoholism
    assessment, 512, 513*t*–514*t*, 514
    management, clinical, 514–516
    presentation, clinical, 510–512, 511*t*–512*t*
    prevalence, 506
  anorexia, 201*t*
  breast cancer, 392
  chlorpropamide, 363
  coronary heart disease, 164
  dementia, 66*t*
  depression, 479

  gout, 286
  hypoglycemia, 366
  nutritional issues, 225*t*, 230*t*, 236*t*
  polypharmacy, 50
  urinary incontinence, 275*t*
Alcoholics Anonymous (AA), 516
Aldomet, 275*t*
Alendronate, 299
Alert-Care products for preventing falls, 351*t*
Alimed products for preventing falls, 352*t*–353*f*
Alkylating agents, 103*t*
Allegra, 108
Allerest, 275*t*
Allergic rhinitis, 107–108
Allergy and nutritional issues, 231*t*
Allopurinol, 288
Allylamines, 465, 465*t*
Al-Anon, 516
Alpha-adrenergic blockers, 275*t*
Alpha-glucosidase, 363, 364
Alpha-1 antitrypsin, 120, 127
Alprazolam, 416
Aluminum hydroxide, 225*t*
Alzheimer's disease (AD), 6
  case studies, 591–593, 601
  dementia, most commonly diagnosed, 57
  depression, 479
  diagnosis, differential, 58*t*–61*t*
  diagnosis, DSM-IV, 65*t*
  sleep disorders, 82
Amantadine, 3–4, 143, 318
Ambien, 83*t*
American Alzheimer's Association, 69
American Association of Retired Persons (AARP), 46
American Cancer Society (ACS), 2, 389, 396
American College of Physicians, 7
American College of Sports Medicine, 31, 32
American Diabetes Association (ADA), 359

American Dietetic Association, 37
American Foundation for
    Urologic Disease, 17
American Heart Association
    (AHA), 2, 164
American Lung Association, 137
American Nurses Association,
    548–549
Amikacin sulfate, 103*t*
Aminoglycoside antibiotics, 103*t*
Amiodarone, 175, 366
Amitriptyline, 52*t*, 415, 482*t*
Amoxapine, 482*t*
Amoxicillin, 105, 109, 206*t*, 278
Amoxil, 105
Amphetamines, 225*t*, 275*t*
Ampicillin, 109, 144
Anacin, 275*t*
Analgesics, 103*t*, 105, 109, 236*t*
    See also Pain
Androgens, 391
Anemias
    age-related changes, 377
    assessment, 379, 379*f*
    chronic disease, anemia of
        (ACD), 381
    hypothyroidism, 371
    macrocytic, 382–383
    microcytic, 379–381
    normocytic, 381–382
    nutritional issues, 232*t*,
        234*t*–235*t*
    presentation, clinical, 378–379,
        378*t*
    prevention, 377
Angina
    assessment, 169
    decubitus, 167
    education, client, 171
    management, clinical, 169–171
    nutritional issues, 231*t*
    presentation, clinical, 167–168,
        168*t*
Angioplasty, 172
Angiotensin-converting enzyme
    (ACE) inhibitors, 164,
    173, 181*t*, 185, 236*t*
Angular cheilitis, 431, 432*f*
Animal dander and asthma, 134*t*
Anorexia, 245, 246
    age-related changes, 199–200
    assessment, 200
    case study, 583
    collaboration and referral,
        200–202
    management, clinical, 200, 201*t*
    nutritional issues, 231*t*
    setting-specific issues, 200
Antabuse, 363

Antacids, 225*t*, 236*t*
Anterior cerebral artery, 313, 314*t*
Antiarrhythmics, 175, 236*t*, 275*t*
Antibiotics
    bronchitis, acute, 144
    debridement, 460
    diarrhea, 217
    diverticulitis, 219
    nutritional issues, 236*t*
    otitis externa, 105
    pressure ulcers, 463
    sinusitis, 109
    sty, 99
    urinary tract infections, 278
    venous ulceration, 447
    See also individual antibiotic
Anticholinergics
    asthma, 137, 139*t*
    bronchodilators, 125
    dementia, 66*t*
    glaucoma, 95
    Parkinson's disease, 321
    xerostomia, 114
Anticoagulation therapy, 375
Anticonvulsants
    nutritional issues, 236*t*
    osteoporosis, 298
    pain, neuropathic, 415–416
    seizures, 336, 337*t*–338*t*
    tinnitus, 106
Antidepressants
    anxiety, 487
    depression, 79
    glaucoma, 95
    nutritional issues, 236*t*
    sleep disorders, 84
    smoking cessation, 38
    suicide, 481–484, 482*t*
    tricyclic, 107, 226*t*, 246, 415,
        489
Antidiarrheal medications, 217
Antifungal drugs, 465*t*
Antihistamines, 66*t*, 95, 107–108,
    145, 225*t*
Antihyperglycemic agents, 363
Antihypertensive agents, 66*t*, 275*t*
Antimalarials, 103*t*
Antipsychotic medications, 78, 236*t*
Antipyretic analgesics, 144
Antiseizure medications, 66*t*
Antispasmodics, 219
Antithyroid drugs, 374–375
Anxiety
    age-related changes, 485–486
    assessment, 486–487
    management, clinical, 487–489
    presentation, clinical, 486, 486*t*
    rebound, 519
    situational, acute, 41

Anxiolytic sedatives, 416
Aortic stenosis, 168
Apathetic thyrotoxicosis, 373–375
Aplastic anemia, 382
Apnea-hypopnea events, 80
Appendicitis, 214*t*
Aqueous production, 95, 96
Aricept, 68
Artane, 321
Arterial ulcers of the lower
    extremities, 438*t*–439*t*
Arteries, cerebral, 313, 314*t*–315*t*
Arthritis
    acute gout, 287
    monarticular, 285
    osteoarthritis, 283–285
    See also Rheumatoid arthritis
Arthrography, 113
Ascorbic acid, 228*t*
Aspiration, 249
Aspirin
    cerebrovascular accident, 316
    coronary heart disease, 164,
        165–166
    hyperthyroidism, 375
    myocardial infarction, 173
    nutritional issues, 225*t*, 236*t*
    pain, 407
    preventive care, 5–6
    urinary system, 275*t*
Assessment. *See specific condition/
    disorder/disease/symptom*
Assistive devices for support/
    balance or ease of
    movement, 331
Asteatotic eczema, 427–429
Astemizole, 108
Asthma
    assessment, 129, 131
    education, client, 137,
        141*f*–142*f*, 143
    management, clinical, 131–137,
        132*t*, 133*f*, 134*t*–135*t*,
        138*t*–140*t*
    nutritional issues, 231*t*
    pathophysiology, 129
    presentation, clinical, 129
    severity, 129, 130*t*
Atherosclerosis, 162, 179, 188–
    189
Ativan, 416
Atrial fibrillation
    assessment, 175
    cardiac and noncardiac causes,
        174
    management, clinical, 175–177
Atrophic vaginitis, 260, 261, 265*t*
Atropine, 66*t*, 275*t*
Atrovent, 125, 137

Audiograms, 330
Audiometer, 19
Augmentation therapy, 127
Augmentin, 105
Auricle, 100
Autogenic training, 43*f*
Autolytic debridement, 461
Autonomy, 546–547, 553
Aversive conditioning and
 smoking cessation, 40
AV node dysfunction, 176
Axid, 204*t*
Axillary dissection, 393–394
Azathioprine, 292*t*
Azmacort, 135
Azoles, 465, 465*t*
Azulfidine, 292*t*

B

Bacillus proteus, 105
BACTEC_R system, 150
Bacterial conjunctivitis, 93
Bactrim, 105, 109, 145, 278
Balance/control disorders,
 324*t*–325*t*
 See also Dizziness
Balloon dilation, 280
Barbiturates, 107, 298, 518
Basal cell carcinomas, 17, 400,
 402
Basal energy expenditure, 241
Baseline bone mineral density
 (BMD), 298–300
Bath oil, 429
Beck Depression Inventory, 479
Beclomethasone, 135, 135*t*
Bed-Check Corp. products for
 preventing falls, 351*t*
Behavioral indications of
 alcoholism, 511
Behavioral indicators of
 prescription drug abuse,
 519, 520*t*
Behavior modification strategies
 for smoking cessation,
 38–41
 See also Counseling for health
 promotion behaviors
Bell's palsy, 339–341
Beneficence and nonmaleficence,
 548–549
Benign positional vertigo (BPV),
 326, 328, 331–332
Benign prostatic hyperplasia
 (BPH), 16, 82, 279–280
Bentyl, 275
Benzodiazepines, 52, 66*t*, 85, 488,
 517–519, 517*t*
Benztropine mesylate, 321

Bereavement. *See* Grief and loss
*Bereavement, Reactions, Consequences
 and Care,* 474
Best interest decisions, 548
Beta blockers
 angina, 170–171
 coronary heart disease, 164
 dementia, 66*t*
 glaucoma, 95, 96
 hyperthyroidism, 375
 myocardial infarction, 173
 nutritional issues, 236*t*
Betadine, 436
Betagan, 95
Beta-adrenergic antagonists, 366
Beta-lactam/lactamase inhibitor,
 145, 147
Beta₂-agonists, 138*t*–139*t*
Betaxolol, 95
Bethanechol, 204*t*
Bethesda System, 15
Betoptic, 95
Biaxin, 206*t*
Bigeriden, 321
Bile acid resins, 166*t*
Biofeedback, 275, 276*t*
Biotin, 228*t*
Bismuth subsalicylate, 206*t*, 217
Bitolterol, 138*t*, 139*t*
Bladder record, the completion
 of a, 266
Blepharitis, 92
Blepharochalasis, 92
Blood pressure, 7, 8*t*, 9
Blood tests, 330
Blood urea nitrogen (BUN), 200
Body composition, 221–222
Body mass index (BMI), 222
Body measurement, 9–10
Boils, 108
Bone, 110, 298–300
 See also Musculoskeletal system
Bowel obstruction, 214*t*
Bowel training program, 215*t*, 216
Braden Scale for predicting
 pressure sore risk,
 451*f*–452*f*
Bradykinesia, 319*t*
Brain stem evoked response
 audiometry (BERA), 330
Brain stem infarction, 324*t*
Brainstorming and clinically
 managing dementia, 71
Brain tumors, 324*t*
Breast cancer, 6, 13, 299, 392–394
Breathing, diaphragmatic, 44, 128
Breathing and smoking cessation,
 deep, 40
Brethair, 137

Bromocriptine, 85*t*, 321
Bromoquinine, 275*t*
Bromo Seltzer, 275*t*
Bronchitis
 acute, 143–145
 chronic, 120, 121
Bronchodilator therapy, 95,
 123–127, 126*t*
Bulimia, 245
Bulk-forming agents, 216, 219
Bullous pemphigoid, 434–435
Bumetanide, 103*t*
Buprenex, 411*t*
Buprenorphine, 411*t*
Bupropion, 482*t*
Burrow's solution, 436
Buspirone, 489
Butorphanol, 411*t*

C

Cadmium, 390
Caffeine, 275*t*, 332, 487
CAGE screening questionnaire,
 512, 514*t*
Calan, 275*t*
Calcitonin, 299, 305
Calcium, 238*t*, 241, 297, 300
Calcium channel blockers
 angina, 171
 congestive heart failure, 186
 hypertension, 181*t*
 myocardial infarction, 173
 nutritional issues, 236*t*
 sleep disorders, 82
 urinary system, 275*t*
Calories, 241, 330, 361
Cancer
 anorexia, 201*t*
 breast, 299, 392–394
 case study, 416–417
 cervical, 396–397
 colorectal, 397–399
 delirium, 395
 introduction, 389
 lung, 395–396
 prostate, 389–391
 screening
  breast, 13
  cervical/uterine and ovarian,
   13–15
  colorectal, 15–16
  oral cavity and pharyngeal,
   17
  prostate, 16–17
  skin, 17–18
 skin, 400–402
Candida infections, 431–432
Capacity, 547
Capsaicin, 436

Carbamazepine, 106, 338*t*, 415
Carbamide peroxide, 101
Carbohydrates, 232*t*, 237
Carbonic anhydrase inhibitors, 96
Carboplatin, 103*t*
Carcinoembryonic antigen
    (CEA), 399
Carcinomas. *See* Cancer
Cardiopulmonary resuscitation
    (CPR), 50
Cardioselective beta blockers, 375
Cardiovascular system
    abdominal pain, 213*t*
    alcohol abuse and dependence,
        511*t*
    angina
        assessment, 169
        education, client, 171
        management, clinical,
            169–171
        presentation, clinical,
            167–168, 168*t*
    atrial fibrillation
        assessment, 175
        cardiac and noncardiac
            causes, 174
        management, clinical,
            175–177
    case studies, 191–196, 595–596,
        600
    congestive heart failure
        age-related changes, 183
        assessment, 184
        education, client, 186
        management, clinical,
            185–186, 185*t*
        presentation, clinical,
            183–184
        setting-specific issues,
            187–188
    control balance disorders, 325*t*
    coronary heart disease
        age-related changes, 161–162
        assessment, 162–163
        education, client, 167
        management, clinical,
            163–166, 166*t*
        rehabilitation, 166
        setting-specific issues, 167
    deep venous thrombosis,
        190–191
    falls, 344*t*
    hypertension
        age-related changes, 178
        assessment, 179
        education, client, 182
        management, clinical,
            179–180, 181*t*, 182
        presentation, clinical,
            178–179

    setting-specific issues, 182
    two types of, 177
    introduction, 161
    myocardial infarction
        assessment, 171–172, 171*t*
        education, client, 174
        management, clinical,
            172–174
    peripheral vascular disease,
        188–190
    refeeding, 252*t*
    sleep disorders, 81
Cardizem, 275*t*
Cardura, 280
Caregivers who are the abusers,
    working with, 539
Carotid artery system, 313, 314*t*
Carpometacarpal (CMC) joint,
    284
Catapres, 275*t*
Cataracts, 92–93
Cathartics, 225*t*
Ceftriaxone sodium, 278
Cellulitis of the external ear, 100
Centers of Disease Control and
    Prevention, 31
Central nervous system
    stimulants, 95
    See also Neurologic system
Central vestibular disorders, 324*t*
Cephalexin, 447
Cephalexin monohydrate, 278
Cephalosporin, 105
Cerebellar ischemia, 324
Cerebrovascular accident (CVA)
    assessment, 312–313, 313*t*–315*t*,
        315
    atrial fibrillation, 174
    case studies, 612–613, 615–616
    falls, 344*t*
    management, clinical, 316–317
    Parkinson's disease
        defining, 317–318
        management, clinical, 318,
            320–322, 320*t*
        presentation, clinical, 318,
            319*t*–320*t*
        rehabilitation, 317
    risk factors for, 312
    seizures, 333
Cerumen impaction, 100–102
Cervical cancer, 13–15, 396–397
Cervical pathology of chest pain,
    168*t*
Cetearyl alcohol, 447
Cetirizine hydrochloride, 108
Chalazion, 93
Character disorders, 493–495
Chemoprophylaxis
    aspirin prophylaxis, 5–6

    hormone replacement therapy,
        6–7
Chemotherapy, 391, 394, 396, 399
Cherry angiomas, 425*t*
Chest wall causes of chest pain,
    168*t*
Chlamydia pneumoniae, 145
Chloramphenicol, 105
Chlordiazepoxide, 52*t*
Chloroquine hydrochloride, 103*t*
Chloroquine phosphate, 103*t*
Chlorpropamide, 52*t*, 363, 363*t*
Choking, 49–50
Cholecystitis, 214*t*
Choledocholithiasis, 209
Cholesterol, 10–13, 11*t*–12*t*, 162,
    164–166
Cholestyramine, 225*t*
Cholinergic agents, 95, 96, 321
Chronic allergic rhinitis, 107
Chronic bronchitis, 120, 121
Chronic gastritis, 208
Chronic gout, 286, 288
Chronic obstructive pulmonary
    disease (COPD), 81–82
    case study, 617–619
    complications, 128–129
    etiology, 120
    incidence, 120
    management, clinical, 123–128,
        124*t*–125*t*, 126*f*, 128*f*
    nutritional issues, 231*t*
    presentation, clinical, 121–123,
        121*f*
Chronic urinary incontinence,
    266, 278
Chronotropic state, 185*t*
Cigarette smoking. *See* Tobacco
    use
Ciliary action, 119
Cimetidine, 66*t*, 204*t*, 225*t*
Cipro, 447
Ciprofloxacin hydrochloride, 278,
    447
Cisapride, 203, 204, 204*t*
Cisplatin, 103*t*
Clarithromycin, 206*t*
Claritin, 108
Clavulanate, 105
*Clinician's Handbook of Preventive
    Services*, 1
Clock Medical Supply products
    for preventing falls, 351*t*
Clofibrate, 225*t*
Clomipramine, 489
Clonazepam, 85*t*, 338*t*
Cloxacillin, 105
Coarctation of the aorta, 179
Cobalamin, 227*t*
Code for Nurses, 548–549

Codeine, 85*t*, 275*t*, 410, 411*t*
Cogentin, 321
Cognex, 68
Cognitive issues
  assessment tool, mental status,
    569–576
  automobile use, 45
  balance/control disorders, 325,
    325*t*
  case study, 87–88
  delirium, 73
    assessment, 77–78
    management, clinical, 78
    presentation, clinical, 74,
      75*t*–76*t*, 76–77
    prevention, 74
  dementia, 58
    age-related changes, 62
    assessment, 62, 65, 66*t*,
      67–68, 67*f*
    diagnosis, differential,
      58*t*–61*t*
    management, clinical, 68–69,
      69*t*, 70*f*, 71–72
    presentation, clinical, 62,
      63*t*–65*t*
    setting-specific issues, 72–73,
      72*f*
  depression, 79
  hypothyroidism, 371
  introduction, 57
  Parkinson's disease, 320*t*
  sleep disorders
    age-related changes, 79–80
    assessment, 80–84, 81*f*, 83*t*
    education, client, 86–87
    management, clinical, 84–86,
      84*t*–85*t*
    presentation, clinical, 80
    therapies, cognitive-behavioral,
      481, 487–488
  urinary incontinence, 265*t*
Colchicine, 225*t*
Cold treatments and rheumatoid
    arthritis, 291
Collaborative/interdisciplinary
    involvement, 71
  See also specific condition/disorder/
    disease/symptom
Colles' fracture, 301–303, 301*f*
Color discrimination, 91
Colorectal cancer, 15–16, 397–399
Coma, hyperglycemic
    hyperosmolar nonketotic
    (HHNK), 369–369
Combination drug therapy, 293
Communal and individual rights
    and responsibilities,
    balancing, 553–554

Communicating effectively with
    emergency services
    personnel, APNs, 174
Communication and clinically
    managing dementia, 69,
    71
Communication disorder, 168
Complete blood count (CBC). *See*
    assessment *under specific*
    condition/disorder/disease/
    symptom
Complex partial seizures, 334,
    334*f*
Compression, 440–441
Compumed, Inc. products for
    preventing falls, 353*f*
Computed tomography (CT),
    302, 304, 306, 315, 330,
    520
Conductive hearing loss, 102
Confusion, 57, 73–74
    See also Delirium
Confusion: Prevention and Care
    (Wolanin & Phillip), 57
Congestive heart failure (CHF)
    age-related changes, 183
    assessment, 184
    case study, 615–616
    education, client, 186
    management, clinical, 185–186,
      185*t*
    presentation, clinical, 183–184
    setting-specific issues, 187–188
Conjunctivitis, 93–94
Constipation
    age-related changes, 210, 260
    management, clinical, 215–216,
      215*t*
    narcotics, 414
    presentation, clinical, 210–211,
      215
    urinary incontinence,
      264*t*–265*t*, 267
Consultation and clinically
    managing dementia, 71
Consumer Nutrition Hotline of
    National Center for
    Nutrition and Dietetics,
    37
Contact dermatitis, 430
Continuing care and diabetes,
    366–368
Continuity and clinically
    managing dementia, 71
Control/balance disorders,
    324*t*–325*t*
    See also Dizziness
Coordination and automobile
    use, 46
Cope, 275*t*

Coping technique, negative, 42
Cordarone, 370
Coronary artery bypass graft
    (CABG), 169–171
Coronary heart disease (CHD),
    10–12, 11*t*
    age-related changes, 161–162
    assessment, 162–163
    education, client, 167
    management, clinical, 163–166,
      166*t*
    rehabilitation, 166
    setting-specific issues, 167
Corticosteroids
    asthma, 134–136, 135*t*, 136,
      137, 139*t*–140*t*
    Bell's palsy, 341
    chronic obstructive pulmonary
      disease, 126–127
    contact dermatitis, 430
    gout, 287
    hyperglycemia, 366
    nutritional issues, 225, 236*t*
    rheumatoid arthritis, 291
    stasis dermatitis, 447
Cortisporin, 105
Cosmetics, 421–422
Cough, 121, 144
Coumadin, 176, 316
Counseling for health promotion
    behaviors
    injury prevention
      household injuries, 46–47,
        48*f*–49*f*, 49–50
      motor vehicle accidents,
        44–46
    nutrition, 33, 34*f*–35*f*, 35, 36*f*,
      37
    physical activity, 30–33
    polypharmacy, 50–51, 52*t*
    smoking cessation, 37–41,
      38*t*–39*t*
    stress management, 41–44,
      42*f*–44*f*
Cranberry juice, 279
Creatinine, 241
Creativity and clinically managing
    dementia, 71
Crioapophyseal joints, 289
Cromolyn, 136
Cuprimine, 292*t*
Cupulolithiasis theory, 331
Cyclandelate, 52*t*
Cyclobenzaprine, 52*t*
Cyclopentolate, 275*t*
Cyclophosphamide-doxorubicin-
    fluorouracil (CAF), 394
Cyclophosphamide-methotrexate-
    fluorouracil (CMF), 394
Cyclospasmol, 52*t*

D

Dakin's solution, 460
Dalmane, 52*t*
Danger, client in imminent, 537–538
Darvon, 52*t*, 85*t*, 275*t*, 407, 413*t*
Debridement, 445*t*–446*t*, 460–461
Debrox, 101
Decongestants, 109, 275*t*
Deep venous thrombosis (DVT), 190–191, 437
Degenerative disorders, 66*t*, 303
Dehydration, 248
Delegated autonomy, 546–547
Delirium, 73
    alcoholism, 510
    angina, 168
    assessment, 77–78, 577
    cancer, 395
    case study, 586, 605–607
    congestive heart failure, 184
    management, clinical, 78
    narcotics, 414–415
    presentation, clinical, 74, 75*t*–76*t*, 76–77
    prevention, 74
    sleep disorders, 82
    urinary incontinence, 261
    See also Dementia
Delusional depression, 479–480, 484
Dementia, 57
    age-related changes, 62
    angina, 168
    assessment, 62, 65, 66*t*, 67–68, 67*f*
    case studies, 587–591, 594–597, 599–600, 614–615
    comparison of acute confusion/depression and, 75*t*–76*t*
    depression, 79
    diagnosis, differential, 58*t*–61*t*
    eating disorders, 244–245
    light therapy, 86
    management, clinical, 68–69, 69*t*, 70*f*, 71–72
    presentation, clinical, 62, 63*t*–65*t*
    setting-specific issues, 72–73, 72*f*
    See also Delirium
"Dementia Care: Creating a Therapeutic Milieu," 73
Demerol, 275*t*, 407, 412*t*
DeMorgan's spots, 425*t*
Dental erosion, 202
Dentin, 110
Deoxyribonucleic acid (DNA) probe technology, 150

Depen, 292*t*
Dependence, substance, 508–509, 508*t*, 518–519
Depression
    age-related changes, 478
    anorexia, 201*t*
    assessment, 479
    cognitive issues, 79
    comparison of acute confusion/dementia and, 75*t*–76*t*
    delusional, 479–480, 484
    dementia, 58*t*–61*t*
    eating disorders, 245–246
    Geriatric Depression Scale, 567
    mania, 480
    presentation, clinical, 478
    prevalence, 477
    risk factors, 479
    See also Suicide
Depth perception, 91
Dermatitis
    contact, 430
    medicamentosa, 429
    perineal, 218
    seborrheic, 320*t*, 430
    stasis, 447
Dermatoses
    dermatitis medicamentosa, 429
    lichen simplex chronicus, 430–431
    seborrheic dermatitis, 430
    stasis dermatitis, 447
    xerosis, 427–429
Desipramine, 482*t*
Desyrel, 84
"Determine Your Nutritional Health," 33, 37
Dexamethesone, 316, 416
Dexfenfluramine, 229
Dexterity and urinary incontinence, 264*t*
Dextroamphetamine, 482*t*, 483, 484
Diabetes, 230*t*–231*t*, 350*t*
    age-related changes, 60
    assessment, 361
    case studies, 599–600, 615–616
    management, clinical, 361–368, 363*t*, 366–367*t*
    presentation, clinical, 360
    prevention, primary, 360–361
    setting-specific issues, 368–369
    three types of, 359–360
    ulcers of the lower extremities, 438*t*–439*t*
Diabetes Control and Complications Trial (DCCT), 366
Diabetic ketoacidosis (DKA), 368
Diabetic retinopathy, 94

Diabinese, 52*t*
Diagnostic and Statistical Manual of Mental Disorders (DSM-IV), 62, 478, 491, 508, 508*t*, 509
Diagnostic studies. *See specific condition/disorder/disease/symptom*
Diamox, 96
Diaphragmatic breathing, 128
DIAPPERS mnemonic, 261, 263, 265
Diarrhea, 216–217, 251–252*t*
Diastolic dysfunction, 183–184
Diazepam, 52*t*, 337*t*
Dicloxacillin, 99
Dicyclamine, 275
Diet. *See* Nutritional issues
Dietary Guidelines for Americans, 33, 35
Digital rectal exam (DRE), 15, 16
Digoxin, 176, 185–186, 375
Dilantin, 415
Dilatation of the urethra, 280
Dilaudid, 410, 411*t*
Diphtheria, 4–5
Diproprionate, 135, 135*t*
Dipyridamole, 52*t*
Dipyridamole-thallium test, 163
Direct autonomy, 546–547
Direct observation therapy (DOT), 152
Disease-modifying antirheumatic drugs (DMARDs), 293
Disequilibrium, 323
    See also Dizziness
Disopyramide, 66*t*
Displaced Colles' fracture, 302–303
Disseminating herpes, 436
Distal interphalangeal (DIP) joint, 284
Distribution of metabolites, 509
Disulfiram, 363
Ditropan, 275
Diuretics
    congestive heart failure, 185
    dizziness, 332
    gallbladder disease, 209
    gout, 286
    hyperglycemia, 366
    hypertension, 181*t*
    nutritional issues, 236*t*
    xerostomia, 114
Diverticulitis, 214*t*, 218–219, 233*t*
Diverticulosis, 233*t*
Dizziness, 322
    age-related changes, 323
    assessment, 326, 327*f*–329*f*, 328–330

case study, 616–617
management, clinical, 330–332
presentation, clinical, 323,
    324t–325t, 326
setting-specific issues, 322–323
Docusate sodium, 216
Dolophine, 412t
Donepezil, 68
Dopa decarboxylase inhibitors, 320
Dopamine, 321
Doppler ultrasound, 190
Doxazosin, 280
Doxepin, 84, 482t
Doxycycline, 109
D-penicillamine, 292t
Dressings and wound
    management, 442t–443t,
    461–462
Dristan, 275t
Driver education programs, 46
Drugs. *See* Medications; Substance
    abuse issues; *individual
    drug*
Dry eye syndrome, 96
Dual x-ray absorptiometry
    (DEXA), 298, 299
Duodenal ulcers, 205
Dysphagia, 114, 246–248
Dyspnea, 121, 127

E

Ears
    age-related changes, 100
    audiograms, 330
    control/balance disorders, 325
    disorders, common
        acoustic neuroma, 100
        cellulitis of the external ear,
            100
        cerumen impaction, 100–102
        hearing impairment,
            102–104
        mastoiditis, 104
        otitis externa, 104–105
        otitis interna, 105
        otitis media, 105
        ototoxicity, 104–105
        tinnitus, 105–106
        tympanic membrane
            perforation, 106–107
        tympanosclerosis, 107
    falls, 347t–348t
Eating disorders
    bulimia, 245
    case study, 583
    dementia, 244–245
    depression, 245–246
    dysphagia, 246–248
    See also Anorexia; Malnutrition;
        Nutritional issues

Ectropion, 94
Eczema, asteatotic, 427–429
Edema
    facial, 617
    hip, about the, 306
    nutritional issues, 232t
    refeeding, 251t
    venous insufficiency, 437, 439
Education, client
    abuse and neglect, 538–539
    alcoholism, 515
    angina, 171
    asthma, 137, 141f–142f, 143
    Bell's palsy, 340, 341
    breast cancer, 394
    cancer, 391
    congestive heart failure, 186
    coronary heart disease, 167
    cosmetics, 422
    diabetes, 367, 368
    gastroesophageal reflux
        disease, 203
    health promotion for the
        elderly, 27
    hormone replacement therapy,
        7
    hypertension, 182
    hyperthyroidism, 374–375
    injuries, preventing, 50
    iron deficiency, 381
    myocardial infarction, 174
    polypharmacy, 51
    prescription drug abuse, 522
    rheumatoid arthritis, 291
    seizures, 339
    skin, 421
    sleep disorders, 86–87
    urinary tract infections, 279
    vertebral compression fracture,
        304
    *See also specific condition/disorder/
        disease/symptom under*
        Preventive care
Elavil, 52t
Eldepryl, 321
Electrical stimulation therapy,
    275, 276t–277t
Electrocardiographic recordings
    (ECGs), 123, 163, 203,
    315, 514, 520
Electroconvulsive therapy (ECT),
    484–485
Electroencephalograms (EEGs),
    514, 520
Electromyography stimulation,
    341
Electronystagmography, 330
Elevated creatine phosphokinase
    (CPK), 371

Elevating the extremity and
    venous ulceration,
    440–441
Emphysema, 120
Enamel, tooth, 110
Encephalopathies, 66t
Endocrine and hematologic
    systems, 82
    anemias
        age-related changes, 377
        assessment, 379, 379f
        macrocytic, 382–383
        microcytic, 379–381
        normocytic, 381–382
        presentation, clinical,
            378–379, 378t
        prevention, 377
    case study, 384–386
    diabetes
        age-related changes, 360
        assessment, 361
        management, clinical,
            361–368, 363t, 366t–367t
        presentation, clinical, 360
        prevention, primary, 360–361
        setting-specific issues,
            368–369
        three types of, 359–360
    falls, 350t
    introduction, 359
    leg ulcers, 440t
    thyroid disorders
        age-related changes, 370
        hormone production, 369
        hyperthyroidism, 373–375
        hypothyroidism, 370–372
        nodules, thyroid, 376–377
    urinary incontinence, 263
Endoscopic retrograde
    cholangiopancreatograp
    hy (ERCP), 209
Endurance, physical, 222
Enema, tap water, 216
Energy needs, 237
Enoxaparin, 191
Enteral nutrition
    access, 248
    complications, 249, 250t–252t,
        252–253
    prescriptions, 248–249
Entex LA, 108, 109
Entropion, 94
Environment, the
    asthma, triggers for, 132, 134t
    dementia, clinically managing,
        71
    skin, 421, 428
Enzymatic debriding agents,
    445t–446t
Epileptics, 333

Epistaxis, 108
Equanil, 52*t*
Erythema, 105, 430
Erythrocyte sedimentation rate
    (ESR), 322, 381
Erythromycin, 105, 144, 145
Escherichia coli, 217, 278
Estazolam, 83*t*
Estramustine phosphate, 391
Estrogen
    breast cancer, 6, 394
    coronary heart disease, 164
    gallbladder disease, 209
    lipid-lowering agent, 166*t*
    minimum effective dose, 7
    osteoporosis, 299
    photoaging, 422
    uterine cancer, 14
Ethacrynate sulfate, 103*t*
Ethacrynic acid, 103*t*, 225*t*
Ethambutol, 152
Ethical issues
    information, where to go for,
        555–556
    introduction, 545–546
    key concepts, 555
    nursing, core ethical concepts in
        beneficence and
            nonmaleficence, 548–549
        conclusions, 555
        patient-based principles,
            546–548
        planning, responsibilities for
            advance care, 549–550
    setting-specific issues
        home-based services,
            550–551
        hospital settings, acute,
            551–552
        managed-care environments,
            554
        nursing homes, 552–554
Ethosuximide, 338*t*
Exacerbations
    asthma, 137, 143
    chronic obstructive pulmonary
        disease, 128–129
    hypotension, 332
    urinary incontinence, 278
Examination, physical. *See specific
    condition/disorder/disease/
    symptom*
Excedrin, 275*t*
Excretion, 509–510
Exercise
    asthma induced by, 134*t*
    constipation, 216
    coronary heart disease, 166
    diabetes, 361, 362
    dizziness, 331

health promotion for the
    elderly, 30–33
    osteoarthritis, 285
    osteoporosis, 301
    rheumatoid arthritis, 291
    smoking cessation, 40
See also Activities of daily living
    (ADL)
Expectations and clinically
    managing dementia, 71
Extracorporeal shockwave
    lithotripsy (ESWL), 209
Extrapyramidal movement
    disorders, 318
Exudate absorbers, 443*t*–444*t*
Eyes
    age-related changes, 91–92
    Bell's palsy, 339–341
    case study, 115–116
    disorders, common
        blepharitis, 92
        blepharochalasis, 92
        cataracts, 92–93
        chalazion, 93
        conjunctivitis, 93–94
        diabetic retinopathy, 94
        ectropion, 94
        entropion, 94
        glaucoma, 94–96
        keratoconjunctivitis, 96
        macular degeneration, 96
        pinguecula, 97, 97*f*
        presbyopia, 97
        pterygium, 97, 98*f*
        ptosis, 97
        retinal detachment, 97–98
        retinal vein occlusion, 98, 99*f*
        sty, 98–99
        subconjunctival hemorrhage,
            99
    falls, 347*t*

F
Facial edema, 617
Facial paralysis, 339–341
Falls, 46–47
    assessment, 342–343, 344*t*–350*t*
    case study, 584, 598–599
    management, clinical, 343,
        351*f*–354*f*, 354
    presentation, clinical, 341–342
Famciclovir, 436
Family
    abusers, working with
        family/caregivers who
        are the, 539
    alcoholism and family therapy,
        516
    home care, 551
    values, 530

Famotidine, 204*t*, 206
Fat in the diet, 237
Fecal incontinence, 217–218
Fecal occult blood (FOB), 15
Fentanyl, 411*t*, 414, 415*t*
Ferrous sulfate, 380
Festinant gait, 319*t*
Fexofenadine, 108
Fibric acid derivatives, 166*t*
Fibrocystic disease, 392
Fibroepithelial polyp, 423*t*
Film dressings, 442*t*–443*t*
Financial/material abuse/neglect,
    530, 535–536
Finasteride, 280, 464
Fish and cholesterol, 164
Flavoxate, 275
Flexeril, 52*t*
Flexibility exercises, 32
Florinef, 332
Flovent, 135
Fludrocortisone, 332
Flunisolide, 135, 135*t*
Fluorouracil, 399
Fluorouracil-doxorubicin-
    cyclophosphamide
    (FAC), 394
Fluoxetine, 482*t*, 488
Flurazepam, 52*t*
Fluticasone, 135, 135*t*
Fluvoxamine, 482*t*
Foam dressings, 443*t*
Folic acid, 86, 227*t*, 234*t*, 238*t*,
    383
Food and Drug Administration
    (FDA), 50, 299, 300, 365,
    523
Food Guide Pyramid, 33, 36*f*
Fosamax, 299
Fractures. *See* Musculoskeletal
    system
Functional Activities
    Questionnaire, 67
Functional status, 21–22, 22*t*
Functional urinary incontinence,
    267*t*, 277
Fungal skin conditions. *See*
    Parasitic and fungal skin
    conditions
Furosemide, 103*t*, 225*t*
Furuncles, 108

G
Gabapentin, 416
Gallbladder disease, 209–210
Gastritis, 208–209
Gastroenteritis, acute, 214*t*
Gastroesophageal reflux disease
    (GERD), 85, 202–204

Gastrointestinal system (GI)
  abdominal pain, 210, 211*f*,
    212*t*–214*t*
  alcohol abuse and dependence,
    511*t*
  anorexia
    age-related changes, 199–200
    collaboration and referral,
      200–202
    management, clinical, 200,
      201*t*
    setting-specific issues, 200
  case study, 219, 596
  chest pain, 168*t*
  constipation
    age-related changes, 210
    management, clinical,
      215–216, 215*t*
    presentation, clinical,
      210–211, 215
  corticosteroids, 136
  diarrhea, 216–217
  diverticulitis, 218–219
  falls, 348*t*
  fecal incontinence, 217–218
  gallbladder disease, 209–210
  gastritis, 208–209
  gastroesophageal reflux
    disease, 202–204
  introduction, 199
  metformin, 364
  nutritional issues, 222, 231*t*,
    232*t*
  peptic ulcer disease
    age-related changes, 204–205
    assessment, 205
    management, clinical,
      205–208, 206*t*, 207*f*–208*f*
    presentation, clinical, 205
  sleep disorders, 82
Gastrostomy tubes, 248
Gawthorne-Cooksey exercises, 331
Generalized anxiety disorder, 486*t*
Generalized seizures, 334, 334*f*
Genitourinary system (GU)
  abdominal pain, 213*t*
  age-related changes, 259–260
  alcohol abuse and dependence,
    511*t*
  benign prostatic hyperplasia,
    279–280
  case study, 280–282
  falls, 348*t*
  introduction, 259
  pathophysiology problems
    urinary frequency, 260–261
    urinary incontinence
      assessment, 266–267,
        268*f*–272*f*
      case study, 584–585, 600

DIAPPERS mnemonic,
  261, 263, 265
  management, clinical, 271,
    273*f*–274*f*, 274–275,
    275*t*–277*t*, 277–278
  symptoms and subtypes,
    262*t*–263*t*
  transient or acute,
    factors/causes of, 261,
    264*t*–265*t*
  urinary tract infections, 82,
    278–279, 585
Gentamicin, 225*t*, 463
Gentamicin sulfate, 103*t*
Geriatric Depression Scale (GDS),
  479
Giant cell arteritis (GCA), 322
  age-related changes, 295
  assessment, 295
  clinical findings, 294*t*
  constitutional symptoms of,
    295
  management, clinical, 295–296,
    296*t*
  polymyalgia rheumatica
    grouped with, 294
Glare from windows and polished
  floors, 92
Glaucoma, 94–96
Glimepiride, 363*t*
Glipizide, 363*t*
Global Deterioration Scale, 62,
  63*t*–64*t*, 65
Global Utilization of Streptokinase
  and Tissue Plasminogen
  Activator for Occluded
  Coronary Artery Trial
  (GUSTO), 172
Glucose intolerance, 350*t*, 359,
  360
  See also Diabetes
Glyburide, 363*t*
Glycerin suppository, 216
Gold, 292*t*
Gout
  age-related changes, 286
  assessment, 286–287
  definition of, 285
  management, clinical, 287–288
  presentation, clinical, 286
Granulocytosis, 374
Grave's disease, 374
Grief and loss
  advanced practice nurses,
    476–477
  age-related changes, 474
  presentation, clinical, 474, 475*t*
  risk factors, 474–476
Guide to Clinical Preventive Services,
  The, 1

Guinine sulfate, 103*t*
Gums, 110
Gynecologic system and
  abdominal pain, 213*t*

H

Haemophilus influenzae, 143–145,
  147
Halcion, 83*t*
Hallpike-Dix maneuver, 326,
  329–330
Haloperidol, 491
Hamilton Depression Rating
  Scale, 479
Hands and smoking cessation,
  substitute activities for,
  40–41
Harmonic acceleration testing,
  330
Harris Benedict equation, 241
Hashimoto's thyroiditis, 374
H_2-blocker therapy, 203, 236*t*, 285
Head positioning exercises, 331
Healing process and venous
  uclers/wound
  management, 462–463
Health belief model (HBM),
  29–30
Health habits, poor, 42–43
Health promotion for the elderly
  case study, 53–54
  counseling for health
    promotion behaviors, 30
  injury prevention
    household injuries, 46–47,
      48*f*–49*f*, 49–50
    motor vehicle accidents,
      44–46
  nutrition, 33, 34*f*–35*f*, 35, 36*f*,
    37
  physical activity, 30–33
  polypharmacy, 50–51, 52*t*
  smoking cessation, 37–41,
    38*t*–39*t*
  stress management, 41–44,
    42*f*–44*f*
  introduction, 27–28
  learning principles, adult,
    28–29
  teaching considerations for the
    older adult, 29–30, 30*t*
  See also Preventive care
Hearing
  acuity, 19–20, 20*f*, 30*t*, 45
  impairment, 102–104
  See also Ears
Heart disease and nutritional
  management, 231*t*
  See also Cardiovascular system

Heat treatments and rheumatoid
    arthritis, 291
Heberden's nodes, 284
Heimlich maneuver, 50
Helicobacter pylori, 204–205, 206*t*,
    208, 209
Helidac therapy, 206*t*
Hematologic system. *See*
    Endocrine and
    hematologic systems
Hemolytic anemia, 382
Heparin, 298
Hepatic hydroxymethylglutaryl
    coenzyme A (HMG
    CoA), 165, 166*t*
Herpes zoster, 324*t*, 435–437
High-density lipoprotein (HDL),
    10, 12, 165
Hip, osteoarthritis of the, 284
Hip fracture, 305–306, 305*t*,
    597–598
Hismanal, 108
Histamine H$_2$-receptor
    antagonists, 204*t*, 206
History. *See specific condition/
    disorder/disease/symptom*
HIV (human immunodeficiency
    virus), 151
Home-based services, 128, 317,
    322, 367, 550–551
Homeopathic remedies, 85–86
Home Safety Checklist for Older
    Adults, 47, 48*f*–49*f*
Hormone replacement therapy
    (HRT), 6–7, 165, 298,
    299
Hospital settings and ethical
    issues, 551–552
Household injuries, 46–47,
    48*f*–49*f*, 49–50
Hutchinson's sign, 436
Hydralazine, 186
Hydration level, 267
Hydrocephalic disorders, 66*t*
Hydrochloride, 108, 217
Hydrocolloids, 442*t*
Hydrocortisone, 105
Hydrogels, 444*t*–445*t*
Hydromorphone, 410, 411*t*
Hydrophilic muccoloid, 216
Hydrotherapy, 460–461
Hydroxychloroquine, 292*t*
Hydroychloroquine sulfate, 103*t*
Hypercalcemia, 260
Hypercholesterolemia, 371
Hyperglycemia, 360
    coma, hyperglycemic
        hyperosmolar nonketotic
        (HHNK), 368–369
    complications of, acute, 368

corticosteroids, 136
drugs associated with, 366
refeeding, 250*t*
Hypericum, 482*t*
Hyperkalemia, 232*t*, 250*t*
Hyperphosphatemia, 232*t*
Hypertension (HTN)
    age-related changes, 178
    allergic rhinitis, 108
    assessment, 179
    case study, 615–616
    cerebrovascular accident, 312
    coronary heart disease, 163
    corticosteroids, 136
    diastolic dysfunction, 183
    dizziness, 332
    education, client, 182
    epistaxis, 108
    gout, 285, 286
    hearing loss, acute unilateral,
        102
    life-style modifications, 9*t*
    management, clinical, 179–180,
        181*t*, 182
    obesity, 221
    presentation, clinical, 178–179
    screening and early detection, 7
    setting-specific issues, 182
    sleep disorders, 81
    tinnitus, 106
    two types of, 177
Hyperthermia, transurethral,
    280
Hyperthyroidism, 175, 373–375
Hypertriglyceridemia, 286
Hypertrophic cardiomyopathy,
    168
Hyperuricemia, 286
Hypoalbuminemia, 238
Hypocalcemia, 251*t*
Hypoglycemia, 175, 362, 364, 366
Hypokalemia, 250*t*
Hypomagnesemia, 251*t*
Hypophosphatemia, 250*t*
Hypotension, 106, 325*t*, 332
Hypothyroidism, 370–372, 374,
    375, 381
Hypoxia, 175
Hysterectomy, 7
Hytrin, 280

I

Ideal body weight (IBW), 222
Imipramine, 275, 482*t*, 489
Immune system and nutritional
    issues, 235, 237, 242
Immunizations
    influenza, 3–4, 128
    pneumonia, 4, 128

tetanus and diphtheria, 4–5
    therapy, immunization, 137
Immunoglobulin A, 119
Immunologic response,
    decreased, 119
Imuran, 292*t*
Incapacitated autonomy, 547
Incontinence
    fecal, 217–218
    urinary. *See* pathophysiology
        problems *under*
        Genitourinary system
        (GU)
Individual and communal rights
    and responsibilities,
    balancing, 553–554
*Individualized Dementia Care:
    Creative, Compassionate
    Approaches* (Rader), 73
Individual needs and clinically
    managing dementia, 71
Indomethacin, 52*t*, 103*t*
Infection
    abdominal pain, 213*t*
    anorexia, 201*t*
    dementia, 66*t*
    gout, 285–286
    leg ulcers, 440*t*
    nosocomial, 239
    urinary incontinence, 264*t*
Inflammatory bowel disease, 214*t*
Influenza, 3–4, 143
Inhalation therapy, 123–127, 126*t*,
    134–137, 135*t*
Injury prevention
    household injuries, 46–47,
        48*f*–49*f*, 49–50
    motor vehicle accidents, 44–46
    wound management, 5. *See also*
        Pressure ulcers and
        wound management
Inotropic state, 185*t*
Insight-oriented psychotherapy, 481
Insomnia, 84*t*, 85
Institutionalized elderly, 239
Instrumental activities of daily
    living (IADL), 21, 22*t*,
    67, 184, 333, 565–566
    See also Activities of daily living
        (ADL)
Insulin and insulin analogues,
    363, 365–366, 366*t*
    See also Diabetes
Intal, 136
Integumentary issues
    case studies, 466–470
    hair, 464
    nails, 464–466
    See also Skin
Intercritical gout, 286

Intergenerational expectations, confusion regarding, 551
Internal carotid artery, 313, 314*t*
International Study of Infarct Survivors, The Fourth (ISIS-4), 173
Interpersonal therapies, 481
Intertrigo, 431–432
Iodine, 228*t*
Iodine, radioactive (I¹³¹), 375
Ipratropium bromide, 125, 137, 139*t*
Iridotomy, laser, 96
Iron, 228*t*, 238*t*
Iron deficiency anemia, 379–381
Irrigation and cerumen impaction, 101
Irritable bowel syndrome, 233*t*
Ischemia, 162, 324*t*
Isocarboxazid, 482*t*
Isolated systolic hypertension (ISH), 177
Isoniazid (INH), 152
Isoxsuprine, 52*t*
Itraconazole, 465

J

Jejunostomy tubes, 248
Joint National Committee Fifth Report on Detection, Evaluation and Treatment of High Blood Pressure in 1993, 177, 179
Judgment, substituted, 547–548
Justice in congregate settings, defining, 554

K

Kanamycin sulfate, 103*t*
Keflex, 447
Keratoconjunctivitis, 96
Keratosis, actinic and seborrheic, 424*t*–425*t*
Ketoconazole, 430
Klebsiella pneumoniae, 278
Klonopin, 85*t*
Knee, osteoarthritis of the, 284
K⁺-sparing diuretics, 185
Kyphosis, 304

L

Laboratory data. *See specific condition/disorder/disease/symptom*
Labyrinthectomy, 332
Labyrinthine trauma, 324*t*
Labyrinthitis, acute, 324*t*

Lactic Dehydrogenase (LDH) level, 382
Lacunar infarcts, 313, 315
Lanolin, 447
Lansoprazole, 203, 204*t*
Laparoscopic cholecystectomy, 209
Laryngeal obstruction and rheumatoid synovitis of the cricoapophyseal joints, 289
Laryngitis, viral, 114
Laser iridotomy, 96
Laxatives, 210, 216, 236*t*
Learning principles, adult, 28–29
Left ventricular function (LV), 169
Left ventricular hypertrophy (LVH), 168
Legionella, 145, 147
Legislation
    Omnibus Budget and Reconciliation Act, 354, 549
    Patient Self-Determination Act (PSDA) of 1990, 549, 550
Leg ulcers, 440*t*, 446*t*
Lesions
    noduloulcerative, 400
    Norwegian scabies, 433
    skin, noncancerous, 422, 423*t*–426*t*
    sun-induced, 421
    See also Cancer; Tumors
Leucovorin, 399
Leukotriene inhibitors/modifiers, 136
Levamisole, 399
Levobunolol, 95
Levodopa, 225*t*, 321
Levodopa-benserazide, 320
Levodopa-carbidopa, 320
Levo-Dromoran, 414
Levoprome, 412*t*
Levorphanol, 412*t*
Levorphanol tartrate, 414
Levothyroxine, 371–372
Librium, 52*t*
Lichen simplex chronicus, 430–431
Life expectancy, 1
Life-style modifications, 9, 9*t*
    coronary heart disease, 166
    dizziness, 332
    hypertension, 179–180
    osteoporosis, 301
Light therapy, 86
Lipid-lowering agents, 166*t*
Lipoproteins, 10–12, 162, 164, 165, 364

Lips, 109
Lithium, 82, 366, 484
Lithium carbonate, 246
Liver function, 241, 364, 509, 511*t*
Loop diuretics, 103*t*, 181*t*
Loperamide, 217
Loratadine, 108
Lorazepam, 337*t*, 416, 488
Lovenox, 191
Lower esophageal sphincter (LES), 202
Lower leg edema, 437
Low-density lipoprotein (LDL), 10, 12, 162, 164, 165, 364
Low-molecular-weight heparin (LMWH), 191
Lumbar fractures, 304
Lumpectomy, 393
Lung cancer, 395–396
    See also obstructive lung diseases *under* Respiratory system
Luteinizing hormone, 391
Lymphadenopathy, 105
Lymphedema, 440*t*
Lymphocytes, 242

M

Macrocytic anemias, 382–383
Macrolides, 145, 147
Macular degeneration, 96
Madopar, 320
Magellan products for preventing falls, 354*f*
Magnesium, 238*t*
Magnesium hydroxide, 414
Magnetic resonance imaging (MRI), 113, 302, 304, 306, 315, 514, 520
Malnutrition
    age-related changes, 235, 238*t*
    assessment, 239, 240*t*, 241–242
    chronic disease, 235
    collaboration and referral, 243
    immune system, 235, 237
    management, clinical, 242–243
    presentation, clinical, 237–239
Mammography, 393
Managed-care environments, 554
Management, clinical. *See* Medications; *specific condition/disorder/disease/symptom*
Mania, 480, 484
Mastectomy, 393
Mastoiditis, 104
Meclizine hydrochloride, 330–331
Medicare, 243

Medications
  alcoholism, 514
  allergic rhinitis, 107–108
  angina, 170–171
  angular cheilitis, 431, 432*f*
  anorexia, 201*t*
  anxiety, 488–489
  asthma, 134–137, 135*t*,
      138*t*–140*t*
  atrial fibrillation, 176–177
  Bell's palsy, 341
  benign prostatic hyperplasia, 280
  bronchitis, acute, 144
  bullous pemphigoid, 435
  cerebrovascular accident, 316
  cerumen impaction, 101
  character disorders, 494
  chemoprophylaxis
    aspirin prophylaxis, 5–6
    hormone replacement
        therapy, 6–7
  chronic obstructive pulmonary
      disease, 123–127, 126*t*
  cognitive or affective change,
      causing, 66*t*
  congestive heart failure,
      185–186
  coronary heart disease,
      165–166, 166*t*
  cross-tolerance/dependence, 519
  deep venous thrombosis, 191
  delirium, 74
  dementia, 68–69, 69*t*, 70*f*, 71–72
  depression, 479
  diabetes, 362–366, 363*t*, 366*t*
  diarrhea, 217
  dizziness, 330–331
  gastroesophageal reflux
      disease, 203–204, 205*t*
  glaucoma, 95, 96
  gout, 287–288
  hair, 464
  hearing loss, 102, 103*t*
  herpes zoster, 436
  hypertension, 180, 181*t*
  hyperthyroidism, 374–375
  hypothyroidism, 371, 372
  iron deficiency, 380–381
  malnutrition, 243
  myocardial infarction, 173
  nails, 465, 465*t*
  nutritional states influenced by,
      222, 225*t*–226*t*
  osteoarthritis, 285
  osteoporosis, 298, 299
  otitis interna, 105
  otitis media, 105
  pain, 405, 407, 410, 411*t*–413*t*,
      414–415
  Parkinson's disease, 318, 321

  peptic ulcer disease, 205–208,
      206*t*, 207*f*–208*f*
  pneumonia, 145, 147
  polypharmacy, 50–51, 52*t*, 507
  rheumatoid arthritis, 292, 293,
      293*t*
  schizoaffective disorder, 491–492
  seizures, 336, 337*t*–338*t*
  sleep disorders, 82, 83*t*, 84–86,
      85*t*
  smoking cessation, 38
  suicide, 481–484, 482*t*
  temporal arteritis, 322
  tinnitus, 106
  tuberculosis, 152–153
  urinary incontinence, 261,
      265*t*, 271, 275, 275*t*
  xerosis, 429
  xerostomia, 113
  See also Immunizations;
      Prescription drug use;
      individual drug
Melanoma, 18, 401, 402
Melatonin, 86
Memory-enhancement drugs, 68
Ménière's disease, 324*t*, 332
Meningitis encephalitis, 324*t*
Menopause, 7, 14, 260, 297
Mental status assessment tool,
    569–576
Meperidine, 412*t*
Meperidine hydrochloride, 407
Meprobamate, 52*t*
Mesenteric artery ischemia, acute,
    214*t*
Mesylate, 85*t*
Metabolic disorders
  alcohol abuse and dependence,
      511*t*
  anorexia, 201*t*
  encephalopathies, 66*t*
  leg ulcers, 440*t*
  See also Endocrine and
      hematologic systems
Metacarpophalangeal (MCP)
    joint, 288
Metatarsophalangeal (MTP) joint,
    284
Metformin, 363*t*, 364–365
Methadone, 275*t*, 412*t*, 414
Methimazole, 374
Methocarbamol, 52*t*
Methotrexate, 292*t*, 399
Methotrimeprazine, 412*t*
Methylphenidate, 482*t*, 483, 484
Methylprednisolone, 139*t*
Metoclopramide, 203–204, 204*t*
Metronidazole, 206*t*, 463
Metropolitan Life Insurance
    Company, 10

Michigan Alcohol Screening Test
    (MAST), 512, 513*t*
Microcytic anemia, 379–381
Micronutrient supplementation,
    229
Midcerebral artery, 313, 314*t*
Migral, 275*t*
Milk of Magnesia, 414
Miltown, 52*t*
Minerals, 237
Mini-Mental State Exam (MMSE),
    45, 65, 67, 77, 559–562,
    594
Minipress, 275*t*, 280
Minoxidil, 464
Misuse of a substance, 507–508
Mites, 134*t*, 432
Mixed hearing loss, 102
Mixed urinary incontinence,
    262*t*, 267*t*, 277
Mobility and urinary
    incontinence, 264*t*
Monitoring
  cerebrovascular accident, 316
  glucose levels, 367
  pain, 407, 408*f*–409*f*
  prescription drug abuse, 521
  pulmonary function, 131–132,
      141*f*
  secretions, 247
Monoamine oxidase inhibitors
    (MAOIs), 107, 246, 321,
    483
Moraxella catarrhalis, 144, 145, 147
Morganella morganii, 278
Morphine, 275*t*, 410, 411*t*
Mortality
  atrial fibrillation, 174
  cancer, 389, 390
  cardiovascular disease, 161
  cerebrovascular accident, 312
  cervical cancer, 396
  colorectal cancer, 399
  hip fractures, 305–306
  hypertension, 177
  mastectomy, 393
  myocardial infarction, 173
  obesity, 221
  pneumonia, 148
  pressure ulcers, 448
  seizures, 333
Motor vehicle accidents, 44–46
Mouth
  age-related changes, 109–110
  aphthous ulcers, 110
  black tongue, 110
  candidiasis, 110–111
  geographic tongue, 111
  herpes simplex, 111–112
  leukoplakias, 112

oral cavity and pharyngeal
  cancer, 17
periodontal disease, 112–113
sialadenitis, 113
temporomandibular joint
  dysfunction, 113
Multiple sclerosis, 324*t*
Muscle
  Bell's palsy, 341
  genitourinary system and age-
    related changes, 260
  relaxants (drugs), 52
  relaxation exercises, 42*f*
  strengthening exercises, 32–33
  tone, 271
  wasting, 232*t*
Musculoskeletal system
  agility, 30*t*
  case study, 307–308
  falls, 346*t*
  fractures
    Colles' fracture, 301–303, 301*f*
    hip, 305–306, 305*t*, 597–598
    vertebral compression
      fracture, 303–305
  giant cell arteritis
    age-related changes, 295
    assessment, 295
    clinical findings, 294, 294*t*
    constitutional symptoms of,
      295*t*
    management, clinical,
      295–296, 296*t*
    polymyalgia rheumatica
      grouped with, 294
  gout
    age-related changes, 286
    assessment, 286–287
    definition of, 285
    management, clinical,
      287–288
    presentation, clinical, 286
  osteoarthritis, 283–285
  osteoporosis
    assessment, 297–299
    defining, 296–297
    management, clinical,
      299–301
  polymyalgia rheumatica
    age-related changes, 295
    assessment, 295
    clinical findings, 293, 293*t*
    constitutional symptoms of,
      295*t*
    giant cell arteritis grouped
      with, 294
    management, clinical,
      295–296, 296*t*
  rheumatoid arthritis
    age-related changes, 288

assessment, 289–290
management, clinical,
  290–291, 292*t*, 293
presentation, clinical,
  288–289
Mycobacterium tuberculosis, 145,
  147, 150
Mycostatin, 432
Mydriatics, 95
Myelin disorders, 66*t*
Myocardial infarction (MI)
  aspirin, 5
  assessment, 171–172, 171*t*
  education, client, 174
  management, clinical, 172–174
Myocarditis, 168

N
Nails, 464–466
Nalbuphine, 412*t*
Narcotics
  antihistamines, 107
  chronic obstructive pulmonary
    disease, 127
  herpes zoster, 436
  pain, 405, 407, 410, 411*t*–413*t*,
    414–415
Nasogastric/jejunostomy tubes,
  248
National Academy of Sciences, 10
National Cancer Institute, 37, 396
National Center for Nutrition and
  Dietetics, 37
National Cholesterol Education
  Program, 11
National Institutes of Health
  (NIH), 84, 163–164
National Safety Council, 47,
  48*f*–49*f*, 49
Nausea
  opioid administration, 415
  refeeding, 252*t*
Near vision, 91
Neck. *See* Throat and neck
Nedocromil sodium, 136
Nefazadone, 482*t*
Neglect. *See* Abuse and neglect
Nembutal, 52*t*
Neomycin, 105, 226*t*, 447
Neomycin sulfate, 103*t*
Neoplastic disorders, 66*t*
Netilmicin sulfate, 103*t*
Neuroleptic medications, 66*t*,
  487, 489, 491, 492, 494
Neurologic system
  age-related changes, 311–312
  alcohol abuse and dependence,
    511*t*
  assessment, 579–581
  Bell's palsy, 339–341

case study, 355–356
cerebrovascular accident
  assessment, 312–313,
    313*t*–315*t*, 315
  management, clinical,
    316–317
  rehabilitation, 317
dizziness, 323
  age-related changes, 323
  assessment, 326, 327*f*–329*f*,
    328–330
  management, clinical,
    330–332
  presentation, clinical, 323,
    324*t*–325*t*, 326
  setting-specific issues,
    332–333
falls, 345*t*–346*t*
  assessment, 342–343,
    344*t*–350*t*
  management, clinical, 343,
    351*f*–354*f*, 354
  presentation, clinical,
    341–342
Parkinson's disease
  defining, 317–318
  management, clinical, 318,
    320–322, 320*t*
  presentation, clinical, 318,
    319*t*–320*t*
seizure disorders
  age-related changes, 333
  assessment, 335–336
  education, client, 339
  management, clinical, 336,
    337*t*–338*t*
  presentation, clinical,
    333–335, 334*f*
temporal arteritis, 322
Neuronal losses, 62
Neuropathology and dementia,
  59*t*–60*t*
Neurotin, 416
Niacin, 166*t*, 227*t*
Nicotine replacement therapy, 38,
  39*t*
Nicotinic acid, 166*t*
Night vision, 91
Nikolsky's sign, 434
Nitrates, 170, 181*t*
Nitrogen mustard, 103*t*
Nitroglycerin (NTG), 167
Nizatidine, 204*t*, 206
Node dysfunction, AV, 176
Nodules, thyroid, 376–377
Noduloulcerative lesions, 400
Nondisplaced Colles' fractures,
  302
Nonmaleficence and beneficence,
  548–549

No-Doz, 275*t*

Nonpharmacologic measures. *See* management, clinical *under specific condition/ disorder/disease/symptom; specific condition/disorder/ disease/symptom*

Nonsteroidal anti-inflammatory drugs. *See* NSAIDs (nonsteroidal anti-inflammatory drugs)

Norflex, 52*t*

Norfloxacin, 278

Normocytic anemias, 381–382

Nortriptyline, 246, 482*t*

Norwegian scabies, 433

Nose and sinuses

  age-related changes, 107

  disorders, common

    allergic rhinitis, 107–108

    epistaxis, 108

    furuncles, 108

    polyps, 108

    sinusitis, 109

Nosocomial infection, 239

NSAIDs (nonsteroidal anti-inflammatory drugs)

  anemias, 377

  asthma, 136

  colorectal cancer, 16

  gout, 287

  hearing loss, 103*t*

  nutritional issues, 236*t*

  osteoarthritis, 285

  pain, 410

  peptic ulcer disease, 206–207, 207*f*–208*f*

  rheumatoid arthritis, 291

  temporomandibular joint dysfunction, 113

  vertebral compression fracture, 304

Nubain, 412*t*

Numorphan, 413*t*

Nursing homes and ethical issues, 552–554

Nutritional issues

  anorexia, 201

  bowel training program, 215–216

  breast cancer, 392

  cancer, 390

  case studies, 253–257

  cholesterol, 164

  congestive heart failure, 186

  coronary heart disease, 166

  diabetes, 361–362, 368, 369

  eating disorders

    dementia, 244–245

    depression, 245–246

    dysphagia, 246–248

  enteral nutrition

    access, 248

    complications, 249, 250*t*–252*t*, 252–253

    prescriptions, 248–249

  gout, 287

  health promotion for the elderly, 33, 34*f*–35*f*, 35, 36*f*, 37

  hypertension, 182

  introduction, 221

  malnutrition

    age-related changes, 237, 238*t*

    assessment, 239, 240*t*, 241–242

    chronic disease, 235

    collaboration and referral, 243

    immune system, 235, 237

    management, clinical, 242–243

    presentation, clinical, 237–239

  management, nutrition

    age-related changes, 221–222

    assessment, 222, 223*f*–224*f*, 225*t*–228*t*

    clinical management, 228–229, 230*t*–236*t*

    collaboration and referral, 229, 235

    osteoporosis, 300–301

    Parkinson's disease, 321

    pressure ulcers, 459, 460*t*

    vitamin B$_{12}$, 383

Nutrition Interventions Manual for Professionals Caring for Older Americans, 37

Nutrition Screening Initiative in 1992, The (NSI), 33, 223*f*–224*f*

Nystagmus, 323, 326, 329

Nystatin, 432

O

Obesity, 9, 10, 221, 285, 360

  See also Nutritional issues

Objective tinnitus, 106

Obsessive-compulsive disorder, 486*t*

Occupational therapy (OT), 291, 316, 321

Ointments, 428–429

Olanzapine, 491

Omeprazole, 203, 204*t*, 206*t*

Oncology care. *See* Cancer

Onychomycosis, 464–466

Open-angle/chronic simple glaucoma, 95

Open reduction and internal fixation (ORIF), 305, 306

Opiates, 275*t*, 412*t*, 414, 415, 518

Oral cavity and pharyngeal cancer, 17

Oral hypoglycemic agents (OHAs), 363–364

Oral stimuli and smoking cessation, 40–41

Orphenadrine, 52*t*

Orthopedic surgery, 291

Osteoarthritis, 283–285

Osteomalacia, 232*t*

Osteomyelitis, 463

Osteoporosis

  assessment, 297–299

  chronic obstructive pulmonary disease, 129

  corticosteroids, 136

  defining, 296–297

  management, clinical, 299–301

  nutritional issues, 233*t*–234*t*, 239

Otitis externa, 104–105

Otitis interna, 105

Otitis media, 105

Ototoxic drugs, 102, 103*t*

Ototoxicity, 104

Ovarian cancer, 13–15

Overflow and urinary incontinence, 262*t*–263*t*, 267*t*, 277

Over-the-counter medications (OTCs), abusing, 523–524

Oxazepam, 488

Oxycodone, 413*t*

Oxygen therapy, 125*t*, 127

Oxymorphone, 413*t*

Oxyphenbutazone, 103*t*

P

Pacemakers, 175, 332

Paclitaxel, 394

Pain

  abdominal, 210, 211*f*, 212*t*–214*t*

  adjuvant analgesics, 415, 416

  age-related changes, 402–403

  anticonvulsants, 415–416

  assessment, 403–405, 406*f*–409*f*

  chest, noncardiac causes of, 168*t*

  controlling, three concepts essential for, 405

  gout, 287

  herpes zoster, 435, 436

  monitoring, 407, 408*f*–409*f*

narcotics, 405, 407, 410,
    411*t*–413*t*, 414–415
non-narcotic analgesics, 407,
    410
osteoarthritis, 283
osteoporosis, 233*t*
pressure ulcers, 457, 459
rest, 189
rheumatoid arthritis, 291
sleep disorders, 82
steroids, 416
tricyclic antidepressants, 415
underreporting of, 45
venous ulceration, 439
Pancreas and alcohol
    abuse/dependence, 511*t*
Pancreatitis, 214*t*
Panic disorder, 486*t*, 608–610
Panthothenic acid, 227*t*
Pap smears, 14–15, 397
Paraneoplastic disorders, 66*t*
Paranoia, 594
Parasitic and fungal skin
    conditions
angular cheilitis, 431, 432*f*
bullous pemphigoid, 434–435
herpes zoster, 435–437
intertrigo, 431–432
scabies, 432–434
Parkinson's disease
case study, 613–614
control/balance disorders, 325,
    325*t*
defining, 317–318
depression, 479
management, clinical, 318,
    320–322, 320*t*
neuroleptics, 492
presentation, clinical, 318,
    319*t*–320*t*
seborrheic dermatitis, 430
Parlodel, 85*t*, 321
Paroxetine, 482*t*
Paroxysmal nocturnal dyspnea,
    121
Partial seizures, 334, 334*f*
Paternalism, 549
Patient-based principles, 546–548
Peak flowmeters, 132, 133*f*
Pelvic examination, 14
Pelvic muscles, 260, 267, 271,
    273*f*–274*f*, 274–275,
    276*t*–277*t*
Penicillamine, 226*t*, 292*t*
Pentamidine, 366
Pentazocine, 52*t*, 413*t*
Pentobarbital, 52*t*
Pepcid, 204*t*
Peptic ulcer disease (PUD)
age-related changes, 204–205

assessment, 205
management, clinical, 205--208,
    206*t*, 207*f*–208*f*
presentation, clinical, 205
Pepto-Bismol, 217
*Pep Up Your Life: A Fitness Book for
    Seniors,* 33
Percutaneous transluminal
    coronary angioplasty
    (PTCA), 169–173
Perforation and abdominal pain,
    213*t*
Pergaloid, 85*t*
Pergolide, 321
Pericardial effusion, 168
Pericarditis, 168
Perineal dermatitis, 218
Periodic leg movement (PLMS), 82
Peripheral neuropathy, 362
Peripheral vascular disease, 169,
    188–190
Peripheral vestibular disorders,
    324*t*
Peripheral vision, 91
Permar, 321
Permax, 85*t*
Peroxide, 460
Perphenazine, 494
Persantine, 52*t*
Personal health behaviors, 27
    See also Health promotion for
    the elderly
Personalities, difficult, 493–495,
    611–612
Pharmacologic measures. *See*
    Medications; *individual
    drug*
Pharyngeal cancer, 17
Pharyngitis, viral, 114–115
Phenelzine, 482*t*, 483
Phenobarbital, 226*t*, 338*t*
Phentermine-fenfluramine
    combinations, 229
Phenylbutazone, 103*t*, 366
Phenylporparolamine, 108
Phenytoin, 226*t*, 298, 337*t*, 366,
    415
Phobias, specific or social, 486*t*
Photoaging, 421, 422
Physical abuse/neglect, 529–530,
    533–534
Physical activity. *See* Exercise
Physical examination. *See specific
    condition/disorder/disease/
    symptom*
Physical self-maintenance scale,
    563–564
Physical therapy, 316, 321
Pick's disease, 58*t*–61*t*

Pill rolling and Parkinson's
    disease, 319*t*
Pilocarpine, 96
Pinguecula, 97, 97*f*
Pinna, 100
Pirbuterol, 137, 138*t*
Pityrosporum ovale, 430
Planning, responsibilities for
    advance care, 549–550
Platelet-inhibiting drugs, 165–166
Pneumonia, 4
assessment, 146–147
atrial fibrillation, 175
incidence, 145
management, clinical, 147–148,
    148*t*, 149*f*
pathophysiology, 145
presentation, clinical, 146
prevention, 146
setting-specific issues, 150
Pollen, 134*t*
Pollutants, 119, 120
Polymyalgia rheumatica (PMR)
age-related changes, 295
assessment, 295
clinical findings, 293*t*
constitutional symptoms of, 295
giant cell arteritis grouped
    with, 294
management, clinical, 295–296,
    296*t*
Polymyxin, 105
Polypharmacy, 50–51, 52*t*, 507
Polyps, 108
Polysomnography, 84
Polyuria secondary to
    hyperglycemia, 260
Posey products for preventing
    falls, 351*f*–352*f*
Position sense disorder, 325*t*
Positive reinforcement and
    smoking cessation, 40
Posterior cerebral artery, 314*t*
Postmenopausal bleeding, 14
Postprandial hyperglycemia, 364
Posttraumatic stress disorder, 486*t*
Postural reflexes and Parkinson's
    disease, 319*t*–320*t*
Postvoid residual urine (PVR),
    267
Potassium, 236*t*, 383
Povidone iodine, 436, 460
Practitioner-related factors
    contributing to
    prescription drug use
    problems, 521
Prazosin, 280
Prealbumin, 241–242, 459
Prednisolone, 140*t*
Prednisone, 140*t*, 296

Preload, 185*t*
Premature ventricular
    contractions (PVCs), 170
Presbycusis, 102, 105
Presbyopia, 97
Prescription drug use, 516
    assessment, 520
    management, clinical, 521–523
    presentation, clinical, 517–520,
        517*t*–518*t*, 520*t*
    See also Medications
Presentation, clinical. *See specific
    condition/disorder/disease/
    symptom*
Pressure Sore Status Tool, 450,
    455*f*–456*f*
Pressure ulcers and wound
    management, 447
    age-related changes, 448
    assessment, 448–450, 449*f*, 450*t*,
        451*f*–452*f*, 453*t*–454*t*,
        455*f*–456*f*
    management, clinical, 459–463,
        461*t*, 465*t*
    nutrition, 459, 460*t*
    pain, 457, 459
    presentation, clinical, 448
    relief, pressure, 454, 457
    setting-specific issues, 463
Prevacid, 204*t*, 206*t*
Preventive care
    abuse and neglect, 536
    anemias, 377
    barriers to, 2
    case study, 22–25
    chemoprophylaxis
        aspirin prophylaxis, 5–6
        hormone replacement
            therapy, 6–7
    delirium, 74
    diabetes, 360–361
    enteral nutrition, 249,
        250*t*–252*t*, 252
    immunizations
        influenza, 3–4
        pneumonia, 4
        tetanus and diphtheria, 4–5
    influenza, 143
    introduction, 1, 2*t*
    pain, 405
    pneumonia, 146
    pressure ulcers, 454
    screening and early detection
        blood pressure, 7, 8*t*, 9
        body measurement, 9–10
        cancer
            breast, 13
            cervical/uterine and
                ovarian, 13–15
            colorectal, 15–16

oral cavity and pharyngeal,
    17
prostate, 16–17
skin, 17–18
cholesterol, 10–13, 11*t*–12*t*
functional status, 21–22, 22*t*
hearing, 19–20, 20*f*
thyroid disease, 18–19
vision, 20–21
tuberculosis, 151
See also Health promotion for
    the elderly
Prilosec, 204*t*, 206*t*
Primadone, 338*t*
Primary hypertension, 177
Primary prevention, 2*t*
Prinzmetal's angina, 167, 172
Probenecid, 288
Procainamide, 66*t*
Procardia, 275*t*
Progestin, 6, 299
Prokinetic agents, 203, 204*t*
Prolastin, 127
Proliferative retinopathy, 362
Promethazine hydrochloride, 331
Promotility medications, 204*t*
Propecia, 464
Propoxyphene, 52*t*, 85*t*, 413*t*
Propoxyphene napsylate, 407
Propulsid, 204*t*
Propylthiouracil (PTU), 374
Proscar, 280
Prosom, 83*t*
Prostate cancer, 16–17, 389–391
Prostatectomy, 391
Prostate gland, 16, 82, 260,
    279–280
    See also Benign prostatic
        hyperplasia (BPH)
Prostate-specific antigen (PSA),
    16–17, 390, 391
Prosthetic replacement, 306
Protein, 228*t*, 235, 237, 241–242,
    459, 460*t*
Proteus mirabilis, 278
Proteus vulgaris, 278
Proton pump inhibitors, 203,
    204*t*, 206
Protriptyline, 482*t*
Proventil, 137
Providencia species, 463
Proximal interphalangeal (PIP)
    joint, 284, 288
Pseudoephedrine, 487
Pseudomonas, 105, 447, 463
Psychiatric Nursing (Wilson &
    Kneisl), 490, 495
Psychiatric symptomology
    anorexia, 201*t*
    case study, 603–605

chest pain, 168*t*
dementia, 60*t*–61*t*
dizziness, 332
eating disorders, 245–246
falls, 348*t*–349*t*
paranoia, 594
sleep disorders, 82
urinary incontinence, 263
See also Depression;
    Psychosocial issues
Psychodynamic psychotherapies,
    481
Psychologic abuse/neglect, 530,
    535
Psychosocial issues
    anxiety
        age-related changes, 485–486
        assessment, 486–487
        management, clinical,
            487–489
        presentation, clinical, 486,
            486*t*
    case study, 498–500
    conclusion, 495–498
    depression
        age-related changes, 478
        assessment, 479
        delusional, 479–480
        mania, 480
        presentation, clinical, 478
        prevalence, 477
        risk factors, 479
    grief and loss
        advanced practice registered
            nurse, 476–477
        age-related changes, 474
        presentation, clinical, 474,
            475*f*
        risk factors, 474–476
    introduction, 473–474
    personalities, difficult, 493–495
    schizophrenia
        age-related changes, 489–490
        assessment, 490–491
        case study, 593
        presentation, clinical, 490
        schizoaffective disorder,
            491–492
    suicide
        age-related changes, 480
        assessment, 481
        management, clinical,
            481–485, 482*t*
        risk factors, 480
    See also Psychiatric
        symptomology
Psychostimulants, 483
Psychotherapy, 481
Pterygium, 97, 98*f*
Ptosis, 97

Pulmonary issues
  abdominal pain, 213*t*
  chest pain, noncardiac causes
    of, 168*t*
  function tests, 123, 124*t*
  See also Respiratory system
Pulse oximetry, 123
Purified protein derivative (PPD),
    151
Pyrazinamide, 152
Pyridoxine, 227*t*

Q

Quality-of-life issues, 390
Quinidine, 66*t*

R

Race
  giant cell arteritis and
    polymyalgia rheumatica,
    295
  hip fractures, 305
  osteoporosis, 297
Radiation treatment, 391, 394,
    396, 399
Radioactive iodine (I^{131}), 375
Radiofrequency catheter ablation,
    175
Radiographs, 306
Radio Shack products for
    preventing falls, 353*f*
Radiotherapy, 393
Raintech products for preventing
    falls, 354*f*
Raloxifene, 300
Ranitidine, 204*t*, 206, 206*t*
Reaction time, 30*t*
Rebound anxiety, 519
Rebound hypoglycemia, 250*t*
Recommended daily allowances
    (RDA), 222, 227*t*–228*t*,
    229, 237, 300
Recreational substance use, 50
Red blood cells, 380, 382
  See also Anemias
Refeeding edema, 251
Referral and collaboration with
    appropriate mental
    health providers, 496,
    496*t*
Reflex urinary incontinence, 263*t*
Regitine, 275*t*
Reglan, 204*t*
Rehabilitation
  alcoholism, 515–516
  cardiovascular system, 166
  cerebrovascular accident,
    316–317
  herpes zoster, 436
  prescription drug abuse,
    522–523

Reinforcement, 29
*Relaxation & Stress Reduction
    Workbook, The* (Davis), 489
Relaxation techniques, 40, 42*f*,
    43–44, 44*f*, 86
Reliance Urinary Control Insert,
    278
Renal system
  gout, 285
  nutritional issues, 232*t*
  sleep disorders, 82
Resignation and abuse, 531
Respiratory system
  acute diseases
    bronchitis, 143–145
    influenza, 143
    pneumonia, infectious,
      145–150
    tuberculosis, 150–153
  alcohol abuse and dependence,
    511*t*
  case study, 153–158
  classification of respiratory
    diseases, 120
  introduction, 119
  narcotics and respiratory
    depression, 414
  obstructive lung diseases. *See*
    Asthma; Chronic
    obstructive pulmonary
    disease (COPD)
  sleep disorders, 81–82
Resting tremor and Parkinson's
    disease, 319*t*
Restless leg syndrome (RLS), 80,
    82, 85
Restoril, 83*t*
Rest pain, 189
Restraints and urinary
    incontinence, 265
Reticulocyte count, 381
Retinal detachment, 97–98
Retinal vein occlusion, 98, 99*f*
Retinopathy, diabetic, 94
Retrograde filling test, 439
Retropulsion and Parkinson's
    disease, 319*t*
Rheumatoid arthritis
  age-related changes, 288
  assessment, 289–290
  management, clinical, 290–291,
    292*t*, 293
  presentation, clinical, 288–
    289
Rheumatrex, 292*t*
Rhinorrhea, 107, 299
Riboflavin, 227*t*
Ridaura, 292*t*
Rifampin, 152

Rigidity with cogwheeling and
    Parkinson's disease, 319*t*
Risperidone, 491, 495
Robaxin, 52*t*
Rosacea, 426*t*

S

Safety as a major concern in
    home-based care, 551
Salicylates, 103*t*, 366, 410
Saline soaks with mild steroid
    ointment, 447
Saliva, excess, 202
Sarcoptes scabies var hominis mite,
    432
Scabies, 432–434
Scandinavian Simvastatin Survival
    Study, 165
Schizoaffective disorder, 491–492
Schizophrenia
  age-related changes, 489–490
  assessment, 490–491
  case study, 593
  presentation, clinical, 490
  schizoaffective disorder,
    491–492
Sclerosing basal cell carcinoma, 400
Screening and early detection
  blood pressure, 7, 8*t*, 9
  body measurement, 9–10
  cancer
    breast, 13
    cervical/uterine and ovarian,
      13–15
    colorectal, 15–16
    oral cavity and pharyngeal, 17
    prostate, 16–17
    skin, 17–18
  cholesterol, 10–13, 11*t*–12*t*
  functional status, 21–22, 22*t*
  hearing, 19–20, 20*f*
  thyroid disease, 18–19
  vision, 20–21
Seborrheic dermatitis, 320*t*, 430
Seborrheic keratosis, 424*t*–425*t*
Secobarbital, 52*t*
Seconal, 52*t*
Secondary hypothyroidism, 370
Secondary prevention, 2*t*
Second Expert Panel on the
    Diagnosis and
    Management of Asthma
    in 1997, 143
Second-hand smoke, 120, 134
Secretion monitoring, 247
Secure Care products for
    preventing falls, 353*f*
Sedatives, anxiolytic, 416
  See also pain *under* Medications

Seizure disorders
  age-related changes, 333
  alcoholism, 510
  assessment, 335–336
  education, client, 339
  management, clinical, 336,
    337–338*t*
  presentation, clinical, 333–335,
    334*t*
Seldane, 108
Selective estrogen receptor
    modulators (SERMs), 300
Selective serotonin reuptake
    inhibitors (SSRIs), 79,
    482–483, 488
Selegiline hydrochloride, 321
Selenium lotions, 430
Self-determination, 546–547
Self-monitoring and smoking
    cessation, 40
Senile lentigos, 423*t*
Senile purpura, 426*t*
Senna, 414
Senokot, 414
Sensorineural hearing loss, 102
Sensory deficits control/balance
    disorders, 325*t*
Sensory neuropathy and
    automobile use, 45
Sepsis, 463
Serevent, 136
Sertraline, 482*t*, 489
Service Merchandise products for
    preventing falls, 354*f*
Setting-specific issues
  abuse and neglect, 539–540
  anorexia, 200
  cerumen impaction, 102
  congestive heart failure,
    187–188
  coronary heart disease, 167
  dementia, 72–73, 72*f*
  dermatitis medicamentosa, 429
  diabetes, 368–369
  dizziness, 332–333
  ethical issues
    home-based services,
      550–551
    hospital settings, acute,
      551–552
    managed-care environments,
      554
    nursing homes, 552–554
  hearing loss, 104
  hypertension, 182
  hyperthyroidism, 375
  hypothyroidism, 372
  pneumonia, 150
  pressure ulcers, 463
  scabies, 433

Sexual abuse, 529, 534–535
Shingles, 435–437
Sick sinus syndrome, 171
Sideroblastic anemia, 382
Sigmoidoscopy, 16
Silver Foxes (Simmons), 33
Silver sulfadiazine, 463
Simple partial seizures, 334, 334*f*
Sinarest, 275*t*
Sinemet, 85*t*, 320, 321
Sinequan, 84
Sinusitis, 109
  See also Nose and sinuses
Skin
  age-related changes, 419, 420*t*
  assessment, 419, 421, 421*t*
  cancer, 17–18, 400–402
  chronic obstructive pulmonary
    disease, 129
  cosmetic effects, 421–422
  dermatoses
    contact dermatitis, 430
    dermatitis medicamentosa,
      429
    lichen simplex chronicus,
      430–431
    seborrheic dermatitis, 430
    xerosis, 427–429
  environmental and photoaging
    changes, 421
  introduction, 419
  noncancerous
    lesions/conditions, 422,
      423*t*–426*t*
  parasitic and fungal conditions
    angular cheilitis, 431, 432*f*
    bullous pemphigoid, 434–435
    herpes zoster, 435–437
    intertrigo, 431–432
    scabies, 432–434
  pressure ulcers and wound
    management, 447
    age-related changes, 448
    assessment, 448–450, 449*f*,
      450*t*, 451*f*–452*f*,
      453*t*–454*t*, 455*f*–456*f*
    management, clinical,
      459–463, 461*t*, 465*t*
    nutrition, 459, 460*t*
    pain, 457, 459
    presentation, clinical, 448
    relief, pressure, 454, 457
    setting-specific issues, 463
  pruritus, 422, 427, 428*t*
  venous ulceration
    assessment, 437, 438*t*–440*t*,
      439–440, 441*f*
    management, clinical,
      440–441, 442*t*–446*t*, 447
    presentation, clinical, 437
    stasis dermatitis, 447

Sleep disorders
  age-related changes, 79–80
  apnea, sleep, 80
  assessment, 80–84, 81*f*, 83*t*
  case study, 116–117
  education, client, 86–87
  management, clinical, 84–86,
    84*t*–85*t*
  presentation, clinical, 80
  vertebral compression fracture,
    304
Sleep hygiene, 86
Smoke, second-hand, 120, 134
Smoking cessation, 37–41,
    38*t*–39*t*, 127, 166
Snoring, 80
Snyder Electronics products for
    preventing falls, 352*t*
Soap, 428, 430
Sodium, 238*t*
Solganal, 292*t*
Soma, 52*t*
Sound, decreased sensitivity to, 100
Speculum exam, 397
Speech, ability to discriminate,
    100
Spine, osteoarthritis of the, 284
Spinocerebellar disorders, 325*t*
Sputum sample, 147
Squamous cell carcinomas, 17,
    400–402
St. John's Wort, 483
Stadol, 411*t*
Staphylococcus aureus, 105, 108,
    147, 447
Stasis dermatitis, 447
Steroids, 66*t*, 298
  angular cheilitis, 431, 432*f*
  anxiety, 487
  cerebrovascular accident, 316
  herpes zoster, 436
  pain, 416
  pruritus, 427
  xerosis, 429
  See also Corticosteroids
Stimulants, 95
Stool impaction, 264*t*–265*t*, 265
  See also Constipation
Stool softeners, 216
Streptococcus pneumoniae, 4,
    143–145
Streptomycin, 152, 153
Streptomycin sulfate, 103*t*
Streptozocin, 399
Stress
  management, 41–44, 42*f*–44*f*
  protein status, 459
  urinary incontinence, 262*t*,
    267*t*, 276*t*–277*t*

Stroke Prevention in Atrial
    Fibrillation, The (SPAF),
    176
    See also Cerebrovascular
        accident (CVA)
Sty, 98–99
Subclinical hypothyroidism, 371
Subconjunctival hemorrhage, 99
Subjective tinnitus, 106
Substance abuse issues
    age-related changes, 509–510
    alcoholism
        assessment, 512, 513*t*–514*t*, 514
        management, clinical,
            514–516
        presentation, clinical,
            510–512, 511*t*–512*t*
        prevalence, 506
    case study, 525–527
    control/balance disorders, 325*t*
    defining the problem
        adverse drug reactions,
            507–509, 508*t*
        causative factors, 506–507
        diagnosis, 507
        incidence and prevalence,
            506
        recognition, lack of, 505
    introduction, 505
    over-the-counter medications,
        523–524
    prescription drug use, 516
        assessment, 520
        management, clinical,
            521–523
        presentation, clinical,
            517–520, 517*t*–518*t*, 520*t*
Substance use, recreational, 50
Substituted judgment, 547–548
Sucralfate, 206
Sudafed, 108, 275*t*
Sudden hearing loss, 102–103
Sugar lactulose, nonabsorbable,
    216
Suicide
    age-related changes, 480
    assessment, 481
    case study, 607–608
    management, clinical, 481–485,
        482*t*
    risk factors, 480
Sulfasalazine, 292*t*
Sulfonamides, 366
Sulfonylureas, 363, 363*t*
Sun-induced lesions, 421
Superficial basal cell carcinoma,
    400
Supplementation, vitamin/
        mineral and herbal
    dysphagia, 248

increasing use of, 229
macrocytic anemia, 383
malnutrition, 243
osteoporosis, 298
pressure ulcers and wound
    management, 459, 460*t*
side effects, nutrition-related,
    236*t*
Support groups/systems, 30*t*, 43,
    128, 137, 523
Surgeon General, U.S., 31
Surrogate decision making, 552
Symmetrel, 318
Sympathomimetics, 125, 136
Synopsis of Psychiatry (Kaplan), 490
Synovial fluid aspirate, 290
Synovitis, 290
Systolic blood pressure (SBP), 177
Systolic dysfunction, 183

T
Tachycardia, 108
Tacrine, 68
Tagamet, 204*t*
Talwin, 413*t*
Tamoxifen, 394
Tapazole, 374, 375
Tap water enema, 216
Tardive dyskinesia, 493
Teaching considerations for the
        older adult, 29–30, 30*t*
Teach Your Patients About Asthma,
    137
Tegretol, 415
Temazepam, 83*t*
Temporal arteritis, 322
Temporomandibular joint (TMJ),
    106, 113
Terazosin, 280
Terbinafine, 465
Terbutaline, 137, 138*t*
Terfenadine, 108
Tertiary prevention, 2*t*
Testosterone, 299
Tetanus, 4–5
Tetanus immune globulin (TIG),
    5
Tetracycline, 144, 206*t*, 226*t*
Theophylline, 125–126, 136, 366
Thiamine, 227*t*, 238*t*
Thiazides, 181*t*, 185, 209, 286
Thioridazine, 491, 494
Throat and neck
    age-related changes, 114
    disorders, common
        dysphagia, 114
        laryngitis, viral, 114
        pharyngitis, viral, 114–115
Thrombolytics, 172
Thyroglobulin, 369

Thyroid disorders
    age-related changes, 370
    anxiety, 487
    falls, 350*t*
    hormone production, 369–370
    hyperthyroidism, 373–375
    hypothyroidism, 370–372
    nodules, thyroid, 376–377
    sleep disorders, 82
Thyroidectomy, 375
Thyroid gland
    function studies, thyroid, 241
    screening and early detection,
        18–19
    supplementation, 298
Thyroid-stimulating hormone
        (TSH), 19, 369–373
Thyrotoxicosis, 373–375
Thyrotropin-releasing hormone
        (TRH), 369
Thyroxine (T_4), 369–371, 373,
    374
Ticlopidine, 165
Tigan, 52*t*
Tilade, 136
Time management and stress, 43
Timolol, 95, 96
Timoptic, 95
Tinea unguium, 464–466
Tinnitus, 105–106
Tiredness, 616–617
Titration, 405, 414
Tobacco use
    chronic obstructive pulmonary
        disease, 120
    respiratory irritant, 119
    second-hand smoke, 120, 134
    smoking cessation, 37–41,
        38*t*–39*t*, 127, 166
Tobramycin sulfate, 103*t*
Tofranil, 275
Toileting programs, 276*t*
Tolazamide, 363*t*
Tolbutamide, 363, 363*t*
Tolerance, drug, 518–519
Tomography, 113
Tonometer, 21
Total iron-binding capacity
        (TIBC), 380
Total lymphocyte count (TLC), 242
Toxic encephalopathies, 66*t*
Tranquilizers, 106, 107
Transferrin, 241, 242
Transient ischemic attack (TIA),
    312
Transrectal ultrasound (TRUS),
    16, 391
Transurethral hyperthermia, 280
Transurethral incision of the
        prostate (TUIP), 280

Transurethral resection of prostate (TURP), 280
Tranylcypromine, 482*t*
Traumatic disorders, 66*t*
Trazodone, 84, 482*t*
Tremulous motions, 319*t*
  See also Parkinson's disease
Trendelenburg test, 439
Tretinoin, 422
Triazolam, 83*t*
Tricyclic antidepressants (TCAs), 107, 226*t*, 246, 415, 489
Triglycerides, 364
Trihexphenidyl, 321
Triiodothyronine (T$_3$), 369, 370, 373
Trimethobenzamide, 52*t*
Trimethoprim-sulfamethoxazole, 105, 144, 145, 147, 278
Trimipramine, 482*t*
Troglitazone, 363*t*, 365
Tropicamide, 275*t*
Tube displacement, 249
  See also Enteral nutrition
Tuberculosis
  assessment, 150–151, 151*t*
  extrapulmonary, 153
  incidence, 150
  management, clinical, 151–153
  prevention, 151
Tumors
  brain, 324*t*
  leg ulcers, 440*t*
  prostatic, 390
  See also Cancer; Lesions
Tylenol, 84, 105, 144
Tympanic membrane perforation, 106–107
Tympanosclerosis, 107

U
Ulcers
  disease, ulcer, 214*t*
  duodenal, 205
  peptic ulcer disease
    age-related changes, 204–205
    assessment, 205
    management, clinical, 205–208, 206*t*, 207*f*–208*f*
    presentation, clinical, 205
Ultrasound, 16, 190, 377, 390
Understanding Difficult Behaviors: Some Practical Suggestions for Coping with Alzheimer's Disease and Related Illnesses (Robinson), 73
Unilateral hearing loss, 102–103

Upper respiratory infections (URIs), 134, 143
Urecholine, 204*t*
Uremia, 232*t*
Urge and urinary incontinence, 262*t*, 267*t*, 275, 276*t*–277*t*
Uric acid, 287
Urinary problems. *See* pathophysiology problems *under* Genitourinary system (GU)
Urispas, 275
Uterine cancer, 13–15

V
Vaccines. *See* Immunizations
Vaginitis, atrophic, 260, 261, 265*t*
Valium, 52*t*
Valproic acid, 337*t*, 415–416
Values, family, 530
Valvular disorders, 325*t*
Vanceril, 135
Vancomycin hydrochloride, 103*t*
Vascular disease
  arterial ulcers of the lower extremities, 438*t*–439*t*
  dementia, 58*t*–61*t*, 66*t*
  giant cell arteritis, 322
  gout, 285
  leg ulcers, 440*t*
  peripheral, 169, 188–190
Vascular systems, brain perfused by two major, 313
Vasculitis, 440*t*
Vasodilators, 95, 106
Vasopressors, 95
Vasovagal attacks, 325*t*
Venlafaxine, 482*t*
Venous lakes, 425*t*
Venous ulceration
  assessment, 437, 438*t*–440*t*, 439–440, 441*f*
  management, clinical, 440–441, 442*t*–446*t*, 447
  presentation, clinical, 437
  stasis dermatitis, 447
Ventolin, 137
Ventricular aneurysm, 163
Vertebral compression fracture, 303–305
Vertebrobasilar artery system, 313, 315*t*, 324*t*
Vertigo, 323, 324*t*, 326, 328–329
Vestibular schwannoma, 100
Vestibular system disorders, 323, 324*t*–325*t*, 326
  See also Dizziness

Viral laryngitis, 114
Viral pharyngitis, 114–115
Visual acuity, 20–21, 30*t*, 45
  See also Eyes
Vitamins
  A, 227*t*, 460*t*
  B, 86, 230*t*
  B$_1$, 227*t*, 238*t*
  B$_2$, 227*t*
  B$_3$, 227*t*
  B$_5$, 227*t*
  B$_6$, 227*t*
  B$_{12}$, 227*t*, 238*t*, 382–383
  C, 228*t*, 238*t*, 279
  D, 227*t*, 238*t*, 297, 300
  E, 86, 227*t*
  K, 227*t*, 238*t*
  pressure ulcers and wound management, 460*t*
  recommended daily allowances, 237
Vivarin, 275*t*
Voiding intervals/habits, 267
Vomiting
  case study, 598–599
  opioid administration, 415
  refeeding, 252*t*
von Willebrand factor, 295

W
Walking, regular, 362
Walk-pain-rest cycle, 189
Water, 228*t*, 237
Water brash, 202
Waterpicks, 461
Weight issues, 9–10, 166, 235, 238, 320*t*
  See also Nutritional issues
Wellness care and health maintenance. *See* Health promotion for the elderly; Preventive care
Wernicke-Korsakoff syndrome, 510
White blood cells, 123, 383
White coat hypertension, 178
Withdrawal and substance abuse issues, 518
Wound healing/management, 5, 239, 440, 453*t*–454*t*
  See also Pressure ulcers and wound management; Venous ulceration
Wound Ostomy and Continence Nursing Association (WOCN), 448

X

Xanax, 416
Xerosis, 427–429
Xerostomia, 113–114
X-ray, chest, 123, 147, 163, 200, 241, 287
Xylocaine, 436

Y

Yesavage Geriatric Depression Scale, 79

Z

Zafirlukast, 136
Zantac, 204*t*, 206*t*
Zileuton, 136

Zinc, 228*t*, 390, 460*t*
Zinc soap, 430
Zollinger-Ellison syndrome, 206
Zolpidem, 83*t*
Zung Self-Rating Depression Scale, 479
Zyban, 127
Zyrtec, 108